Assisted Living Administration

The Knowledge Base

Second Edition

James E. Allen, PhD, MSPH, CNHA is
Associate Professor (retired) of Health Policy and Administration in the
Department of Health Policy and Administration
School of Public Health
University of North Carolina at Chapel Hill
He is a licensed North Carolina nursing home administrator.

The UNC-CH Long Term Care Administration Teaching Resources Program

This program makes available to students and course instructors relatively complete sets of materials for classroom use and for preparation for becoming a nursing home administrator.

Five key elements for this preparation are:

1. The text, *Nursing Home Administration,* 4th. ed, Springer Publishing Company, 2003.

2. *Nursing Home Federal Requirements: Guidelines to Surveyors and Survey Protocols*, 5th. ed., Springer Publishing Company, 2003 user friendly rendering of the Health Care Finance Administration's State Operations Manual, Provider Certification.

3. *The Licensing Exam Review Guide in Nursing Home Administration,* 4th ed., Springer Publishing Company, 2003 – 864 practice questions.

4. *The Five-Step Administrator-in-Training Internship Program* plus *AIT Self-Assessment Tool* available through the national association of state boards.

Instructor's Guide -- 20 case studies plus several hundred questions for classroom use available to course instructors. Instructors: write to the author, James E. Allen.

Correspondence courses for licensure preparation – used by over a dozen state licensing boards.

For further information write to the above address,
Or call 1-800-458-8125 or fax 919-933-6825.

Assisted Living Administration

The Knowledge Base

Second Edition

James E. Allen, PhD, MSPH, CNHA

 ***Springer Publishing Company***

Springer Publishing Company, Inc.
536 Broadway
New York, NY 10012-3955

Cover design by Joanne Honigman
Acquisition Editor: Sheri Sussman
Production Editor: Jeanne Libby

04 05 06 07 08 /5 4 3 2 1

Library of Congress Cataloging-in-Publication Data

Allen, James E. (James Elmore), 1935-
Assisted living administration : the knowledge base / James E. Allen. –2nd ed.
p. ; cm.
Includes bibliographical references and index.
ISBN 0-8261-1516-0
1. Congregate housing--United States--Administration. 2. Older people—Home care—United States. 3. Older people—Housing—United States. 4. Community health services for older people—United States. I. Title.
HD7287.92.U5A44 2204
362.16'0973--dc22

2004008870
CIP

Printed in the United States of America by Integrated Book Technology

Contents

Part Two Assisted Living Facility Organizational Patterns; Human Resources **91**

Part Three Assisted Living Facility Financing, Business Operations **185**

List of Figures

List of Tables

Introduction

New Industry. Assisted living is a new segment of health care which burst upon the American landscape in the late 1980s. Ten thousand assisted living facilities operated in the early 2000s with more opening every month.

Population Served. Assisted living facilities serve the health care market segment of persons who no longer are able to live independently, who need help with the activities of daily living, but do not need the 24-hour a day nursing care provided in nursing facilities.

New Knowledge Base. Recognizing that assisted living is a major new health care phenomenon, the National Association of Boards of Examiners for Long Term Care Administrators (NAB) in 1996 began a two-year job analysis of the practice of assisted living facility administration. In November, 1997 the NAB's study task force recommended five areas in which the assisted living administrator should be knowledgeable:

1. organizational management
2. human resources management
3. business and financial management
4. physical environment management
5. resident care management

In June, 1998 the NAB began offering a national examination covering these five knowledge areas, known as the Domains of Practice, for persons wishing to become professional assisted living administrators.

The five NAB Domains of Practice are explored in this text. Each of the five parts of the text focuses sequentially on the five domains of practice recommended to the assisted living administrator.

Domains of Practice. In this text *Part One* covers Domain 1: organizational management, *Part Two* explores Domain 2: human resources management, *Part Three* presents Domain 3: business and financial considerations, *Part Four* summarizes Domain 4: the laws and issues surrounding physical environment management, and *Part Five* focuses on Domain 5: resident care.

Part One:
Industry Overview, Management, Governance, and Leadership

The reader is introduced to the assisted living industry through an overview description of the industry. The industry is defined and described, and forces creating the need for the assisted living industry are analyzed.

The management and marketing skills needed by the assisted living administrator are presented here. Skills needed such as planning, organizing, staffing, directing, controlling, evaluating, innovating and marketing are explored along with such topics as policy making, leadership, communication skills, and organizational values.

Part Two
Assisted Living Facility Organizational Patterns; Human Resources

Various organizational patterns the assisted living facility may take are explored. Several models are presented. Extensive data on the assisted living industry are provided. Skills needed by the assisted living administrator to identify personnel needs, recruit, train, and retain employees are described.

Part Three
Assisted Living Facility Financing, Business Operations

An extensive description of the financial aspects of the assisted living industry is followed by a presentation of the basic financial concepts important to managing an assisted living facility. The accounting process, financial statements, and concepts such as depreciation and budgeting are explained. This knowledge base is augmented with a section exploring concepts related to the legal system, risk management, insurance, wills, and estates.

Part Four
The Assisted Living Facility Environment: The Long-Term Care Continuum: Laws and Regulations

Numerous laws and regulations affect the day-to-day operation of assisted living facilities. These laws are summarized following an introduction to the long-term care organizations with which assisted living facilities interact such as nursing homes, home health agencies, and hospitals.

Part Five
Assisted Living Facility Resident Care

After presenting the aging process and theories about why we age, the scope of health care issues affecting the assisted living facility are described. A brief explanation of the healthcare-related impacts of aging is provided. Finally, a number of resident care policy issues are explored such as defining and maintaining quality of care in the assisted living facility.

The reader may choose to read the sections in any sequence.

PART ONE

INDUSTRY OVERVIEW, MANAGEMENT, GOVERNANCE AND LEADERSHIP

1.0 The Assisted Living Industry: An Overview

1.0.1 Defining Assisted Living

ASSISTED LIVING: A PHILOSOPHY OF SERVICE

Population Served

Assisted living is that part of the long-term care continuum that serves the rapidly expanding population of persons who no longer are able to live independently in a residence but who do not need the 24-hour-a-day nursing services provided in nursing homes.

A Philosophy of Service

Assisted living is a philosophy of service that focuses on maximizing each resident's independence and dignity (AAHSA, 1997; ALFA, 1998). The assisted living philosophy emphasizes flexibility, individualized supportive services, and health care. Involvement of the community, as well as the residents' family, neighbors, and friends, is encouraged. The availability of staff to meet scheduled and unexpected care needs is a major aspect of assisted living caregiving.

No Single National Definition

There is no single, nationally agreed on definition. Additional perspective can be gained from the following definitions offered by (a) the two national assisted living associations, (b) the U.S. Department of Health and Human Services, (c) an astute industry analyst, and, (d) in April, 2003, the Assisted Living Workgroup in its report to the US Senate Special Committee on Aging (2003, p. 12).

National For-Profit Association Definition. The Assisted Living Federation of America (ALFA) defines assisted living as a combination of housing, personalized supportive services, and health care designed to meet the individual needs of persons who require help with the activities of daily living but who do not require the skilled medical care provided in a nursing home (ALFA, 1998). The activities of daily living generally are considered to include eating, bathing, dressing, getting to and using the bathroom, getting into or out of a bed or chair, and general mobility.

National Not-for-Profit Association Definition. The American Association of Homes and Services for the Aging (AAHSA) defines assisted living as a program that provides and/or arranges for daily meals, personal and other supportive services, health care, and 24-hour oversight for persons residing in a group residential facility who need assistance with the activities of daily living (AAHSA, 1997).

U.S. Department of Health and Human Services Definition. The Department of Health and Human Services defines assisted living as a residential setting that provides either routine general protective oversight or assistance with activities necessary for independent living for mentally or physically limited persons (Sirrocco, 1994).

Industry Analyst's Definition. Peter Martin (1997), an industry analyst, has defined assisted living as a combination of housing and personal support services available 24 hours a day designed to aid elderly residents with activities of daily living, such as bathing, eating, personal hygiene, grooming, and dressing. The assisted living setting is residential and promotes resident self-direction and participation in decisions that emphasize independence, individuality, privacy, and dignity.

The US Senate's Special Committee on Aging's definition **(April, 2003)** is "Assisted living is a state regulated and monitored residential long-term care option. Assisted living provides or coordinates oversight and services to meet the residents' individualized scheduled needs, based on the resident's assessments and service plans and their unscheduled needs as they arise.

Part A: Services and Regulations

Services that are required by state law and regulation to be provided or coordinated must include but are not limited to:

- 24-hour awake staff to provide oversight and meet scheduled and unscheduled needs
- Provision and oversight of personal and supportive services (assistance with activities of daily living and instrumental activities of daily living)
- Health services
- Social services
- Recreational activities
- Meals
- Housekeeping and laundry
- Transportation

A resident has the right to make choices and receive services in a way that will promote the resident's dignity, autonomy, independence, and quality of life. These services are disclosed and agreed to in the contract between the provider and resident. Assisted living does not generally provide ongoing, 24-hour skilled nursing.

Part B: Private Units
Assisted living units are private occupancy and shared only by the choice of residents (for example, by spouses, partners, or friends).

Part C: Levels of Care
A state must establish at least two assisted living licensure categories, based on the types and severity of the physical and mental conditions of residents that the assisted living residence is prepared to accommodate. The licensure category shall determine licensure requirements relating to important concerns such as staffing levels and qualifications, special care or services, participation by health care professionals and fire safety.

(US Senate Special Committee on Aging, 2003)

It must be noted, however, that of the nearly 50 organizations voting on the above definition, unqualified support for Part A was given by only 18, for Part B by 7, and by Part C by 11. About a dozen organizations, including significant assisted living associations, opposed the definition. (US Senate Special Committee on Aging, 2003, p. 15).

Age Range of Assisted Living Services

Assisted living serves a broad range of the elderly population (70 to 90+ years of age), becoming, in effect, a bridge between active retirement living and, for some, care in a nursing facility (Martin, 1997).

Now Part of the Continuum of Health Care

Assisted living facilities are part of the continuum of long-term care services available to the aging population.

1.0.2 Prevalence Of Assisted Living Facilities

Phenomenon beginning in the 1990s

Assisted living, as we know it today, is a phenomenon of the 1990s.

Ten Thousand Facilities

A fully accurate count of assisted living facilities in the United States is unavailable. The best estimates are that, in 1997, assisted living facilities numbered 8,000 to 10,000 (Sirrocco, 1994). By 2003 the number of facilities was more likely approaching 10,000. The *Senior Housing Construction Report*, 2003, estimated that, by their definition of assisted living (high end facilities), there were 6,150 properties containing 717,000 living units (*American Seniors Housing Association, 2003*).

Focus of This Text

This text focuses on these approximately 8,000 to 10,000 facilities in the United States (of approximately 30 or more units each), which offer assistance with the activities of daily living (ADLs) following the philosophy of offering 24-hour services promoting resident self-direction and participation in decisions that emphasize independence, individuality, privacy, and dignity.

Unique Focus on the ADLs

Assisted living facilities offer less complex services than those provided by nursing homes' 24-hour medically complex nursing care, but more complex services than those offered by residential care facilities (which provide no assistance with ADLs). Assisted living facilities focus on providing residents with assistance in performing these activities.

Typically, these facilities are members of either the national for-profit or national not-for-profit assisted living associations.

A national study for the US Department of Health and Human Services (DHHS) estimated 11,459 assisted living facilities nationwide with approximately 611,000 bed and 520,000 residents (*A National Study of Assisted Living for the U.S. Department of Health and Human Services*, 1999) identified four categories of assisted living facilities:

Low privacy and low service	59%
High privacy and low service	18%
High service and low privacy	12%
High privacy and high service	11%

Source: (*A National Study of Assisted Living for the U.S. Department of Health and Human Services,* 1999).

Note that most of the assisted living facility units built since 1996 have been high privacy and high service.

EXPLOSION OF ASSISTED LIVING FACILITIES

Confluence of Powerful Forces

The explosion of assisted living facilities onto the long-term care scene in the United States results from the confluence of a variety of powerful forces that are shaping long-term care, such as powerful demographic trends and the public's emphatic desire for better and more cost-effective living options for the elderly.

Since 1990 the total number of assisted living facilities has risen dramatically, whereas the total number of Medicare/Medicaid-certified nursing homes (15,300) has remained relatively flat. A nursing home is a facility with three or more beds that is either licensed as a nursing home, certified as a nursing facility under Medicare or Medicaid, identified as a nursing care unit of a retirement center, or determined (by Medicare, Medicaid, or a state government) to provide nursing or medical care (Sirrocco). Meanwhile, the number of hospitals in the United States has shrunk, from 6,000 in 1980 to 5,300 in 2003.

Variety of Assisted Living Settings

Assisted living facilities may be stand alone, part of a continuing care retirement community, attached to or within a nursing facility, part of a housing complex, or part of a hospital the combinations are almost limitless.

THE BROADER CONTEXT OF SENIOR LIVING FACILITIES

Several industry segments offer a wide range of long-term care services. The basic segments, moving from least intense to most intense caregiving, are independent living settings, congregate care facilities (CCFs), assisted living facilities (ALFs), and nursing facilities (NFs).

Independent Living: Absence of Health Services

Independent living covers a broad range of settings in which persons, as a matter of preference and lifestyle, move into adult communities that impose age restrictions and offer social activities, and often, increased security. The lack of any health services characterizes independent living settings. Size may range from a single building, to a large campus of buildings, to entire "city" settings. Sun City, Arizona, is an independent living setting with over 100,000 persons age 55 and over living in duplex condominiums and similar housing. Sun City, as an organization, offers an array of social activities in large centers housing recreational and hobby facilities for residents. The independent living target population is generally age 75 or younger.

Congregate Living: Absence of Health Services, But Assistance with Activities Outside the Facility

Congregate care is an industry segment between independent living and the health-related services of the assisted living facility. Congregate care facilities provide social activities, security, and nonhealth-related services such as meals, housekeeping services, and transportation. The target population is typically persons ages 75 to 82+. The focus is companionship, organized social activities, and some personal care of a temporary nature. Congregate care facilities typically assist residents with the instrumental activities of daily living (IADLs): activities such as preparing meals, doing housework, shopping, and keeping health care appointments.

Assisted Living: Focus of This Work

Assisted living facilities are the next step up in intensity of care. These facilities generally serve 30 or more residents and offer help with both the IADLs mentioned previously and the ADLs: eating, bathing, dressing, getting to and using the bathroom, and getting into or out of a bed or chair. Assisted living facilities vary, from stand-alone facilities to a floor in a congregate care facility, a part of a continuing care retirement community (CCRC), or a section of a nursing facility. The target population is age 83 and over. Applicants to independent and congregate care facilities are making a lifestyle choice, whereas applicants to assisted living facilities generally are driven more by a need for assistance with the activities of daily living than by personal choice.

Nursing Homes

Nursing facilities offer the highest acuity level of long-term care and are characterized primarily by the need for 24-hour nursing care. Few, if any, persons enter a nursing facility as a matter of choice.

Hospitals

Hospital services are normally defined as short-term care (under 30 days). Although hospitals are not part of the long-term care continuum, they complete the continuum of intensity of caregiving, offering the most intense and expensive level of care.

Inappropriate Placement

Reimbursement decisions by third-party payers, unavailability of assisted living facilities as an option until just a few years ago, and resident preferences have resulted in residents being cared for at inappropriate levels. Until recently, Medicaid reimbursed almost exclusively for care in nursing homes, tilting health care toward nursing home placement when a less intense level, such as assisted living, would have more appropriately met residents' needs and preferences. Some board-and-care homes, seeking to retain high-level occupancy, have provided care to residents needing the intensity of health care offered by nursing facilities. Finally, residents' decisions to "age in place" in the least institutionalized setting has resulted in a complex caregiving picture.

Providers Who Bridge IADLs and ADLs

Providers in this category are known variously as residential care facilities, adult congregate living facilities, rest homes, homes for the aging, personal care homes, catered living facilities, retirement homes, homes for adults, adult foster care, board and care, domiciliary care homes, community residences, and the like. In 2003 these types of independent living facilities totaled approximately 20,000.

These providers, which typically are smaller (defined as fewer than 30 residents), may also provide assistance with the activities of daily living.

Assisted living is the appropriate caregiver between congregate care and nursing home care. We turn now to a closer look at the assisted living industry.

ASSISTED LIVING RESIDENT PROFILE

This section explores some of the characteristics of those who choose assisted living. Table 1.1 lists the typical statistics of the residents in such facilities. Table 1.2 identifies the variety of units available in assisted living facilities by geographic region. The typical assisted living facility resident is a woman in her 80's who needs assistance with an average of three ADLs. The assisted living resident profile is not unlike the nursing facility resident profile, which is also about 80% female, even fewer with spouses, but with heavier health care needs. It will be argued later in this text that as the acuity level of assisted living facility residents increases over the next several years, the health-related services offered in assisted living facilities will more and more resemble the sophistication of care offered at nursing facilities. These are identified below as level 1 facilities (minimum assistance), level two facilities (moderate assistance to residents with the ADLs) and level 3 facilities (considerable assistance).

These data depict buildings with ample private spaces for residents. Some units have over 800 square feet. The average of 40% common space suggests that recreation areas and other areas used in congregate living are available to residents, minimizing the institutional feel associated with nursing homes and hospitals.

TABLE 1.1 Assisted Living Facility Resident Profile in Percent

Resident profile	National average
Female	78
Male	22
Age of female residents	84
Age of male residents	82
With spouse in facility	3
Number of ADLs Requiring Assistance	3

AMENITIES IN ASSISTED LIVING

The following amenities are becoming standard in the industry (Martin, 1997):

- emergency call systems in rooms
- locking doors
- room for personal furnishings
- personal telephone
- kitchen area
- pets allowed
- individualized heating and air conditioning units
- wheelchair accessibility

TABLE 1.2 Characteristics of Assisted Living Facilities Across the U.S.

	U.S.	Northeast	Southwest	Midwest	West
Number of Units	58	73	51	32	88
Size of building (sq ft)	47,000	78,000	35,000	27,000	50,000
Common space	40%	43%	33%	50%	40%
Semi-private (sq ft)	321	311	306	270	410
Studio (sq ft)	306	284	304	291	343
One bedroom (sq ft)	481	444	501	534	487
Two bedroom (sq ft)	638	670	675	687	731
Refrigerator in room	67%	67%	52%	61%	80%
Private toilet	80%	90%	78%	46%	76%
Private shower	80%	90%	78%	46%	76%
Private tub/bath	34%	36%	27%	31%	37%

Source: Coopers & Lybrand LLP, "Overview of the Assisted Living Industry Report," cited in P. Martin (1997), *The Assisted Living Industry*, p. 53. New York: Jeffries.

NATIONAL OCCUPANCY RATES AND SIZE OF ASSISTED LIVING FACILITIES

The occupancy rate for the estimated 8,000 to 10,000 assisted living facilities in 1997 was believed by one study group to be as high as 93% and in 2002 as high as 94% (*The State of Seniors Housing*, American Seniors Housing Association, 2002) This compares favorably to the estimated 86% occupancy rate for board and care homes and the estimated 92% occupancy rate for nursing facilities. However, according to the National Investment Center for the Seniors Housing and Care Industries (NIC) the average occupancy rate reported by the NIC for the fourth quarter of 2002 was 85%, falling to 83.5% in the first quarter of 2003 (*Provider,* September, 2003, p. 19).

The actual occupancy rates nationally most likely varied greatly with the likelihood that on average the occupancy rates for most chains and owners more nearly approached 83 to 85% rather than the more optimistic 94% estimated in *The State of Seniors Housing*. Assisted living facilities averaged 60 units per facility, compared to an average of 15 beds for board and care homes, and 106 beds for nursing homes (Sirrocco, 1994, pp. 1–8). The assisted living facility's 60 units will contain more or fewer "beds" depending on the number of semi-private, studio, and one- and two-bedroom units. By 2002 the median number of beds in surveyed assisted living facilities had risen to 80 (American Seniors Housing Association, 2002, p. 18).

1.0.3 Forces Creating the Need for Assisted Living Facilities

A number of social phenomena are creating the need for assisted living:

- an aging population
- exploding population numbers
- healthier older persons
- financial capacity to purchase services
- growing public resources
- increase in number of elderly who are single
- attitudinal changes
- aging caregivers
- attitudes toward nursing homes
- new health care technologies
- commitment to "aging in place"

AN AGING POPULATION

People are living longer. In the United States, for example, life expectancy at the beginning of the 20th century was 47 years. Today it is 75 years and rising.

Potential Life Span

Death from infectious diseases and other causes in the past has meant that all but a few persons were failing to achieve their potential life span. Public health engineering developments beginning in the late 19th century, combined with advancements in modern medicine in the 20th century, have enabled more people to live into their 80s and 90s.

Age 100 Less Newsworthy

A few years ago, when a resident of a long-term care facility reached 100, a call to the local newspaper brought a reporter and a story in the next day's edition. Today such a call to the local newspaper produces at most a yawn. In 1940 the percentage of persons age 65 who were expected to live to age 90 was 7%. Currently it is 25% and is expected to be 42% by the year 2050 (Martin, 1997, p. 30).

Changing Definitions of "Old"

Even the definition of "old" is changing. A few years ago persons characterized as "old" were classified as 65 and over. Increasingly, older persons are referred to as the "young old" (age 65–74), the "middle old" (age 75–84), and the "old-old" (age 85 and over).

Growing Need for Assistance Among the Aging Population

Table 1.3 lists the percentage of the general population, by age, in need of assistance with activities of daily living. Table 1.4 gives assisted living needs, by activity type, for those over 85 years of age. The U.S. General Accounting Office found that in 1993 approximately 7 million seniors needed assistance with ADLs (Martin, 1997, p. 31). By the year 2020, this number is expected to double, to 14 million. About half of all seniors 85 and over currently need assistance with daily living—the type of services for which the assisted living facility is designed.

TABLE 1.3 Persons by Age Needing Assistance with Activities of Daily Living

Age	Percentage of population
15-64	2
65-69	9
70-74	11
75-79	20
80-84	31
85 and over	50

Source: U.S. Census Bureau.

TABLE 1.4 Need for Assistance Among the 85+ Population

Activity	Percentage of population
Eating	4
Getting out of chair	7
Toileting	11
Dressing	12
Bathing	17
Walking	25
Going outside	27
ADLs	35
ADLs or IADLs	57

Source: U.S. Census Bureau; Martin, 1997, p. 31.

EXPLODING POPULATION NUMBERS

The Baby Boomer Generation

The U.S. population is both aging and expanding in terms of absolute numbers. The post–World War II baby boom population is aging. Its numbers caused enormous expansions, first in the elementary schools, then progressively the high school, college, and available work force populations. Now this population bulge is beginning to reach retirement age and is causing a matching need for rapid expansion of long-term health care facilities, especially assisted living facilities (Martin, 1997, p. 29).

HEALTHIER OLDER PERSONS

Improved Quality of Life

Older people are living healthier lives. At the same time that the life expectancy is rising almost yearly, older people are experiencing an improved quality of life. In the past, living into old age meant living with increasingly debilitating multiple chronic diseases; hence the need for more nursing homes.

Today, due to improved health care, people who are living longer increasingly enjoy a higher level of physical and social health; hence the need for more assisted living facilities. Fewer need 24-hour nursing care; more simply need help with ADLs during their 60s and 70s. However, even these healthier persons, as they reach their late 70s and early 80s, find more and more health and other obstacles to living independently.

Need for Assisted Living Facilities

In 1993, 7 million older persons needed assisted living facility services. By the year 2020, 14 million older persons are expected to need assisted living facility services (Martin, 1997, p. 30). The typical assisted living resident is, as mentioned, female, age 83 to 85, single or widowed, who needs assistance with two or three ADLs.

FINANCIAL CAPACITY TO PURCHASE SERVICES

Private Resources

A number of economic forces have resulted in financial security for a larger proportion of the elderly needing assistance with ADLs. Livable retirement income for the average American is a fairly recent phenomenon and is based on the development of private-sector lifetime pensions in the second half of the 20th century. Today most American workers have some form of private pension, providing them with buying power. Increasingly, however, as health care costs continue to escalate, companies are scaling back their retirement benefit packages. Thus, while the first baby boomers to retire in the year 2010 may have retirement benefits, the proportion able to count on retirement benefits to fund their later years will begin to shrink after 2020.

Value of Home Ownership

Home ownership contributes to the financial solvency of older Americans as well as the assisted living market. Seventy-seven percent of aging Americans own their own homes, with an equity value of over $1.5 trillion (Martin, 1997, p. 34). The median net household worth of Americans age 65 and over in 1993 was $86,423 (Martin, 1997, p. 34). As Table 1.5 shows, a significant portion of aging Americans have both a steady income from a private pension and a nest egg from the sale of their home. The typical assisted living resident had an average of $200,000 of financial resources in 1997 (Martin, 1997, p. 52).

Despite the above rosy picture, in 2001 the average resident net worth was:

$100,000 to $300,000 6.2%
$ 50,000 to $ 99,999 14.8%
$ 0 to $ 49,999 78.9%
(Source: *American Senior Housing Association*, 2001)

Given that the yearly costs of living in an assisted living facility can range from $30,000 to over $50,000 the net worth of most seniors would be used up within one to two years.

TABLE 1.5 Asset Ownership of Households, 1993: 65 Years and Over

Age	65-69	70-74	75 and over	Total
No. of households	6.0 million	5.5 million	9.0 million	20.5 million
Median net worth	$92,500	$95,700	$77,600	$86,300

Source: U.S. Census Bureau; Martin, 1997, p. 34.

GROWING PUBLIC RESOURCES

Social Security was passed in 1935 to enable the often destitute aging population to have a steady flow of income throughout old age. Today Social Security provides somewhere between $5,000 and $15,000 in income to persons age 65 and over, typically resulting in modest discretionary buying power if combined with other sources of income.

Medicare and Medicaid

The demand for assisted living facilities is greatly expanded by the availability of Medicare Part B financial support to pay for what might be otherwise prohibitively expensive health care for aging Americans.

The long-term care industry, at its current size, was created by Medicare and Medicaid legislation in 1965 and 1966, respectively. Medicare and Medicaid policies determine the size and shape of the long-term and acute-care industries. This theme will be developed throughout this book. Medicare pays for the health care of many assisted living residents using Medicare-reimbursed home health care agencies. Medicaid pays for 73.7% of the care in nursing facilities.

To understand Medicare and Medicaid reimbursement policies is to understand how the health care industry developed and the future directions it will take over the next few decades. Consider the following dominating influences exercised by Medicare and Medicaid.

Impact of Medicare and Medicaid

Medicare pays for the greater portion of health care costs of assisted living residents. Payment comes primarily through use by assisted living residents of home health care agency personnel who make visits to residents in assisted living facilities. Medicare typically pays for 80% or more of all home health care agency charges. Changes in Medicare policies on home health care agency reimbursements directly affect the economics of the assisted living facility.

Medicare also pays for hospice care. Increasingly, assisted living facilities, as well as nursing homes, are engaging hospice agency personnel for the terminally ill. Entering a hospice program may permit an assisted living resident to remain in the facility rather than being transferred to a hospital or nursing home.

Prospective Payments

Medicare determines, by its reimbursement policies, where care is given and the way reimbursement is received. When, in 1983, legislation in Congress authorized Medicare to prospectively pay for care based on a diagnosis related groups scheme, the shape of health care in the United States was dramatically affected.

Hospitals were suddenly faced with caps on their Medicare-covered elderly patient income. A chain reaction has ensued. Under current prospective payment mechanisms, hospitals have strong incentives to discharge Medicare patients quicker and sicker. In short, the hospitals have shifted to nursing homes much of the subacute care previously provided in the hospital.

This practice has dramatically changed the patient mix in nursing homes. The nursing home of today increasingly treats medically complex patient who are older and sicker. This directly affects the assisted living facility resident mix. Many Medicare recipients who, 10 years ago, would have been placed in what were then called intermediate nursing care facilities are now residing in assisted living facilities. In summary, the acuity level in both assisted living facilities and nursing facilities is rising.

Other Forces

As the agricultural era ended, the United States became increasingly urbanized. The elderly were traditionally cared for in the intergenerational farm home in the agricultural setting. Today's typical urban family is geographically dispersed. The "children" scatter throughout the country in pursuit of job opportunities. Increasingly, there are fewer and fewer caregivers available to aging Americans. The assisted living facility helps fill this gap.

INCREASE IN NUMBER OF ELDERLY WHO ARE SINGLE

In 1960, 7% of elderly individuals lived alone, compared to 30% who lived alone in 1997 (Martin, 1997, p. 31). This reflects the fact that women are outliving men by an average of almost 7 years, the higher divorce rates, and current lifestyle choices: more people are choosing not to marry. Census data indicate that in 1993, 32% of women age 65 to 74 were likely to live alone, increasing to 57% of women age 85 and over. In 2001 this was reflected directly by the resident gender in assisted living facilities: 25% men, 75% women (*American Senior Housing Association*, 2001, p. 11).

ATTITUDINAL CHANGES

End to Intergenerational Dependence

In the agricultural setting depending on the younger generation to care for elderly parents and grandparents was typical. Today, urban parents increasingly desire to avoid being dependent on their children, either financially or for the activities of daily living.

Today's Retirees

Today retirees want to maintain their personal independence as long as possible. They are better educated, have become accustomed to being independent, and generally have the means to remain so. In this urbanized setting, depending on one's children is no longer a positive value. Women, who traditionally provided assistance to aging parents, are now, as often as not, wage earners. Fewer and fewer have the time or inclination to assume the role of caregiver for their and their spouses' aging parents. The assisted living facility thus is an increasingly viable alternative.

AGING CAREGIVERS

Those who, a few decades ago, were the caregivers are themselves becoming in need of care. As the average age of residents in long-term care facilities approaches 90, the "children" who traditionally provided care to aging parents are in their 60s—often candidates themselves for assisted living.

ATTITUDES TOWARD NURSING HOMES

Few, if any, aging adults wish to become candidates for placement in nursing facilities. No one wants to fit the profile of the typical nursing facility resident: frail, 87 years old, with two or three chronic illnesses, an inability to perform several of the activities of daily living, widowed, on Medicaid, taking five or six medications daily, and, often as not, dying. Federal and state regulators have ensured that nursing facility living is highly institutionalized. Public preference creates powerful incentives for assisted living facilities in which the resident can "age in place."

NEW HEALTH CARE TECHNOLOGIES

New technologies allow procedures once performed only in the acute-care hospital setting to be accomplished in persons' homes or in an assisted living facility. Intravenous feeding and even kidney dialysis are increasingly commonplace services provided by the home health care agencies. The ability to bring these new, formerly hospital-bound technologies to residents in an assisted living facility permits assisted living residents to bypass the traditional stay in a nursing facility. An assisted living resident experiencing an acute episode may enter the hospital for acute care, then return directly to the assisted living facility with the aid of high-tech in-unit care provided by the local home health care agency.

COMMITMENT TO "AGING IN PLACE"

Life care communities, often called continuing care retirement communities, have offered their residents the luxury of "aging in place." Consequently, there has been a veritable explosion of life care communities across the United States over the past few decades. However, life care communities, for the most part, are available only to well-to-do individuals who can afford from $50,000 to $250,000 and up for the lifetime occupancy fee and $1,500 to $3,000 and up for the monthly maintenance fee. Assisted living facilities, in contrast, normally do not charge any entry fee, but often have higher monthly maintenance fees than life care communities. As more and more retirees seek the opportunity to "age in place" in a quality care setting, the assisted living facility becomes the location of choice.

1.0.4 Clouds on the Horizon

Lest the reader begin to think that assisted living administration will be a comfortable niche characterized by low competition in the long-term care market of the future, the following must be considered.

THIRD-PARTY PAYERS DICTATE THE CHANGING SHAPE OF REIMBURSEMENT FOR LONG-TERM CARE

Medicare will pay for less and less even though the nation's ability to provide assistance and health care in the later years of life will improve. The new technologies are too costly. Rationing has already become a health care fact of life for many Americans. As Medicare continues to squeeze hospitals, nursing homes, and home health care agencies, the amount of health care available to assisted living residents through home health care agencies and other Medicare funding will continue to shrink, placing an economic squeeze on assisted living facility residents' dollars even though Medicare has begun paying for some drug costs of seniors.

MEDICAID

Increasingly states are seeking Medicaid waivers which allow them use Medicaid funds to supplement monthly payments of assisted living residents. To the extent this phenomenon continues to occur more and more assisted living residents will be Medicaid recipients whose typical reimbursement rate is at or often below actual costs of care. Medicaid funding will bring additional government regulations and inspections.

LONG-TERM CARE INSURANCE: VERY SLOW TO GROW

Thus far, the average assisted living facility resident typically is unable to afford private long-term care insurance protection. Assisted living facilities cannot count on continued availability of either generous public funding or private insurance. The federal Health Insurance Portability and Accountability Act of 1996, which became effective January 1, 1997, made long-term care insurance more attractive through favorable tax treatment. However, the inclusion of assisted living insurance within long-term care insurance has been slow. Industry experts expect that it may be 2008 before this type of insurance becomes a significant assisted living payment source (*Assisted Living Business Week,*

1998). The proportion of assisted living monthly bills being paid by long-term care insurance by the year 2010 may not be for more than around 10 to 15% of residents.

THE SHAPE OF THE HEALTH CARE INDUSTRY CHANGES DAILY

The roles expected of hospitals, nursing homes, home health care agencies, hospices, and the assisted living industry will continue to undergo dramatic metamorphoses. For instance, along with the general population, the elderly are being placed in managed care organizations for their health care. What far-reaching implications this will have on the economics of the assisted living facility can only be the subject of conjecture.

CONGRESS: BURNED BY THE ELDERLY

The elderly forced Congress to repeal the Medicare Catastrophic Health Care Act of 1987. Since the elderly of the nation so vehemently attacked Congress for this legislative effort in health care for the elderly, Congress has shown little inclination to undertake further legislation favoring this age group.

SHRINKING DISCRETIONARY RETIREMENT INCOME

The number of applicants to assisted living facilities who have adequate retirement income is likely to shrink over the coming decades. Companies have scaled back on pension benefits. The current generation entering assisted living facilities may be the only group to have comfortable pensions that can fund their lifetime stays in such facilities. Today's workers' retirement benefits come more often as 401(K) funds rather than funded pension plans in which the worker gains vested rights to a lifetime pension. Workers who shift jobs sometimes cash out their 401(K) funds to buy a new car or to pay for a child's college education. Fewer and fewer assisted living facility applicants will come with guaranteed lifetime income.

GOVERNMENT REGULATIONS

Many analysts feel that the maturing assisted living facility industry may in the future be overburdened with government regulations. Currently, compared to the nursing home industry, the assisted living industry is largely unregulated. Massive federal and state regulations followed the growth of the nursing home industry from the early 1950s to the present. The nursing home industry of today is increasingly one of close public scrutiny, regulations, and decreasing funding levels. The same fate may await the assisted living industry. In 1997, 13 states licensed assisted living facilities and 12 states had task forces developing recommendations for regulations (Martin, 1997, p. 49). During the years 2000 to 2002 nearly fifty national organizations (the Assisted Living Workgroup appointed by the US Senate Special Committee on Aging) struggled to reach a consensus on such topics as definition, oversight, medication management, staffing, and operational models for assisted living. Little consensus, however, was reached. Most state governments are passing assisted living regulations. Whether the US Congress will follow suit is unclear, but is not likely before perhaps 2010.

FUTURE SOLVENCY OF SOCIAL SECURITY AND MEDICARE/MEDICAID

Fund solvency is a matter of national debate. It is just these funds on which the lifeblood of the assisted living facility depends.

OVERSUPPLY OF ASSISTED LIVING FACILITIES

Unrestricted building is already leading to a predictable oversupply of assisted living facilities in some states. The U.S. real estate market goes through periods of building, with its resulting temporary lowering of occupancy rates during the catch-up period when supply outstrips demand. This has happened in the hospital industry and, in many parts of the US has happened in the assisted living facility industry. The only barrier to entry is capital that is needed to sustain the heavy start-up costs and the 1.5 to 3.0 years often needed to reach the break-even occupancy level, estimated to be 70% to 75% or more of capacity (Martin, 1997, p. 48). During 2000 to 2003 increased competition due to an oversupply of assisted living facilities lengthened the time needed to reach the break-even point, which in turn led to overall lower occupancy rates, more costly pricing incentives resulting in pressures on the profit margin.

TURNOVER RATE RISKS

In an era of overbuilding, turnover rates may become a problem. In the typical assisted living facility the annual resident turnover rate averaged 25% to 40% in the late 1990s (Martin, 1997, p. 49). In the average 100-bed facility this means 25 to 40 units must be remarketed each year. In conditions of an oversupply of facilities there may be longer lulls between new residents. By 2002 the average annual resident turnover rate for assisted living residents had increased to 52% (*American Senior Housing Association*, 2002).

CONTINUING FAST PACE

The only certainty is that change in the assisted living industry will move at a fast pace over the coming decades. Change, and ways to respond to it, is a major topic in the rest of Part One.

In Part Two we will describe the role in the long-term care continuum played by assisted living and the organizational pattern of a typical 100-bed assisted living facility. We turn now to an examination of the administrative tasks facing the assisted living administrator.

1.1 Administrative Tasks Performed by the Assisted Living Aministrator

The skilled administrator of an assisted living facility is a person capable of giving life to the assisted living philosophy of care by organizing the resources and finances available to best meet the needs of the residents. In successfully accomplishing this, the assisted living administrator makes innumerable decisions.

Assisted living management involves decision making. What the administrator does for the assisted living facility is make decisions about what ought to happen in the facility.

Although by now there is an extensive literature describing the field of management theory, authors have returned again and again to a basic set of activities as the best explanation of what administrators do (Dale, 1969; Drucker, 1954).

Luther Gulick an early-20th-century author, defined the administrator's tasks as

- Planning
- Organizing
- Staffing
- Directing
- Coordinating
- Reporting
- Budgeting

Several decades later Ernest Dale (1969), in his textbook *Management: Theory and Practice,* differed only slightly in his description. He agreed on the importance of the first four tasks but consolidated the last four under three rubrics: controlling, innovating, and representing.

We will discuss current management concepts (such as total quality management) in detail later in this section. Very briefly, this is what an assisted living administrator must accomplish: (Figure 1.1)

Forecasts: Projects trends and needs that the facility management must meet in the future.

Plans: Decides what needs to be done and makes a set of plans to accomplish it.

Budgets: Projects costs and establishes categories, with dollar amounts for each.

Organizes: Once a plan has been made, decides how to structure a suitable organization to implement the plan, to put it into action. This will include the number of people needed for the staff and the materials with which to build or to work.

Staffs: Attempts to find the right person for each well-defined job.

Directs: Provides direction (preliminary training and ongoing supervision) through communication to each employee who thereby learns what is expected of him or her.

Evaluates: Judges the extent to which the organization is accomplishing its goals.

Controls quality: Takes steps to ensure that the goals are accomplished and that each job is done as planned.

Innovates: Leads the staff to develop new ideas that enable the facility to enhance its attractiveness to the community served.

Markets: Ensures that the facility successfully attracts and admits the persons it seeks to serve.

The assisted living facility administrator is responsible for ensuring that all of these activities are accomplished by the facility. Ensuring that forecasting, planning, organizing, staffing, directing, evaluating, controlling, innovating, and marketing is successfully accomplished is providing leadership to the facility (Argenti, 1994).

An approach to leadership of particular value in the assisted living facility setting is leading by walking around (LBWA). LBWA allows the administrator to see for himself or herself that facility resources and finances are successfully being used to best meet the needs of the residents and that the assisted living philosophy is being successfully implemented. This is a part of the quality assurance process (discussed later in this section).

The administrator's job is to ensure that the appropriate employees do the tasks of the organization at an acceptable quality level. Many volumes have been written about managing because it is one of the more complex tasks in modern society. Three professors (Christenson, Berg, & Salter, 1980) at the Harvard Graduate School of Business Administration, in the eighth edition of their text *Policy Formulation and Administration,* state that what administrators do is ask three questions: Where are we now? Where do we want to go? and How do we get there?

FORECASTING
PLANNING
ORGANIZING
STAFFING
DIRECTING
EVALUATING
CONTROLLING
INNOVATING
MARKETING

= LEADING
(Managing by Walking Around)

...ensuring quality.

FIGURE 1.1 Conceptual depiction of the management functions of the facility administrator.

GOVERNING BODY

The administrative process begins with a governing body. The facility must have a governing body, or designated persons functioning as a governing body, that is legally responsible for establishing and implementing policies regarding the management and operation of the facility. The governing body in turn appoints the administrator, who meets any state requirements for qualification (and any continuing education requirements) and is responsible for the management of the facility.

DISCLOSURE OF OWNERSHIP

Most states have regulations requiring assisted living facilities to disclose selected data and information specific to the ownership of the facility. Typically, persons with an ownership interest must be reported to a state agency responsible for licensing the facility. This information usually includes the officers, directors, agents, and managing employees, as well as the corporation, association, or other company responsible for the management of the facility.

LICENSURE OF FACILITY

In most states each facility must be licensed under applicable state and local law. Normally, applicable licenses, permits, and approvals must be available for inspection upon request. The facility must operate and provide services in compliance with all applicable federal, state, and local laws, regulations, and codes and with accepted professional standards and principles that apply to professionals providing services in such a facility (e.g., state and local laws, regulations, and codes relating to health, safety, and sanitation).

Accepted professional standards and principles include the various practice acts and scope of practice regulations in each state and current, commonly accepted health standards, established by national organizations, boards, and councils.

A DETAILED LOOK AT WHAT ASSISTED LIVING ADMINISTRATORS DO

We have described in very general terms what administrators do. What is actually involved in forecasting, planning, organizing, staffing, directing, evaluating, controlling, innovating, and marketing? Consider the following basic functions of the administrator:

Forecasting (projecting trends into the future): The administrator forecasts the economic, social, and political environment expected for the organization and the resources that will be available to it.

Planning (deciding what is to be done): The administrator decides what is to be accomplished, sets short- and long-term objectives, then decides on the means to be used for achieving them.

Budgeting (deciding acceptable costs): All facilities must operate on plans that have been translated into budgets that are realistic yet functional.

Organizing (deciding the scheme of the organization and the staffing it will require): The administrator decides on the structure the organization will take, the skills that will be needed, and the staff positions and their particular duties and responsibilities. This includes coordinating the work assignments (i.e., the interrelationships among the departments and their workers).

Staffing (the personnel function): The administrator attempts to find the right person for each defined job.

Directing (providing daily supervision employing good communication, people, and skills): The administrator provides day-to-day supervision of subordinates, makes sure that subordinates know what results are expected, and helps the staff to improve their skills. In short, the administrator explains what is to be done, and the employees do it to the best of their abilities.

Evaluating (compares actual to expected results): The administrator determines how well the jobs have been done and what progress is being made to achieve the organization's goals as stated in its policies and plans of action.

Controlling quality (takes necessary corrective actions): The administrator revises policies, procedures, and plans of action and takes necessary personnel actions to more nearly achieve the facility goals.

Innovating (the effective administrator is always an innovator): The administrator develops new ideas, combines old ideas to form new ones, searches for useful ideas from other fields and adapts them, and acts as a catalyst to stimulate others to be creative.

Marketing (identifies and attracts the persons to be served): The administrator ensures that the facility identifies the group(s) of persons to be served and successfully attracts and serves the residents it seeks. In today's competitive world marketing is a major function within the assisted living setting.

These are the basic functions of administrators. The reader may wish to use other words to describe these functions, or even improve on the model. Certainly, administrators do much more than has been described above (see, e.g., Pressman & Wildavsky, 1974). However, if forecasting, planning, organizing, staffing, directing, evaluating, controlling, innovating, and marketing are not successfully accomplished, the minimum leadership responsibilities of an assisted living facility administrator have not been fulfilled. The skilled assisted living administrator is capable of providing leadership that accomplishes each of these tasks in a manner that meets both facility financial needs and resident care needs.

In *A Passion for Excellence,* Tom Peters and Nancy Austin (1985) describe management's role as care of customers, constant innovation, turned-on people, and leadership. They observe that in both the for-profit and not-for-profit sectors, superior performance, over the long haul, depends on two things: taking exceptional care of clients (residents in the facility) via superior service and superior quality of care; and providing constant innovation.

Peters and Austin observe that financial control is vital, but that one does not sell financial control, but rather a quality service or product (in this case, well cared for residents). A facility seldom sustains superior performance merely by having all the units full; the superior facility sustains superior performance through innovation in ways to serve residents and promote market development. Efficient management of the budget is vital in any organization, whether a university or an assisted living facility; yet a great organization is never characterized by the remark "It has a good budget." Just as the superb university is superb only by virtue of its success in serving its ultimate customers, the students, the superb assisted living facility is superb only by virtue of its success in serving its ultimate customers, the residents.

The authors advocate a management model based on what they call "a blinding flash of the obvious." Giving every employee the space to innovate, at least a little. Answering the phones and fulfilling residents' requests with common courtesy. Doing things that work (giving quality care). Listening to residents and asking them for their ideas, then acting on them. Soliciting staff input, then, as appropriate, implementing it. Wandering around: with residents, staff, visitors. Obvious, right? But the obvious must not be so obvious or more would practice it. All of these are "people" skills, based on an ability to facilitate communication among staff and residents.

To achieve a "blinding flash of the obvious" in the assisted living facility environment, the administrator normally must cultivate good "people" skills (communicate successfully with both residents and staff) to achieve excellence in service to the facility residents. "People" skills will be discussed in more depth later in this section.

1.1.1 Levels of Management

Two additional concepts are worth noting at this point: upper/middle/lower levels of management and line-staff relationships. The administrator of a large assisted living facility might assign some of these responsibilities to others.

The administrator need not personally perform each of the management tasks, but rather must ensure that these tasks are successfully carried out. To accomplish this, management is often divided into three layers: upper, middle, and lower (Katz & Kahn, 1967).

UPPER-LEVEL MANAGEMENT (THE FACILITY ADMINISTRATOR)

The upper-level administrator is responsible for the overall functioning of the facility, normally interacting directly with the board of directors and/or the owners. This person is responsible for formulating policies that will be applied to the entire facility. The assisted living facility administrator is an excellent example of upper-level management (Mintzberg, 1979).

MIDDLE-LEVEL MANAGEMENT (THE DEPARTMENT HEAD)

Middle-level administrators report to upper-level administrators and at the same time interact significantly with lower-level managers. A good example in the assisted living facility is the director of health who reports to the facility administrator and in turn has administrators—for example, a night supervisor—reporting to him or her.

The middle-level administrator normally does not make policies affecting the entire facility, as does the facility administrator. However, the middle-level administrator does make decisions of policy for administrators responsible to him or her. The middle-level administrator must have good communication skills to deal successfully with both the administrator of the facility and the lower-level workers.

The emergence of assisted living facility chains has implications for the type of management role local assisted living facility administrators are being assigned. Some chains allow local facility administrators wide latitude in decision making, in which case the local administrator functions primarily as an upper-level administrator. In other chains, decision making is more centralized at the corporate level, in which case some dimensions of the local administrator's role more nearly resemble that of the middle-level administrator.

LOWER-LEVEL MANAGEMENT (RESIDENT CARE COORDINATOR)

As a rule, lower-level administrators have direct supervisory responsibilities for the staff who do the actual work (e.g., the personal care or health aide who physically takes care of the resident in his or her unit). The health care aide supervisor is a good example of lower-level management in an assisted living facility. At this level administrators deal directly with those at the middle level but not with administrators at the upper tier. That is, they are expected to conduct their business through the channel of their middle-level administrators.

If the health care assistant wants a change in a policy, he or she will discuss the matter with the health supervisor, who in turn will bring it to the attention of the administrator, should this be desirable. The middle-level administrator might also make a policy decision without consulting upper-level management (e.g., to change the activities schedule to accommodate additional resident needs that have been identified).

1.1.2 Line-Staff Relationships

Line-staff relationships constitute a second important concept in understanding management functions. A person who is empowered by the administrator to make decisions for the organization is said to have line authority. A person is said to have a staff role if he or she is advisory to the administrator and does not have authority to make decisions for the organization (Robey, 1982).

A LINE POSITION

The administrator must assign to other employees some of the decision-making authority to accomplish the work of the organization. Such employees are line administrators. They are empowered to make decisions on behalf of the administrator. The resident care coordinator is a line position. Therefore, decisions by the resident care coordinator have the same force as if the administrator had made them. The administrator still remains responsible for all decisions made on his or her behalf by persons to whom decision-making authority has been delegated.

A STAFF POSITION

A staff position, on the other hand, is an advisory role. None of the administrator's authority to make decisions on behalf of the facility is delegated to persons in a staff position. An accountant in the business office is an example of a staff position. Persons who are paid consultants, such as a local pharmacist or a registered dietitian, hold staff positions. These persons are expected to advise the administrator or appropriate others in the facility on what to do, but they have been given no authority by the administrator to make decisions on behalf of the facility.

Again, life in the assisted living facility is seldom this uncomplicated. A large number of assisted living facilities in the United States are operated by chains, with corporate staff who often visit or are assigned to assist a facility for a short period of time. Technically, these corporate representatives may be there only to advise, but facility staff are hardly free to ignore such "advice." Some chains expect their corporate staff to function more nearly as consultants to local facilities they visit; other chains want them to function as if they exercised line authority in their area of expertise while in one of that chain's facilities. Or, again, when the facility is functioning smoothly, the corporate representative might be comfortable with a "take it or leave it" approach to advice given, but in times of crisis that same representative might come in and exercise direct line authority in the day-to-day operation of that facility.

We turn now to a more detailed discussion of some of the activities and skills involved in the management functions. We will begin to explore some of the complexities of these functions.

1.2 Forecasting

Administrative success belongs to those who successfully prepare for the future. In the assisted living facility industry, the late 1990s and early 2000s belong to administrators who can anticipate and successfully prepare for rapid change. The shape of the assisted living industry changes almost daily as new facilities with new features filling newly created market niches are opened.

TREND ANALYSIS

After several decades of older persons having few if any alternatives to entering a rest home or nursing facility, assisted living facilities have developed quickly to begin to fill this gap in service needs.

Forecasting involves trend identification and analysis. Clues to the future are present in trends that the alert administrator can observe. The skill needed in forecasting is the ability to predict accurately the future implications for the assisted living facility of new trends to which the current environment may offer clues. For example, there is a trend toward public assistance programs paying for assisted living resident care. The federal government is actively studying various reimbursement methods. Alert administrators in states using evolving reimbursement approaches can estimate the likelihood that such a method may be adopted in their state.

One apparent certainty is that conventional perceptions of the assisted living facility's roles will continue to evolve in the American health care system. In the past, developments occurred more incrementally, at a slower pace. In today's world, the rate of transformation in the health care field is exponential, shifting so rapidly that it is ever more difficult to predict the shape of the assisted living facility industry, from year to year, as Congress and states modify, sometimes radically, the reimbursement approaches in long-term health care settings.

THE CHANGING CORE

Consider the following. Every 10 years, one fourth of all current knowledge and accepted practices in the health care and other industries will be obsolete. The life span of new technologies is down to 18 months, and decreasing (Kriegel, 1991, p. xvi). Estimates are that people under 25 can expect to change careers every decade and jobs every 4 years, either by choice or because the industry in which they work will disappear and be replaced by others yet unimagined. The "core" business of the assisted living facility of the late 1990s may be entirely different from one in the 21st century. In Part Two we discuss three levels of assisted living services that offer increasingly sophisticated health-related services as residents age in place.

As Kriegel (1991) has observed, assisted living facility administration is a new and unpredictable world, an arena in which we have not played before. The rules will be different. The game itself is changing: The assisted living facility we went to work for 3 years ago may have changed dramatically in the types of services offered. Everything is moving faster in the health care field. New technologies are replacing current technologies ever faster. What the assisted living facility administrator needs to know to act effectively is changing. Relying on the "tried and true," observes Kriegel, is dangerous because what was tried yesterday is no longer true today. Assisted living facilities that continue to rely on conventional formulas for success will both miss opportunities for new markets and find themselves in the backwash of the long-term care industry as it metamorphoses into constantly new permutations.

The truth is, for the first time in human history the capacity exists to provide more expensive and effective long-term health care than any nation, including the United States, may be able to afford. The roles possible for assisted living facilities, hospitals, nursing homes, home health care agencies, managed care organizations, and other providers are not fixed and will remain so over the next few decades as society struggles to absorb elder services and elder health care costs and technologies.

CHANGE ITSELF

Change at a laser-fast pace will continue. As one chief executive officer has observed, mankind's cumulative knowledge has doubled over the last decade and will double again every 5 years (Kriegel, 1991, p. 1). In health-related fields, such as the long-term care industry, of which assisted living is a segment, this may occur more rapidly. The U.S.

Congress's Office of Technology has warned that the rate of development is too fast for proper monitoring of the effects and will threaten the foundations of even the most secure American businesses (Kriegel, 1991, p. 2). Assisted living workers are learning new skills daily. Even so, almost as soon as rules are established, they become obsolete.

Survival in the assisted living facility industry will depend on the ability to forecast the future and to learn entirely new ways of thinking, behaving, motivating, and communicating in the assisted living facility. Survival will depend on an ability and willingness to change, something both owners and staff do with great reluctance.

1.3 Planning

1.3.1 Why Plan?

AN INTEGRATED DECISION SYSTEM

The purpose of planning is to provide an integrated decision system that, based on the changes forecast by the administrator, establishes the framework for all facility activities (Dale, 1969; Levey & Loomba, 1973; Rogers, 1980). Plans, in essence, are statements of the organizational goals of the facility.

A MEANS OF COPING WITH UNCERTAINTY

Plans are a means of coping with the uncertainty of the future (Katz and Kahn, 1967; Levey & Loomba, 1973). All organizations must deal with the outside world in order to survive. Inevitably, events beyond the control of the assisted living facility will shape the range of options available to the facility and set the context within which it will be obliged to function.

A plan is a prediction of what the facility's decision makers believe they must do to cope with the future. A carefully developed plan makes it possible to compare what actually happens to what was expected to happen. The plan may then be altered to achieve the set goals when external conditions change. For example, if the plan called for the new assisted living facility to attain full occupancy after 12 months' operation and it is only three fourths full, revisions to the plan may be in order.

Break-it Thinking

It is important to have a plan. Sometimes, however, it is even more important to abandon it. As Kriegel (1991) has observed, change is coming at such a fast pace that today's innovations are tomorrow's outworn models. He observes that, if it ain't broke today, it will be tomorrow. Kriegel cites an architect who finds the pace of change so fast that he feels like a gunfighter dodging bullets and an electronics administrator who does little besides come up for air in the momentary lull before the next storm (p. 3). The assisted living facility administrator within the next few years is likely to be faced with regulations from the federal and state governments and new financial approaches. We will explore ways to make an ally of change in Part 1.6.3.

1.3.2 Steps in Planning

PHASE ONE: DECIDE WHAT OUGHT TO BE DONE

Few people have the opportunity to plan for an organization from the very outset. Typically, in the assisted living facility field, an individual is hired as the administrator of an existing facility. For the purposes of illustration, however, let us follow the planning process that might occur in the creation of a new facility.

Suppose that one is asked by the regional vice president of a midsize publicly traded for-profit chain of assisted living facilities to evaluate a medium-sized community (about 50,000 residents) for the purpose of recommending or advising against the building of an assisted living facility there. Assume that sufficient funds are available if the decision is favorable. The assumption is further made that, if a new facility is built, the person doing this assessment would serve as its administrator.

This individual must appraise the present competitive, economic, and political environment in that community. We will not attempt to provide a complete checklist for arriving at an assessment of a community, but among the major planning considerations might be the following factors.

Governmental Permission

Numerous governmental bodies must grant permission to build a facility. Zoning requirements, building codes, and local fire codes must be met. If permission to build or similar governmental permission to build a new assisted living facility is needed, the likelihood of obtaining this must be an early consideration. Will approval of all required state and local government permits be forthcoming (Boiling et al., 1983; Miller, 1982)? What is the political climate in the town? Is the proposed assisted living facility likely to be welcomed, or if not, would permits probably be delayed, disapproved, or interpreted so strictly that costs rise unacceptably?

Competition

What is the level of unmet need for assisted living facility units in the community and its environs? How many competitors are there? What are their present and projected unit capacities? Is there enough unmet need for new units to expect that a new assisted living facility would fill up sufficiently quickly (typically, a 1-year start-up period is anticipated) and maintain the desired level of occupancy (typically, 95% or more for an assisted living facility) over an extended period of at least 5, preferably 10, years? What expansion plans do present facilities have? Are other competing assisted living facilities apt to be built over the next 3 to 5 years? One market researcher (Mullen, 1998) recommends four steps for uncovering proposed or planned projects:

1. In each town within what you believe to be your primary market area personally check the records in three departments: planning, zoning, and building. All three are necessary, some projects bypass planning and go directly to zoning, whereas others obtain zoning permits but have no plans to build.
2. Ask existing facility operators what they know about proposed or planned projects.
3. Visit and query local senior citizens groups or Area Agency on Aging personnel.
4. Check local newspapers' archives for stories about developers' intentions to build new assisted living units.

Typically, the primary market area is considered to be 10 to 13 miles from the propose project's site (slightly greater area in rural zones). Generally, if a developer has purchased land and started the zoning process, that project is highly likely to go forward.

What is known about local hospitals? Are they likely to enlarge, shrink, or stay the same? Are hospitals themselves in the process of building assisted living units, or expecting to do so? What is known about local home health care agencies? If the facility chose to utilize the home health care agency to provide the health care–related needs of its residents, would the agency be able to provide quality care? Is there an active hospice agency? As the residents age in place, would the home health care agency serve any residents in the facility who sought their services?

Economic Considerations

Are the expected residents apt to have the present and future income needed to keep the occupancy level high and with the desired mix of residents? Currently, over 90% of all assisted living care is private pay. Based on the company's projected daily charges for care, would the facility, if built, be competitive with charges by its competitors? Will the community and its surrounding area maintain or improve its economic condition over the next several years? What are the public and third-party reimbursement trends in this community and state?

Market Considerations

The evaluator must visualize the desired roles of the proposed assisted living facility in this environment. The considerations mentioned amount to conducting a needs assessment for the proposed assisted living facility. The perceived unmet needs will influence the role planned for the proposed facility. Unmet need, however, is not the sole criterion. The company may seek to create new markets for assisted living facility care not currently existing in that community. Increasingly, the assisted living facility census is made up of a profile of several types of residents. Assisted living facility care is now more frequently characterized by niche marketing, in which facilities offer identifiable increasingly specialized types of care (e.g., including an Alzheimer's or dementia unit).

PHASE TWO: SET SHORT- AND LONG-RANGE OBJECTIVES

Let us assume that a decision to build a new 100-bed facility has been made. The next step is to develop broad goals, objectives, and plans that will direct the efforts. A broad goal might be to build in keeping with the architecture of the community in a location convenient to the local hospital or other community resources.

From a set of broad goal statements such as these, more specific objectives and plans can be developed. A short-range objective (Kotter, 1982) might be to have a 60-bed facility in operation within 18 months, and, as a long-range objective, perhaps a new wing of 60 dementia units within 5 years.

PHASE THREE: DECIDE ON THE MEANS TO ACHIEVE THE OBJECTIVE

The next logical step is to translate broad planning goals into functional efforts on a more detailed basis. It is at this stage that allowable cost levels are determined, detailed plans for the building drawn, and the building site purchased. Specific decisions must be made: for example, will any Alzheimer's or dementia unit be included as a wing of a single building or as a separate building?

The planning process has moved from the general to the specific: from broad goals to architectural plans that are detailed enough to direct every person connected with the project. In this way, broad goals are translated into detailed behaviors for everyone who takes part in realizing these goals.

Planning for Next Year

We have used planning for a new facility as an example because this demonstrates the entire planning process. Most planning is shorter range (done for the next year). As a practical matter, this planning is usually accomplished when the budget for the next fiscal year (next 12 months) must be developed. An extensive example of the steps of planning for the next fiscal year through the budgeting process is given in Part Three.

Once plans have been crystallized, the next step is to put them into effect, to make them operational. This is the process of giving plans an organizational form. The form depends on the administrator's perceptions of the organization's structure, in particular, and behavior of the organization, in general.

Plan to Change Your Plans

No matter how carefully we plan, at any moment circumstances can change. The three main sources of residents today may be entirely different tomorrow. Perhaps this is why administering an assisted living facility will remain a challenging job—nothing remains stagnant in the health care field. Alas, the availability of residents with the ability to pay privately for their care will inevitably shrink, requiring many assisted living facilities to seek new funding combinations.

Consider Kriegel's (1991) experiences in teaching people how to prepare mentally for difficult rock climbing. Looking up the mountain from the bottom one mentally constructs a plan to reach the top. Once the climb begins, however, the view becomes different. Other, more promising routes to the top begin to appear. The climber can thus change the route. Mountain climbers come to expect that no matter how well they plan from the bottom of the mountain, they can count on running into the unexpected on the ascent. To those who enjoy finding new ways and improving current modes of doing things in the assisted living facility, this is an exciting prospect, an opportunity for creativity. Assisted living facility administrators who learn to deal with the unexpected, even to thrive on it, will endure in the profession.

The management guru Peter Drucker (1954) observed that no other area offers richer opportunities for successful innovation than the unexpected. Today, for example, the federal government does not regulate the assisted living industry. But all this could change overnight for the assisted living industry as it changed overnight for the nursing home industry when the *Federal Conditions of Participation* were imposed in 1970.

Successful assisted living facility administrators will assume that once they begin to implement any plan they will meet new people, receive new information, learn of new developments, and see possibilities about which they could not have known at the outset. The unexpected cannot be controlled. In the assisted living facility industry of today, uncertainty and surprise, from both the public and private sectors, are normal. What can be controlled is one's attitude toward the unanticipated. If one accepts that change is integral to living, one can look forward to it and be ready to take advantage of the new opportunities it offers. Accepting the inevitability of change is an attitude that will serve the administrator well.

1.4 Organizing

Organizing is a method of ensuring that the work necessary to achieve a goal is broken down into segments, each of which can be handled by one person (Dale, 1969). There must be no duplication of work. Efforts are then directed toward accomplishing the goal by dividing the work so that each job can be done by one person, and providing a means for coordinating the jobs done by different people—the task of the administrator.

Descriptions are written for each job. A job list for each position usually includes the following:

- the objectives (result to be accomplished)
- the duties and authorities of the position
- its relationship to other positions in the organization

As a rule, an organizational manual containing all job descriptions and perhaps several charts is prepared.

Gulick and Lyndall (1937) noted that job analysis consists of answering the following questions:

- What does the worker do? (worker functions)
- How does the worker do it? (methods and techniques)
- What aids are necessary? (machines, tools, equipment)

- What is accomplished? (products, services produced)
- What knowledge, skills, and abilities are involved? (qualifications)

Organizing is the first step in implementing of a plan. It is the process of translating plans into combinations of money, materials, and people.

All administrators organize their facilities according to some theory of organization. Their understanding of organization is reflected in their day-to-day and year-to-year direction. For some administrators, this is a very thoughtful process; for others, it is quite superficial. Nevertheless, all of them apply their concept of organization through their behavior in daily decision making.

SYSTEMS

Organizations are systems of interactions among the three available inputs: people, materials, and money (Robey, 1982).

A great deal has been written in recent decades about systems theory. This literature appeared after World War II and has paralleled the development of computer applications to management tasks (Boling et al., 1983; Katz & Kahn, 1967; Levey & Loomba, 1973). The systems concept is primarily a way of thinking about the task of managing any organization. It offers the administrator a framework for visualizing the internal and external environment of the organization.

A system has been defined as an organized or complex whole, an assembling or combining of things or parts forming a complex or single whole. Stated more simply, the idea of systems helps us to figure out how things are put together. How, for example, do all of the employees in the assisted living facility relate to each other, to the community, and to the rest of the world that affects them?

Systems theory is a tool for making sense out of our world by helping to make clearer the interrelationships within and outside the organization. The administrator uses systems theory to determine what is going on inside the facility and between the facility and the larger outside community.

1.4.1 Description of the Organization as a System

Systems descriptions vary from completely nonmathematical to highly sophisticated mathematical models (George, 1972; Mintzberg, 1979). The model we present does not require quantification, although numerical weights could be given to each of its elements (DeGroot, 1970; Zmud,1983).

OVERVIEW

In Figure 1.2, we illustrate a systems model that may be useful to the assisted living facility administrator in daily management of the facility. This model consists of the following elements: inputs, processor, outputs, control, plans of action, feedback and environment. (For an equally simplified model, see Miller, 1982, pp. 4015–4018; see also Robey, 1982, pp. 134–135).

Organizations such as assisted living facilities use inputs to get work done, which results in outputs. The outputs are evaluated by the residents, their significant others, and the public, which then react, and the facility receives feedback. The outputs are also evaluated by the administrators and compared to what was sought. If the results, or outputs, do not conform to organizational policy and action plans, the administrators take control actions to bring the outputs into line with those planned. All of these activities occur within the constraints placed on the organization from the external environment.

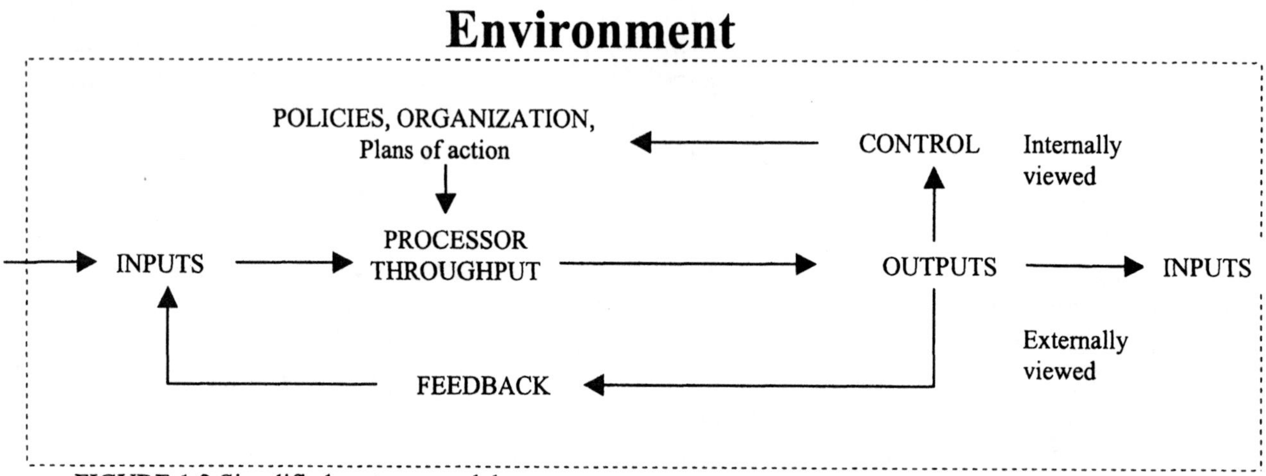

FIGURE 1.2 Simplified systems model.

INPUT

The input in any organization can be described as three elements: money, people, and materials. Input involves elements the facility administrators can change and use to advantage.

How Can Input Be Increased?

A primary concern of the system's administrator is, how input can be renewed and increased. To accomplish this, organizations take in resources. Just as the human body must have oxygen from the air and food from the environment, the assisted living facility must constantly draw renewed supplies of energy from other institutions, people, and the material environment.

As residents die or move to a nursing facility setting, more residents must be admitted into the facility if it is to continue to function. As food is consumed in the dining rooms, more food supplies must be brought in, so that the work of the facility (caring for residents) may continue. As employees leave for other jobs, new staff must be recruited. As the month's cash income is spent paying the facility bills, more revenue from residents must be brought in.

PROCESSOR

The processor is the work the organization accomplishes. Organizations transform the energy (input) available to them, just as the human body converts starch and sugar into heat and action. The assisted living facility cares for residents, helping them achieve the activities of daily living. Work is completed. Input is reorganized (e.g., food supplies are blended into recipes for the next meal). This is sometimes called the throughput. It is the actual work that the organization performs.

The assisted living facility takes its input (staff, money, and materials) and reorganizes it into active caring for residents. In essence, what assisted living facilities do is take money resources from residents and other sources and use those funds to hire staff and provide materials needed (buildings, units, food, etc.) to meet resident needs.

OUTPUT

The results of the work (caring for residents) that assisted living facilities do are the output, the product of the work accomplished by the organization. The organization exports some product (service) to the environment.

An assisted living facility produces services for residents. These services may take many forms, such as improved mobility as the output of a physical therapy visit or improved self-feeding as the output of a restorative feeding program for residents who may have experienced a stroke. Assisted living facilities provide an increasing variety of output.

The usefulness of thinking about the administrative tasks within a systems framework will become more evident as we describe the complex ramifications of the work of assisted living facilities (resident care) that is produced for the community. Later on in this section we will examine a number of additional insights provided by viewing organizations as systems.

CONTROL OF QUALITY

Control will be discussed at greater length below. For the purposes of exploring the systems diagram in Figure 1.2, it will be described only briefly here. Control is a most important tool available to administrators in the process of keeping the organization on course. It is the corrective action taken after evaluation of output by the organizational decision makers.

In the assisted living facility the administrator exercises control of quality by comparing the actual care provided residents with the care called for in the organizational policies and plans of action. This, in our view, is at the very heart of what administrators do. Just as important, every assisted living facility administrator has the responsibility to compare the ultimate financial results with the expected financial results. We deal with this in depth in Part Three.

Put simply, control of quality is the process of asking if the work accomplished by the facility is up to expected standards and, if not, taking corrective actions to remedy the problem. Here we are discussing the actual standards the organization has established for itself through its policies and plans of action.

POLICIES AND PLANS OF ACTION

Policies and plans are discussed in greater depth elsewhere in this text. For the purpose of illustrating the system configuration we use, let us simply refer to policies and plans of action as the guidelines the administrator uses to compare the output (e.g., actual resident care or financial results achieved) with the expected (i.e., the policies and plans of action developed and put into operation by the facility). As the arrows in Figure 1.2 indicate, the administrator uses the organization's policies (broad statements of goals and procedures) and plans of action, which are the more specific procedures designed to govern the implementation of the policies.

There are many areas in which assisted living facilities must develop and implement their own policies and plans for action. One such area is food services: Every facility develops policies by which it hopes to control the quality of food served its residents.

To summarize, administrators compare the results obtained with the results expected, then take steps to reorganize the inputs and/or reorganize the processor (the work itself) to more nearly achieve the desired standards.

FEEDBACK

Feedback is a form of control, but feedback is used here to refer to the external responses to the output (resident care provided, etc.) by the assisted living facility.

Assisted living facility outputs have many dimensions, such as roles played in long-term care in the community.

External Feedback

Feedback is normally expressed through reactions in the community about quality of work (outputs) being produced. This appears in

- word of mouth evaluations
- newspaper articles and radio and TV commentary
- the reputation enjoyed by the facility's staff that leads potential employees to consider it as a desirable or undesirable place to work
- the number of potential residents applying for admission to the facility

The reader can add to the list. All of these elements constitute what is referred to in Figure 1.2 as the environment.

ENVIRONMENT

The environment consists of all relevant external forces that affect the assisted living facility.

Defining the Environment

Defining the relevant environment of one's organization is perhaps the most complex and least obvious aspect of viewing organizations as systems. The environment consists of opportunities and constraints. One way to conceptualize this is to ask two questions:

1. Does it relate meaningfully to my objectives? If, so it is an opportunity.
2. Can I do anything about it? If not, it is a constraint.

If the answer to the first question is yes and the second question is no, it is a constraint in the relevant environment. If the answer to both questions is yes, it is an opportunity for the facility.

From the systems perspective, the entire world is interconnected in one large network. The challenge is to identify the aspects of the external world that now affect or may eventually affect the facility in its attempt to achieve objectives, such as serving residents and making a profit. This is the first step in the management process: forecasting.

The environment is both a set of constraints within which the facility must operate and a set of opportunities that the facility administration may seize (Pfeiffer & Salanick, 1978).

Some easily recognizable constraints in an assisted living facility's environment might be

- state or local regulations
- the number of other facilities operating in the area
- the availability of qualified applicants for positions to be filled in the facility
- the availability of foods at affordable prices
- increasingly, for some facilities, insurance company and other third-party payers' practices and reimbursement policies
- availability and costs of money
- inflation or deflation rates

Some recognizable opportunities might be

- the opportunity to identify and serve niches in care needs
- the increasing number of frail elderly who will need ADL and IADL assistance
- pressures for increased number of facilities due to the aging of the "baby boom" population explosion (1945–1965) that followed World War II

1.4.2 Identifying Systems

The outputs of one system normally become the inputs for the next system (Levey & Loomba, 1973), for example, the relationships that normally exist among hospitals, nursing homes, assisted living facilities, home health care agencies, and hospice providers.

WHO DEFINES THE SYSTEM?

The selection of what is to be viewed as the system is left entirely to the discretion of the person who describes or analyzes it. This may be one of the more subtle concepts in systems theory. The fact is that the user decides what to designate as a system for his or her own purposes. For example, the chief executive officer of a large assisted living facility chain is accustomed to thinking of the several hundred facilities as the system. The individual assisted living facility administrator may conceive of the departments operating in the facility as the system. The housekeeping supervisor may consider his or her area as the system. Because the groups studying the number of assisted living facilities have used different definitions, the number of facilities believed operating has varied significantly.

One of the virtues of the systems concept is that it is almost infinitely adaptable to the needs of the individual user. Anybody can define any set of interrelationships as the system for purposes of description or analysis. All of us use systems analysis in our everyday thinking about the interrelationships of things around us. The systems theory described here is an analytic tool that the administrator can use to solve organizational problems as they arise.

1.4.3 Additional Characteristics of Systems

Social science researchers have identified several characteristics of systems that the reader may find useful as analytical tools.

The output of each system furnishes the stimulus for repeating the cycle (Katz & Kahn, 1967). In the case of health care facilities, the successfully cared for resident (the desired outcome of the assisted living facility's efforts) furnishes the source of more inputs: Other persons apply for admission to the facility to replace the resident who has died. The new resident brings renewed energy in the form of a renewed source of continuing income to the facility and thereby furnishes a renewal of the capacity of the facility to continue to pay employees and provide services.

The administrator can view the assisted living facility as a dynamic system whose essence is the cycle of activities (providing care to residents, making sufficient income) for which he or she is responsible.

ORGANIZATIONAL GROWTH

An assisted living facility and similar social organizations can grow indefinitely.

Scientists speak of the entropic process, a universal law of nature that holds that all organisms move toward death. All of us, for example, realize that one day we will die because one of our vital systems comes to a halt.

In sharp contrast, an assisted living facility or chain not only does not have to die, but it can keep on growing, with no time constraints, as long as it receives more energy from the environment than it consumes. In this way organizations can be said to acquire negative entropy (Robey, 1982).

Organizations tend to try to grow. Theorists refer to this as the tendency of organizations to maximize the ratio of imported to expended energy. One social scientist (Miller, 1982) observed that the rate of growth of an organization, within certain ranges, is dramatic if it exists in a medium that makes available unrestricted amounts of additional inputs. The significance for administrators is that organizations, unlike people, are not subject to disintegration as long as they can keep adding to their resources. Between the early 1990s and the present, the number of assisted living facilities has grown almost exponentially in response to the rapid increases in the number of aging Americans who need and can pay for assistance with the activities of daily living. Growth may be qualitative (better care) or quantitative (a larger resident census or more facilities being added to the chain).

MAXIMIZING BASIC CHARACTER

Another important aspect of organizations is that, as they grow, they attempt to accommodate the world around them to meet their own needs (Katz & Kahn, 1967). For example, in planning for an extended care system, the assisted living facility associations place themselves at the heart of the system by seeking to help residents age in place over an extended period of time. The American Hospital Association, on the other hand, envisions the American health care system with hospitals at its core. The insurance companies are similarly convinced of their own strategic importance at the very center of such a system.

RESISTING CHANGE

Once in place, organizations become creatures of habit and develop a tendency to resist change. There can be a strong effort to keep the current pattern of relationships with others from changing at all. Organizations that have become set in their ways will try to maintain the status quo:

1. Any internal or external situation that threatens to force a change in the organization is countered by employees seeking to retain their old patterns and modes of operation. For example, the assisted living facility faced with a "disruptive employee" agitating for change may instead dismiss him or her, thus resisting change (Bradley & Calvin, 1956).

2. Administrators, when confronted with external changes that might affect the organization, will try to ignore them. For example, if their resident census declines while

it increases in nearby assisted living facilities, the tendency will be to find excuses rather than to examine if the other facilities are offering better services.

3. Resisting change, many organizations will attempt to cope with external forces by acquiring control over them. For example, if an assisted living facility chain is losing residents to a competing group of facilities, the chain might attempt to acquire those other facilities rather than remedy its own situation (Katz & Kahn, 1967).

Assisted living facilities and assisted living facility chains can fall from leadership. How can this happen? A Massachusetts Institute of Technology study on productivity attributes this to "a deep reservoir of outmoded attitudes and policies" at most organizations (Kriegel, 1991, p. 3).

Rapid and unanticipated changes are a permanent fixture of the administrative landscape of today. This textbook is about learning to appreciate that change brings opportunities.

WE'VE ALWAYS DONE IT THAT WAY

Once firmly in place, systems, policies, procedures, plans, organizational approaches, and assumptions become the standard operations of the facility, its sacred cows. They are sacrosanct because it has "always" been done this way. Creativity is thus stifled and competitive strength weakened. Today, anything that remains unchallenged or untouched for very long can become the sacred cow of tomorrow. Sacred cows are difficult to round up for a variety of reasons. They may be untouchable because some of the owners want it that way, or are the administrator's special concerns, or relate to one area's closely guarded turf.

A corporate executive officer of Quad Graphics (Kriegel, 1991, p. 119) identified the following sacred cow areas:

- **Budgets:** Consider eliminating budgets—use computer files to give you an up-to-the-moment report.
- **Plans:** Consider that using plans is like firing a cannonball at a castle—only today's markets are moving targets.
- **The pyramid:** Push functions down the pyramid—let the department head run the department
- **The Purchasing Department:** Sell the purchasing department—let departments buy and be accountable for the supplies they need.
- **Personnel:** Let personnel departments go—let each administrator hire, then be responsible for, employees.
- **Residents:** Let everyone interact with the customers—welcome the residents' children and others into the facility.
- **Quality control:** Reject any quality control department—make everyone responsible for quality.
- **The time clock:** Discard the time clock—if the employees can't be trusted to work their shift, don't hire them.
- **Levels:** Eliminate levels—it's hard to build a team among unequals.

Conclusion: You can't move fast if you're following a herd of sacred cows. Paper trails represent people trying to keep tabs on others, all this when the real purpose of systems as we have described them is to empower, not control, people, to liberate staff to experiment with new ways to meet residents' needs, not to tie them down.

ORGANIZATIONS GROW INCREASINGLY COMPLEX

New organizations tend to be simple at their start, then become more and more complex as they grow. The human personality is similar. As infants we have few perceptions. As we grow, we begin to build ever more complex and complicated perceptions of the world around us. The personality we develop is a system with no physical boundaries. A social organization such as an assisted living facility is also a system with no physical boundaries (Allport, 1962; Katz & Kahn, 1967).

Just as the human personality becomes progressively more sophisticated, so social organizations move toward the multiplication and elaboration of roles with greater specialization of functions. For example, the small rest homes of a few decades ago are giving way to increasingly larger and more sophisticated facilities offering a broad array of services.

The organization of American medicine provides another illustration. In 1870, 80% of all American physicians were general practitioners. Only a few were specialists. Today, with the explosion of medical technology, the reverse is true: About 80% of American physicians are specialists, and only 20% are general practitioners. As was bound to happen, today one must become a 3-year trained specialist to become a general practitioner, who today is called a family practice specialist.

The trend of assisted living facilities being combined into increasingly larger chains has led to a number of different management jobs. Middle- and upper-level positions are now available in corporate assisted living facility management offices. In 1994 only four assisted living providers managed 2,000 or more units. Three years later 10 providers managed 2,000 or more units.

SUMMARY

In the process of looking at organizations we have suggested that thinking of organizations as systems is a useful approach to the task of understanding how an assisted living facility operates. The systems model is a way to visualize the inputs (money, materials, and people) that are available to administrators. The way in which administrators configure and use money, materials, and people will depend on their beliefs about how organizations function.

1.5 Staffing

Staffing is hiring the right persons for the jobs in the organization. It is one of the most difficult tasks the administrator and his or her middle-level managers face because it is seldom possible to predict from an interview and recommendations how a person will work out on the job. The number of variables is almost infinite, and many of them are difficult to recognize beforehand.

One thing is quite clear: The success of the assisted living facility depends directly on adequate staffing. Assisted living care is helping older adults live as independently as possible. The interactions between residents and staff determine the quality of life in the facility. Physical facilities are important, but once they are in place at a minimally adequate level, the resident's satisfaction varies directly with his or her satisfaction with the staff performance.

The administrator may choose to delegate coordination of the hiring process to a personnel director or assign it to the individual middle-level manager with the advice and consent of the administrator. For this reason, we mention the staffing function at this point. The reader is referred to Part Two for a detailed discussion of staffing tasks.

In Part Two we offer a model of three levels of staffing for assisted living facilities in which personnel costs move from 35% of revenue at level 1 (lower level of ADL assistance) to 55% of revenues in level 3 (higher level of ADL assistance).

1.6 Directing

Directing is the process of communicating to employees what is to be done by each of them and helping them to accomplish it. An earlier step, organizing, included breaking down the work necessary to achieve the organizational goals into work assignments that can be handled by one person. Directing is an aspect of the organizational activity in which the actual work is done.

Several important management concepts will be included under this heading:

- policymaking
- decision making
- leadership
- power and authority
- communication skills
- organizational norms and values
- additional related concepts

Directing involves reference to each of these key concepts to arrive at the goal of a successful program.

1.6.1 Policymaking

The ultimate goal of the administrator is to design a program in which every member of the organization makes the same decisions given the same set of circumstances. To this end, the administrator attempts to persuade the entire staff to carry out their responsibilities exactly as he or she would like them to.

PURPOSE AND FUNCTION

It is impossible for the administrator to be everywhere at once, 24 hours a day, throughout the facility. It is possible, however, for the administrator to make policies that direct the activities of the employees everywhere in the facility 24 hours a day. The purpose and function of these policies is to communicate to each employee as exactly as possible what the management expects in any situation on the job.

It is, of course, neither possible nor desirable to establish policies for every conceivable situation. However, an administrator can provide guidelines or policies that become the framework within which the employee decides what to do in each situation requiring action on behalf of the assisted living facility. In his book *Principles of Management*, G. R. Terry (1969) defined policy as a verbal, written, or implied overall guide that sets up boundaries supplying the general limits and direction in which action will take place.

Policies are used to help keep decisions within the areas intended by the planners, since they provide for some consistency in what employees decide in particular situations usually under repetitive conditions. Policies reveal the facility administrator's intentions with respect to the behavior of employees, residents, and the public. They are decided before the need for employee knowledge arises. A simple illustration might be useful.

It is not possible for management to know when, where, or even whether a fire will break out in the facility. By developing a complete set of procedures for personnel to follow in case of fire, however, the administrator is able to communicate before the occasion arises precisely what each employee in the facility must do if a fire should occur.

Quality of Life

There are nationally available policy statements available to assisted living facilities to use in developing and modifying their own policy statements in such areas as the quality of life expected in the facility. The following policy has been developed by the federal government for long-term care providers, such as assisted living facilities, rest homes, domiciliary homes, and nursing homes, to consider in its *Federal Requirements and Guidelines to Surveyors* (June 1995), transmittal no. 274.

> This facility will care for its residents in a manner and in an environment that promotes maintenance or enhancement of each resident's quality of life. The facility will create and sustain an environment that humanizes and individualizes each resident.

In their interactions with residents, staff should carry out activities so that residents maintain and enhance their self-esteem and self-worth. Examples include the following:

- As needed, assisting residents to dress as they wish and to be groomed (e.g., hair combed and styled, beards shaved/trimmed, nails cleaned and clipped) to suit their individual taste.
- As needed, assisting residents to dress in their own clothes appropriate to the time of day and individual preferences.
- As needed, assisting residents to attend activities of their own choosing.
- As needed, labeling each resident's clothing in a way that respects his or her dignity.
- Promoting resident independence and dignity in dining: providing a pleasant dining room experience with attention to each resident's wishes.
- Respecting residents' private space and property (e.g., staff will always knock on residents' doors and await a response before entering unless responding to the emergency call light, which is increasingly a standard safety feature in the assisted living facility).
- Respecting residents' social status—speaking respectfully, listening carefully, treating residents with respect (e.g., addressing each resident using the a name of the resident's choice and not excluding residents from conversations or discussing residents in community setting).
- Addressing residents as individuals when providing care and services.

To determine if staff are meeting the standards reflected in a facility's policy on quality of life, the administrator may ask the following questions:

- Do staff show respect for residents?
- When staff interact with a resident, do staff pay attention to the resident as an individual?
- Do staff respond in a timely manner to the residents' requests for assistance?
- In group activities, do staff focus attention on the group of residents? Or do staff appear distracted when they interact with residents? For example, do staff continue to talk with each other while doing a task (such as making a bed) for a resident as if he or she were not present?

Policy on self-determination and participation

Each resident has the right to choose activities, schedules, and health care consistent with his or her interests and to interact with members of the community both inside and outside the facility.

To determine if staff are meeting the standards established in the facility's policy on self-determination and participation, the administrator should

- Observe how well staff know each resident and what aspects of life are important to him or her.
- Determine if staff make adjustments to allow residents to exercise choice and self-determination. For residents needing assistance in dressing, for example, a personal

care aide may choose to put clothes on the resident rather than wait for the resident to dress himself or herself. This contributes to what is sometimes referred to as "learned helplessness" and is in contrast to the facility's stated policy on self-determination.

POLICIES VS. PROCEDURES

The reader may have noticed the use of the word procedures above, rather than policies. Writers in the field of management use the terms policies and procedures, to indicate movement from generalized statements of intention (policies) to specific (procedures) for carrying out those policies or plans of action.

Consider the following examples, which move from the general to the specific, setting forth behaviors the administrator wishes the employees to exercise.

Example of Policies and Procedures

Fire preparedness. General goals or objectives may be stated for the facility. In the area of fire preparedness it might be: "Our goal is to have our facility employees completely prepared to take appropriate action in case of fire." The administrator might then draw up a general policy statement indicating that the head of the housekeeping area should develop a step-by-step plan of action for every area to follow in case of fire. This plan is a set of procedures highly detailed and specific actions that each employee would be expected to follow in case of fire.

Notice in this example that at each level the degrees of freedom within which decisions can be made are reduced. The head of housekeeping can develop a variety of configurations for employee responsibilities, but by the time the individual employee becomes involved, the degrees of freedom have nearly vanished. The responsibility in case of fire has moved from the general goal, fire preparedness, to a detailed set of instructions or procedures to be followed. "The moment you hear the fire alarm, proceed immediately to station J on the Blue wing and report to the person in charge" is an example of a procedure.

Food Preparation

The board of directors might set a policy goal of offering an outstanding selection of first-quality food to the residents of the facility. It becomes the responsibility of each progressively lower level of management to actually implement this policy. The food service director must take this communicated policy or goal and develop a series of policies for decision making by the kitchen staff that result in the actual service of an outstanding selection of first-quality food to the residents.

General policies are developed at each level of management. Normally, the amount of specificity increases at each lower level. The food service director, for example, may announce a policy to the food service employee responsible for salads that there be a sufficient variety with specified proportions of crisp, fresh lettuce every evening. The supervisor may then write out a step-by-step set of procedures for the kitchen worker who prepares salads.

The set of steps the salad worker is to follow at 4:00 P.M. each afternoon, beginning, perhaps, with removing the lettuce from the refrigerator, is an example of a set of procedures. The broad policy of excellence in food service promulgated by the administrator has now been translated into a set of procedures or individual steps for the salad worker in the kitchen to follow at 4:00 P.M. each afternoon to assure the crispness of the lettuce to be served each evening. Sounds simple, but ask the residents; too few assisted living facilities succeed in serving a sufficient variety of salads with crisp lettuce. Interesting salads 365 days a year is but one of hundreds of complex tasks that must be successfully accomplished each 24 hours.

SUMMARY

Policies serve as general statements that guide or channel subordinates' thinking as they make decisions. Policies limit the area within which a decision is to be made and seek to ensure that it will be consistent with the overall objectives. Policies tend to decide issues beforehand by establishing the framework and scope of the actions.

The decisions made at each level of management establish the framework for decision making at each successively lower level of management, generally with progressively less and less discretion to do so. However, each level of management does participate in the policy-making process, and policies are made at every level of management.

When do policies become procedures? Sometimes these are separated by a fine line that is hard to distinguish. Generally, a policy is a statement that contains some degree of freedom, some further need for interpretation. Procedures are step-by-step instructions on how a specific task is to be carried out.

1.6.2 Making a Decision

Although decision making can be synonymous with managing, it is difficult to define. G.L.S. Shackle (1957) defined *deciding* as the focal creative psychic event in which knowledge, thought, feeling, and imagination are fused into action (see also Dale, chap. 23). Both Dale and Shackle point out the impossibility of a useful formula for decision making. Inevitably, we are left with an imprecise definition of the process. Even so, administrators do make numerous decisions every day.

To make the "right" decision in a given situation is often difficult. It is the assisted living facility administrator's job to ensure that all employees make the right decisions for the organization as often as possible.

We define a successful administrator as a person who is able, on balance, to make enough right decisions for the organization and *no* disastrously wrong ones.

1.6.3 Leading

Organizations that thrive over an extended period of time depend on effective leaders -- persons who have foresight combined with an ability to guide the organization to successfully take advantage of the opportunities the future offers.

THE GREAT LEADERSHIP THEORY OF HISTORY

Just as a satisfactory description of *deciding* is elusive, so is a definition of *leading*. One proposal is "the great leadership theory of history," which suggests that history is "made" or measurably influenced by individuals who become leaders. Whatever one might think of their accomplishments, Alexander the Great, Genghis Kahn, Confucius, Joan of Arc, George Washington, Abraham Lincoln, Margaret Sanger, and Winston Churchill, to name only a few, assumed leadership roles that affected the course of history.

Leadership in the business world is no less crucial to the success of organizations. Between the years 1915 and 1973, for example, Thomas Watson, Sr. and Thomas Watson, Jr. provided leadership to an organization, International Business Machines Corp. (IBM), that came to dominate the computer world only during their tenure because this father and son had foresight (successfully predicted the future) combined with an ability to guide the organization to successfully take advantage of opportunities.

It was not until being discharged from a job he had held for 14 years that Tom Watson, Sr. joined a company that manufactured scales, meat slicers, time clocks, and punch cards for data sorting. He envisioned that these punch cards could revolutionize the future. He borrowed money and renamed the company. At the time, 1924, his son, Tom Watson, Jr., commented, "What a big name for a pip-squeak company that makes meat grinders." International Business Machines Corp. had just been born.

The health care industry has its own share of successful leaders. William McWhorter, for instance, was given responsibility for 103 hospitals that, in 1987, Hospital Corporation of America believed to be irreversibly unprofitable. Through his personal leadership these hospitals became both profitable and a major leader in the hospital industry.

The leadership provided to the assisted living facility by the administrator, resident care coordinator, and other administrators is no less critical to the success or failure to thrive of each assisted living facility.

THE ADMINISTRATOR AND THE RESIDENT CARE COORDINATOR

There is scant research literature to prove the assertion that leadership by the administrator and the resident care coordinator is key to the success of any assisted living facility. Even in the absence of such data, however, there is a broad consensus among observers of the industry that quality care in an assisted living facility does depend on its administrators' being able to exercise good leadership skills. When IBM's leadership changed after 60 years under the Watsons the giant lost its leadership position. IBM had ridden the wave of change with them at the helm. When the Watsons led IBM it usually was ranked in *Fortune* magazine's annual survey of America's Most Admired Corporations as number one. Lou Gerstner, IBM president, stated several times in the mid-1990s that he did not have to have a vision to lead the corporation. By 1995, out of the 500 ranked companies, IBM had dropped from the most admired to the 281st most admired corporation. Leadership counts. The Watsons inspired IBM to six decades of greatness with a vision. Vision, it seems, also counts.

Through forecasting, planning, organizing, staffing, directing, evaluating, controlling quality, innovating, and marketing decisions the administrator is providing leadership to the assisted living facility. We will next examine the various styles of leadership.

LEADERSHIP BY WALKING AROUND

One effective style, mentioned earlier, is leading by walking around (LBWA). When walking around and observing such things as staff interaction with residents and with families, volunteers, and other employees, the administrator can personally evaluate the quality of resident services being rendered. This is also an opportunity to see if the residents are having any problems and to physically inspect the building and equipment.

LBWA provides an opportunity for the staff to speak with the administrator informally. It allows time to observe what is going on and to let the staff know the administrator is interested in them, the residents, and the facility.

In this way, the administrator receives a daily update on the real world of the facility—in the rooms, hallways, work areas, and rest rooms. This positions the administrator to uncover problems before they become major irritants. Administrators who do not take the initiative to keep informed about facility affairs on a daily basis often become involved in a style of management known as fire fighting. Once small issues become hot issues a lot of time must be spent extinguishing flames.

In making daily rounds the administrator can do naive listening, gaining raw impressions of what is happening in the facility, sensing how things are going. Not enough time available to get the paperwork done, meet all the other administrator requirements, and still be able to walk daily around the facility, taking its pulse? Consider Sam Walton, the founder of Wal-Mart Corp., who visited every one of his stores at least once a year when he had only 18 stores. By the early 1990s he owned over 800 stores and was still visiting each one at least once a year, riding cross-country with Wal-Mart truck drivers, having donuts at 3:00 A.M. He thought the checkout clerk to be the most important employee. Until his death in the early 1990s, every clerk knew that sometime each year Mr. Sam might be the next customer waiting in the line, observing how the customer ahead of him was being treated. The resident care aide is like the checkout clerk and needs to know that the administrator cares about the details of the job.

The future doesn't just happen: Leaders like Tom Watson, Sam Walton, and the local assisted living facility administrator dream it, shape it, sculpt it.

MAINTAINING THE CHAIN OF COMMAND

Walking around the facility, talking with residents, visitors, and staff, appears to violate the traditional concept of chain of command. The administrator is there to hear about problems firsthand and to communicate firsthand. Ed Carson, a former airlines chairman who used the LBWA management style, took lots of notes on scraps of paper but never told people down the line what to do or change. He never corrected on the spot what he disliked. He did, however, promise to get back to the parties involved in a few days. He then discussed each situation with his department head and charted with him or her a course of action to resolve any problem. After a few days he would check back to see if appropriate action had indeed been taken. He was practicing what he called "visible management" (Peters, 1985, p. 386).

The basic benefits LBWA are listening (finding out what's happening on the firing line), teaching (communicating the facility's values), and facilitating. Through LBWA the administrator can facilitate the work of employees by asking naive questions, finding out what is frustrating the staff, then running interference and knocking down small hurdles for them. Meeting residents' needs is what the assisted living facility is about. Only the facility that pays excessive attention to details can achieve excellence in resident care. Quality of care is staff paying attention to the details that lead to excellent care as they emulate their administrator.

A LEADERSHIP STYLE

The challenge for the administrator is how to achieve employees' compliance with management's goals. Once the owners or directors have set forth the mission statement (goals and objectives of the facility), the administrator's work begins. The search for personnel who will implement the plans made by the organization's chief decision makers can then be undertaken.

Riding the Waves of Change

Deciding on the approach to leading is one of the more important decisions administrators ever make. Kriegel (1991) compares leading an organization to riding the waves of change. The time to change is when you don't have to, he asserts, when you are on the crest of a wave, not when you are in the trough. In the world of resident care delivery administration, the surf is up. Waves of change are coming from government, third-party payers, and the residents and their families.

The best surfers (assisted living facility administrators) are not necessarily the best swimmers (best management theoreticians). The best surfers are persons with the following mind-set.

Passion Rules. Catching and riding a wave may seem simple, but it requires effort to master it. Many wannabes look and act the part—they have the correct equipment and stylish outfits, they know all the right jargon—but they spend most of their time on the beach just talking about surfing. The best surfers spend their time out in the water, rough or calm, looking for the next wave. They are totally committed to surfing, in body, mind, and spirit.

No Dare/No Flair. Good surfers constantly push their limits, continuously trying new moves, going for bigger and bigger waves. They know that no two waves are ever the same, so that each one is ridden a little differently. Keeping ahead of the wave involves risk taking, constantly challenging yourself and those around you.

Expect to Wipe Out. For every successful ride there will likely be two or three wipeouts. A changing ocean with its dynamic wave patterns and shapes is a source not of fear but of challenge that provides the thrill of surfing. Successful surfers know that if they do not wipeout several times each day they are playing it too safe to keep improving.

Don't Turn Your Back on the Ocean. Surfers know that they are dealing with an environment beyond their control. They understand that uncertainty and unpredictability are part of the game. They respect the ocean and its power, never taking it for granted. They never turn their backs on the ocean.

Keep Looking "Outside." The outside waves are those on the horizon. It is important to pay attention to the wave closest to you and also to what is coming. First, there may be a bigger and better wave coming in on the horizon. Second, the wave on the horizon may crash over you as you come up for air after riding the wave nearest you.

Move Before It Moves You. Surfing is forecasting and planning for the future. You have to begin moving yourself while that big wave is still on the horizon or it will surge by you, leaving you in its trough.

Never Surf Alone. It is not smart to tackle the complexities of life alone. One needs backup help when emergencies arise. By pooling one's knowledge and insights surfers can learn about and get more exotic spots, trade tips, and techniques that work. It is also a lot more fun to have a friend along to "talk story" with as you navigate the complexities of the assisted living facility operations. Having someone to share your hopes, dreams, and frustrations leads to more creativity, joy, and effectiveness.

As Kriegel (1991) has suggested, the future is coming at us like enormous waves of change in set after set, and they are getting bigger. The surf is up in the assisted living industry, the hospital industry, the home health care industry, and the managed care industry. The future belongs to those who decide to ride, to those who welcome the unexpected.

While president of General Electric, John F. Welch became widely regarded as the leading master of corporate change by shedding 200,000 employees while tripling GE's market value between 1981 and 1993. He believed that every business must be fast and adaptable to survive. People ask, he observed, if the change is over at GE. He responds that change has just begun, that it is never ending. Change, he asserts, is a continuing process, not an event. He sees the administrator's job as listening to, searching for, and spreading ideas—the process of exposing people to good ideas and role models (Welch). As observed by Dennis Kodner in the *Journal of Long Term Care Administration,* the days of "business as usual" in the long-term care industry are over. He foresees that success in today's world depends on understanding where the industry is heading, having a vision of the future, and developing the capacity to implement change as an ongoing aspect of managing a facility. Facilities that resist change and continue to function in isolation may survive but will not thrive in the 21st century.

FIRE IN THE HEART

To be a successful assisted living facility administrator over a sustained period of years requires that one be excited and passionate about the profession. Top performers in all fields have one thing in common: passion. Their drive and enthusiasm for assisted living facility administration are what distinguishes them. As numerous executive recruiters have observed, "The thing that makes the difference between a good administrator and an inspiring, dynamic leader goes beyond competence. It's passion. That is the single quality that is going to lift a person head and shoulders above the rest" (Kriegel, 1991, p. 13).

Passion brings complete commitment to one's work. And it's contagious. An administrator enthusiastic about the work can inspire excitement in employees. Knowledge of the field, competence, and experience make a good administrator, but a greater commitment provide the edge necessary in today's assisted living facility.

Of course, passion is not a scientifically measurable component of assisted living facility administration, but then management is not exactly a science. What the assisted living facility administrator needs is a fire in the heart for continuously improving the quality of the daily life of each resident.

A Continuum of Leadership Styles

In *Leadership and Organization,* Tannenbaum, Wechsler, and Massarik (1961) outlined a continuum of leadership styles, ranging from manager-centered to employee-centered leadership. Several dimensions are portrayed in Figure 1.3.

Manager-centered leadership						Employee-centered leadership
Use of authority by manager				Areas of freedom for employees		
manager decides and announces decision	manager sells, persuades acceptance	Manager presents ideas & invites questions	Manager present tentative decision	Manager presents problem, takes suggestions, makes decision	Manager defines the limits, tells group to make decision	Manager permits employees to function within policies set by manager
1	2	3	4	5	6	7
Manager retains a high degree of control				Manager shares decision making		

FIGURE 1.3 Range of Decision-Making Strategies Open to the Manager

Manager-Centered Leadership. Under manager-centered leadership, the manager retains a high degree of control and uses authority extensively.

Position 1. The manager simply makes the decision, then announces it (autocratic style).
Position 2. The manager attempts to convince the employees of the value of the decision made.
Position 3. The manager presents ideas and invites questions, in effect engaging the employees actively in the decision-making process.

Employee-Centered Leadership. Under employee-centered leadership, the manager shares decision-making responsibilities with employees.

Position 4. The manager presents a tentative decision, subject to change; the employees are further involved in the decision-making process itself.
Position 5. The manager presents the problem requiring a solution, invites suggestions, then makes the decision.
Position 6. The manager permits the subordinates to make the decision and function within the limits defined by the manager (laissez-faire leadership style).

DECIDING HOW TO LEAD

At least the following three levels of considerations should be taken into account by the administrator who is selecting the leadership style for a particular situation

First level: Forces in the administrator

- his or her own values
- his or her confidence in the middle-level managers
- his or her own feelings of security or insecurity

Second level: Forces in the employees. The facility administrator can permit greater freedom to staff who

- have a need for independence (e.g., the resident care coordinator)
- are ready to assume responsibility for decision making
- are interested in the problem and consider it important (take resident care seriously)
- understand and agree with the mission statement or goals of the facility
- have the necessary knowledge and experience
- are prepared and expect to make decisions (e.g., a skilled chef)

Third level: Forces in the organization

- expectations of the organization's management (position taken by the corporation or the board)
- ability of subordinates to function as a group
- the problem itself
- time constraints

THREE LEVELS OF LEADERSHIP SKILL REQUIREMENTS

We have already discussed three levels of management— upper, middle, and lower—each with its own particular skill requirements. Figure 1.4, adapted from Katz and Kahn (1967) shows three different levels of leadership skills.

The Upper-level Administrator

The assisted living facility's top echelon is primarily responsible for creating and changing the organization's structure.

The Middle-level Administrator

The head of dietary or head of housekeeping, for instance, is responsible for development of more specific policies that interpret administration policy implications for their areas.

The Lower-level Administrator

The resident care coordinator who supervises a specific group of health care workers/health assistants has the responsibility of applying the policies provided by the director of health to the hour-by-hour care given.

As Figure 1.4 suggests, different skills are needed at the three distinct levels of management.

CHARACTERISTICS OF THE EFFECTIVE LEADER

Katz and Kahn (1967) have characterized an effective leader as a person who

- mediates and tempers the organizational requirements to the needs of persons in a manner that is organizationally enhancing (e.g., through the Family and Medical Leave Act provisions, the facility assists employees having family crises through unplanned time off and other support)
- promotes group loyalty and personal ties (working for the facility becomes a personally satisfying experience)
- demonstrates care for individuals (knows each employee by name and something about that employee's interests)
- relies on referent power (respect from employees and residents) rather than the power of legitimacy and sanctions alone (discussed below)

Type of Leadership Process	Appropriate Organizational Level	Abilities and Skills: Cognitive	Abilities and Skills: Affective
Origination: change, creation, and elimination of structure	Top Echelons	System perspective	Charisma, referent power
Interpolation, supplementing and piecing out of structure	Intermediate levels: pivotal roles	Subsystem perspective: two-way orientation upwards and downwards	Interpersonal relations skills
Operational use of existing structure	Lower levels	Technical knowledge and ability to apply the system of rules	Equity in use of rewards and sanctions

FIGURE 1.4. Three levels of skill requirements for managers.

Tannenbaum and colleagues. (1961) concluded that a successful leader is a person who is keenly aware of relevant forces in the situation, understands himself or herself and the individuals with whom he or she is dealing, and is able to behave appropriately vis-à-vis the situation, making decisions where needed and sharing the decision-making where appropriate. They consider the successful leader as being neither strong nor permissive, but rather as endowed with a strong "instinct" for determining appropriate personal behavior and acting accordingly.

Day-to-Day Leadership Requirements

In the daily administration of the typical long-term care facility the administrator will face a variety of situations with different leadership needs. Recognition of appropriate leadership behavior for any specific situation is a valuable insight; the capacity to use different leadership styles is an accomplishment. Much of the flexibility the administrator can exercise in distinctive leadership styles depends on how comfortable he or she is in wielding power and authority in the management of the facility.

Charismatic Leadership

Although charismatic leadership cannot be consciously chosen by the administrator, it is worth mentioning here. This quality has been described by Max Weber as a magical aura with which people sometimes endow their leaders. It appears when a group has an emotional need for a person who, they feel, will make the right decision for them. The acts of charismatic leaders are typically unexamined. Their followers do not scrutinize their acts as they would those of their immediate supervisors. Charisma is not an objective assessment by the followers and normally requires a psychological distance between the followers and the leader. When charisma is assigned to a leader, the power and authority of the organization is enhanced.

1.6.4 Power and Authority

Power is the ability to control the behavior of others. A person has power when he or she is able to make other people do what he or she wants them to. One writer says this is the ability to motivate someone to do something that they would otherwise not do (Argenti, 1994). The administrator of an assisted living facility has the power to order employees to act to implement the goals of the facility as expressed in the policies and plans.

Webster's New World Dictionary gives 14 definitions for the word *power.* An additional half-dozen synonyms indicate that power denotes the inherent ability or the admitted right to rule, govern, determine, control, regulate, restrain, and curb. Power is a complex concept in our culture.

The administrator has the power (from the board or the ownership) to tell employees what to do and to expect them to do it. It is well known that although an organization theoretically provides equal legitimating power to all administrators at the same level, the administrators do not in fact remain equal. For example, a board of directors controlling five assisted living facilities, in theory, delegates equal authority to the administrators to act on its behalf in the five facilities. Some of these five administrators might have firm control over employee behavior, whereas others might be having difficulty convincing employees to do what they request. Why?

TYPES OF POWER

Power is a reciprocal relationship. The board of directors or the owners can confer power on the administrator, but the employees and residents must accept that power as if it is to be meaningful. This does not imply disrespect or chaos. The concept of authority or power is more complicated than the mere announcement that power has been given to the administrator by the board or the owners.

French and Raven (1960), Robey (1982), and others have identified five types of power: legitimate, reward, punishment (coercive), referent, and expert. It is important for administrators to be familiar with these types of power and their applications.

Legitimate Power

This describes authority given to a particular position and is associated with the person's position in the organization. Organizations expect each person to yield to the appropriate authority of others. The administrator has more legitimate power, than the head of marketing and activities and so on. When employees or residents respond to legitimate power their actions are motivated by the level or position of the administrator, not to any characteristic of that person.

Reward Power

The fact that reward is a second type of power is testimony to the mundane reality that employees do not always respond correctly. Administrators are given reward power to induce or persuade employees or residents to do what the administrator asks. If not, certain desired approvals may be withheld. For example, if the administrator has authority to give a 15% year-end cash bonus to the three supervisors who have best achieved the facility's goals (translation: those who most often responded acceptably to the administrator's instructions), then he or she has reward power.

Punishment Power

Also known as coercive power, this type exists when the employee believes that the administrator has the ability (and inclination) to punish unacceptable behaviors. The ultimate punishment power is firing the employee or requiring the resident to leave the facility, but there are many intermediate, less drastic means. The employees who do not observe the administrator's rules for functioning in the facility may receive a written warning, a copy of which is placed in the personnel file. Use of punishment power is normally a last resort, used after other types of power have failed. Extensive use of punishment power leads to distrust and fear, which clearly are not conducive to quality resident care.

Referent Power

Power to influence is often based on liking or identifying with another person. When the employees like the administrator and identify with him or her, they are more apt to do what the administrator wishes. Referent power exists to the degree employees and residents identify with the administrator. Employees who do not admire an administrator or do not identify with him or her are more difficult to control.

Expert Power

Power can derive from recognition by the employees and residents that the administrator is very skillful, has had considerable training, and is quite knowledgeable in the field of assisted living facility administration. For the nurse, this acknowledgment comes from the registered nurse license; for the physician, the license to practice medicine.

POWER FROM OUTSIDE THE ORGANIZATION

It is important to note that expert and referent power, to the extent they are present in the facility, are additions to the power of organizationally given rewards and punishments because expert and referent power cannot be conferred by the organization. There is literally an increase in the amount of power or control that can be exerted over the personnel and residents, and it is a persistent factor in increased organizational performance.

Expert and referent power can be substituted for power based on punishment. This can mean fewer negative or undesired or unintended organizational consequences. It is desirable to promote referent power in addition to, or instead of, power based on rewards and punishment or organizational dictates. Remember, the goal of the administrator is to motivate the members of the organization to achieve the organization's goals.

Expert and referent power are available to all members of the staff. Referent power, in particular, depends on personal and group characteristics and is available to peers (persons at the same level) in the organization. Peer influence is often more readily accepted than influence from superiors. If, for example, one of the personal care aides is particularly skillful in creating a cheerful atmosphere in the facility, his or her leadership through referent power gives the assisted living facility greater control over the quality of life achieved.

THE ADMINISTRATOR'S POWER IS REAL

Administrator's do have power over other people's lives. Christensen, Berg, and Salter (1980) characterized the power of the chief administrator as potentially "irresponsible" (p. 49), not necessarily because of the use of power in any particular decision or even because of the motives of the administrator, but because those affected by the decisions (the employees, residents, and even the board or owners) very often have little or no real immediate voice in the making of some decisions (e.g., when to finally tell employees that the cumulative effect of their behaviors renders them unfit to work at that facility). This can be especially true when most of the power is centralized in the office of the administrator. The task of achieving control over the behavior of the professional employees is a complicated one, requiring tact and ingenuity on the part of the administrator.

1.6.5 Communication Skills

Directing is the process of communicating the organizational objectives to the staff, residents, and their significant others. *Communication* is the exchange of information and the transmission of meaning.

Communication is essential for the survival of any social system, such as the assisted living facility. The skills of the administrator in communicating what is to be accomplished and the manner in which it is to be carried out have much to do with the success of the administrator in achieving the plan for the facility. Unless the plans of action are successfully communicated to the staff, the plans will, at worst, not be implemented at all, or at best, only partially carried out.

Steps in the communication process are: (1) someone initiates it, (2) it is transmitted from its source to its destination, and (3) it has an impact on the recipient. Unless and/or until a communication has made its intended impact on the recipient, it has, for all intents and purposes, not taken place.

COMMUNICATION = INFORMATION = POWER

Communication is the transmission of information, and information is power because it provides sounder bases for judgments. The informed person is on sounder ground and therefore is more powerful. The withholding of information is also a form of power, inasmuch as the person with the information is in a superior position to make decisions. Good communication is sometimes described as active listening, that is, listening with intensity, acceptance, empathy, and a willingness to assume responsibility for understanding the speaker's complete message (Argenti, 1994).

SYSTEMS OF COMMUNICATION

Organizations are described as having at least two systems of communication: the formal and the informal communication process.

The *formal communication process* closely resembles the formal organizational structure of the assisted living facility (Dale, 1969). An example would be the administrator sending memoranda to the area heads, such as housekeeping or the kitchen.

The *informal communication process* exists in nearly every organization. The social groups within the facility define the informal communication process (Dale, 1969; Mintzberg, 1979). Housekeeping workers chatting in their lounge communicate informally and exchange much important information in the course of their casual conversation.

Communication is the flow of information in the organization, which social scientists describe as flowing upward, downward, and horizontally. As the words themselves suggest, *upward communication* flows from subordinates upward to the next levels or administration. *Downward communication* flows from upper-level management to lower-level members of the staff. Horizontal communication is information flowing between peers or persons of equal rank or status.

The closer a person gets to the organizational center of control, the more pronounced the emphasis is on the exchange of information. Administrators process information and use it in their decision making. Communicating is at the heart of the management process.

Communicating is an art that administrators must master. Communications between administrators and personnel are full of subtleties and shades of meaning. Most communication also has numerous levels of meaning and function and is essential to building a relationship. Any act of communication may answer a question at the moment, but it has different meanings for the persons involved. Administrators need to be aware that there are many barriers to full, clear communication. Seldom does any single communication have only one level of meaning (Kotter, 1982).

BARRIERS TO COMMUNICATION

Agenda Carrying

Each person carries his or her own agenda into every communication situation, preoccupied with his or her own concerns and life experiences. Each individual filters what is communicated by means of his or her own perceptions.

Selective Hearing

Persons hear selectively; that is, they tend to hear what they want to hear, thereby filtering out the unpleasant. A supervisor may wish to communicate to a personal care aide dissatisfaction with one aspect of the aide's performance. To soften the effect, the supervisor may first praise the employee for some other work. The employee may hear the praise and effectively screen out the criticism.

Differences in Knowledge Levels

Persons who have only sketchy knowledge about a topic may process information quite differently from persons who may be more knowledgeable. That is, degrees of sophistication vary among listeners, and the "information" they process from a single communication may differ significantly.

The Filter Effect

The administrator may be told what the employees believe he or she wants to hear. It is not easy to give bad news to a superior when one already knows such news is not welcome. Ancient Greek tales recount how frequently the messenger bringing bad news to the king was killed. The implications of this reaction have not been lost on most organizational members.

It seems that no matter how much middle- and upper-level administrators insist they want to hear bad as well as good news, the employees filter the information toward the known bias of the next level of management. When there are several layers of management through which unwelcome news must filter, the upper management may receive little accurate information.

Subgroup Allegiance

Each one of the subgroups in the organization (e.g., kitchen workers, housekeepers, residents on a hall) demands allegiance from its members. Tangible and intangible rewards are given in each group, so when a communication arrives, it is interpreted in light of the goals and needs of each subgroup and usually not from the viewpoint of the organization as a whole.

Jay Jackson, in "The Organization and Its Communication Problems" (1960), concluded that

- people communicate far more with members of their own subgroup than with others
- people prefer to communicate with someone of higher status than themselves
- people try to avoid having to communicate with those lower in status than themselves
- people will communicate with those who will help them achieve their goals—higher-status persons have power to create either gratifying or depriving experiences
- people communicate with those who can make them feel more secure and avoid those who make them anxious

Status Distance

The assisted living facility staff interact with a broad range of professional and nonprofessional groups. At the top of the status ladder is, perhaps, a resident's physician by whose orders some staff services are directed. It is difficult for lower-level employees to communicate upward. The personal care aide may feel uncomfortable in telling the resident's physician during a visit information about the resident the physician should be told. The administrator must be aware of the status sensitivities of these many groups and be capable of successfully fostering the needed communication among all of them.

Language Barrier

Doctors and health care workers speak "medicalese." Pharmacists speak yet another language, and physical therapists have their own jargon. Because of this, the personal care aide may not really understand what the doctor or nurse just said; the kitchen worker may not understand what the consulting dietitian directed.

Self-Protection

People often fail to communicate information that might reflect badly on them, their friends, or the organization (translation: The administrator should check that the accident report portrays what actually occurred).

Information Overload

The abundance of information flowing in the facility may produce an information overload that results in the staff's compromised ability to distinguish among communications requiring particular attention. The maintenance person, for instance, may fail to distinguish a maintenance request that should receive immediate attention because of the number of such requests.

Others

The administrator must bear in mind that all communication is multidimensional, needing appropriate interpretation to be of use.

In sending out a memorandum to employees or engaging in any communication, the administrator must take into account that its effect depends at least on the following:

- feelings and attitudes of the parties toward each other
- expectations
- how well the subordinates' needs are being met by the organization—if the assisted living facility is supportive, employees receiving administrative communications may be less defensive and more problem-oriented, that is, readier to absorb the communication and comply with the organization's request

1.6.6 Organizational Norms and Values

DEVELOPING LOYALTY TO FACILITY GOALS

Administering an organization such as an assisted living facility is a complicated process. We have discussed some of the problems encountered by administrators as they attempt to lead employees to do the tasks required. One of the impediments to accomplishing this is that the organization can never count on the individual employee's undivided attention. This is known as the concept of partial inclusion, or the segmental involvement of people in the job role.

LIMITATIONS ON EMPLOYEE PARTICIPATION

The assisted living facility defines behaviors that require only a portion of a person's 24-hour day. The facility asks only that during each shift employees perform the tasks or roles prescribed for them and that they have agreed to do (Pfeffer & Salanick, 1978). Unavoidably, however, the whole person must be brought into the work situation (Katz & Kahn, 1967). To deal with this, the employee is asked to set aside the non-job aspects of life while at work. This is literally a depersonalizing demand, which most employees find difficult to accomplish, so informal "organizations within the organization" develop in defense of personal identity.

The result is that people behave less as members of the assisted living facility and more in terms of some compromise of their many commitments. For example, when asked about the sources of satisfaction from their jobs, employees often rate their interpersonal relationships with their fellow employees as the most important aspect of their work. Association with the residents follows, with the goals and values of the assisted living facility itself tending to be somewhat low on the list of employee motivation. Administrators and supervisors engage in a constant struggle to gain loyalty from employees for the goals of the facility.

There is yet another important limitation to employees' full participation. People tend to interpret the facility as a whole from the viewpoint of their particular section of the organization. This is another reason why upper-level administrators who collect information only from their immediate subordinates may never know what is actually taking place.

People tend to exaggerate their importance to the organization as a whole. Loyalties develop to the work area rather than to the whole facility. This is a major source of conflict among work areas. The personal care workers view the organization from their unique perspective, as do those in maintenance, food service, and other areas.

To enable staff to accomplish necessary work, organizations develop and specify roles (job descriptions) that are carefully prescribed forms of behavior associated with the tasks the organization wants performed. *Roles* are standardized patterns of required behavior (Katz & Kahn, 1967). The health aide is told very clearly what his or her role is during the 8 hours on the job.

Connecting Roles to Norms

To build loyalty, organizations try to identify roles and impart to persons the norms, or values, of the organization, general expectations for all employees.

Professional standards for personal care workers and health aides are examples of such norms. They are behavior patterns to which all members of the group are expected to adhere. Respecting the personal privacy of residents would be an example of such a norm. Sam Walton, by standing in a checkout line in all his Wal-Mart stores each year, was constantly teaching and reinforcing an important norm: ensure that checkout is a pleasant experience, thus stimulating the customer to feel favorably toward Wal-Mart.

Norms are justified by *values,* which are more generalized statements about the behavior expected from staff members. Values furnish the rationale for the normative requirements. Treating all residents with respect for their rights as individuals is an example of a broad value statement, justifying the more specific norm that health personnel ought to respect each resident's personal privacy. For Sam Walton, building customer loyalty and repeat business might be the general value under which he established a pleasant checkout experience as a norm to be enforced.

System norms and values are attempts to connect employees with the system so that they remain within system values while carrying out their role assignments. It could be said that norms and values furnish "cognitive road maps" (ways to think about the organization and its goals). Norms help personnel adjust to the system.

Justification of the Facility

Another contribution of organizational norms and values is the moral or social justification for the activities of the assisted living facility. This is often put in the form of a *mission statement* for the facility—defining the purposes and values held by the facility. The mission statement often appears at the front of the personnel handbook; it becomes the first impression the prospective employee has of the purposes of the facility.

The administrator demonstrates what is important—the values that actually guide the day-to-day behavior of staff—by the way he or she behaves, to what he or she gives attention. If the administrator constantly moves around the facility to check that each resident is enjoying a high quality of life, the employees will probably follow suit. Likewise, if the administrator instead concentrates on getting paperwork done and saving money, the staff will do the same.

Dreams, Vision, and Goals

Another way to conceptualize values, norms, and roles is to equate them to dreams or visions, goals or behaviors (mentioned elsewhere in this text). A dream or vision is a motivating abstract or belief. People are more motivated by and able to accept a vision or dream held by a leader. Dr. Martin Luther King, Jr., for example, could not have motivated the unprecedented number of demonstrators who took part in the March on Washington, DC, by telling them that he had a goal, or even a well-devised plan of action. Rather, he moved them by telling them that he had a dream of equality for all Americans. A dream or vision of constantly improving the daily life experiences of residents and staff in an assisted living facility can motivate.

Specific goals, such as having a full activities program, are secondary to the dream. Goals give employees specific targets to shoot for and provide feedback, but goals must be guided by something larger—a dream or vision that inspires. Each goal is a step toward a dream.

In the field of assisted living administration, a new approach that has emerged in recent years is the "Eden" concept, which holds that plants, animals, and children should be woven into the daily life of a facility. The vision here is of a fully interactive environment that provides maximum stimulation for every resident. The specific goal in such a program may be to have x number of plants in place by such and such a date.

Most assisted living facility corporations publish mission statements that resemble a list of goals more than a vision or dream—for example, "We seek to be the provider of choice for each community in which we have a facility." This is fine for the corporate honchos but not very motivating to the health assistants in their day-to-day struggles to provide care. Deming has observed that goal statements from the corporate level seldom motivate. Many local facilities have corporate goal statements in large print on well-designed posters on the walls, but these may not be their own goals. Each facility must also generate its own vision of what it is seeking to do.

WHY ORGANIZATIONS NEED ADMINISTRATIVE LEADERSHIP

Once all the plans have been developed and staff hired and trained, why doesn't the organization run smoothly? Although there are a number of dimensions to any answer to this question, we will discuss only a few that seem especially relevant.

All organizational designs are imperfect (Demski, 1980). Differences between the organizational chart, the written policies, and the organization's actual functioning are easily seen. It is commonly recognized that the new worker, after being instructed by the supervisor, turns to group members to learn what the job requirements really are.

Actual behavior, the actual functioning of the organization, is infinitely more complex, inconclusive, and variable than the plan. An illustration of this is organizational sabotage. Any worker who wants to sabotage the facility can do so by merely following organizational law to the letter—doing what is formally stipulated, no more and no less.

Assisted living facilities, like all organizations, need administrative leadership to cope with the constantly changing external environment that requires internal adjustments. When, for example, three new assisted living facilities open in an area and one's own occupancy rate drops from 92% to 72%, organizational leadership is in order.

Organizations also need leadership to accommodate to the changes constantly occurring within them. Employees retire or find work elsewhere, the needs of staff and residents change, conflicts develop, physical systems break down, and decisions to repair or replace are called for.

As Kriegel (1991) has pointed out, change is here to stay. To meet current challenges it is necessary to constantly adapt. J. B. Fuqua has observed that whether you feel you have reached the top or are still climbing, you cannot stay still (Kriegel, 1991, p. 73). The old saying "If it ain't broke, don't fix it" needs to be changed to "If you don't fix it all the time, it will break."

1.6.7 Related Concepts

We turn now to several other related concepts worth reviewing in any consideration of attempts by administrators to direct the efforts of the organization.

FACILITY CULTURE

Facility culture is the overall style or atmosphere of a facility. This culture governs how people relate to each other in the organization. Corporate (facility) culture is important to the organization's survival. The corporate culture at IBM, for example, changed dramatically from Tom Watson, Sr. and Tom Watson, Jr.'s commitment to "respect the individual" once they retired (Argenti, 1994).

DELEGATION

The concept of *delegation* is to permit decisions to be made at the lowest possible level. Such authority is given to middle-level and lower-level administrators, allowing them to make decisions for the organization, as appropriate. The essential issue is the determination of the nature of the decisions to be made at whatever level (Meal, 1984; Mintzberg, 1979).

Delegating can be both beneficial and disadvantageous. At optimum operation, delegation channels decision making to staff members who are best informed and most skilled to make a particular decision or set of decisions.

The negative aspect of this practice is that since the middle-level workers have only a partial view of the organization, they consciously or unconsciously may make decisions in a manner that maximizes their area of the organization, to the possible detriment of the facility as a whole.

Ultimate responsibility cannot be delegated. The chief administrator is held accountable for the acts of all employees working under facility auspices.

UNITY OF COMMAND

The concept of unity of command emphasizes the importance of each person being accountable to only one supervisor (Simon, 1960). Because it is functionally difficult for any employee to answer to two administrators, the facility must be organized to assure this relationship.

SHORT CHAIN OF COMMAND

This principle asserts that there should be as few levels of management as possible between the chief administrator and the rank and file (Dale, 1969). Certainly, for the communication purposes of upper-level management, this seems a good principle to follow. It minimizes the number of interpreters through whom information for upper-level administrators must be sifted.

BALANCE

Advocates of the principle of balance (Dale, 1969) assert that there is a need for continual surveillance to maintain balance among the following:

- size of the various work areas
- standardization of procedures and flexibility
- centralization and decentralization
- span of control and short chain of command

MANAGEMENT BY OBJECTIVES (MBO)

This approach emphasizes setting specific, jointly developed goals with a time period for goal achievement and performance feedback (Argenti, 1994). The theory is to create a process of participation beginning with the lowest levels of workers whose recommendations are constantly moved upward until final selection of the goals to be put into place is made by upper management.

While MBO, in theory, meaningfully involves lowest-level employees/administrators in recommending organizational goals, the real effect is to shift power upward (Swiss, 1983). This occurs because it is the upper-level administrators who actually make the final choice among (and modify if necessary) recommendations from the lower levels.

MANAGEMENT INFORMATION SYSTEM (MIS)

The term *management information system* (MIS) originally came into the literature as a description of computer-based information processing systems available to managers (Dearden & McFarlan, 1966). Withington (1966) defined MIS as the study of how the organization communicates and processes information to maximize the effectiveness of management and to further the objectives of the organization.

The point recognized in MIS is that the administrator needs a constant rationalized and organized flow of information in order to make appropriate decisions. In Levey and Loomba's view (1973), developing an MIS is as simple as

- determining one's need for information
- identifying the sources of information
- deciding on the amount, form, and frequency of information needed
- choosing the means of information processing
- implementing the system

Under the headings of the individual work areas of the assisted living facility discussed below, we will offer some ideas on appropriate management information systems for the work areas individually and the assisted living facility as a whole.

MANAGEMENT BY EXCEPTION

Every day the administrator receives numerous verbal and written reports, which usually contain routine information about the functioning of the facility. One way administrators can effectively use allocate some of their time is by giving attention to exceptions to the plan. If the census, the number of meals served, or the projected costs are within the plan, for example, there may be no need for action. There are multitudes of detailed tasks being accomplished in acceptable fashion by the staff every day. What merits the administrator's attention are the exceptions to the policies and plans of action originally established for the organization.

The budget is one of the more useful tools for spotting exceptions (Gordon & Stryker, 1983). Getting information about the amount of money that has been spent in the last quarter is a reasonably exact control measurement. As long as any department is spending within the agreed-on budget there may be no need for the administrator's attention. Whenever a departmental budget falls short or exceeds the amounts allocated to it, however, the administrator should give attention to the exception and take whatever steps may be necessary to bring expenditures back within the budgeted limits. The health care staff having to hire unexpected numbers of "pool" personal care workers for weekends (workers hired by the day from an agency that supplies temporary help), for example, is a frequent cause of budget overage. However, too little expenditure by personal care areas or by, for example, food service might be as much a cause for alarm as too great an expenditure. In the first case the facility might be short on the required number of health personnel hours planned per day; in the second case the quality of food being purchased and prepared might be unsatisfactory.

Management by exception does not mean that the routine and within-specification behaviors of the facility remain unexamined. It is the routine behaviors of the organization that are being examined for deviations from the norm.

PERT/CPM

Program evaluation and review technique (PERT) and critical path method (CPM) are control tools showing the relationship among the activities that make up a project. The renovation of a wing of a facility, for example, may be mapped out with time estimates for completion of each necessary step, the critical path, which aids in allocating resources.

CONCEPTS OF EFFICIENCY AND EFFECTIVENESS

Efficiency is the ability to produce the desired effect with a minimum of effort, expense, or waste. It can be measured by the ratio of effective work to the energy expended in producing it. In systems terms, this simply means getting the maximum output with the minimum input.

Effectiveness is the power or ability to bring about the desired results. An assisted living facility that sets a goal of achieving excellence in resident care and then does so is said to be effective.

The facility, however, may not be efficiently achieving excellence of resident care. The home, for example, may be employing a large number of health care workers and aides to accomplish excellence in resident care as its residents age in place and the facility moves from being a level 1 (lower level of ADL assistance) provider to a level 3 (higher level of ADL assistance) provider. Yet studies in personnel reveal that when more people are placed on a work shift than are needed, the quality of care is not necessarily improved. The staff may simply divide the work up to lighten the load for everyone or take more frequent breaks and not actually give additional attention to the residents. In this case, the too heavy staff/resident ratio may lead to both inefficiency and ineffectiveness.

The solution is to assign the optimum number of staff known to be needed to provide excellent in care to a specified number of residents, then manage their time so that the amount of work and quality are optimized. In this way, the administrator achieves both efficiency (the desired effect with a minimum of effort, expense, or waste) and effectiveness (the desired results). Given enough resources and appropriate consultation, almost any assisted living facility administrator can achieve effectiveness. What is essential today is to be both effective and efficient. As a practical matter, if the administrator is given a staffing choice, staff may work both more efficiently and more effectively when they perceive the facility to be slightly understaffed than when slightly over staffed, leading them to, perhaps subconsciously, relax their level of effort.

SUMMARY

In this section, we have examined a number of concepts: policy making, decision-making styles, power, authority, need for communication skills, norms, and values. We have touched lightly on a number of concepts guiding the administrator in attempts to direct the efforts of the assisted living facility and have indicated that the administrator, in providing day-to-day guidance for the staff, ensures that they know what is expected of them.

Having done this, the administrator may be tempted to rest on past efforts. This could be a fatal error in judgment. We have demonstrated that organizations are volatile systems that may or may not respond to the administrator's direction. The only way an administrator can be certain that the assisted living facility is in fact making appropriate progress toward implementing its policies and plans of action is by comparing the outputs (results of organizational work) with the intended results. This is the process of comparing and controlling quality.

1.7 Comparing and Controlling Quality

Because all organizational designs are incomplete, the quest for quality is frustratingly elusive, both in industry and in the health care setting. The quest for quality in the assisted living facility is especially challenging because of its organizational complexity.

Even so, or perhaps because of this circumstance, the most valuable functions administrators perform for the facility are comparing (evaluating) and controlling the quality of facility outputs. *Comparing* is judging the extent to which actual results of the facility's efforts achieve the outcomes proposed in the plans. *Controlling* is successfully taking the steps necessary to adjust the policies and plans of action to more satisfactorily achieve stated goals.

One problem in controlling quality is that it obliges the administrator to take sometimes unpleasant corrective actions to keep the facility on target. This may involve advising staff members that the work result is not suitable or informing department administrators that the actual outputs (level of performance) are unsatisfactory. This is invariably an awkward business and avoided by administrators who hope the situation will correct itself or that the problem will simply disappear. But matters usually get worse and require attention.

TOTAL QUALITY MANAGEMENT

Definition

Total quality management (TQM) is difficult to define precisely because it is a philosophy of total organizational involvement in improving all aspects of quality of service. There is no single set of steps that has gained broad acceptance as the TQM methodology. However, the basic definition is to improve constantly and forever the system of production and service. This definition implies that it is too expensive to maintain quality by inspections and more efficient to produce quality in the first place. To achieve TQM, responsibility for quality is ultimately placed with the workers who actually produce the service or product. This is sometimes called quality at the source. In this scheme the quality departments are focused on training employees in quality control and implementing the quality control concepts throughout the organization. Employee empowerment in decision making, the use of teams in the organization, the use of individual responsibility for services, and customer service are characteristics of most TQM efforts (Argenti, 1994).

According to the American Hospital Association, TQM is a customer-driven approach that applies the scientific method to improve organizations' systems (Melvim & Siniotis, 1992). The focus on quality is total, including every aspect of an organization—its services, products, suppliers, business procedures, management systems, and human resources. Total quality management is a process of continuous improvement, a process of continuously striving to exceed customer expectations. Problems in the organization are viewed as problems of processes used, not of individuals within the organization—processes that can be improved using TQM approaches.

Six Factors for Success

The following factors are viewed as keys to a successful total quality management program.

1. **Visionary leadership.** The CEO, along with middle- and lower-level administrators, offers a vision statement regarding quality of service and sets goals. Employees are empowered to implement TQM, evaluate and recognize TQM progress, promote commitment to customers, and serve as role models of TQM behavior. The CEO and administrators act as coaches, not bosses. Coaching implies mentoring employees, helping them to develop needed skills to perform their jobs.
2. **Commitment to customers.** This involves anticipating, meeting, and exceeding customers' expectations (in this case, residents') and linking reward systems to customer satisfaction.
3. **Trained teams.** In a TQM program, the entire workforce must participate in teams, applying TQM in their daily work. Administrators act as trainers. Quality is the leading agenda item at all meetings.

4. **Physician involvement.** Physicians are involved in TQM training so that they function as TQM enablers for the health staff.
5. **Processes.** In TQM a process is put in place for planning and organizing the overall management of the facility. Having an improvement process solves specific problems, improves specific processes, and maintains these changes over time.
6. **Avoiding a separate TQM system.** The TQM is made the sole management process in the organization.

Experience suggests that it takes 5 to 10 years to fully implement a TQM program. The three steps to accomplish this transformation are

1. Direct TQM through the quality implementation plan.
2. Educate on quality to empower people.
3. Align management systems to integrate and sustain TQM.

J. M. Juran (cited in Melvin & Siniotis, 1992), an important figure in the managing for quality movement, summarizes the process this way:

1. **Quality planning.** Decide who the customers are and what their needs are; features that respond to their needs, along with processes to respond.
2. **Quality control.** Evaluate the actual output; compare output to expected output; act on the difference.
3. **Quality improvement.** Establish the needed infrastructure; identify improvement projects; establish project teams. Train, motivate, and empower the teams to diagnose the causes, find remedies, and maintain gains.

1.8 Innovating

The effective administrator is always an innovator. Innovating is the process of bringing new ideas into the way an organization accomplishes its purposes.

The process of innovating is the result of the administrator's study of the changes that are constantly occurring in the organization itself and the environment in which it functions. Innovating is an act of leadership. It is the administrator's role to be the sensor of the organization for those external and internal changes that will have an impact on its well-being.

The administrator is not necessarily the innovator, but he or she does have the task of ensuring that innovation occurs within the organization. To achieve this, the administrator can develop new ideas, combine old ideas into new ones, borrow and adapt ideas from other fields, or stimulate others to develop innovations (Dale, 1969).

To focus on the resident and his or her family or significant others is to be in constant contact with the changing needs of residents. Nearly all staff have contacts with residents and their families or significant others. If practical innovation is sought from all staff, the staff must become outwardly focused adaptive sensors, listening and adapting to changing needs.

An assisted living facility's staff will innovate only if the administrator intentionally introduces changes in the organization that are responses to changes perceived in the environment and encourages others to do the same. Innovation is the process of finding new solutions to creating a good quality of life for residents and staff. Not all new solutions will work. However, the administrator must encourage and praise new solutions that fail as well as new solutions that succeed; otherwise staff will stop suggesting new solutions.

Innovation requires being in constant touch with the new—new requirements, new employment trends, new benefits, new resident activities. To be innovative is to respond flexibly to changes in the environment. Most organizations fight innovation. Hospitals, for instance, fought the introduction of birthing suites until women arranged to be delivered outside the hospital in homelike suites. In response, more and more hospitals have added this amenity to their list of services.

The American health insurance industry grew out of an innovation developed by one hospital administrator in Texas. During the depression of the 1930s, the administrator of Baylor University Hospital, recognizing the eroding economy and faced with a drastically reduced cash flow, devised a plan to create a regular cash flow to the hospital from the one group left who had a steady income: schoolteachers paid from public taxes. For 50 cents a month, teachers were offered up to 14 days of prepaid hospital care per year. The teachers bought the idea, and the U.S. health insurance industry was born.

Innovators tend to be survivors of change. The future belongs to those organizations that are successful in constantly innovating over time. The early years of the 21st century hold promise to innovators in the assisted living facility industry.

1.9 Marketing the Assisted Living Facility

1.9.1 The Turn to Marketing

Why, one might ask, should the assisted living facility administrator be concerned with marketing? High occupancy rates seem guaranteed as the American population rapidly ages and the baby boomers become retirees. Many assisted living facilities currently have resident waiting lists. The proportion of Americans who will need assisted living facility care is expected to increase yearly at least through the middle of the 21st century. A number of factors are coming together, however, that may threaten any seeming guarantee of high occupancy rates.

NARROWED PROFIT MARGINS

While today most assisted living facility revenue is from private paying residents, the ability of an assisted living facility to survive economically may be affected by an increasing variety of pressures such as expected changes in state and federal reimbursement policies the types of services offered by the facility, and the sources of resident payment.

Facility costs can be expected to increase in response to the additional regulatory requirements established by the Americans with Disabilities Act, the Family Medical Leave Act and the more rigorous universal precautions requirements. Over the next 10 years, as the original assisted living facility populations age in place, and if present trends toward increasing acuity of care continue, some assisted living facilities will be forced to staff up toward nursing home levels. We describe this process in Part Two as moving from a level 1 to a level 3 assisted living facility.

ALWAYS MESS WITH SUCCESS

The most cogent reason for marketing the assisted living facility is that if you don't mess with your success, your competitor will. It is easy to be blinded by short-term success. Yet whenever a facility feels it has achieved premier status as the best caregiver in the community, whenever it starts taking its success for granted, it will lull itself into complacency and slack off.

Good isn't good enough. Good-enough assisted living facilities abound. Simply doing a good job of marketing the facility will not yield the edge necessary to succeed in today's pressure-packed health care marketplace. Good only puts you with the rest of the pack.

1.9.2 The Marketing Concept

DEFINITION OF MARKETING

The American Marketing Association defines *marketing* as the process of planning and executing the conception, pricing, promotion, and distribution of ideas, goods, and services to create exchanges that satisfy both individual and organizational objectives (Kinnear & Bernhardt, 1986). The assisted living facility is in the business of marketing services. Nearly half of every dollar spent by U.S. consumers is spent on services (Berkowitz, Kerin, & Rudelius, 1986).

GOALS VS. NEEDS

Why is it increasingly necessary to pay special attention to the fit between the goals of the assisted living facility and the needs of the persons it seeks to serve? The simple answer: to ensure that the facility will stay in business.

STEPS IN MARKETING

The steps in marketing are described by Levey and Loomba as

- conducting an audit
- analyzing market segmentation
- choosing a marketing mix
- implementing the plan

The goal of the assisted living facility is to discover the needs and desires of potential customers and to satisfy them through product design and price, delivering appropriate and competitively viable services (Kotler & Clarke, 1987; Star, 1989). This is market-centeredness, focusing primarily on customer needs, wants, perceptions, preferences, and satisfaction. Satisfaction is defined as a state felt by a resident when a service has fulfilled his or her expectations (Kotler & Clarke, 1987). Health care services, such as assisted living services, are increasingly a buyer's market. Long-term customer satisfaction with the manner in which the facility is being run is one of the major factors in keeping an assisted living facility at or near capacity (Peters & Austin, 1985).

1. 9. 3 Developing a Marketing Strategy

NEED FOR A MARKETING STRATEGY

A *marketing strategy* involves selecting a target market or markets, choosing a competitive position, and developing an effective marketing mix to reach and serve the identified customers (Kotler & Clark, 1987).

A *market* is all the persons who have an actual or potential interest in using the facility's services. A facility may select among several market coverage strategies. It may concentrate on one market or market segment, for example, choosing to serve only private paying residents (*market concentration*). The facility may decide to offer only one service for all markets, for example, serving only Alzheimer's residents, regardless of their funding source (*product concentration*). The facility may opt for *market specialization,* that is, serving only one market segment, such as persons who need only one type of cooking (e.g., kosher). Or it may prefer to work in several product markets, for example, serving both Alzheimer's and other residents with various related dementias (*selective specialization*).

CREATING NEW MARKETS, NEW NICHES

Tom Peters (1987) distinguishes between market sharing and market creation. Persons using the market share mentality focus on how they can attain a desired share of the present market. Market creators attempt to create a new market.

Survival for both individual facilities and assisted living facility chains is becoming increasingly tied to specializing in market niches in which the facility can gain a reputation for excellence, in order to keep census at the needed levels (90% to 95% occupancy). In recent years assisted living facilities have made inroads into other health services. By vertically integrating their services or by contracting with home health care agencies, they have expanded their market by allowing residents to "age in place." This allows residents who enter with only minor care needs to remain in a facility, additional health care services or provided or imported on an as-needed basis. Similarly, assisted living facilities may expand downwards by catering to more nearly independently living adults, thus serving wider age range.

One assisted living chain, Diversified Senior Services, Inc., defines its market as publicly subsidized units for persons who cannot afford the monthly rents of most large assisted living facility chains (*Assisted Living Business Week,* 1998). The focus is on not-for-profits, which creates eligibility for tax-exempt bond financing. Diversified Senior Services specializes in 60-unit facilities placed in smaller markets with populations of about 75,000—smaller cities and towns.

STEPS IN DEVELOPING A MARKETING STRATEGY

Step One: Conducting an Audit

The first step in developing a marketing strategy is to conduct an audit. *Auditing* is the process of identifying, collecting, and analyzing information about the external environment. Markets are characterized as potential, available, qualified, served, and penetrated. The *potential market* is all individuals who express some level of interest in a defined market offer. Removing those who are interested but unable to pay defines the *available market,* that is, persons who have interest, the funds, and access to the market offering. The *qualified market* is those persons who have interest, financial means, and access and qualify (e.g., meet the requirement for 24-hour-a-day assistance). The *served market* is that part of the qualified market the facility makes an effort to attract. Those who are admitted to or served by the facility constitute the *penetrated market*—the persons actually consuming the services offered.

As part of an audit, it is necessary to estimate the extent of demand for a service the facility might offer. *Total market demand* is the total volume of services that would be bought by a defined available number of persons in a specific geographic area in a defined time period in a stated marketing environment under a specific marketing program (Kotler & Clarke, 1987). *Market forces* is the number of services the facility could expect to be purchased under such a specific marketing plan.

In forecasting future demand, Kotler and Clarke (1989) suggest the facility examine three categories: (1) uncontrollable environment factors such as the economy, technological changes, reimbursement formula changes, and broad changes in the health care system (e.g., the emergence of managed care), (2) new competition from other providers (e.g., new facilities, new services, and new marketing budgets), and (3) intraorganizational factors such as the condition of the facility, possible new services, and promotional efforts programs. Forecasts may be based on what people say they will do, are actually doing, or have actually done in the past.

Consider the following estimates of the U.S. Census Bureau:

	1995	2050
American population age 65+	33 million	80 million

According to the U.S. Census Bureau in 1995, persons age 65 and over comprised 4% of the total population. By the year 2050 they are projected to comprise 20% of the population, a 400% increase. Persons age 85 and over comprised 1% of the U.S. population in 1995 according to the U.S. Census Bureau, and are expected to comprise 5% of the U.S. population in 2050—again, a 400% increase. The potential market for assisted living facility care appears to remain strong into the third and forth decades of the 21st century. The extent to which retirees will be able to privately pay for assisted living care is increasingly under a cloud, however. Only a modest proportion of these seniors will be able to afford the +/- $4,000 monthly fees over an extended period of time.

Other Forces at Work. Restrictions in some states on expansion of nursing home beds, limiting construction to state-approved facilities, are expected to result in a significant decrease in the number of nursing home beds per 1,000 for the 85+ population. From a peak in 1986 of 690 beds per 1,000 persons age 85 and over, the U.S. Census Bureau estimates that the number will shrink to 350 nursing home beds per 1,000 persons after 2,000. This constitutes a marketing opportunity for the assisted living industry.

Cost containment by government and private industry to slow the usage and costs of health care services also creates marketing opportunities for the assisted living industry. In an era of cost consciousness the lower costs of assisted living when compared to nursing homes or medium to high levels of home health care become marketing opportunities for the assisted living industry. However, assisted living monthly fees are beginning to approach those of the nursing facilities due to the increasing need for staff to assist assisted living residents with the activities of daily living.

Changes in Family Dynamics. In general, Americans are less and less able and less and less willing to be the primary caregivers of their aging parents. Studies suggest that a few decades ago 72% of persons caring for seniors were unpaid female relatives (Martin, 1997, p. 33). In 1915, 20% of women worked outside the home; by 1993 over 50% of women worked outside the home (Martin, 1997, p. 33). These trends lead to fewer and fewer at-home caregivers available to aging parents. Expectations have shifted dramatically. At the beginning of the 20th century parents expected to be taken care of in the home by their adult children. At the beginning of the 21st century both parents and adult children are increasingly seeking to live their own lives independent of each other. The assisted living facility is positioned to meet the needs of aging persons who need assistance formerly provided by their children in a multigenerational family home setting.

As can be seen in Table 1.6 few (15%) seniors who move from senior living arrangements return to live with relatives, the largest proportion going to assisted living.

Consumer Preference for Less "Institutionalized" Care. The assisted living industry delivers its services primarily under a social model compared to the more institutionalized heavily medical model of the skilled nursing facility. As Martin has observed, aging is perceived as a fact of life, not a disease. The assisted living model can be more homelike than the nursing facility, which must meet much more extensive construction requirements that have forced the appearance of over-institutionalization of the nursing home setting.

Step 2: Analyzing Market Segmentation

Analyzing *market segmentation* is using the audit information to divide the potential persons served into identifiable subgroups. An assisted living facility chain might segment the market it seeks by geography: region of the country, urban/rural, population density, climate, and so on.

Table 1.6 Destinations of Seniors Who Move from Senior Apartments: Who Are the Competition?

Other senior apartment	7%
Active adult community	1%
Congregate senior housing	1%
Assisted Living Facility	**28%**
CCRC	2%
Skilled Nursing Facility	18%
With relatives	15%

For all seniors (including assisted living) in a survey conducted by the American Senior Housing Association in 2002, 64% of residents had moved from within 10 miles, 87% had moved from within 25 miles(*The Senior Apartment*, 2001, p 12).

Markets can be segmented by demographic characteristics such as age, family size, sex, educational level, occupation, and religion. Psychographic social classes can be used (e.g., lifestyle and personality). Individuals who are by nature gregarious and thrive on extensive personal interactions, for example, are good candidates for application to assisted living communities. In addition, behavior tendencies can be used to segment markets such as benefits sought (e.g., life care benefits), user status (within age limits and able to pay), readiness stage (e.g., persons over a certain age, retired, and actively seeking a caregiver). The assisted living industry enjoys the opportunity to develop numerous markets.

Markets for Assisted Living. When independent living is no longer an option, the assisted living facility may become the alternative of choice. Assisted living generally provides a homelike environment with private units furnished by the residents, approaching to the degree possible, the comfort, independence, and privacy aspects of a single-family residence (Table 1.7).

Table 1.7 Overall Market Segmentation of the Senior Living Continuum

	Supply*			
	1997	2001		
Larger facilities (30+ residents)	300,000	625,000		
Smaller facilities (<30 residents)	440,000	525,000		
Total estimated	740,000	1,150,000		
	Potential Demand			
Age	85+		75-84	
	1997	2001	1997	2001
Seniors not in nursing facilities	2,815,000	3,444,800	8,442,750	9,171,980
Potential transfers from nursing facilities	295,500	319,860	95,100	102,930
Total estimated	3,110,500	3,764,660	8,537,850	9,274,910
Supply/demand imbalance	4.2x	4.2x	11.5x	8.1x

*Total units in assisted living facilities.
Source: Martin (1997). *The Assisted Living Industry.*

Step 3: Choosing a Marketing Mix

Choosing a market mix consists of deciding what types of residents to approach and in what proportions. Most facilities find it useful to identify specific groups of persons being sought to serve.

Most facilities will consciously choose a *product mix,* that is, the set of all product lines and items the facility intends to offer. A *product line* in the assisted living facility setting is a set of services within the product mix that are closely related due to functional similarity (e.g., being made available to the same type of persons or marketed through the same channels). A *product item* is a distinct unit within a product line that is distinguishable by purpose and, usually, some other characteristic.

Serving Specific Groups: The Alzheimer's or Dementia Niche. A number of assisted living facilities choose a market mix that includes traditional assisted living arrangements combined with specialized care units, such as dementia units, either in the same building or on the same campus. According to an *Assisted Living Federation of America* survey, 29% of assisted living facilities in 1996 had a dedicated dementia unit in 1996 (Martin, p. 36). By 2002 the proportion of assisted living units with skilled nursing Alzheimer's and specialty care had risen to 31% of all facilities (American Senior Housing Association, 2003, p. 19).

The Alzheimer's Association estimates that the population identified as suffering from Alzheimer's disease will grow from 4 million in the 1990s to 14 million by 2050 if no cure or effective treatment is found (Martin, 1997). Current estimates range as high as 47% of persons age 85 and over to be afflicted with either Alzheimer's disease or a similarly dementing condition (Martin, 1997). A significant proportion of older persons suffer some form of dementia or disease process, which may offer marketing niches for assisted living facilities.

Reasons for Entry. Typically, persons entering assisted living facilities do so because they are unable to live independently either at home or in a congregate living setting. Typically, they need help with three of the ADLs (discussed in Part Five). In one survey "Overview of The Assisted Living Industry," see Martin, p.54), the referral sources for assisted living facilities were found to be

- 25% family members
- 15% hospitals
- 11% physicians
- 8% yellow pages or the media
- 8% aging agencies
- 7% current residents
- 6% nursing facilities
- 6% drive by the facility
- 3% trustee or legal adviser
- 1% churches
- 10% other

Geographical Parameters. On average, nearly 60% of assisted living residents are within 10 miles of family members. This suggests that residents choose to be in a facility as close to family as possible. Since most assisted living facilities have been located in urban and suburban areas, perhaps for this very good marketing reason, it is not surprising that distance from family is typically short (as shown in Table 1.8).

Table 1.8 Living Distance of Families from Assisted Living Facilities

Distance from families	National average (%)
Under 5 miles	34
5-10 miles	25
10-20 miles	16
20-50 miles	12
More than 50	13

Source: Coopers & Lybrand, "Overview of the Assisted Living Industry," 1996. Cited in Martin (1997).

The Assisted Living Workgroup Report to the U.S. Senate Special Committee on Aging (April, 2003, p. 269) recommends the following be required elements of contracts and agreements:

1. The term of the contract
2. Billing and payment policies and procedures
3. Services provided in the basic fee
4. Fee schedule for a la carte costs or tiered pricing system not included in the basic fee
5. Policy for changing fees
6. Advance notice of fee change policy
7. Entrance fee security deposit, or other fees, if charged
8. Circumstance for refunds
9. Policies during a resident's temporary absence
10. Process for initial and ongoing assessments and resident's right to participate in it
11. Physical exam requirements
12. Third party services uses, e.g. health services: how arranged, paid for etc.
13. All conditions for involuntary transfer
14. Complaints resolution process
15. Termination process for resident to follow who wishes to leave
16. List of resident rights as detailed in statutes affecting the facility

Discharge Planning. The likelihood of having vacancies through discharges each month is an important element in each facility's marketing strategy. Reasons for discharge, like most of the data on the assisted living industry, is a moving target. The only clear trend is for later and later discharge. In the early 1990s the average length of stay was one to two years. In the late nineties the average length of stay had stretched to over two years. There are reasons for believing the average length of stay will continue to lengthen:

- some facilities are attracting residents at an earlier age
- aging Americans are living healthier into old age
- assisted living facilities are increasingly offering higher-health-care-acuity services
- the growing marketing commitment to residents' preference for "aging in place" will lead facilities to seek to serve residents longer

A national survey of destinations of residents who are discharged from assisted living facilities revealed the pattern in Table 1.9.

This would continue a trend for residents to die in lower health care intensity settings. In recent years hospitals have increasingly discharged terminally ill patients to the less expensive and less high-tech nursing home setting. As assisted living facilities provide for residents to "age in place," end-of-life care will become a more frequent reality in the assisted living setting. In many cases this will involve the assisted living facility staff with assistance from a local hospice agency.

Table 1.9 Destinations of Residents Who Are Discharged from Assisted Living Facilities provide end-of-life care.

Living Facilities

Destination	Percentage of residents discharged
Nursing home	36
Death	31
Hospital	12
Move in with relatives	5
Move to another assisted living facility	4
Unknown	12

Source: Coopers & Lybrand, "Overview of the Assisted Living Industry." 1996. Cited in Martin (1997).

Step 4: Implementing the Plan

Implementing the marketing plan is the process of managing organizational behaviors and outreach activities to attract residents with the identified characteristics in the proportions desired.

Creating awareness among potential consumers that the services exist, assisting them in deciding, and ensuring that they are satisfied with the quality of services provided by the facility is the process of *marketing implementation*. An ongoing evaluation of the effectiveness of the marketing efforts is necessary.

The Marketing of Services

Assisted living facilities are primarily in the business of marketing services. A service is an activity or benefit that one person can offer to another that is intangible and does not result in ownership of anything (Kotler & Clarke, 1987).

According to Berkowitz et al. (1986) services have four characteristics that differentiate them from durable goods (e.g., cars or television sets): intangibility, inconsistency, inseparability, and inventory.

First Characteristic of Service: Intangibility. Services cannot be touched, sat in, or driven like a car: They are intangible. Health care that the resident expects will be given in an assisted living facility cannot be directly experienced before entering the facility. Assisted living facilities can, however, make services appear more tangible, for example, by running a television advertisement portraying attentive care being given to a resident at the facility.

Inconsistency. Marketing services differs from marketing tangible goods such as a car because the quality of service can be inconsistent from day to day, or even shift to shift. Quality that endures over time can be built into a car through consistent assembly line procedures and materials quality checks, but the service received at the hands of the staff on any given day can vary widely depending on the mood of each employee.

Inseparability. The third characteristic of marketing services is that the consumer does not separate the service from the deliverer of the service or the setting in which the service is given. The assisted living facility may be giving excellent care, but if the bathrooms smell bad and are dirty the residents' and visitors' perceptions of the facility, including their perceptions of quality of care, are affected. The services given and the service provide are inseparably linked in the consumer's mind.

Inventory. Idle production capacity (i.e., the presence of an unoccupied unit in an assisted living facility) is the fourth characteristic of service marketing. Inventory carrying costs of empty assisted living facility units is high: Empty units may cost as much as 70% of the costs of occupied units due to fixed and semi-variable costs (discussed in Part Three).

Construction Trends

Watching construction trends is the key to estimating available and needed inventory. Supply and demand have had powerful impacts on construction during the years 1997 through 2003.

Table 1.10 Senior Housing Construction: Total Properties by Type (1997-2003)

	1997	1998	1999	2000	2001	2002	2003
Senior Apartments	**31**	**38**	**41**	**32**	**52**	**44**	**77**
Independent Living	**77**	**89**	**103**	**93**	**65**	**43**	**51**
Assisted Living	**294**	**460**	**403**	**164**	**89**	**43**	**71**
Continuing Care (CCRCs)	**33**	**27**	**44**	**31**	**24**	**20**	**23**

Source: American Seniors Housing Association, *Seniors Housing Construction Report,* (2003), p.14.

As can be seen in Table 1.10, for three of the four segments of the industry, construction remained relatively stable with minor upwards and downwards trends with the exception of the assisted living industry construction, which peaked dramatically in 1997, 1998, and 1999, and plunged in 2002 to 10% of the construction in 1998. The minor up tick in construction in 2003 suggests that the oversupply may have been absorbed by the market.

Consumer Decision Making

Marketing texts (e.g., Berkowitz et al., 1986) typically characterize consumer decision making as

1. problem recognition
2. information search
3. alternative evaluation
4. purchase decision
5. post purchase evaluation

Kotler and Clarke (1987) describe consumer decision making as:

1. need arousal (trigger factors such as a hospital episode)
2. information gathering
3. decision evaluation
4. decision execution
5. post-decision assessment

The decision for a person to enter an assisted living facility is often a complex one shared by several participants. According to Kotler and Clarke (1987), the decision-making unit typically consists of

1. the initiator (e.g., the daughter, who suggests looking into assisted living facility care)
2. influential friends (e.g., acquaintances already in local assisted living facilities)
3. the decider, the person who ultimately forces some part of the decision (e.g., the daughter who decides she can no longer provide the assistance needed)
4. the *buyer,* the person who will pay the bills, if not the resident himself or herself
5. the *user,* the person who will be the new resident or assisted living facility service user

Consumer decisions are based on their perceptions of whether the service provided by the assisted living facility will meet their needs (Goldsmith & Leebow, 1986; Kotler, 1986; Peters & Austin, 1985). Research suggests that physicians typically have a major influence on resident decisions (Smith, 1984). Recommendations from local physicians can provide the facility with a sustainable advantage (Ghemawal, 1986).

Effective Marketing Tools

Conducting personal tours through the facility is one of the most effective marketing tools (Butler, 1986; Skelly, 1986). During a visit the potential client, as well as the adult children or close friends of the prospective resident, can gather impressions on which they will make judgments of the facility. Often subliminal perceptions become the key factor. Subliminal perceptions are factors of which the decision maker is not consciously aware. These may include the general appearance of the facility, the absence of odors, the friendliness of the staff, and the appearance of the residents (Robertson, Zielinski, & Ward, 1984).

As one writer has put it, image is credibility (Peterson, 1986). Numerous ways of creating a positive image for the facility in the community are available. Developing a community advisory board, hosting neighborhood open houses, publicizing enthusiastic families and volunteers, sponsoring lectures for residents and community members on topics of general interest to older persons, and cosponsoring community events such as local arts festivals are but a few of the avenues available to facilities (Anderson, 1986; Jerstad & Meier, 1986; Kotler & Clarke, 1987; Ruff, 1986; Sweeney & Lewis, 1986; USDHHS, Administration on Aging, 1985).

ADVERTISING

Many facilities have begun to advertise their services. Advertising consists of non-personal forms of communication conducted through paid media with a clear sponsorship (Kotler & Clarke, 1987). The purpose of advertising is to motivate the target audience to move through the following buyer readiness states toward actual use of facility services:

- cognitive (aware that the facility is available)
- affective (favorable image of facility when comparing it to alternatives)
- behavioral (conviction, for example, fill out an application and place a move-in deposit)

Assisted living facilities are increasingly focused on serving the customer (Hauser, 1984; Rosenberg & Van West, 1984). A key point to remember is that the move to assisted living is driven more by need for health care assistance than by lifestyle choice. Assisted living meets the needs of persons who can no longer live independently.

The Pre-Move-In Screening Process recommended to the U.S. Senate Special Committee on Aging (*Assisted Living Workgroup Report*, April, 2003) is:

- Information and discussion of assisted living residence contract including resident and family expectations and resident rights, responsibilities and move in/out criteria
- Information and discussion on rate structure with full disclosure of rate charges.
- Written information regarding advance directives (e.g. living will, durable power of attorney, and/or do not resuscitate

- History and physical exam
- Evaluation of the resident's ability to self administer medications
- Evaluation of the ADLs and IADLs and risk factors such as falls, weight loss, elopement, self-neglect, abuse, exploitation
- Assessment of cognitive abilities and behavioral issues.

REFERENCES

Allport, F. H. (1933). *Institutional behavior.* Chapel Hill: University of North Carolina Press.

_______. (1962). A structuronomic conception of behavior. *Journal of Abnormal and Social Psychology,* 3–30.

American Association of Homes and Services for the Aging. (AAHSA). (1997). *Assisted living.* Washington, DC: Author.

American Hospital Association. (1990a). *Hospital statistics, 1989–1990.* (1990). Chicago: Author.

American Hospital Association. (1990b). *Trends among U.S. registered hospitals.* Chicago: Author.

American Senior Housing Association. (2003). *Senior Housing Construction Report: 2003.* Washington, DC: Author.

American Senior Housing Association. (2002). *State of Seniors Housing.* Washington, DC: Author.

American Senior Housing Association. (2001). *The Senior Apartment.* Washington, DC: Author.

Anderson, C. C. (1986). Local arts festival raises facility to new heights. *Provider, 12*(4), 50–55.

Argenti, P. A. (1994). *The portable MBA desk reference.* New York: Wiley.

Arnold, E. (1921). *The soul and body of an army.* London: Edward Arnold Publishers.

Assisted Living Business Week (1998). *2*(2, 5, 7, 11), 7–54.

Assisted Living Development Monitor (1998, January 19). *2*(1), 1–2.

Assisted Living Federation of America. (ALFA). (1998). *Assisted living.* Fairfax, VA: Author.

Barnard, C. I. (1938). *The functions of the executive.* Cambridge, MA: Harvard University Press.

Berkowitz, E. N., Kerin, R. A., & Rudelius, W. (1986). *Marketing.* St. Louis: Times Mirror/Mosby College Publishing.

Bertalanffy, L. von. (1967). Der Organismus als Physikalishes System Betrachtet. In D. Katz & R. L. Kahn (Eds.), *The social psychology of organizations.* New York: Wiley.

Black, H. C. (1979). *Black's law dictionary* (5th ed.). St. Paul, MN: West.

Boling, T. E., et al. (1983). *Nursing home management.* Springfield, IL: Charles C Thomas.

Bradley, D. F., & Calvin, M. (1956). Behavior: Imbalance in a network of chemical transformations. In *General systems yearbook of the Society for the Advancement of General Systems Theory 1.*

Burton, W. C. (1980). *Legal thesaurus.* New York: Macmillan.

Butler, R. L. (1986). Nursing homes gain consumer confidence. *Provider, 12*(11), 48.

Buttaro, P. J. *Home study program in principles of long term health care administration.* Aberdeen, SD: Health Care Facility Consultants.

Califano, J. A., Jr. (1986). *America's health care revolution.* New York: Random House.

Childe, V. G. (1972). *Man makes himself.* New York: New American Library. Englewood Cliffs, NJ: Prentice Hall.

Christensen, C. R. Berg, N. A., & Salter, M. S. (1980). *Policy formulation and administration* (8th ed.). Homewood, IL: Richard D. Irwin.

Dale, E. (1969). *Management: Theory and practice.* (2nd ed.). New York: McGraw-Hill.

Davis, W. E. (1985). *Introduction to health care administration.* Bossier City, LA: Publicare Press.

Dearden, J., & McFarlan, F. W. (1966). *Management information systems: Text and cases.* Homewood, IL: Richard D. Irwin

DeGroot, M. H. (1970). *Optimal statistical decisions.* New York: McGraw-Hill.

Demski, J. S. (1980). *Information analysis.* (2nd ed.) Reading, MA: Addison-Wesley.

Dobbs, D. B. (1971). *Law of remedies.* (4th ed.). St. Paul, MN: West.

Drucker, P. F. (1954). *The practice of management.* New York: Harper & Row.

Federal Requirements and Guidelines to Surveyors. (1995, June). Transmittal no. 274. Washington, DC: U.S. Department of Health and Human Services.

Fine, S. H. (1984, June 16). The health product: A social marketing perspective. *Hospitals,* pp. 66–68.

Focus on retirement. (1998, March 9). *The Wall Street Journal,* p. 22.

French, J. R. P., Jr., & Raven, B. H. (1960). The bases of social power. In D. Cartwright & A. Zander (Eds.), *Group dynamics: Research and theory* (2nd ed.). Evanston, IL: Row, Peterson.

George, C. S., Jr. (1972). *The history of management thought* (2nd ed.). Englewood Cliffs, NJ: Prentice-Hall.

Ghemawat, P. (1986). Sustainable advantage. *Harvard Business Review, 64*(5), 53–58.

Gifis, S. H. (1975). *Law dictionary.* Woodbury, NY: Barron's Educational Series.

Gilbert, A. (1965). *Machiavelli: The chief works and others.* Durham, NC: Duke University Press.

Glueck, W. F. (1982). *Personnel; a diagnostic approach* (3rd ed.). Plano, TX: Business Publishers.

Goldsmith, M., & Leebov, W. (1986). Strengthening the hospital's marketing position through training. *Health Care Management Review, 11*(2), 83–93.

Gordon, G. K., & Stryker, R. (1983). *Creative long term care administration.* Springfield, IL: Charles C. Thomas.

Gulick, L., & Lyndall, (Eds.). (1937). *Papers on the science of administration.* New York: Institute of Public Administration.

Hamel, G., & Prahalad, C. K. (1994). *Competing for the future.* Boston, MA: Harvard Business School Press.

Hauser, L. J. (1984, September 1). Ten reasons hospital marketing programs fail. *Hospitals,* pp. 74–77.

Hayes, J. L. (1969). In E. Dale (Ed.), *Management: Theory and practice* (2nd ed.). New York: McGraw-Hill.

Health care TV advertising up 40% for first half of 1986. (1986, October 20). *Hospitals,* pp. 16.

Inguanzo, J. M., & Harju, M. (1985, January 1). Creating a market niche. *Hospitals,* pp. 62–67.

Jackson, J. (1960). The organization and its communication problems. In A. Grimshaw & J. W. Hennessey, Jr. (Eds.), *Organizational behavior: Cases and readings.* New York: McGraw-Hill.

Jerstad, M. A., & Meier, P. (1986). Advisory board a valuable "two-way link" to community. *Provider, 12*(11), 60–63.

Johnson, L. (1994). TQM: A process for discovering. *LTC Administrators, 28*(1), 1, 10.

Kapp, M. B. (1987). *Preventing malpractice in long-term care: Strategies for risk management.* New York: Springer.

Katz, D., & Kahn, R. L. (1967). *The social psychology of organizations.* New York: Wiley.

Keen, P. G. W., & Woodman, L. A. (1984). What to do with all those Mircos. *Harvard Business Review, 84*(5).

King, H. (1963, June). Effective marketing can maintain census. *Contemporary Administrator,* pp. 39–41.

Kinnear, T. C., & Bernhardt, K. L. (1986). *Principles of marketing* (2nd ed.). Glenview, IL: Scott, Foresman.

Kotler, P. (1986). Megamarketing. *Harvard Business Review,* 64(2), 117–124.

Kotler, P., & Clarke, R. N. (1987). *Marketing for health care organizations.* Englewood Cliffs, NJ: Prentice-Hall.

Kotter, J. P. (1982). *The general managers.* New York: The Free Press.

Kretch, D., & Crutchfield, R. (1948). *Theory and problems of social psychology.* New York: McGraw-Hill.

Kriegel, R. J. (1991). *If it ain't broke.* New York: Warner.

Levey, S., & Loomba, N. P. (1984). *Health care administration: A managerial perspective* (2nd ed.). New York: Lippincott.

Levey, S., & Loomba, N. P. (1973). *Health care administration: A managerial perspective.* Philadelphia: Lippincott.

Likert, R. (1961). *New patterns of management.* New York: McGraw-Hill.

_______. (1967). *The human organization: Its management and value.* New York: McGraw-Hill.

Martin, P. (1997). *The assisted living industry.* New York: Jeffries and Co.

Meal, H. C. (1984). Putting production decisions where they belong. *Harvard Business Review, 84*(2).

Melvin, M. M., & Siniotis, M. K. (1992). *Total quality management.* Chicago: American Hospital Publishers.

Midgett, M. (1984). Skilled nursing facility marketing. In W. J. Winston (Ed.), *Marketing long-term care and senior care services* (pp. 77–81). New York: The Haworth Press.

Miller, A. (1998, March 23). *Assisted Living Business Week, 2*(11).

Miller, D. B. (Ed.). (1982). *Long term care administrator's desk manual.* Greenvale, NY: Penel Publishers.

Miller, D. B., & Barry, J. T. (1979). *Nursing home organization and operation.* Boston: CBI.

Miller, J. G. (1955). Toward a general theory for the behavioral sciences. *American Psychologist, 10.*

Mintzberg, H. (1979). *The structuring of organizations: a synthesis of the research.* Englewood Cliffs, NJ: Prentice-Hall.

Orlikoff, J., Fifer, W., & Greeley, H. (1981). *Malpractice prevention and liability control for hospitals.* Chicago: American Hospital Association.

Peters, T. (1987). *Thriving on chaos.* New York: Harper & Row.

Peters, T., & Austin, N. (1985). *A passion for excellence: The leadership difference.* New York: Random House.

Peterson, S. (1986). Take note: Image is as image does. *Provider 12*(11), 36–39.

Pfeffer, J., & Salancik, G. R. (1978). *The external control of organizations.* New York: Harper & Row.

Pressman, J. L., & Wildavsky, A. B. (1974). *Implementation.* Berkeley: University of California Press.

Prosser, W. L. (1973). *Laws of torts.* St. Paul, MN: West.

Quality Care Advocate. (September/October, 1989). Washington, DC: National Citizens' Coalition for Nursing Home Reform.

Rice, J. A., & Taylor, S. (1984, February). Assessing the market for long-term care services. *Healthcare Financial Management,* pp. 32–46.

Riffer, J. (1984, June 16). The patient as guest: A competitive strategy. *Hospitals,* pp. 48–55.

Robertson, T. S., Zielinski, J., & Ward, S. (1984). *Consumer behavior.* Palo Alto, CA: Scott, Foresman.

Robey, D. (1982). *Designing organizations.* Homewood, IL: Richard D. Irwin.

Rogers, W. W. (1980). *General administration in the nursing home* (3rd ed.). Boston: CBI.

Rosenberg, L. J., & Van West, J. H. (1984, November–December). The collaborative approach to marketing. *Business Horizons,* pp. 29–35.

Ruff, K. A. (1986). Families and friends can help educate. *Provider, 12*(11), 46–47.

Scanlon, W. J., & Feder, J. (1984, January). The long-term care marketplace: An overview. *Healthcare Financial Management,* pp. 18–36.

Shackle, G. L. S. (1957). *Uncertainty and business decisions: a symposium* (2nd ed.). Liverpool, England: Liverpool University Press.

Showalter, J. (1984). *Quality assurance and risk management: A joinder of two important movements.* Journal of Legal Medicine, 5, 497.

Simon, H. A. (1960). *The new science of management decision.* New York: Harper & Row.

Sinioris, M. E., & Butler, P. (1983, June 1). Basic business strategy: Responding to change requires planning, marketing, and budgeting strategies. *Hospitals,* p. 57.

Sirrocco, A. (1989). Nursing home characteristics: 1986 inventory of long-term care places. *Vital Health Statistics, 14*(33).

Sirrocco, A. (1994, February 23). *Nursing homes and board and care homes.* Advance Data, No. 244. Washington, DC: U.S. Department of Health and Human Services.

Skelly, G. (1986). Is food service a part of your marketing strategy? *Provider, 12*(11), 58–60.

Smith, S. M. (1984). Family selection of long-term care services. In W. J. Winston (Ed.), *Marketing long-term and senior care services* (pp. 101–113). New York: The Haworth Press.

Star, S. H. (1989). Marketing and its discontents. *Harvard Business Review, 89*(6), 148–154.

Sweeney, M., & Lewis, C. (1986). Neighborhood nursing home program opens the right doors. *Provider, 12*(11), 70–71.

Swiss, J. E. (1983). Establishing a management system: The interaction of power shifts and personality under federal MBO. *Public Administration Review, 43*(3).

Tannenbaum, R., Wechsler, I., & Massarik, F. (1961). *Leadership and organization.* New York: McGraw-Hill.

Terry, G. R. (1969). *Principles of management.* Homewood, IL: Richard D. Irwin.

Ting, H. M. (1984, May). New directions in nursing home and home healthcare marketing. *Healthcare Financial Management,* pp. 62–72.

Troyer, G. T., & Salman, S. L. (1986). *Handbook of health care risk management.* Rockville, MD: Aspen.

U.S. Department of Health and Human Services. (1999, December). *National Study of Assisted Living for the Frail Elderly.* Results of a national survey.

U.S. Senate Special Committee on Aging. (2003, April 29). *Assisted Living Workgroup's final report.*

USDHHS Administration on Aging. (1985). On finding, training, and keeping volunteers from dropping out. (USDHHS Publication No. 348). Washington, DC: Author.

Weissert, W. G., et al. (1989). Models of adult day care: Findings from a national survey. *The Gerontologist, 29*(5).

Wildavsky, A. (1964). *The politics of the budgetary process.* Boston: Little, Brown.

Williams, S. J., & Torrens, P. R. (1980). *Introduction to health services.* New York: Wiley.

Winston, W. J. (Ed.) (1984). *Marketing long-term and senior care services.* New York: The Haworth Press.

Wrapp, H. E. (1984). Good managers don't make policy decisions. *Harvard Business Review, 84*(4).

Zitter, M. (1989). Outline can help hospitals success with seniors' care. *Modern Healthcare, 19*(52).

Zmud, R. W. (1983). *Information systems in organizations.* Dallas: Scott, Foresman.

PART TWO

ORGANIZATIONAL PATTERNS AND HUMAN RESOURCES

2.0 Organizational Patterns of the Assisted Living Facility

ROLE OF THE ASSISTED LIVING FACILITY

An Emerging Need

Assisted living is a term that first emerged in the 1980s and 1990s to describe a new style of personal care available to the rapidly expanding population of older persons. Previously, the need for personal care had been limited primarily to small board and care homes or in nursing homes.

The Continuing Care Retirement Communities, themselves a phenomenon of the 1970s and 1980s, typically built only a combination of residential units and nursing home units—the need for assisted living had not yet been identified. As the residents of the life care communities aged in place, it became obvious that a level of care between independent living units and the nursing center was needed (Table 2.1). Life care communities began building assisted living units as transitional care units when their regular residents were no longer able to perform all the activities of daily living but did not need the 24-hour-a-day nursing care available in the nursing units.

The emergence of the large number of freestanding assisted living facilities in communities across the nation represents, on a national scale, the need recognized within the life care communities.

Today, assisted living facilities may be freestanding, part of a life care community, or part of a hospital or nursing home chain. There are perhaps as many as one million aging Americans already living in assisted living facilities (Assisted Living Business Week, 1998).

Table 2.1 Percentage of Assisted Living Facility Residents Requiring ADL Assistance

Activity	Percentage of Residents
Eating	10
Transferring	15
Toileting	33
Dressing	46
Medication reminder	50
Bathing	64
Medication dispensing	70

Source: Martin, p. 51; Coopers & Lybrand "Overview of the Assisted Living Industry."

ASSISTED LIVING SERVICE MODELS

Direct Services, Contracted Services

Two broad service models have emerged: direct services and contracted services. Under the direct service model much of the health care–related care is provided by in-house staff. Under the contracted service model nearly all health care–related care is provided by outside agencies such as the local home health agency or nurse or other health care pool agencies.

Typically, the contracted services model is not required to be licensed because no health care-related services are provided by the staff (Table 2.2). This text focuses primarily on the direct service model, which normally will be licensed and provide in-house some type of health care-related services to residents.

Typical Services

Assisted living residences typically offer the following types of services:

- organized group and individual social and recreational activities including health promotion and exercise programs
- three meals a day in a dining room setting; snacks, other nutritional needs
- assistance with Activities of Daily Living such as eating, bathing, dressing, toileting and walking
- 24–hour health-related care including medication management and, typically, dementia needs
- planned participation in community programs including transportation needs; shopping assistance
- housekeeping services
- laundry services

Table 2.2 Instrumental Activities of Daily Living Typically Included in Assisted Living

Preparing meals	Managing money/maintaining finances
Housekeeping	Linen and laundry services
Social activities	Maintaining the utilities
Transportation	Escort services
Barber/beauty shop	Wellness programs (including physical, occupational, and speech therapies)

ORGANIZATIONAL PATTERN FOR A 60–UNIT AND A 100–UNIT FACILITY

Size Variations

Assisted living facilities vary in size from a few to a few hundred units. Some chains prefer smaller facilities of perhaps 60 units. Other chains are building larger-sized units to take advantage of the economies of scale. The typical assisted living facility built in recent years has approximately 100 units. This is not surprising. The nursing home industry discovered that the economies of scale are best met at about 120 units. Because some chains, however, choose to specialize in smaller, more personal facilities of 30 to 60 units, we illustrate here both a 60–unit facility and a 100–unit arrangement.

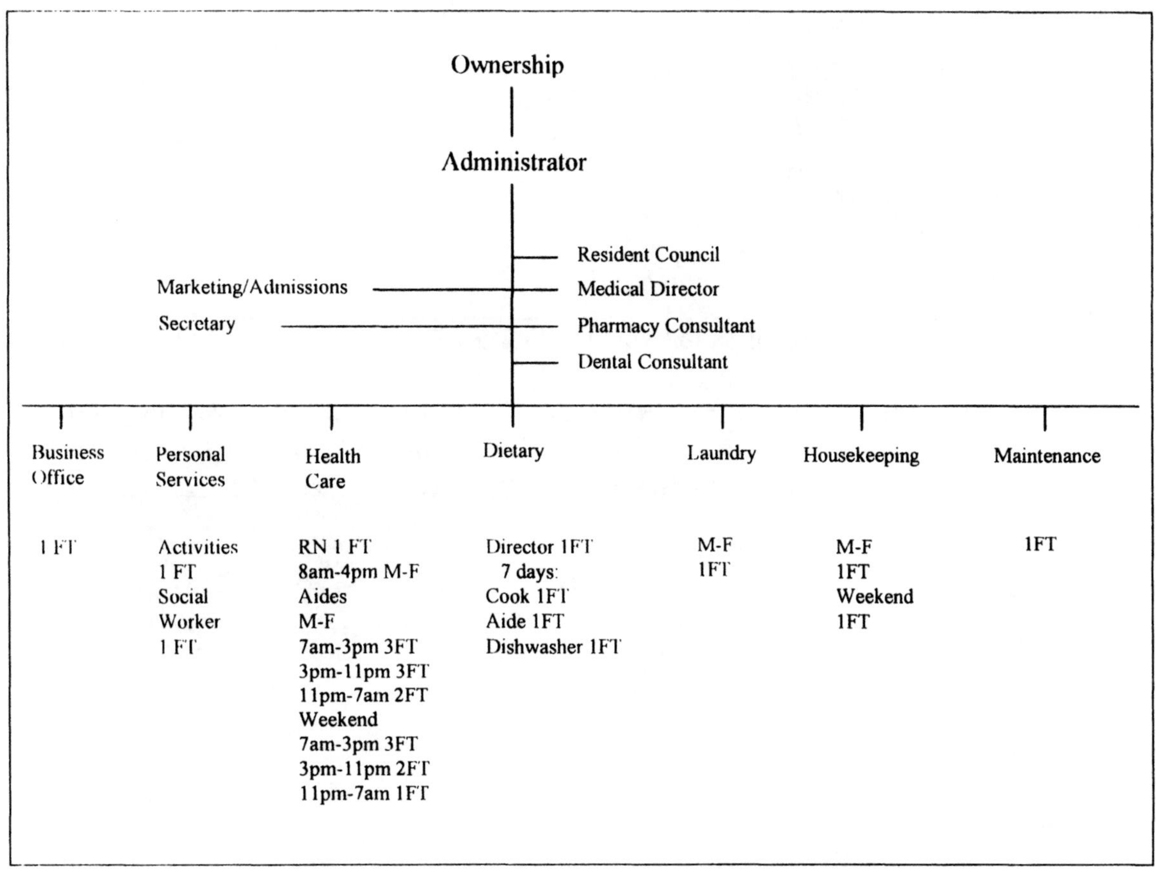

FIGURE 2.1(A) Organizational pattern and staffing levels for a 60-unit facility.

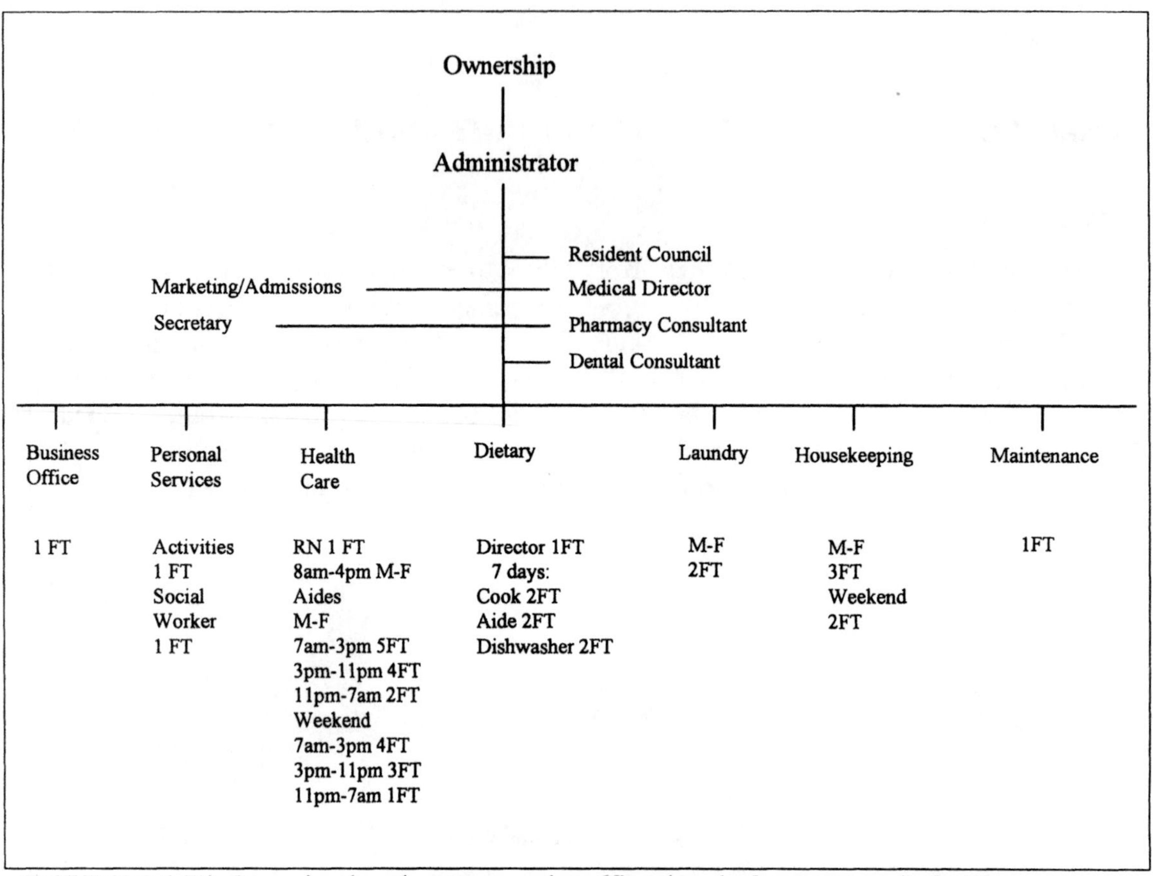

FIGURE 2.1(B) Organizational pattern and staffing levels for a 100-unit facility.

The smaller facility is designated the Jordan Lake Assisted Living Facility (Figure 2.1(A)), the larger, the Kerr Lake Assisted Living Facility (Figure 2.1(B)). As can be seen in both figures the work of a facility has been divided into the traditional areas of

- marketing/admissions
- business office
- personal services
- health care
- dietary
- laundry
- housekeeping
- maintenance

In this model all area heads report directly to the administrator.

Workable Variations

Numerous workable variations on this model exist. In both Figures 2.1(A) and 2.1(B) line authority is given to the administrator leading to several functional or work areas. The administrator has responsibility, directly or indirectly, for all of the facility.

A variant of this model, more suited to a larger facility of perhaps 200 residents, is to group several of these functions under middle-level managers who report to the administrator. One such arrangement is to appoint additional middle-level managers (Miller, 1982) who are directors of

- Personal services (e.g., volunteers, transportation, barbers, and beauticians)
- Administrative services (e.g., marketing/admissions, business office, clerical staff, and personnel)
- Health care services (all health care activities)
- Housekeeping
- Laundry
- Maintenance
- Food services
- Therapy services (usually done on an outpatient basis, e.g., physical, occupational, and speech therapy)

In the typical 60- to 100-bed assisted living facility the administrator will have eight or nine areas reporting directly to him or her.

Assumptions About the Facilities

These facilities can be either for-profit or not-for-profit, freestanding or part of a small or large chain. The staffing is heavier than will currently be found at many assisted living facilities. This is intentional. These facilities are designed to care for the resident populations expected in 2000 to 2007, which are anticipated to need increasingly heavier health care. The rationale for each of the positions is discussed under the separate department/function headings below. Wages for each staff position are presented in Table 2.3(A) and Table 2.3(B). How these wages fit within the income and expense flow of the facility is given in Table 2.4(A) and Table 2.4(B).

Facility Size and Monthly Rates

Just a quick glance at the bottom lines of these two facilities demonstrates that the fixed and semivariable costs of a facility can dramatically affect profitability. The figures in these tables suggest that the small incremental costs of serving 100 residents when compared to serving 60 residents significantly improve profitability in the 100–unit facility.

How to Staff. The decision on how to staff an assisted living facility depends on many variables. An overarching consideration is the level of residents' capacities to perform the activities of daily living. Changes in activities capabilities will normally result in altered staffing patterns. Admission of several heavier care residents may lead to employment of an additional experienced health care staff person. The two facilities described here are assumed to have an average level of resident ability to perform ADLs.

TABLE 2.3 (A) Staff and Consultants Budget for 60-Unit Jordan Lake Assisted Living Facility (based on a 2,000-hour work year per full-time employee)

Department/Area	Hourly wage	Annual wage	Total
Administrator	22.50	45,000	
Office manager	9.50	19,000	
Mkt/Admissions	7.50	15,000	
Recep/Secy	6.75	13,500	92,500
Personal Services			
Social worker	12.50	25,000	
Activities director	14.50	29,000	54,000
Health Care			
Registered nurse	19.00	38,000	
CNAs	(rate 6.90)	(each 13,800)	
Weekdays			
7-3 3 aides			
3-11 2 aides			
11-7 2 aides		110,400 total M-F	
Weekends			
7-3 3 aides			
3-11 2 aides			
11-7 1 aides		33, 120 total Sa-Su	181,520
Dietary			
Supervisor	10.50	21,000	
Aide	6.25	12,500	
Dishwasher	6.25	12,500	
Cook	8.75	17,500	
			63,500
Sa.-Su.	(same staffing)		25,400
Laundry			
Aide	6.50	13,000	
			13,000
Housekeeping			
Weekdays 1 FT	6.50 each	13,000 each	
Weekends 1 FT	6.50	5,200	18,200
Maintenance	9.00	18,000	18,000
Regular Staff plus			Total: 466,120
Benefits @ 20%			93,224
Total personnel cost			559,344
Medical director	350 month	4,200	4,200
Pharmacist	16.00 hr x 8 hrs mo.	1536	1536
			Total: 565,080

TABLE 2.3 (B) Staff and Consultants Budget for 100-Unit Kerr Lake Assisted Living Facility (based on a 2,000-hour work year per full-time employee)

Department/Area	Hourly wage	Annual wage	Total
Administrator	22.50	45,000	
Office manager	9.50	19,000	
Mkt/Admissions	7.50	15,000	
Recep/Secy	6.75	13,500	92,500
Personal Services			
Social worker	12.50	25,000	
Activities director	14.50	29,000	54,000
Health Care			
Registered nurse	19.00	38,000	
CNAs	(rate 6.90)	(each 13,800)	
Weekdays			
7-3 5 aides			
3-11 4 aides			
11-7 2 aides		151,800 total M-F	
Weekends			
7-3 4 aides			
3-11 3 aides			
11-7 2 aides		49,680 total Sa-Su	239,480
Dietary			
Supervisor	10.50	21,000	
Aide	6.25	12,500	
Aide	6.25	12,500	
Dishwasher	6.25	12,500	
Dishwasher	6.25	12,500	
Cook	8.75	17,500	
Cook	8.75	17,500	106,000
Sa.-Su.	(same staffing)		34,000
Laundry			
Aide	6.50	13,000	
Aide	6.50	13,000	26,000
Housekeeping			
Weekdays 2 FT	6.50 each	13,000 each	
Weekends 1 FT	6.50	5,200	31,200
Maintenance	9.00	18,000	18,000
Regular Staff plus			Total: 601,180
Benefits @ 20%			120,236
Total personnel cost			721,416
Medical director	400 month	4,800	4,800
Pharmacist	16.00 hr x 8 hrs mo.	1536	1536
			Total: 727,752

TABLE 2.4 (A) Income and Expense Statement for 60-Unit Jordan Lake Assisted Living Facility

Variables	Month	Year	Total
Expenses			
Salaries	46,612	559,344	
Raw food @4.00 per day per resident	7,300	87,600	
Supplies	7,200	86,400	
Capital equipment	800	9,600	
Utilities	6,560	78,720	
Telephone/e-mail	250	3,000	
Insurance	3,600	43,200	
Capital costs			
Mortgage payments	14,700		
(principle and interest)	25,666		
Depreciation	11,900		
Total capital costs		627,192	
Uncollectibles	750	9,000	
Total expenses			1,504,056
Income			
Average $2,160/mo. at average 93% occupancy	200,880		1,451,520
Income (loss) before taxes			52,536

Assumptions: 60 units, monthly fee = average of $2,160, occupancy rate = 93%, construction costs = $4.9 million (bank line loan 20% equity/80% debt @ 8.5% interest rate), depreciation period = 40 years.

TABLE 2.4 (B) Income and Expense Statement for 100-Unit Kerr Lake Assisted Living Facility

Variables	Month	Year	Total
Expenses			
Salaries	54,746	727,752	
Raw food @4.00	12,166	146,000	
Supplies	12,000	144,000	
Capital equipment	800	9,600	
Utilities	8,200	98,400	
Telephone/e-mail	250	3,000	
Insurance	4,000	48,000	
Capital costs			
Mortgage payments	21,000		
(principle and interest)	36,666		
Depreciation	17,000		
Total capital costs		679,992	
Uncollectibles	1,250	15,000	
Total expenses			1,871,744
Income			
Average $2,160/mo. at average 93% occupancy	200,880		2,410,560
Income (loss) before taxes			538,816

Assumptions: 100 units, monthly fee = average of $2,160, occupancy rate = 93%, construction costs = $7.0 million (bank line loan 20% equity/80% debt @ 8.5% interest rate), depreciation period = 40 years.

Pricing Assisted Living Services

A variety of pricing strategies have evolved in the assisted living industry. Here a system in which the facility assigns points on a scale of 1 to 5 for each of the activities of daily living to represent the amount of staff time needed to care for each resident is presented.

Level One Facility. Level 1 is a light-care facility. In this model the average care burden placed on the staff averages assistance with one to three of the activities of daily living (generally including eating, bathing, dressing, getting to and using the bathroom, getting into or out of a bed or chair, and mobility). The typical resident needs help with three ADLs. Staffing costs are expected to be at least 35% of total revenues in the Level 1 facility.

Level Two Facility. Level 2 is a medium-care facility. In this model the average care burden placed on the staff averages four of the activities of daily living mentioned above. Staffing costs are expected to be about 45% of total revenues in the Level 2 facility.

Level Three Facility. Level 3 is a heavy-care facility. In this model the care burden placed on the staff is from four to five ADLs. Staffing costs may average or exceed about 55% of total revenues in the Level 3 facility.

Variations in Acuity Patterns

The caregiving burden placed on staff, hence the number of employees needed to provide an adequate number of hours of resident care each day, will determine the total staff needs. A facility may have 70% lightcare residents (help with 1 to 3 ADLs) plus 30% heavy-care residents (help with all ADLs) and require similar total staffing to a facility with nearly all medium-care residents (help with 3 or 4 ADLs). Each facility or corporation must devise a scale to measure the total care burden that determines its total staffing needs. Financial aspects are discussed in detail in Part Three. Here we present this matter only in an introductory manner.

We turn now to consideration of the organizational work to be accomplished by each work area and associated staffing requirements.

THE ADMINISTRATOR'S ROLES

We have demonstrated that the administrator is responsible for ensuring that all work is accomplished according to policy at an acceptable level of quality.

The managerial goal of the assisted living administrator is that personnel in every unit arrive at a level of daily performance that reflects a passion for quality. This goal is more easily articulated than accomplished. The multitude of resident care functions to be achieved in the assisted living setting, given the typical level of financing, can seem overwhelming.

To summarize briefly, consider the following as an initial description given in no particular order of priority. It is the responsibility of the administrator to:

- ensure a satisfactory quality of care and of life for residents and staff
- advocate for the residents and, as needed, the staff and the facility
- monitor and control all the subsystems in the facility
- develop and manage the budget
- manage the interface between the facility and its many constituencies, including the outside community
- monitor and manage the human resource functions
- coordinate or ensure coordination of the work of all areas and functions in the facility
- provide stimulus on a daily basis to activities that implement the facility's goals and mission
- forecast and lead the facility to a successful future
- assist all staff and residents to understand the nature and value of change
- interface with the local community, owners, inspectors, public representatives, third-

party insurers, hospitals, fire inspectors, and the myriad of other persons, groups, and functions necessary to the survival of the facility
- communicate with staff, residents, and others
- empower work area heads and staff to accomplish their work
- facilitate the functioning of the facility by walking around and similar management approaches
- set the tone for the facility in matters of dress, taste, compassion, and concern by word and behavior
- mediate territorial and jurisdictional disputes among staff, residents, and owners

Administrator salaries in 1999 ranged between 31,400 – 130,000 according to the Housing the Elderly Report, 1999 Staff Compensation Survey.

EDUCATION REQUIREMENTS FOR ASSISTED LIVING FACILITY ADMINISTRATORS

The requirements for becoming an assisted living facility administrator are shown in Table 2.5. As can be seen, requirements vary dramatically from state to state. For the most part, they reflect the earlier requirements for persons expected to manage the bed and board homes of yesteryear.

In practice, the educational requirements for the assisted living facility administrator will be market driven. Fifty years ago few hospital administrators held a master's degree in health care administration. Today, without at least a master's degree, one need not bother to get into the long line of applicants for the position of hospital administrator. There are no educational or other requirements for hospital administrators. In fact, the only health care administrators who must be licensed are nursing home administrators, and in some states some states, assisted living facility administrators. Whether assisted living facility administrators will be routinely required to hold licenses similar to a nursing home administrator has yet to be determined.

The assisted living facility industry itself will, at least initially, determine the educational and other qualifications necessary for the successful applicant for the position of administrator. As can be seen in Table 2.5, 20 states require continuing education for assisted living facility administrators.

Assisted Living Workgroup Report to the U.S. Senate Special Committee on Aging (April, 2003, p. 321), recommended the following:

- Be a licensed nursing home administrator or complete a state-approved course and pass a state-approved exam
- Study at least: philosophy of assisted living, management, resident services, clinical services, environmental management, finance, personnel regulations.
- 18 hours of continuing education per year.
- Education:
    - High school diploma + 4 years experience
    - Associate's degree + two years experience
    - Bachelor's degree + one year experience

TABLE 2.5 Requirements for Assisted Living Facility Administrators

State	Initial Licensure	Annual Continuing Education (hours/per year)
Alabama	Well trained	6
Alaska	"Sufficient" not specified	18
Arizona	County-approved program	6/18/12 *depending on licensed level of care
Arkansas	H.S./ certification program	Yes
California	Certification program (40+ hours) + Exam	20
Colorado	30 hours operator training program	
Connecticut	RN & BSN + 2 years experience (or AA/Diploma)	
Delaware	Nursing home admin. license	
Florida	H.S. GED or equiv.	6
Georgia		16
Hawaii	ALF admin course	6+
Idaho	Admin course; exam	12
Illinois		
Indiana	H.S.	
Iowa	age 21 and "qualified"	
Kansas	60+ residents—college degree <60 residents—high school degree + training	Required for administrators only
Kentucky	H.S. (21 yrs. old) demonstrated management or administrative ability	
Louisiana	Various combinations of education & experience	12+
Maine	Training program	10
Maryland	H.S. or equivalent or other appropriate education/experience	Periodic course update
Massachusetts	BA or experience	10
Michigan	Be 21, be "competent"	
Minnesota		
Mississippi	H.S. or GED	
Missouri	Licensed nursing home administrator	
Montana	H.S. or GED	6
Nebraska		
Nevada	H.S. or equivalent; examination 40 hour program	8
New Hampshire	H.S. plus additional education and experience (Varies according to facility size)	12
New Jersey	H.S. or equivalent; exam	10
New Mexico	H.S. or equivalent; exam	
New York	H.S. or equivalent and experience	30

North Carolina	Some college or as approved	15
North Dakota	BA and NHA license, or experience	12
Ohio	NHA or BA or BS or 2000 hours experience or 100 hours post H.S. education in gerontology	9+
Oklahoma	NHA or certificate of training	
Oregon	H.S. or equivalent; 40 hour course	20
Pennsylvania	H.S. or GED and 40 hours training	6
Rhode Island	44 hours course work; or RI nursing home licensure (New rules to be promulgated in 2003)	"Responsible Adult" 24 hours/day
South Carolina	H.S. or equivalent; 12 months experience; examination	12
South Dakota	Health Professional or H.S. equivalent and training	
Tennessee	H.S. or GED	12
Texas	H.S. or equivalent (more if large facility)	12
Utah	Various combinations of education and experience	
Vermont	State-approved certification course or required education and /or experience	12+
Virginia	H.S. or GED and 1 year post-secondary ed. or supervisory caregiver exp. (w/some exceptions)	20
Washington	H.S. + 2 yrs. caregiving experience or national certification	
West Virginia	H.S. or equivalent; new: A.A. in related field	10+
Wisconsin	H.S. or equivalent	12
Wyoming	Exam	
D.C.	H.S. or GED	12

Assistant Administrator/Administrative Assistant

An assistant administrator has line authority to represent the administrator, can make decisions on his or her behalf, and is usually assigned some area or areas to oversee. An administrative assistant, on the other hand, has no line authority, cannot make decisions for the facility, and does not represent the administrator except in an information gathering, or processing manner. The administrative assistant is a staff position.

In the assisted living facility of 100 units there tends not to be enough organizational room for an assistant administrator; 300 or more units would call for such a position. The appointment of an assistant administrator or administrative assistant depends on the personality of the administrator. Assistant administrator salaries ranged between $33,540 and 72,000 in 1999 according to the Housing the Elderly Report, 1999 Staff Compensation Survey.

Secretary

Generally, the facility secretary works in the administrator's office, in an area shared with the receptionist/telephone/Internet/e-mail operator/manager. As a rule, the administrator has several advisory persons or groups. Any advising physician and resident council fit into this slot. Other consultants, such as the medical director, pharmacist, or dentist, and any other advisory committees might appear here. The administrator's office is responsible for keeping on file the original of several types of information (e.g., reports of any inspection teams, work area reports, and other important documents).

In the typical assisted living facility the duties assigned the secretary will vary widely. Often the secretary will have functions such as being the receptionist, word processor, telephone attendant, first responder to some resident needs (e.g., for cash from their account), copier manager, and a variety of other assignments, depending on facility needs and the individual's qualifications.

PROFESSIONAL STANDARDS OF PRACTICE AND THE ASSISTED LIVING FACILITY

Do professional standards of practice exist for the assisted living facility? This is a complicated question. In essence, professional standards of practice are dictated by most states. This is demonstrated in Tables 2.6 and 2.7, which summarize the states' staffing requirements and staff education requirements for assisted living facilities. The reader will note that staffing and staff education requirements vary considerably from state to state. For the most part, the requirements, on the surface, do not appear to be well developed or consistent from state to state.

TABLE 2.6 Staffing Requirements for Assisted Living Facilities

State	Staff: Resident Ratio	Required Hours	Licensed	Other Qualifications
Alabama	1:6	1 + staff 24 hours/day	RN consultant	Initial and refresher training in specified areas
Alaska				Sufficient Language skills
Arizona				Contin'g ed.; training
Arkansas	Varied	1 + staff 24 hours/day	RN available 24 hrs/day in level 2	Licensed staff in level 2
California	Variable	1 + staff 24 hours/day		10 hours initial in-service training, 4 hours/year (ADL caregivers)
Colorado		1+ staff on site		Education and/or experience for those w/direct care responsibilities
Connecticut		Required hours for SALSA only	RN on call or on site	
Delaware				
Florida	Varies w/number of residents	Varies w/number of residents	Required to perform certain tasks	In-service training (direct care)
Georgia	1:15 (waking hours) 1:25 (night)	1+ staff 24 hours/day		Direct care staff 16 hours/year education

Hawaii		Awake 24 hours	LNs, 7 days/week	6+ hours/year in-service education
Idaho		1+ staff 24 hours/day	1 visit/month RN	8 hours/year training (personal assistance staff)
Illinois	Sufficient to meet scheduled & unscheduled resident needs	1 CPR trained staff on duty 24 hours a day		Direct care staff are subject to Heath Care Worker Background Check
Indiana		1+ staff 24 hours/day (more if > 100 residents)	L.N. on-site or on-call	In-service training
Iowa	Sufficient to meet tenant needs	1+ staff 24 hours/day	RN delegation	Training
Kansas				
Kentucky		24-hour staffing		One awake staff member onsite at all times
Louisiana	Sufficient in number and qualification on duty at all times	1 + awake 24 hours/day		Annual training (direct care)
Maine	1:12 (7am-3pm) 1:18 (3pm-11pm) 1:30 (11pm-7am)	> 2 awake 24 hours/day		Direct care: certification course
Maryland		24 hours/day		On-going training
Massachusetts		1 + staff 24 hours/day		6+ hours/year cont. ed.; 54+ hours training (personal care service providers)
Michigan	Sufficient to meet residents needs	1+ staff awake 24 hours/day		Training regarding general resident care, dementia, and resident rights
Minnesota	Must staff to meet resident needs			Orientation and training
Mississippi	1:15 (7am-7pm) 1:25 (7pm-7am)		RN – 8 hrs/day	
Missouri	1:15 (morning) 1:20 (evening) 1:25 (night)		RN 8+ hours/week	
Montana		1+ staff 24 hours/day		Pre-service training (direct care staff)
Nebraska		1+ staff 24 hours/day		12 hours/year training (direct care); orientation
Nevada	1:6 (Alzheimer's facilities only)	1+ awake 24 hours/day if > 20 residents		8 hrs/year training (caregivers)
New Hampshire	Meets the needs of residents	1+ staff 24 hours/day (awake if 17+ residents)		
New Jersey		2+ staff on-site 24 hours/day (1+awake)	RN on call at all times	Training (direct care)
New Mexico	1:15	Variable		In-service training
New York	Variable	Variable, including 24 hours		
North Carolina	Varies w/time of day	Detailed		Variable training requirements for personal care aides.

North Dakota				Continuing education for dietary and activities staff; in-service training
Ohio	One staff 24 hours/day plus sufficient additional staff to meet needs of residents			Successful completion of American Red Cross First Aid Basics; training and continuing education for staff
Oklahoma	Sufficient			Training
Oregon	Variable	24 hr. availability	RN on staff or contract	Pre-service training (direct care staff)
Pennsylvania	Variable			
Rhode Island	Staffing ration required in special care units	"Responsible adult" 24 hours/day	RN visit once every 30 days	Training
South Carolina	1:8/building ("peak" hours) 1:30/building (night)	1+ staff on active duty at all times		Training
South Dakota		Detailed 1+staff 24 hours/day		Training
Tennessee	Certified by TN Board for Licensing Health Care Facilities	1+ staff 24 hours/day	Available as needed	Annual in-service training
Texas		Nightly shift staff immediately available/awake		Direct care: 6 hours ed./year
Utah		24 hours/day (direct care personnel)	CAN (personal care)	Nursing Overview must be provided by an RN
Vermont			Nursing overview must be provided by an RN	12+ hours training/year & dementia care for direct care staff
Virginia		1+ staff awake 24 hours/day	To provide some services	8+ hours/year training (direct care)
Washington	Minimum 1 staff person – must have sufficient trained staff	Minimum 1 staff present when residents are onsite		One staff must be at least 18 yrs. old with CPR and first aid. All staff must pass criminal history background check
West Virginia	Variable	1+staff 24 hours/day	Employ or contract with LN if meds administered	Specific topics must be included for all staff
Wisconsin	Variable for Class C	1+ care staff when residents are present		Caregiver background checks, Initial training; cont. ed. for care staff
Wyoming		1+ staff awake 24 hours (if 8+ beds)	RN, LPN or CAN every shift; must employ or contract with RN	Central registry background check
D.C.		1+ staff/24 hours with first aid and CPR		Training

TABLE 2.7 Staff Education Requirements for Assisted Living Facilities

State	Education	CE (hours)
Alabama	As needed	16
Alaska		
Arizona	16-hr county program	20
Arkansas	Orientation to residents' rights	
California	On-the-job training	
Colorado		
Connecticut	Aides must be CNAs or CHHAs	
Delaware	Be OBRA CAN trained aids	
Florida	One empl. cert. in first aid, HIV/AIDS	
Georgia	Some in-service required	
Hawaii	In-service education	
Idaho	Ongoing training	
Illinois		
Indiana		
Iowa	Sufficient trained staff	
Kansas	In-services: principles of assisted living; fire safety; disaster preparedness; accident prevention; residents' rights; infection control; prevention of abuse, neglect, or exploitation.	
Kentucky		
Louisiana	Adequate training	
Maine	In-service training	
Maryland	Orientation	
Massachusetts	Licensed nurse, qualified CAN, HHA, personal care homemaker or do 54-hr course	6
Michigan	Age 21	
Minnesota		
Mississippi	Appropriate quarterly training	
Missouri		
Montana	Orientation	
Nebraska		
Nevada	Be familiar with regulations	8
New Hampshire	In-services	
New Jersey	Be CNA or CHHA	
New Mexico	Age 18 yrs., have adequate training	
New York		
North Carolina		

North Dakota	Personal care aides, activities dir., reg. therapeutic rec. specialist, certified OT or OT assistant or 2 yrs. of activity experience	12
Ohio	Age 16, first aid training + approved training curse, speak English, observe residents' rights	
Oklahoma	One cert. in CPR, 8 hrs. of initial training appropriate food service supv. training	8
Oregon	Demonstrated ability to provide services	
Pennsylvania	In-services	
Rhode Island	In-services	
South Carolina	Annual in-services	
South Dakota	In-services, infection control training	
Tennessee	Employees to meet needs of residents	
Texas		
Utah	CNA if give care, inservices	
Vermont		
Virginia	CNA certification	12
Washington	Fundamentals of caregiving	15
West Virginia	Orientation, in-services	
Wisconsin	Fire safety, first aid, univ. precautions, emergency plan training	
Wyoming	RN, LPN, or CNA (or contract RN)	

NATIONAL LONG-TERM CARE PROFESSIONAL STANDARDS OF PRACTICE

Pressures

Through pressure brought on Congress over the years the federal government has evolved professional standards of practice regarding resident care in nursing homes. These standards are embodied in the regulations and guidelines developed for such facilities. No matching set of professional standards of practice have ye to be formally placed into effect for home health care agencies, life care communities, assisted living facilities, hospice providers, adult day care centers, or, for that matter, hospitals.

Clear Intent

The intent of Congress is clear: older citizens who are at risk and need few or many services to enable them to live their days in dignity, whether in an assisted living facility, a life care community, or at home receiving home health care services, should be accorded quality care in a professional and dignified manner. The regulations developed and applied specifically to nursing facilities are, in this author's belief, also intended to establish expected standards for all who provide care to the elderly.

Avoiding Regulation

Professional care standards, then, already exist in the long-term-care field. The failure to adhere to professional quality of care standards by the nursing home industry resulted in the imposition of care standards. To the extent the assisted living industry implements the care standards already developed for the long-term-care industry (the *Nursing Home Federal Requirements and Guidelines to Surveyors*), it may avoid being subjected to the heavy regulations, constant inspections, and mandatory fines currently being imposed on nursing homes.

In 2003 the U.S. Senate Special Committee on Aging received staffing recommendations from the 50 organization Assisted Living Workgroup in the areas of:

> Communication; criminal background checks; abuse registry; job descriptions; staff vaccinations; compliance with federal employment laws; verification of employment history; administrator qualifications; workload; awake staff; acting administrator authorization; management recruitment and retention practices; human resources recruitment and retention practices; direct care training and supervision; orientation and performance evaluations (U.S. Senate Special Committee on Aging, 2003, p. 303).

These recommendations may serve as models to state governments or, possibly, the US Congress.

In the following discussion of the various staff areas of the Kerr Lake Assisted Living Facility selected federal requirements are offered as the professional standard that facilities such as Kerr Lake might practice.

MULTIPLE SOURCES OF PROFESSIONAL STANDARDS

Numerous sets of standards that apply to the assisted living facility exist in addition to the nursing facility related standards cited above. There are, for example, the requirements of the Life Safety Code for assisted living facility facilities, the requirements of the Americans with Disabilities Act, Occupational Safety and Health Act (OSHA), and several more.

HEALTH CARE SERVICES

As residents age in place, health care services will become increasingly important in the daily routine of the typical assisted living facility. The scope of care permitted to assisted living facility staff in each state is presented in Table 2.8. Most of these regulations were written for the traditional rest home and are being revised to permit assisted living facilities to provide higher levels of health care. Current statutes permit help with the activities of daily living and assistance in administering medications. Some states specify that outside providers be used for nursing care. This is changing.

Registered Nurse

In Figure 2.1(B) it is recommended that a registered nurse be hired full time. In addition, it is recommended that persons trained as nurse's aides be employed to provide assistance with the activities of daily living. The rationale for employing registered nurses and nurses' aides who are in the state nurse's aide registry is a recognition that, nationally, residents in assisted living facilities already require assistance with three ADLs and are, for the most part, frail, both in terms of physical abilities and health. Registered nurse salaries ranged between $32,230 and 50,000 in 2003.

TABLE 2.8 Scope of Care by Assisted Living Facilities Permitted by State Statutes

State	Scope of Care Permitted
Alabama	Help with ADLs. Temporary RN consultant for periodic illness
Alaska	Help with ADLs. Help with self-medication. Some nursing care if under RN direction.
Arizona	Help with ADLs. Medication administration. Some intermittent nursing.
Arkansas	Supervision of ADLs but not assistance! Cueing self-medications.
California	Help with ADLs. Numerous nursing care procedures such as intermittent oxygen, colsotomy care, injections, care of indwelling catheters.
Colorado	Help with ADLs. Intermittent nursing care, assistance with medications.
Connecticut	Help with ADLs. Nursing care if stable. If "unstable" health care must be provided by outside agencies, e.g. home health agency.
Delaware	
Florida	Help with ADLs. No nursing services. However, with designation as Extended Congregate Care Facility (ECCF) may provide nursing care up to help with three ADLs if provide nursing diagnoses and plans of care, ongoing social and medical evaluation, infection control.
Georgia	Help with ADLs.
Hawaii	Help with ADLs. Nursing assessment, administration of medications, health monitoring.
Idaho	Help with ADLs. Help with medications, no nursing care permitted.
Illinois	Help with ADLs. Permits 24 hour a day intermittent nursing care.
Indiana	
Iowa	Help with ADLs. Registered nurse may monitor and assess.
Kansas	Help with ADLs. Intermittent skilled nursing services permitted.
Kentucky	Help with ADLs. Any health-related services must be arranged for outside.
Louisiana	Help with ADLs. Help with self-administration of drugs.
Maine	Help with ADLs. In-house nurse limited to non-skilled nursing facility type care, home health agency nurse may give full range of care.
Maryland	Help with ADLs. Help with medication administration.

Massachusetts	Help with ADLs. Help with self-administration of drugs. Otherwise, outside providers required.
Michigan	Help with ADLs.
Minnesota	Help with ADLs. Help with self-administration of drugs. Outside providers required for other services.
Mississippi	Help with ADLs.
Missouri	Help with ADLs. Use of outside providers required.
Montana	Help with ADLs. Use of outside providers required. Effective 1994 a facility may be designated a Category B facility and provide direct skilled nursing assistance.
Nebraska	Help with ADLs.
Nevada	Help with ADLs. Medication assistance. May provide medical care via outside providers or, if appropriately skilled, in-house providers.
New Hampsh.	Help with ADLs. Medication administration. Outside provider or appropriately skilled in-house provider.
New Jersey	Help with ADLs. Per facility policy may provide skilled nursing care.
New Mexico	Help with ADLs. May use own nursing staff or outside provider.
New York	
North Carolina	Help with ADLs. Outsider providers needed for nursing or hospice care.
North Dakota	Help with ADLs. Help with medications that are non-prescription.
Ohio	Help with ADLs. May use outside providers or in-house staff to provide necessary nursing and medical care.
Oklahoma	Help with ADLs. Medication administration assistance.
Oregon	Help with ADLs. May add needed services depending on the needs of the residents.
Pennsylvania	Help with ADLs. Assistance with medications.
Rhode Island	Help with ADLs. Help limited to cueing and observation.
South Carolina	Help with ADLs. Medication administration permitted.
South Dakota	Help with ADLs. Medication assistance permitted.
Tennessee	Help with ADLs. Medication assistance permitted.
Texas	Help with ADLs. Medication assistance permitted.
Utah	Help with ADLs. Medication assistance permitted. Intermittent nursing care permitted.
Vermont	Help with ADLs. Medication assistance permitted. Some nursing care under specified circumstances. Moving in direction of increasing nursing care permitted.
Virginia	Help with ADLs. Medication assistance permitted.
Washington	Help with ADLs. Medication assistance permitted. Some nursing permitted, but not nursing care for residents who are bed-bound more than 14 days.
West Virginia	Help with ADLs. Medication assistance permitted. Facility policy may permit some nursing care if intermittent.

Wisconsin	Help with ADLs. Medication assistance permitted. Intermittent nursing care permitted. Nurse and pharmacist must delegate medication administration.
Wyoming	Help with ADLs. Medication assistance permitted. Intermittent nursing services.

The "Sufficient Staff" Requirement

Most state statutes (refer to Table 2.6) require "sufficient staff." This normally is interpreted to mean that each facility must properly staff for the level of care resident acuity level requires. As residents age in place, their acuity level will continue to rise, requiring the skills of a registered nurse and trained nurse's aides to provide the needed nursing diagnoses, plans of care, ongoing social and medical evaluation, and infection control.

Health care services are discussed extensively in Part Five: Resident Care.

MARKETING/ADMISSIONS

Lifeblood of the Facility

The marketing and admissions functions typically are joined in the assisted living facility. In much larger facilities the two functions might be separated. Marketing and admissions are the lifeblood of the facility. The typical finance structure of an assisted living facility is based on a 95% or better occupancy. High occupancy is necessary to cover fixed costs such, as mortgage expenses, utilities, and the like, which do not decrease with lowered occupancy. Everything else can be in place—an excellent staff, an outstanding building—but if the marketing/admissions functions fail, the facility may fail. Assisted living is an increasingly competitive market. Those who market successfully will thrive.

In developing admissions policies, the facility will want to consider the following, which are normally considered to be appropriate policies to ensure residents' dignity.

- Each resident living in the facility will be ensured a dignified existence, self-determination, and communication with and access to persons and services inside and outside the facility in the community.
- The facility staff will extend to each resident the right to exercise his or her rights as a resident of the facility and as a citizen or resident of the United States.
- Exercising rights means that residents have autonomy and choice, to the maximum extent possible, about how they wish to live their everyday lives and receive care, subject to the facility's rules and the rights of other residents.
- *Notice of rights and services.* The facility will inform each resident both orally and in writing in a language that the resident understands of his or her rights and all rules and regulations governing resident conduct and responsibilities during the stay in the facility.

The goal is to ensure that each resident knows his or her rights and responsibilities and that the facility communicates this information prior to or upon admission, as appropriate during the resident's stay, and when the facility's rules change. Marketing director salaries ranged between $24,000 and 52,000 in 2003.

THE BUSINESS OFFICE

In a typical 100-bed facility one full-time and often an additional part-time employee staff the business office. Briefly, the business office

- keeps financial records
- manages accounts receivable and accounts payable
- maintains vendor files
- assists in monitoring the budget
- prepares the payroll
- keeps required records and makes financial reports
- deals with third-party payers
- safeguards and controls resident funds depending on facility policy
- often acts as receptionist and answers the telephone

PERSONAL SERVICES: ACTIVITIES/RECREATION

The activities director can be the most important employee in an assisted living facility. An activities program sufficient to meet the intellectual, psychological, physical, and spiritual needs and preferences of residents is the most essential function the assisted living facility performs for its residents. Health care is also an important function, but even health care is a means to an end: a satisfying social and personal life for each resident of the facility.

The activities coordinator's task is to ensure that the physical, social, and mental well-being of each resident is included in each resident plan of care. The activities director and the social services worker are assigned primary responsibility for attention to the quality of psychosocial life that exists within a facility (Gordon & Stryker, 1983). It is difficult to imagine a more complicated undertaking in shaping the quality of the residents' life.

The administrator may evaluate the activities program by asking, among other questions, if the activities program

- reflects the schedules, choices, and rights of the residents
- offers activities at hours convenient to the residents (e.g., morning, afternoon, some evenings and weekends)
- reflects the cultural and religious interests of the resident population
- would appeal to both men and women and all age groups living in the facility

Qualifications for the person employed as activities director are at the discretion of the facility administrator. An individual with imagination and social leadership skills is critical to the success of the activities program. To the extent that facilities take on the personality of its leaders, the personality of the activities director is as important as the personality of the administrator as a leader who sets the tone of life in the facility.

A safe approach to hiring an activities director would be to follow the guidelines provided for the long-term care field. In other long-term care facility settings the following qualifications are sought. Although these guidelines do not apply to assisted living facilities, they offer a basis for choosing among applicants.

National Guidelines for Activities Director Qualifications

- Is a qualified therapeutic recreation specialist or an activities professional who—
- Is licensed or registered, if applicable, by the state in which practicing, and
- Is eligible for certification as a therapeutic recreation specialist or as an activities professional by a recognized accrediting body, or
- Has 2 years of experience in a social or recreational program within the last 5 years, 1 of which was full time in a patient activities program in a health care setting; or
- Is a qualified occupational therapist or occupational therapy assistant, or
- Has completed a training course approved by the state

Recognized accrediting body refers to those organizations or associations recognized as such by certified therapeutic recreation specialists or certified activity professionals or registered occupational therapists. The best combination is an employee who both meets the above qualification standards and has a personality to which the residents respond enthusiastically.

PERSONAL SERVICES: SOCIAL SERVICES

The typical assisted living facility may or may not have a qualified social worker on staff. Identifying and meeting the social needs of residents is a necessary part of providing the quality of life residents seek when they enter an assisted living facility. A qualified social worker is not required for the assisted living facility, and not even required of nursing facilities under 120 units. However, fulfilling the residents' needs normally served by a qualified social worker is expected of each assisted living facility's staff.

A qualified social worker is an individual with a bachelor's degree in social work or a bachelor's degree in a human services field, including but not limited to sociology, special education, rehabilitation counseling, and psychology, and had one year of supervised social work experience in a health care setting working directly with individuals.

The assisted living facility administrator can use the following checklist of goals for social services in evaluating the extent to which his or her own assisted living facility is meeting social services needs of the residents. This list of goals need not be, in fact cannot be, met by the individual responsible for social services for the residents. It is an all-hands operation jointly achieved by the various staff persons, especially those in health care services.

The goal of social service function in the assisted living facility is to attain or maintain the highest practicable physical, mental, and psychosocial well-being of each resident.Regardless of size, each assisted living facility is expected to provide for the social needs of each resident. This suggests that facilities aggressively identify the need for social services and ensure the provision of these services. It is not required that a qualified social worker necessarily provide all of these services. Rather, it is the responsibility of the facility to identify the social service needs of the resident and ensure that the needs are met by the appropriate staff members.

The following is a checklist of residents' needs to which a social worker or equivalent staff person might respond:

- Making arrangements for obtaining needed adaptive equipment, clothing, and personal items for residents needing help with ADLs
- Maintaining contact with the residents' family (if the resident wishes this service) to keep them up-to-date on any changes in health
- Helping staff to inform residents about each resident's health status and health care choices and their ramifications—whether to bring caregivers into the assisted living facility or to assist the resident to obtain care in the community
- Assisting residents wishing to make contact with organizations in the community and obtaining services from outside entities (e.g., talking books, absentee ballots, community transportation)
- Assisting residents with financial and legal matters (e.g., applying for pensions, referrals to lawyers, referrals to funeral homes for preplanning arrangements) to the extent facility policies encourage this
- Providing or arranging provision of needed counseling services
- Identifying and seeking ways to support residents' individual needs and preferences, customary routines, concerns, and choices
- Building relationships between residents and staff and teaching staff how to understand and support residents' individual needs
- Promoting actions by staff that maintain or enhance each resident's dignity in full recognition of each resident's individuality. This may range from sensitizing the maintenance person to resident privacy needs to working with a new outside agency care provider who may lack training in meeting resident dignity goals
- Assisting residents to determine how they would like to make decisions about their health care and whether or not they would like anyone else to be involved in those decisions
- Finding options that most meet the physical and emotional needs of each resident. As residents age in place, they may need additional assistance in identifying and making and implementing choices
- Meeting the needs of residents who are grieving. Given the average age of over 85 of most residents, loss of friends will be a constant challenge

Furthermore, the social services–oriented staff person can assist the health care staff to be sensitive to the increasing need for attention to factors with a potentially negative effect on physical, mental, and psychosocial well-being, which might include an unmet need for

- Dental/denture care
- Podiatric care
- Eye care
- Hearing services
- Equipment for mobility or assistive eating devices
- Need for control, dignity, and privacy

Types of conditions to which the facility should respond with social services by staff or referral include the following:

- Lack of an effective family/social support system. Some residents will have children and grandchildren constantly assisting them; other assisted living facility residents may have no family or nearby friends to provide a support system
- Behavioral symptoms. Adjusting to group life in an assisted living facility is a new experience for most residents. Problems may manifest themselves behaviorally
- As residents in America's assisted living facilities age in place, an increasingly larger proportion will exhibit symptoms of dementia. If a resident with dementia strikes out at another resident, the facility social worker should evaluate the resident's behavior. For example, a resident may be reenacting an activity he or she used to perform at the same time everyday. If that resident senses that another is in the way of his or her reenactment, the resident may strike out at the resident impeding his or her progress. The facility is responsible for the safety of any potential resident victims while it assesses the circumstance of the resident's behavior
- Presence of a chronic disabling medical or psychological condition (e.g., multiple sclerosis, chronic obstructive pulmonary disease, Alzheimer's disease, or schizophrenia)
- Depression
- Chronic or acute pain
- Difficulty with personal interaction and socialization skills
- Presence of legal or financial problems
- Abuse of alcohol or other drugs
- Inability to cope with loss of function
- Need for emotional support
- Changes in family relationships, living arrangements, and/or resident's condition or functioning

The assisted living facility administrator can use the following questions to judge the extent to which social needs of the residents are being met:

- How do facility staff implement social services interventions to assist the residents in meeting their social goals?
- How do staff responsible for social work monitor each resident's progress in maintaining and, if needed, improving physical, mental, and psychosocial functioning?
- How does the care plan link goals to psychosocial functioning/well-being?
- Have the staff responsible for social work established and maintained relationships with each resident's family, if appropriate?
- Do social services interventions successfully address residents' needs and link social supports, physical care, and physical environment with residents' needs and individuality?

FOOD SERVICES

The Food Standard

Food is an essential ingredient in the quality of residents' life. Satisfaction with the facility is as often influenced by the food as by the quality of health care. Some families feel they may not have enough long-term-care background to judge the adequacy of health care, but most do consider themselves experts in the matter of food. Tasty food is important to a satisfactory quality of life. Hospital food, eaten for a relatively short period of time, can be tolerated. Assisted living facility food, consumed for much longer periods, is subject to much greater scrutiny by both residents and their families or significant others. Food service director salaries ranged between $25,000 and 52,000 in 2003.

24 Hours a Day. The food area's influence extends 24 hours a day. The availability of bedtime snacks, or midnight snacks for insomniac residents, is as much a part of the ambience of the facility as the availability of continuous health care services. This work area is heavily interactive with health care services (e.g., refreshments at social activities) and with most other work areas. The food service depends on other work areas as well: laundry for linens and maintenance to keep the kitchen functioning, for example. Some facilities contract for food service with outside vendors. In this situation, the head of dietary may be an employee of the food service contractor.

Administrator Monitoring. The administrator can monitor food services in a number of ways—randomly walking through the kitchen, eating with residents in the dining hall, assisting with feeding in residents' rooms. Much can be learned by getting a tray and eating its contents under circumstances similar to those experienced by the resident.

Critical Functions. A few of the critical functions surrounding food service are

- achieving any nutritional diet prescribed by the physician and developed by a registered dietitian or registered dietitian consultant
- ensuring tasty food at the right temperature
- doing nutritional assessments
- monitoring weight gains and losses
- monitoring I/O (input/output)
- providing food substitutes as requested
- catering for facility functions and its many visiting groups
- maintaining the kitchen and dining areas according to cleanliness standards

Dietary Guidelines

The following guidelines are recommended for long-term care facilities, such as assisted living facilities.

The facility will provide each resident with a nourishing, tasty, well-balanced diet that meets the daily nutritional and special dietary needs of each resident.

STAFFING GUIDELINES

The facility will employ a qualified dietitian either fulltime, part-time, or on a consultant basis.

If a qualified dietitian is not employed fulltime, the facility will designate a person to serve as the director of food service, who receives frequently scheduled consultation from a qualified dietitian. A qualified dietitian is one who is qualified based upon either registration by the Commission on Dietetic Registration of the American Dietetic Association or on the basis of education, training, or experience in identification of dietary needs, planning, and implementation of dietary programs.

A director of food services has no required minimum qualifications, but will be able to function collaboratively with a qualified dietitian in meeting the nutritional needs of the residents.

A dietitian qualified on the basis of education, training, or experience in identification of dietary needs, planning, and implementation of dietary programs has experience or training that includes:

- Assessing special nutritional needs of geriatric persons
- Developing therapeutic diets
- Developing regular diets to meet the specialized needs of geriatric persons
- Developing and implementing continuing education programs for dietary services and health care personnel
- Participating in resident care planning
- Budgeting and purchasing food and supplies
- Supervising institutional food preparation, service, and storage

SUFFICIENT STAFF

Sufficient support personnel is defined as enough staff to prepare and serve tasty, attractive, nutritionally adequate meals at proper temperatures and appropriate times, with proper sanitary techniques being utilized.

MENUS: MEET NUTRITIONAL NEEDS, BE PREPARED IN ADVANCE, BE FOLLOWED

Menus will meet the nutritional needs of residents in accordance with the recommended dietary allowances of the Food and Nutrition Board of the National Research Council and National Academy of Sciences.

Question to be asked:

- Does the menu meet basic nutritional needs by providing daily food in the groups of the food pyramid system and based on individual nutritional assessment, taking into account current nutritional recommendations?

Note: A standard meal planning guide (e.g., food pyramid) is used primarily for menu planning and food purchasing. It is not intended to meet the nutritional needs of all residents. This guide must be adjusted to consider individual differences. Some residents will need more due to age, size, gender, physical activity, and state of health. There are many meal planning guides from reputable sources (e.g., American Diabetes Association, American Dietetic Association, American Medical Association, and U.S. Department of Agriculture) that are appropriate for use when adjusted to meet each resident's needs.

CONSERVATION OF NUTRITIVE VALUE, FLAVOR, APPEARANCE, ATTRACTIVE, PROPER TEMPERATURE

Goal: to ensure that the nutritive value of food is not compromised and destroyed because of prolonged food storage, light, and air exposure; prolonged cooking of foods in a large volume of water and prolonged holding on steam table, and the addition of baking soda. Food should be tasty, attractive, and at the proper temperature as determined by the type of food to ensure residents' satisfaction.

Food palatability refers to the taste and/or flavor of the food.
Food attractiveness refers to the appearance of the food when served to residents.

Questions to be asked:

- Does food have a distinctively appetizing aroma and appearance, which is varied in color and texture?
- Is food generally well seasoned (use of spices, herbs, etc.) and acceptable to residents?
- Is food prepared in a way to preserve vitamins? (Method of storage and preparation should cause minimum loss of nutrients.)
- Is food served at a preferable temperature (hot foods are served hot and cold foods cold), as discerned by the resident and customary practice? (Not to be confused with the proper holding temperature.)

FOOD PREPARED TO MEET INDIVIDUAL NEEDS

Goal: to ensure that food is served in a form that meets the residents' needs and satisfaction and that each resident receives appropriate nutrition when a substitute is offered.

A food substitute should be consistent with the usual and ordinary food items provided by the facility.

THERAPEUTIC DIETS

Some assisted living facilities provide therapeutic diets for residents upon request of their attending physician. If so, the following guidelines are useful.

Goal: to ensure that the resident receives and consumes foods in the appropriate form and/or the appropriate nutritive content as prescribed by a physician.

Therapeutic diet is defined as a diet ordered by a physician as part of treatment for a disease or clinical condition, or to eliminate or decrease specific nutrients in the diet (e.g., sodium), or to increase specific nutrients in the diet (e.g., potassium), or to provide food the resident is able to eat (e.g., a mechanically altered diet).

Mechanically altered diet is one in which the texture of a diet is altered. When the texture is modified, the type of texture modification will be specific and part of the physician's order. A simple food blender is capable of preparing most mechanically altered diets.

FREQUENCY OF MEALS

Goals:

1. Each resident receives and the facility provides at least three meals daily, at regular times comparable to normal mealtimes in the community.
2. There will be no more than 14 hours between a substantial evening meal and breakfast the following day, except as provided in point 4 below.
3. The facility will offer snacks at bedtime daily.
4. When a nourishing snack is provided at bedtime, up to 16 hours may elapse between a substantial evening meal and breakfast the following day if a resident group agrees to this meal span and a nourishing snack is served.

A *substantial evening meal* is defined as an offering of three or more menu items at one time, one of which includes a high-quality protein such as meat, fish, eggs, or cheese. The meal should represent no less than 20% of the day's total nutritional requirements.

Nourishing snack is defined as a verbal offering of items, single or in combination, from the basic food groups.

ASSISTIVE FEEDING DEVICES

One of the advantages to residents of assisted living facilities is availability of staff who have knowledge of assistive devices, which will enable the residents receiving assistance with eating to enjoy their meals to the maximum extent possible.

The goal is to provide residents with assistive devices to maintain or improve their ability to eat independently (e.g., improving poor grasp by enlarging silverware handles with foam padding, aiding residents with impaired coordination or tremor by installing plate guards, or providing postural supports for head, trunk, and arms).

FOOD: PROCURED FROM SATISFACTORY SOURCES

Sanitary Conditions. The facility will procure food from sources approved or considered satisfactory by federal, state, or local authorities and store, prepare, distribute, and serve food under sanitary conditions.

Goal: to prevent the spread of food-borne illness and reduce those practices that result in food contamination and compromised food safety. Since food-borne illness is often fatal to residents, it can and should be avoided.

Sanitary conditions is defined as storing, preparing, distributing, and serving food properly to prevent food-borne illness. Potentially hazardous foods will be subject to continuous time/temperature controls in order to prevent either the rapid and progressive growth of infections or toxigenic microorganisms such as *Salmonella* or the slower growth of *Clostridium botulinum*. In addition, foods of plant origin become potentially hazardous when the skin, husk, peel, or rind is breached, thereby possibly contaminating the fruit or vegetable with disease-causing microorganisms. Potentially hazardous food tends to focus on animal products, including but not limited to milk, eggs, and poultry.

Improper holding temperature is a common contributing factor of food-borne illness. The facility will follow proper procedures in cooking, cooling, and storing food according to time, temperatures, and sanitary guidelines. Improper handling of food can cause *Salmonella* and *E. coli* contamination. The 1997 FDA Food Code advises the following precautions.

Note: The food temperatures recommended in the 1997 FDA Food Code are target temperatures and give a margin of safety in temperature ranges in order to avoid known harmful contamination.

Refrigerator Storage. Refrigerator storage of food to prevent food-borne illness includes storing raw meat away from vegetables and other foods. Raw meat should be separated from cooked foods and other foods when refrigerated on its own tray on a bottom shelf so meat juices do not drip on other foods. Foods of both plant and animal origin will be cooked, maintained, and stored at appropriate temperatures. These temperatures are better utilized as food hold temperatures rather than the food temperatures as residents receive the food.

Hot Foods. Hot foods that are potentially hazardous should leave the kitchen (or steam table) above 140°F, and cold foods at or below 41°F, freezer temperatures should be at 0°F or below. Refrigerator temperatures should be maintained at 41°F or below. The 1997 FDA Food Code can be used as an authoritative guide on how to prepare and serve food to prevent food-borne illness.

CONTINUOUS QUALITY IMPROVEMENT STEPS THE ADMINISTRATOR CAN TAKE

Food storage. Observe storage, cooling, and cooking of food. If a problem is noted, conduct additional observations to verify findings.

Handwashing. Observe that employees are effectively cleaning their hands prior to preparing, serving, and distributing food. Observe that food is covered to maintain temperature and protected from other contaminants when transporting meals to residents.

Question to be asked:

- Are handwashing facilities convenient and properly equipped for dietary services staff use? (Staff uses good hygienic practices and staff with communicable diseases or infected skin lesions do not have contact with food if that contact will transmit the disease.)

Refrigerated storage. Check all refrigerators and freezers for temperatures. Use the facility's properly sanitized thermometer to evaluate the internal temperatures of potentially hazardous foods with a focus on the quantity of leftovers and the container sizes in which food leftovers are stored.

Food preparation. Use a sanitized thermometer to evaluate food temperatures. In addition, how do kitchen staff process leftovers? Are they heated to the appropriate temperatures? How is frozen food thawed? How is potentially hazardous food handled during multistep food preparation (e.g., chicken salad, egg salad)? Is hand contact with food minimized?

Food service. Using a properly sanitized thermometer, check the temperatures of hot and cold food prior to serving. How long is milk held without refrigeration prior to distribution?

Food distribution. Is the food protected from contamination as it is transported to the dining rooms and residents' rooms?

Observe food storage rooms and food storage in the kitchen. Are containers of food stored off the floor and on clean surfaces in a manner that protects them from contamination? Are other areas under storage shelves monitored for cleanliness to reduce attraction of pests?

Questions to be asked:

- Are potentially hazardous foods stored at 41°F or below and frozen foods kept at 0°F or below?
- Do staff handle and cook potentially hazardous foods properly?
- Are potentially hazardous foods kept at an internal temperature of 41°F or below in cold food storage unit, or at an internal temperature of 140°F or above in a hot food storage unit during display and service?
- Is there any sign of rodent or insect infestation?

DISHWASHING

The 1997 Food Code recommends the following water temperatures and manual washing instructions.

Question to be asked:

- Are food preparation equipment, dishes, and utensils effectively sanitized and cleaned to destroy potential disease-carrying organisms and are they stored in a protected manner?

Machine Dishwashing

1. Hot water:
   a. 140°F wash (or according to the manufacturer's specifications or instructions).
   b. 180°F rinse (160° or greater at the rack and dish/utensils surfaces).
2. Low temperature:
   a. 120°F+25 ppm (parts per million) hypochlorite (household bleach) on dish surface.

Manual Dishwashing

Compartment sink (wash, rinse, and sanitize): sanitizing solution used according to manufacturer's instructions.

a. 75°F+50 ppm hypochlorite (household bleach) or equivalent, or 12.5 ppm iodine.
b. Hot water immersion at 170°F for at least 30 seconds.

PROPER DISPOSAL OF GARBAGE AND REFUSE

Goal: to ensure that garbage and refuse is properly disposed.

Pest free: Is the area pest free? Look for signs of pests such as mice, roaches, rats, and flies.

Questions to be asked:

- Are garbage and refuse containers in good condition (no leaks), and is waste properly contained in dumpsters or compactors with lids or otherwise covered?
- Are areas such as loading docks, hallways, and elevators used for both garbage disposal and clean food transport kept clean, free of debris, and free of foul odors and waste fat? Is the garbage storage area maintained in a sanitary condition to prevent the harborage and feeding of pests?
- Are garbage receptacles covered when being removed from the kitchen area to the dumpster?

Hazard free

Are toxic items (e.g., insecticides, detergents, and polishes) properly stored, labeled, and used separate from the food?

LAUNDRY

Clean linens, clean resident clothes (whether done by the residents themselves or by relatives or the facility), the availability of linens and clothes when needed, and safe and sanitary handling techniques for both soiled and clean linen are areas of responsibility for the head of laundry. Whether it is better to do laundry in-house or to contract with a linen service (known as outsourcing the purchasing of portions of services from outside providers) is a subject of continuing debate. Whatever the decision, there will be procedures for handling linens that the administrator can observe for conformity to recommendations and to facility policies.

HOUSEKEEPING

Importance of good housekeeping

Just as members of the general public make intuitive value judgments about a facility based on its cleanliness and physical appearance, so also will most of the residents themselves and their significant others.

Dirty floors and walls, empty toilet paper holders, yellowing toilets and lavatories, and offensive odors associated with them communicate a message to the residents, staff, and visitors revealing what the facility thinks about itself. Inattention to housekeeping details leads inspectors and the public alike to wonder to what extent this lack of attention carries over to resident care, sanitation in food preparation, and cleanliness of the residents themselves.

The head of housekeeping designs job assignments for the housekeepers. The administrator can tell how effective these schedules are simply by walking around the facility. On these tours the administrator must be able to "see" dirt.

There is a surprising amount of regulation surrounding the housekeeping area, such as the required Material Safety Data Sheets for all chemicals, to which the head of housekeeping and the administrator will give attention.

MAINTENANCE WORK AREA

Distinguishing between maintenance and housekeeping responsibilities is often an issue. If a wall has a hole in it, it is clearly maintenance's job to fix the hole. If that same wall is only dirty and needs washing, it is probably housekeeping's job. Each facility will designate through established policies the respective responsibilities of these two functions. The repair and upkeep of physical systems is clearly the responsibility of maintenance. Maintenance chief salaries ranged between $21,000 and 46,000 in 1999.

Preventive maintenance, anticipating when a machine will need servicing or risk ceasing to function, is a complex task requiring experienced judgment. A well-trained maintenance director can do much to anticipate troublesome, unnecessary breakdowns of equipment. The administrator can participate in the maintenance process by occasionally assuming a maintenance mind-set, then walking through the facility and judging the state of repair of all he or she encounters.

AREAS REQUIRING SPECIAL ATTENTION

The following areas typically require constant attention from the administrator:

- resident care planning and implementation of resident care plans
- successful billing, from recording supplies consumed to required wording for resident charges
- housekeeping vs. maintenance
- food/health care coordination in getting food to residents on a timely basis, at the right temperature, and attractively presented, with attention to accommodating residents' preferences

- differentiating between activities functions and the social work function
- resident advocacy to the staff and families
- health care/housekeeping/laundry coordination

2.1 Identifying the Personnel Functions

Managers in organizations have always performed certain basic personnel functions. These activities include record keeping, employee recruitment and selection, training and development, compensation management, performance evaluations, and often labor relations (Chruden & Sherman, 1980).

The administrator's role in personnel functions includes the following:

- **Record keeping**—ensuring that all necessary information is in the employee's file and that it is kept confidential
- **Recruitment**—assisting work area heads in finding employees for vacant positions
- **Selection**—assisting work area heads in interviewing and assessing job applicants
- **Training and retaining employees**—assisting work area heads in employee orientation, in-service training, and continuing education
- **Compensation management**—assisting work area heads and payroll office in administering salary and the other benefits offered by the facility
- **Performance evaluation**—assisting managers in conducting employee evaluation in conformity with the facility personnel policies
- **Labor relations**—assisting managers in creating a favorable work environment

In a facility of 100 to 150 residents, no full-time personnel director is usually hired. However, some of the typical personnel work area functions are usually given to one employee, who, in effect, serves as a part-time personnel coordinator for the facility. This person is sometimes given the title staff development coordinator. Alternately, assisting the work area managers with personnel matters, such as record keeping and ensuring that employees are offered hepatitis B vaccinations, may be part of the job description of an assistant administrator, an administrative assistant, a staff nurse, or an employee in the business office.

2.2 Planning Employment Needs: Writing Job Descriptions

In Part One we indicated the need for each assisted living facility to break down all work to be accomplished into a set of activities that can be performed by one person. Several definitions provided by the U.S. Employment Service and the U.S. Office of Personnel Management may be useful to review at this point (Ivancevich, Szjlagyi, & Wallace, 1977).

Job analysis: The process of defining a job in terms of tasks or behaviors required and specifying the qualifications of the employee to be placed in that job.

Job description: Information about the job that results in a statement of the job to be done, usually including a list of duties and responsibilities in order of importance. Usually a job description includes the title, the qualifications, to whom the worker is primarily responsible, and the duties or specific expectations (Argenti, 1994; Boling, 1983).

Job specification: A statement of the skills, education, and experience required to perform the work. This is derived from the job description.

Job titles (or job classifications): That which distinguishes one job from all others. Job titles may also indicate the occupational level of the job.

Task: A coordinated and aggregated series of work elements used to produce an output (e.g., making up rooms).

Position: The responsibilities and duties performed by one individual. There are as many positions as there are employees.

Job: A group of positions that are similar in their duties (e.g., laundry, housekeeping, and grounds).

Job family: A group of two or more jobs that have similar duties (Ivancevich et al., 1977).

All the work to be accomplished in operating an assisted living facility will be broken down into a series of tasks. Tasks are grouped together so that they can be performed by one individual.

Job analysis is the process of grouping a series of related tasks into a position. Each position can then be described in terms of the tasks, the behaviors involved, and the education and training needed to perform the job successfully.

POTENTIAL PROBLEMS WITH JOB DESCRIPTIONS

The federal government examines job descriptions and specifications for possible discriminatory effects. Each of the requirements for a job will be necessary for the adequate performance of that job. If, for example, an assisted living facility in an area with an unusually large number of available job applicants requires 2 years of college for applicants for the resident care aide position, it will have to be able to demonstrate why this is essential to perform the job. Because this is a higher educational requirement than usual, the facility is obliged to prove that it did not serve to discriminate against members of a particular group on the basis of sex or ethnic origins.

Once job descriptions have been written and the expected workload of the facility estimated, future employment needs can be forecast.

2.3 Forecasting Future Employment Needs

The planning process begins with a projection of the number of residents and the expected levels of social and health care complexity the facility expects to serve over a period of time, usually during the next 1 to 5 years. This forecast can then be translated into specific personnel requirements for the future period.

TAKING A PERSONNEL INVENTORY

Numerous factors will be taken into account in projecting the present and future availability of qualified personnel.

Several sources of employment information exist. The Employment Security Commission and the Department of Labor gather data that are useful in estimating the future availability of needed employees.

Identifying Trends

Data such as those mentioned help to identify trends. A number of trends are of potential importance.

Competition for Personnel. It is practical to take an inventory of present and planned assisted living and other related facilities that are or will be competing for similarly qualified personnel. For example, if no acute care hospital exists in the geographic area but a large for-profit hospital is expected to be constructed within 2 years, competition may increase dramatically for health aides. Or, similarly, if the local hospital is one of the several area institutions that are downsizing, the labor pool may be suddenly increased.

In-Migration or Out-Migration Patterns in the Labor Supply. Knowledge of whether the worker pool from which employees will be chosen is shrinking or enlarging is important. Statistics are usually available on the local unemployment rate. Unfortunately, for the assisted living facility a low local unemployment rate can have the effect of a noticeable reduction in the quality of applicants, level of job interest, and longevity for positions such as caregiver's aide, housekeeper, and grounds person. This may extend to all positions in the facility.

Wage Scale Movements in the Area. An increasing worker pool may reduce wage scales, whereas a shrinking worker pool may cause the wage scale to rise. The widespread health care shortage of the late 1980s and early 1990s, for example, resulted in rapid increases in health care salaries during those years. Most long-term care providers, such as assisted living facilities, base their wages in large measure, on what the competition is paying.

Affects of Educational Institutions. Educational institutions such as local community colleges are becoming major sources of training for personnel needed by assisted living facilities. Any expected increase or decrease in training activities (e.g., the addition or closing of a nurse assistant program at the local community college) could dramatically affect the availability of labor, especially trained health care aides.

Knowledge of these trends can help planners to take action before an anticipated employment crisis. If a shortage is foreseen, the facility might join with other local health care providers in a program to attract additional health care–related personnel to the area. The availability of activities, dietary, and social services personnel is similarly affected.

2.4 Recruiting Employees

Once the forecast of the resident profile has been translated into specific personnel requirements for the facility, recruitment and selection program can be developed. The forecast assists the administrator in determining the number and types of employees that will be needed, as well as the sources for recruitment.

INFLUENCE OF AFFIRMATIVE ACTION

Since the passage of the Civil Rights Act of 1964, the process of seeking new employees has become more public. Before 1964, facilities could choose employees without scrutiny by government agencies with regard to possible job discrimination based on age, sex, race, marital status, religion, national origin, or handicap (Miller, 1982).

Today government agencies can review for possible legal violations by examining the following: (1) the facility's list of recruitment sources for each job category, (2) recruitment advertising, and (3) statistics on the number of applicants processed by personal category (e.g., sex, age, and race), level and type of disabilities, and job category.

The government may require an assisted living facility chain or an individual facility to recruit qualified employees whose group is not proportionately represented in the present staff. If, for example, there are no African-American caregivers on staff and the government ascertains that the facility does not advertise its job openings at African-American health care schools or in newspapers or other sources normally used by African-Americans seeking jobs, the government may require that an Equal Employment Opportunity program be used by the facility or chain.

Many employers are under pressure to increase the number of minority members and women employed in their facilities, especially at the higher levels from which these groups have traditionally been excluded. Requiring a facility to increase the proportion of minority persons is called *ratio hiring.*

While it has not been a matter of Office of Civil Rights enforcement, disproportionately few male health care workers tend to be hired, probably out of deference to the mostly female assisted living facility population and limited availability of male workers.

In general, the administrator should seek a workforce that is diversified and representative of the community that the facility serves.

The Americans with Disabilities Act has also influenced the hiring process in a number of ways.

INFLUENCE OF THE LABOR MARKET

The labor market is the geographic area from which applicants are to be recruited. Recruitment for a new administrator or director of resident care may be national in scope. The new administrator may be willing to move across the country. When staffing for jobs requiring little skill, however, the scope of the labor market will tend to be a relatively small geographic area surrounding the facility. The new janitor or health care aide is unlikely to be willing, or economically able, to move to accept a position at the facility.

If there is a surplus of labor at recruiting time, the facility may be flooded with applications. If there is a shortage, on the other hand, it may take considerable initiative to find and hire well-trained staff.

Impacts of Transportation

The ease with which employees can commute to the facility will have a direct effect on the geographic area from which the facility can recruit. The absence of an efficient public transportation system, especially for evening and night workers, will oblige the facility to hire only persons who have access to automobiles or can walk to work.

Assisted living facilities in cities sometimes face special problems in finding suitable employees. Population migration to the suburbs generally leaves less-qualified persons available in a city. Some larger institutions around the country have arranged special transportation to and from work for suburban employees in an effort to attract staff.

RECRUITMENT SOURCES

A number of sources for recruitment exist, both within and outside the facility.

Present Employees

The current employees of the facility can be a primary source for filling vacancies. Hiring from among present employees is a policy decision to promote from within. There are a number of advantages to such a policy.

Career Ladders. Career ladders are paths along which an employee can hope to progress. They constitute a major source of employee incentive and satisfaction. Persons entering the facility are encouraged to stay if there is reasonable expectation that, when openings occur, there will be advancement possibilities from within the organization. This practice stimulates employees to develop skills that will be necessary to qualify for promotion.

Job Posting and Job Bidding. A job that becomes available is literally posted on appropriate bulletin boards, and employees are encouraged to bid, or apply, for the job. In this way employees become more aware of the actual requirements of positions and the selection processes for filling vacancies. Advancement of present employees has the obvious advantage of recognizing and rewarding successful workers. It also has benefits for the facility by placing a person who already has some understanding of the organization and is loyal to its policies.

However, hiring from within may slow the process of introducing persons with new ideas and fresh approaches into the facility. There are times when the management may purposely seek to bring in an outsider who will be expected to reorganize or reengineer a work area.

Outside Sources

Unless it is planned to reduce the size of the staff, every vacancy presents the organization with an option to promote from within or hire from without.

A promotion from within might trigger a series of promotions. If the resident care coordinator is promoted to administrator, for instance, the nurse serving the facility will want to be considered for resident care coordinator.

Any vacancy, if filled from within, will eventually result in hiring a new person from an outside source. Some of the more common outside sources are discussed below.

Referrals

Employees, residents, and their significant others are good sources of referrals. Satisfied employees, residents, and their significant others constitute a valuable asset for the recruiting effort.

Employee referrals can be especially beneficial. When a staff member's recommendation is accepted, he or she is receiving special recognition by the facility. In addition, the employee will have a vested interest in assisting the recruit to adjust to the environment and to be productive. However, the facility will be careful to avoid referrals that lead to nepotism (favoring one's family members) or to the formation of closely knit groups or cliques composed of persons who have close outside ties and tend to exclude others. Employee, resident, and family referrals are, in essence, word-of-mouth recommendations that reflect the reputation of the facility in the community.

Advertisements

Advertising in appropriate media, such as newspapers and professional and trade journals, is one of the most common methods for contacting prospective applicants. For registered caregivers, the professional journal may be an appropriate medium; however, local newspapers are the most used source. For health care aides and maintenance staff, the local newspaper will also be an appropriate medium.

Public Employment Agencies

State governments operate local public employment agencies using federal payroll tax rebates from the U.S. Employment Service. Public employment agencies can provide lists of individuals who are unemployed and currently drawing unemployment insurance benefits.

Private Employment Agencies

Agencies in the private sector offer specialized services, more closely matching the needs of the potential employer and employee. Fees are charged.

Most often the employee pays the agency. However, the employer sometimes shares in the fee and occasionally pays it altogether. The facility may also sign a contract with a private employment agency over a period of time. In this case, the contract should be carefully reviewed to avoid unwanted or unintended commitments, such as a fee to the agency for all new employees, whether found by the agency or the employer.

Search Firms

Search firms generally focus their efforts on middle-and upper-level management positions. Clients for search firms normally are employers who agree to pay the search firm for finding a suitable candidate. The search firm operates in a wider geographic area than is normally possible for the employer, and it is able to offer a nationwide inventory. These firms can save employer time and energy by providing extensive screening before any candidate is recommended.

Professional and Industry Organizations

Many professional and industry groups may maintain rosters of their members who are seeking employment. These lists are published in the groups' journals and posted at meetings. Much interviewing, both formal and informal, occurs at association meetings for job openings.

Educational Institutions

Accredited schools are an increasingly important source for assisted living facility personnel. Community colleges and technical institutes are training students to be not only licensed health care aides but also activities directors and heads of dietary.

Unsolicited Applications

A number of unsolicited employment inquiries will arrive at the facility by mail or in person. Although the proportion of such applicants who are suitable may be low, there are nevertheless important reasons for careful attention to them. It is good public relations practice to extend courteous treatment to applicants who approach the facility on their own initiative and to deal with them candidly about the likelihood of employment with the organization.

Some administrators report a tendency for long-term-care employees to seek a change of job every few years. They may be entirely competent people who periodically look for a new work situation while remaining within their field. Such individuals may submit unsolicited applications simply to let a facility know of their availability.

2.5 Hiring Staff

Recruitment is the process of locating prospective staff. Personnel selection is the process of deciding which of the applicants best fits the requirements of the job for which he or she is being considered (Owen, 1984). Often, however, this prospective staff member is evaluated not only for one of several positions the organization has open at that moment but also for anticipated slots expected in the near future.

Through experience, employers have learned that when individuals are carefully selected for clearly defined positions, the result may be faster adjustment to the position, greater job satisfaction, and a minimum number of misfits between applicants and job needs in the organization (Chruden & Sherman, 1980).

MEASURING THE EFFECTS OF LEGISLATION

Employers are directing greater attention to the job selection process. This is because of the often intense scrutiny given employers by the government enforcers of the Civil Rights Act of 1964, the Equal Employment Act of 1972, and, more recently, the Americans with Disabilities Act, which was passed in 1990, took effect in 1992, and fully implemented in July 1994 (see Part Four for a discussion of the act). In an attempt to clarify rules, the Equal Employment Opportunity Commission wrote an interpretation of regulations, referred to as the Uniform Guidelines on Employee Selection Procedures.

The Civil Rights Act of 1964 prohibits discrimination in employment practices on the basis of race, color, religion, sex, or national origin. This act created the Equal Employment Opportunities Commission (EEOC) to implement the provisions of the act. A later amendment, known as the Tower Amendment to Title 7, permitted the use of ability tests in employee selection procedures. Subsequently, the courts and the EEOC have made numerous rulings that determine the construction and use of ability tests.

The Equal Employment Act of 1972 is an amendment to Title 7 of the Civil Rights Act of 1964 and is intended to cover all employers of 15 or more persons and numerous other groups, such as educational institutions. Enforcement machinery was authorized and subsequently set up. Today personnel policy is shaped by the Civil Rights Act and the Equal Employment Act, as well as court decisions and regulations instituted by authorized government agencies. They affect such employment practices as retirement rules and considerations during pregnancy. Both acts are discussed at greater length in Part Four.

In 1987 four federal agencies jointly published a far-reaching document entitled the Uniform Guidelines on Employee Selection Procedures (EEOC, 1978), establishing the standards by which federal agencies determine the acceptability of validation procedures used for written tests and other selections devices. The guidelines require the employer to be able to demonstrate that the selection procedures used are valid in predicting or measuring employee performance in a specific job. They define discrimination as

> the use of any selection procedure which has an adverse impact on the hiring, promotion or other employment or membership opportunities of members of any race, sex, or ethnic group[. Such use] will be considered to be discriminatory and inconsistent with these guidelines, unless the procedure has been validated in accordance with these guidelines. (EEOC, 1978, Sec. 3A)

Adverse impact is defined as occurring whenever the selection rate for any racial, ethnic, or sex group is less than 80% of the rate of the group with the highest selection rate.

If 200 of 1,000 Caucasian applicants are selected (a selection rate of 20%), at least 16% of the minority applicants must be selected. Several court rulings, such as *Griggs v. Duke Power Company* (which we discuss in detail in Part Four), have already clearly established the principle that all personnel tests and activities must avoid having any discriminatory effect, whether intended or unintended.

The Uniform Guidelines have, in effect, become a handbook for decision making in personnel matters. The personnel selection process must now be reported to state and federal compliance agencies, usually on EEOC forms that require accurate data on the actual hiring results of the assisted living facility. As Chruden and Sherman (1980) have observed, what used to be the exclusive concern of the facility administrator can now be carried into the courtroom.

The Federal Equal Employment Opportunity poster should be prominently displayed in an area accessible to staff, applicants, and residents. All advertising must announce the facility's position as an Equal Opportunity Employer.

MATCHING PERSONNEL NEEDS AND APPLICANTS

Finding the right person for a position is a complex task. The employer understandably wants to learn as much about the applicant as possible to determine his or her likelihood of success if hired for a position in the facility (Matheny, 1984).

Methods of Obtaining Information

There are several methods for learning about applicants. Most organizations use written application forms, interviews, and background checks. The search for a new administrator or resident care coordinator, on the one hand, may involve appointing a committee, allowing for lengthy exploration, and conducting extensive interviewing. Filling a vacancy for a personal care aide, on the other hand, is much less complicated. In both cases, however, it is important that all solicited information be demonstrably job related or predictive of success in that position.

Reliability and Validity of Information

Information that is valid and reliable is necessary for making an informed decision about an applicant's skills, knowledge, aptitudes, level of motivation, and likely fit with the organization.

Reliability of the tests, interviews, and other tools used in selecting among applicants refers to the consistency with which the same results are obtained over a period of time and when used by different testers (called inter-rater reliability).

In measuring applicants' abilities, reliability means that an applicant will achieve the same or nearly the same score or results when taking the test at different times (e.g., a week or two apart). If a test were to give differing results from week to week, it would be unreliable, just as a set of scales used to weigh produce in a store will reliably give the same weight week after week every time produce of equal weight is placed on it. Reliability also requires that different applicants with the same skills score the same on the test. If word-processing aptitude is being measured, applicants with the same level of skill will score the same on the test.

A test or selection procedure provides validity when it actually measures what it is intended to measure and does it well. In essence, validity is a measure of how effectively an instrument does its job (Chruden & Sherman, 1980).

Two Types of Validity

Personnel experts have relied on at least two types of validity for several years: content and construct. Content and construct validity are used by government agencies in judging the results of a facility's hiring program.

Content Validity. Content validity is the degree to which a test, interview procedure, or other selection tool measures the skills, knowledge, or performance requirements actually needed to fill the position for which the applicant is applying.

Construct Validity. The extent to which a selection tool measures a trait or behavior perceived as important to functioning in a job is construct validity. Intelligence is an abstract construct that is established by putting together answers to a series of different questions that together yield a measure of the theoretical construct called intelligence.

The following is an example of construct validity: An assisted living facility administrator's requirement of a "friendly facial expression" toward residents is an example of a construct (trait) that the administrator believes is needed for the position. To validate a friendly facial expression as a job requirement, the administrator would have to identify the work behaviors required for the position, identify the constructs (e.g., smiling) that are required, then show by empirical evidence that this selection requirement is truly related to the construct.

It is of real importance for an assisted living facility to require that all staff treat residents in a cheerful or friendly manner, although this directive may be difficult to achieve. In one Fort Worth, Texas, case a federal judge ruled that American Airlines had the right to discharge an otherwise good flight attendant because he did not smile enough. The flight attendant had sued the company, contending that he was a good employee and met all requirements of the job except for the smile. The federal judge upheld American's policy of requiring a friendly facial expression as "essential in the competitive airline industry" ("Now We Know Why They're So Friendly," 1985). Personnel rules do not require that the assisted living administrator put up with staff who do not treat residents respectfully and pleasantly.

APPLICATION FORMS—PRE-EMPLOYMENT QUESTIONS

Employers must avoid questions that might be construed as violating the Civil Rights Act, Title 7, or the Americans with Disabilities Act. Before hiring a person, questions should be avoided that relate to age, sex, race, national origin, education, religion, arrest and conviction records, marital status, credit rating (Title 7), or disabilities (Americans with Disabilities Act and Title 7). The interviewer will review any unsolicited requests for reasonable accommodation under the act. If the applicant is a minor (i.e., under 18 years of age), federal and state child labor laws may specify hours of work, type of work, machinery to be operated, and supervision requirements.

Table 2.9 gives a list of subject areas about which the interviewer is permitted, or not, to ask questions on application forms or in the preemployment interviews under Title 7.

Handicap-related Questions

The Equal Employment Opportunities Commission issued a 49-page notice (915.002) on May 19, 1994, with the goal of clarifying what questions employers may ask that might be related to handicaps as viewed under the Americans with Disabilities Act. This notice made it clear that an employer may ask an applicant about the nature of any need the applicant may have for adjustment to a handicap only after making a job offer. It is only at this point that the employer may consider what reasonable accommodation might be needed. Prior to offering a job it is unlawful to ask such questions as "Do you need a reasonable accommodation to perform the essential functions of the job? If so, what kind?"

In an attempt to clarify which preemployment interview questions are permissible, the EEOC notice offered the following as examples.

Lawful	Unlawful
1. Do you drink alcohol?	How much alcohol do you drink per week?
2. How well can you handle stress?	Do you ever get ill from stress?
3. Are you currently illegally using drugs?	Have you ever been treated fro drug problems?
4. Do you regularly eat three meals per day?	Do you need to eat a number of small snacks at regular intervals throughout the day in order to maintain your energy level?
5. How did you break your leg?	How did you come to use a wheelchair?
6. Do you have a cold?	Do you have AIDS?

INTERVIEWING APPLICANTS

Interviews are used extensively in evaluating job applicants. Each administrator or personnel manager will develop his or her own style and identify information needs during interviews.

Preliminary Interviews

One approach is to use a preliminary interview, which generally involves having the applicant fill out a short questionnaire, after which there is a brief conversation with him or her based on the questionnaire. This serves to screen out unsuitable candidates, using a minimum of time and organizational resources.

TABLE 2.9 Suggestions for Interviews

Inquiries before hiring	Lawful	Unlawful*
1. Name	Name	Inquiry into any title which indicates race, color, religion, sex, national origin, handicap, age, or ancestry.
2. Address	Inquiry into place and length of current address	Inquiry into foreign addresses that would indicate national origin.
3. Age	Age inquiry limited to establishing that application meets any minimum age requirement that may be established by law	A. Requiring birth certificate or baptismal record before hiring. B. Any other inquiry that may reveal whether applicant is at least 40 and less than 70 years of age.
4. Birthplace or national origin		A. Any inquiry into place of birth. B. Any inquiry into place of birth of grandparents or spouse. C. Any other inquiry into national origin.
5. Race or color		Any inquiry that would indicate race or color.
6. Sex		A. Any inquiry that would indicate sex. B. Any inquiry made of members of one sex, but not the other.
7. Religion/creed		A. Any inquiry that would indicate or identify religious denomination or custom. B. Applicant may not be told any religious identity or preference of the employer. C. Request pastor's recommendation or reference.
8. Handicap	Inquiries necessary to determine applicant's ability to substantially perform specific job without significant hazard.	Any other inquiry that would reveal handicap.

Inquiries before hiring	Lawful	Unlawful*
9. Citizenship	A. Whether a U.S. citizen B. If not, whether applicant intends to become one. C. If U.S. residence is legal D. If spouse is citizen E. Require proof of citizenship after being hired.	A. If native-born or naturalized. B. Proof of citizenship before hiring. C. Whether parents or spouse are native-born or naturalized.
10. Photographs	May be required after hiring for identification purposes.	Require photograph before hiring.
11. Arrests and convictions	Inquiries into conviction of specific crimes related to qualification for the job applied for.	Any inquiry that would reveal arrests without convictions.
12. Education	A. Inquiry into nature and extent of academic, professional, or vocational training. B. Inquiry into language. Skills such as reading and writing of foreign languages.	A. Any inquiry that would reveal the nationality or religious affiliation of a school. B. Inquiry as to what mother tongue is or how foreign language ability was acquired.
13. Relatives	Inquiry into name, relationship, and address of person to be notified in case of emergency.	Any inquiry about a relative that would be unlawful if made abut the applicant.
14. Organizations	Inquiry into organization memberships and offices held, excluding any organization, the name or character of which indicates the race, color, religions, sex, national origin, handicap, age or ancestry of its members.	Inquiry into all clubs and organizations where membership is held.
15. Military service	A. Inquiry into service in U.S. Armed Forces when such service is a qualification for the job B. Require military discharge certificate after being hired.	A. Inquiry into military service in named service of any country but United States. B. Request military service records.
16. Work schedule	Inquiry into willingness to work required work schedule.	Any inquiry into willingness to work any particular religious holiday.
17. Other	Any question required to reveal qualifications for the job applied for.	Any non-job related inquiry that may reveal information permitting unlawful discrimination.
18. References	General personal work references not relating to race, color, religion, sex, national origin, handicap, age, or ancestry.	Request references specifically from clergy or any other persons who might reflect race, color, religion, sex, national origin, handicap, age, or ancestry of applicant.

I. Employers acting under bona fide affirmative action programs or acting under orders of Equal Employment law enforcement agencies of federal, state, or local governments may make some of the prohibited inquiries listed above to the extent that these inquiries are required by such programs or orders.

II. Employers having federal defense contracts are exempt to the extent that otherwise prohibited inquiries are required by federal law for security purposes.

III. Any inquiry is prohibited that although not specifically listed above, elicits information as to, or which is not job related and may be used to discriminate on the basis of, race, color, religion, sex, national origin, handicap, age, or ancestry in violation of law.

*Unless bona fide occupational qualification is certified in advance by the State Civil Rights Commission.

Reprinted with permission from Panel Publishers. Miller, Dulcy B, ed. *Long Term Care Administrator's Desk Manual.* Greenvale, NY: Panel Publishers, Inc., 1982. Exhibit 203.H, pp. 2059-2061.

Telephone Interviewing/Screening

The person who will do the interviewing, in setting up interviews with candidates for positions, can elicit over the phone a good bit of information, such as

- present employment
- why candidate is looking for a position, what kind of position is being sought
- candidate's salary requirements
- why candidate left previous positions, past salaries
- number of persons supervised, if a manager, and their job functions

As part of the initial telephone interview, give the candidate information about the facility and set up a follow-up interview if, after the preceding explorations, mutual interest exists.

Interviewing Methods

Interviewing methods vary but generally can be classified into three types according to the degree of structure used: nondirective, in-depth, and patterned.

In the nondirective interview the interrogator refrains from influencing the applicant's remarks. This allows the applicant maximum freedom to ask questions and give information. The interviewer's task is to pay special attention to attitudes, values, or feelings that may be exhibited by the candidate.

This approach maximizes the amount of information the applicant may reveal and is often called an open-ended interview technique. The interviewer asks only broad, general questions such as "Tell me about how you did and how you liked your last job," or "What is it about working in an assisted living facility that attracts you?" or "Where do you want to be in your career in the next 5 years?" There is no prescribed set of questions.

An in-depth interview provides more structure in the form of specific question areas to be covered. This is sometimes called a directed interview. Examples of questions appropriate to the in-depth interview are

- What do you consider your most important skills for this job?
- Tell me about your last job.
- Under what type of supervision techniques do you function best?
- What did you like most about your last job?
- What are your feelings toward older people? What do you like most/dislike most about older persons?

The patterned interview allows the least amount of freedom to both the interviewer and the applicant. All questions are sequential and highly detailed. Generally, a summary sheet will be filled out by the interviewer interpreting the results of the encounter.

Some Approaches

Experts in business management and personnel administration offer the following tips on interviewing:

- Avoid forming strong impressions during the early minutes of the interview.
- Allow the candidate to do most of the talking.
- Don't clue the candidate into precisely what you are looking for early in the interview.
- Ask specific questions about past job behavior.
- Probe for all the information needed.
- Take notes, but not on the application form.
- Use second and third interviews when appropriate.

General Areas for Questions

One major long-term care corporation suggests the following areas as appropriate for follow-up questions during an interview:

Professional Maturity

- What has been the toughest assignment you have ever had and how did you handle it?
- What would you do if [name an adverse situation that an employee in that job might encounter]?
- What actions have you taken if you disagreed with a supervisor's decision?
- What is the impact or role of your work area on your current facility's objectives?

Skill Level

- What are your present job responsibilities?
- What results were achieved in terms of successes and achievements?
- What do you feel you can learn from this position?
- What are your greatest strengths? What areas need improvement?
- What was the biggest contribution you made to your current position?
- How would your references rate your technical competence?
- The ability to solve problems is critical to this position. Please provide an example of how this ability has been important to your success.
- What important trends to you see in your profession?

Character

- What do you consider the most important aspects of a job?
- Where do you see yourself in 2 years? 5 years? 10 years?

- What have you liked best about your present [recent] supervisor(s)? liked least?
- Why should we hire you?
- How successful do you think you have been so far in your career?
- How long would it take you to make a meaningful contribution to this facility?

Research Findings on the Use of Interviews

A good deal of research has been conducted on the reliability and validity of interviews as a tool for judging job applicants. Chruden and Sherman (1980) reported on some of the major findings:

- Structured interviews are more reliable than unstructured interviews.
- When there is a greater amount of information about a job, inter-rater reliability is increased; that is, several interviewers are more likely to come to the same decision.
- Interviews can explain why a person would *not* be a good employee, but not why they *would* be a good one.
- Factual written data seem to be more important than physical appearance.
- Interpersonal skills and level of applicant motivation are best evaluated by an interview.
- Allowing the applicant time to talk provides a larger behavior sample. Also, one can learn more from listening than by talking.
- An interviewer's race affects the behavior of the person being interviewed.

BACKGROUND INVESTIGATIONS

If the interviewer decides the candidate is of interest to the organization, background information can be sought.

It is advisable to obtain from applicants a signed request for references. Increasingly, former employers are reluctant to put any recommendations into writing for fear of lawsuits. Many will only provide information about the date of hire, position(s) held, and date of separation.

Background Checks

Background checks are increasingly important. Grant and Kemme (1993) recommend that, despite most employers' adoption of a neutral policy on employment (e.g., revealing only name, job title, and dates of employment), employers should run such checks. They recommend a screening process consisting of (1) background checks on trustworthiness, honesty, gaps in employment, required licenses, and other relevant information; (2) drug tests (the Americans with Disabilities Act does not protect drug users); and (3) criminal background checks. Here the so-called Business Necessity Rule applies: Employers will consider all job-related circumstances around a conviction to determine if the person would be a safe employee in the facility. Some allowable considerations are (1) time of conviction, (2) nature of conviction, (3) number of convictions, (4) facts of each case, (5) job-relatedness, (6) length of time between conviction and application, and (7) efforts at rehabilitation. Generally, any person convicted of substance abuse becomes a high risk for the facility. Reference requests should be obtained on at least two jobs, preferably the two most recent, or for the past 3 years (whichever is longer). For applicants with no work experience, school, volunteer, or personal references can be used. For health care aide applicants, two basic checks need to be made:

- the state registry to verify current certification and whether the applicant has met training and competency requirements
- the substance abuse registry in every state in which the facility has reason to believe the applicant has worked as a health care aide to determine whether any record of resident abuse or neglect or misappropriation of resident property has occurred

The Privacy Act of 1974 (Public Law 93–579) gave federal staff the right to examine personnel records, including letters of reference. Although not mandated by federal law, the Privacy Act of 1974 seems to have led to a trend for employers to permit staff to review and challenge their personnel files (Chruden & Sherman, 1980).

Negligent hiring lawsuits can be minimized by gathering as much pertinent information as possible about applicants. Discrimination charges can be minimized by focusing on job-related criteria.

Abuse

All health care providers who use certified nursing assistants, including hospitals, nursing homes, home health care agencies, and assisted living facilities, must be vigilant for signs of resident abuse. What may be usual behavior in the home or community setting becomes abuse, especially when dealing with frail elderly.

Before hiring any applicant the facility must assure itself that the applicant has not in the past been abusive. A discussion of what is considered abusive behaviors follows for both prospective and present employees.

The goal is for each resident to be free from abuse, corporal punishment, and involuntary seclusion. The facility is well advised to prevent not only abuse but also those practices and omissions, neglect, and misappropriation of property that, if left unchecked, could lead to abuse.

Residents should not be subjected to abuse by anyone, including, but not limited to, facility staff, other residents, consultants or volunteers, staff of other agencies serving the individual, family members or legal guardians, friends, or other individuals.

Abuse is defined as the willful infliction of injury, unreasonable confinement, intimidation, or punishment with resulting physical harm or pain or mental anguish, or deprivation by an individual, including a caretaker, of goods or services that are necessary to attain or maintain physical, mental, and psychosocial well-being. This presumes that instances of abuse of all residents, even those in a coma, cause physical harm, pain, or mental anguish.

"Verbal abuse" is defined as any use of oral, written, or gestured language that willfully includes disparaging and derogatory terms to residents or their families, or within their hearing distance, regardless of their age, ability to comprehend, or disability. Examples of verbal abuse include, but are not limited to, threats of harm and saying things to frighten a resident, such as telling a resident that he or she will never be able to see his or her family again. What staff members say to residents behind closed doors remains a facility concern.

Sexual abuse includes, but is not limited to, sexual harassment, sexual coercion, and sexual assault.

Physical abuse includes hitting, slapping, pinching, and kicking. It also includes controlling behavior through corporal punishment.

Mental abuse includes, but is not limited to, humiliation, harassment, threats of punishment, and deprivation.

Involuntary seclusion is defined as separation of a resident from other residents or from his or her room or confinement to his or her room (with or without roommates) against the resident's will, or the will of the resident's legal representative.

The facility should not employ individuals who have been

1. found guilty of abusing, neglecting, or mistreating residents by a court of law
2. have had a finding entered into the state nurse's aide registry concerning abuse, neglect, mistreatment of residents, or misappropriation of their property

The facility should ensure that all alleged violations involving mistreatment, neglect, or abuse, including injuries of unknown source and misappropriation of resident property, are reported immediately to the administrator of the facility and, if required, to other officials in accordance with state law through established procedures.

The facility should have evidence that all alleged violations are thoroughly investigated and should prevent further potential abuse while an investigation is in progress.

The results of all investigations should be reported to the administrator or designated representative and to other officials in accordance with state law (including the state survey and certification agency) within 5 working days of the incident, and if the alleged violation is verified appropriate corrective action should be taken.

The goal is to ensure that the facility has in place an effective system that, regardless of the source (staff, other residents, visitors, etc.), prevents mistreatment, neglect, and abuse of residents, and misappropriation of resident's property. However, such a system cannot guarantee that a resident will not be abused; it can only ensure that the facility does whatever is within its control to prevent mistreatment, neglect, and abuse of residents or misappropriation of their property.

Neglect is defined as failure to provide goods and services necessary to avoid physical harm, mental anguish, or mental illness. Neglect occurs on an individual basis when a resident does not receive care in one or more areas (e.g., absence of frequent monitoring for a resident known to be incontinent, resulting in being left to lie in urine or feces). *Misappropriation of resident property* is defined as the patterned or deliberate misplacement, exploitation, or wrongful, temporary, or permanent use of a resident's belongings or money without the resident's consent.

Questions to Be Asked: Actions

- Was the administrator notified of the incident and when?
- Did investigations begin promptly after the report of the problem?
- Is there a record of statements or interviews of the resident, suspect (if one is identified), any eyewitnesses, and any circumstantial witnesses?

- Was relevant documentation reviewed and preserved (e.g., dated dressing that was not changed when treatment record showed change)?
- Was the alleged victim examined promptly (if injury was suspected) and the finding documented in the report?
- What steps were taken to protect the alleged victim from further abuse (particularly where no suspect has been identified)?
- What actions were taken as a result of the investigation?
- What corrective action was taken, including informing the nurse's aide registry, state licensure authorities, and other agencies (e.g., long-term care ombudsman and adult protective services)?

The goal is to prevent employment of individuals who have been convicted of abusing, neglecting, or mistreating individuals in a health care–related setting (e.g., residents of an assisted living facility or patients in a hospital). Facilities should be thorough in their investigations of the past histories of individuals they are considering hiring. In addition to inquiry of the state nurse's aide registry or other licensing authorities, the facility should check all references and make reasonable efforts to uncover information about any past criminal prosecutions.

Found guilty by a court of law applies to situations where the defendant pleads guilty, is found guilty, or pleads nolo contendere.

Finding is defined as a determination made by the state that validates allegations of abuse, neglect, mistreatment of residents, or misappropriation of their property.

An aide or other facility staff found guilty of neglect, abuse, or mistreating residents or misappropriation of property by a court of law should have his or her name entered into the nurse's aide registry, or reported to the licensing authority, if applicable. Furthermore, if a facility determines that actions by a court of law against an employee are such that they indicate that the individual is unsuited to work in an assisted living facility (e.g., felony conviction of child abuse, sexual assault, or assault with a deadly weapon), then the facility should not hire that person, or if a present employee, report that individual to the nurse's aide registry (if a nurse's aide) or to the state licensing authorities (if a licensed staff member, such as a nurse or physical therapist or pharmacist). Such a determination by the facility is not limited to mistreatment, neglect, and abuse of residents and misappropriation of their property, but to any treatment of residents or others inside or outside the facility that the facility determines to be such that the individual should not work in an assisted living facility environment.

Credit Reports

Under the federal Fair Credit Reporting Act (Public Law 91–508), the employer must advise applicants if credit reports will be requested. If the candidate is rejected because of a poor credit report, he or she should be so informed and given the name and address of the reporting credit agency.

Physical Examination

All facility staff must have periodic health examinations to ensure freedom from communicable disease. The practical impact of this stipulation is to seek a preemployment physical to ensure that this is met by new staff. There is debate as to whether requiring a physical before offering a job is permitted or whether one must offer the job, then require a physical before the employee begins work. In essence, all applicants must be informed that a condition of employment will be the preplacement health exam following the conditional job offer.

There are several practical reasons for a physical examination:

1. It establishes the physical capability of the applicant to meet the job requirements (a delicate proceeding given the tenor of the Americans with Disabilities Act).
2. It provides a baseline against which to assess later periodic physical exams.
3. The employment-related physical examination is especially valuable in determinations of claims of work-associated disabilities under workers' compensation laws.
4. The laboratory analyses that are part of the exam can detect the presence of illicit drugs in the applicant.

If the physician determines that the new employee cannot perform the essential functions of the job due to a disability under the definition of the Americans with Disabilities Act, the facility must follow a policy on Reasonable Accommodations for Individuals with Disabilities (described in Part Four). If the physician determines the employee cannot perform the essential functions of the job but does not have a disability under the definitions of the Americans with Disabilities Act, the employee is notified that he or she is not qualified for the position.

Normally, the health file is not considered part of the personnel file due to its confidential nature; only authorized persons may have access to the employee's health record on a "need to know" basis.

.COMPLIANCE WITH THE IMMIGRATION REFORM AND CONTROL ACT

Passed in 1986, this act determines which individuals are legally eligible to work in the United States. This is discussed in Part 4.

THE DECISION TO HIRE

Who should decide which applicant to hire? Not the personnel staff. Generally, the final decision to hire is given to the head of the work area in which the recruit will work. The administrator of the facility can define a role for herself or himself in the final decision making or leave it entirely up to the work area head.

Two Approaches to the Hiring Decision

The hiring decision itself is complex. Two basic approaches have been identified in the literature: the clinical and the statistical.

In the *clinical approach* the decision maker reviews all the information in hand about the match of the applicant and the job, then decides.

In the *statistical approach* the decision maker identifies the most valid predictors, then weights them according to complicated formulas. This method has been shown to be superior to the clinical approach (Meehl, 1954). However, few facilities will normally have enough staff time available to make this practical. A compromise is for the decision maker to rate each applicant for a position on several dimensions, such as test score results, education, experience, and apparent interest level, assigning numerical scores on each dimension to each candidate. The results can provide a systematic set of comparison data for reaching the final decision (Jauch, 1976).

Achieving Construct Validity

It is not enough to establish that an applicant has the technical skills needed for a job. Staff will realize that successful caring for frail, elderly assisted living facility residents is often less dependent on the technical knowledge of the staff than on their compassion for others. Knowing the technique for assisting a resident to use a walker is useless, for example, if the staff member cannot encourage the person to leave the chair. As the assisted living facility population becomes more health care complex, both caring and technical skills become increasingly important. Sensitivity, compassion, and caring have construct as well as technical competence and will increasingly have validity as hiring criteria in the assisted living facility setting of the 21st century.

A number of assisted living facilities choose to hire personal care aides who are not trained as nurse's aides. These facilities furnish their own training program for these personal care aides. This has both advantages and disadvantages. On the one hand, compassionate, caring individuals who seek only part-time work but who choose not to go through nurse's aide training may be some of the best prospective employees available. On the other hand, these persons may be a liability to the facility from the point of view of risk management. The nurse's aide has had publicly specified training in safe resident care techniques, among other areas. The facility that chooses to do its own training program would be well advised to train at least to the level of competency required of the nurse's aide.

Passion Index

In Part One we discussed the need for the administrator to have a passion for the tasks necessary to operating an assisted living facility. It is not just the administrator, however, who needs passion all staff in the facility need to be passionate in carrying out their tasks. Kriegel (1991) described a sales vice president of a large U.S. camera firm who explained who makes the best salespeople (translated here for the assisted living facility). Drawing a vertical line down a flip chart, on the left side the vice president listed basic skills and competencies, such as knowledge of the tasks to be performed, being well informed about what competing facilities were doing, having a good employment record, and having the necessary experience.

On the right side of the chart he wrote "Fire in the heart," commenting that if he had to, he would choose someone with fire than one well trained and well recommended. Staff who have fire, he felt, are more motivated, will work harder, will go the extra mile, and are more resourceful. Health care assistants who have drive and enthusiasm for caring for residents can be taught any technical skills they lack. Applicants who lack fire in their hearts or passion for their work are not so easily taught.

Counting grades

How much should grades count? Do the highest grade point averages in school or on the health care assistant test point consistently to the best candidates? Consider the following findings. Over half of the chief executive officers at *Fortune* 500 companies had a C or C– average in college. Two thirds of U.S. senators come from the bottom half of their class. Three fourths of the U.S. presidents were in the lower half of their school classes. More than half of millionaire entrepreneurs didn't finish college (Kriegel, 1991).

OFFERING THE JOB

Once the successful candidate is chosen, he or she should be informed. Information such as proposed salary, job title and level, starting date, and any other relevant information should be communicated. Normally, a period of time during which the offer may be considered is specified. In every case, the candidate needs to be informed about starting date, pay rate, where and when to report, and the name of his or her supervisor, at the very least.

It is useful to include the personnel handbook with the offer if the applicant has not yet received one. The handbook (discussed later in detail) describes facility policy on a number of matters about which the prospective employee should be made aware as part of his or her own evaluation of the proposed position. It is useful to set a 3-day time limit for the newly hired staff member to complete all paperwork.

Unsuccessful applicants should be informed by letter as soon as the job is filled.

2.6 Training Staff

ORIENTATION

First Day on the Job

The first day on the job can potentially leave a lasting impression (Chruden & Sherman, 1980). It is an opportunity for the facility. The new employee usually brings an initial reservoir of goodwill toward the facility. Enthusiasm and anxiety characterize the first day. A sensitively managed orientation program can help the new employee reduce anxiety and begin to build positive images of the new work environment.

Typical first-day activities can include

- official welcome to the new employee
- introduction to as many of the staff as is appropriate
- tour of the facility, including location of any lockers for safekeeping of personal effects, any staff lounges, rest room, parking arrangements
- instructions on use of any time clock
- safety rules, such as infection control and emergency procedures, especially those concerning fire and staff assignments in case of fire
- explanation of residents' rights
- discussion of contents of the personnel handbook (Rogers, 1980)

There is only one first day on the job for each new employee. Whether the orientation is for the resident care coordinator or a health care aide, it is equally important to the success of the organization. If the place is organized to take notice of the new employee and attempts to meet his or her needs on the first day, this latest member of the staff will be more likely to assist the facility in meeting its needs during the following months and years (Bryan, 1984).

Facilities of 130 units are as capable of a personalized orientation program as those with only 30. In practice, by having a properly constituted personnel process, the larger organization may have a functional advantage over the smaller, where orientation may be left to chance and good intentions without assigned responsibility for this introduction.

Targeted Jobs Tax Credit Program

State and/or federal legislation requires that new employees complete a questionnaire and that the facility call in the information to the qualifying agency on or before the employee's first day on the payroll. When participating facilities comply, valuable tax credits are allowed to the facility.

Using a Checklist

Precisely because orientation is a complex task, the use of a checklist is valuable. Those charged with familiarizing the new staff member with the organization are thereby less likely to overlook any element of the employee's new responsibilities as they review each item on the list (S. Scott, 1983). One researcher suggested that the use of a checklist may help reduce employee turnover by helping each new employee to gain a realistic and clearer set of expectation about the new positions (R. Scott, 1972). Turnover is always expensive. The 1997 assisted living industry survey conducted by the National Center for Assisted Living revealed a 53% average annual turnover rate among assisted living caregivers. Turnover rate can be calculated by dividing the total number of employees by the number of new hires in one year.

One industry consultant group suggests that, to calculate the costs to the facility for each turnover, multiply that employee's monthly salary by 4. Based on this formula, the cost for an aide making $7 an hour is approximately $4,500 (*Assisted Living Business Week,* 1998).

Others consider it advisable that both providers and receivers of the orientation be required to sign each activity on the checklist (Davis, 1985; Rogers, 1980). This maximizes the probability that the orientation will be successfully completed. When this document is placed in the employee's personnel file, the signed orientation form becomes a legal basis for establishing that the information was received. Rogers and Davis both suggest that responsibility for the orientation and its documentation be vested in a single staff member, who is thus accountable for its successful completion from introduction to signed checklist.

THE PERSONNEL POLICY HANDBOOK

The personnel policy handbook, often called the employee's handbook or the staff' manual, is a compilation of the facility policies that directly relate to work conditions. Whereas a job description relates to only one job, the personnel policies are general in nature and cover the entire staff.

Each facility will have its own handbook. Chains generally have sets of policies that apply to all their staff, allowing local facilities to add their own policies within the broader policy guidelines and any requirements specific to state or local government regulations.

The main elements most often included in such a handbook are a statement of general policies, followed by details of benefits and general information relevant to the conditions of employment. The personnel handbook can be considered the rules or terms under which staff are hired and carry out their work.

A typical handbook would be arranged along the following lines.

A. Introduction/welcome to the facility

B. History of background of the facility/mission statement/handbook disclaimer

C. General employment policies

1. Equal opportunity employment (conforming to the Civil Rights Act)/sexual harassment policy, age discrimination policies.
2. Classification of staff into full time and part-time by number of hours worked per week; working hours of the facility.
3. Confidentiality of information about residents and facility matters.
4. Residents' rights statement.
5. Employee's records—confidentiality, employee access policy, usual contents:
   (a) application for employment;
   (b) preemployment checks, letters, records of phone calls;
   (c) credit checks;
   (d) performance evaluations, promotions;
   (e) federal and state withholding certificates;
   (f) correspondence;
   (g) disciplinary actions;
   (h) grievances;
   (i) attendance;
   (j) signatures for receipt of personnel policy manual, orientation activities, and in-service attendance records;
   (k) health-related materials, such as annual physical results, hepatitis B vaccination records, annual tuberculosis tests results, records of injuries or other health-related matters;
   (l) license or certificate verification;
   (m) other relevant materials.
6. Reporting policies—required call-in times prior to shift if unable to come to work.

7. Discipline system—whether a progressive system, and if so, a listing of each rule with a statement of disciplinary action (i.e., the number, if any, of oral and or written warnings before dismissal). For example, failure to follow a dress code may allow an oral warning and one or more written warnings before dismissal, whereas physical abuse of a resident could bring immediate suspension/investigation and, if appropriate after investigation, dismissal.
8. Uniforms or dress code expected for staff.
9. General conduct expected (e.g., proper behavior regarding avoidance of vulgarity, courtesy toward residents, attendance and punctuality, absenteeism, and visitors to staff).
10. Gifts (not permitted from residents, their families, or significant others or sponsors).
11. Eating, drinking, smoking, and kitchen traffic rules.
12. Use of alcohol and illegal drugs.
13. Parking, mail, rest breaks, meal breaks, lost and found, phone calls to staff (a never-ending concern), smoking and use of tobacco policy, employment of relatives, search of staff (package and purse inspection).
14. Destruction of assisted living facility property.
15. Suggestion box, permitted uses of bulletin boards, solicitation/distribution of literature rules.
16. Probationary period, use of anniversary or other dates for personnel reviews, seniority policies.
17. Health requirements and physical examinations.
18. Employee debts, garnishment of wages.
19. Performance ratings, promotion policies and interwork area transfer policies, job postings.
20. Wages and salaries, time cards, pay plan, date procedures for determining payroll calculations, payrolls, deductions, overtime policy, severance pay.
21. Grievance procedures.
22. Hospitalization and first aid treatment.
23. Facility position on unions.
24. Resignation notice and procedures, exit interview.
25. On-the-job injuries policies.
26. In-service education requirements.
27. Reimbursement for specified expenses (e.g., travel, meals, memberships).
28. Confidentiality of company affairs/nondisclosure of information.
29. Family and health care leaves, workers' compensation insurance.
30. Fire and disaster/evacuation plans.
31. Incident reports.

D. Benefits

1. Holidays.
2. Vacations, leave-accumulation policies.
3. Leaves, Family and Medical Leave Act time: sick leave, funeral leave, military leave, maternity leave, jury duty, extended leave.

4. Health benefits, dental benefits.
5. Tax-deferred savings plans (e.g., 401(K) plan).
6. Stock purchase plan (if any).
7. Retirement benefits.
8. Insurance: life insurance, unemployment compensation, occupational disease insurance, disability insurance, long-term-care insurance, other.
9. Shift differential (if paid).
10. Other (e.g., child care benefits, meals at work).
11. Group rates: Chains and groups of facilities can negotiate reduced rates on a variety of items, such as accident insurance, life insurance, and liability policies.

Employee handbooks have been a subject of concern to management in recent years because some courts have held the handbooks to be an enforceable contract between the employer and the employee. Entering disclaimers in the handbook has not prevented staff from successfully suing in court.

TRAINING

As we have noted, directing is the task of ensuring that each work role is successfully communicated to the employee. Directing is the process of communicating to the staff what is to be done, then helping them to perform their role successfully (Givnta, 1984).

Purpose

The purpose of the orientation program is to provide an initial introduction to the new employee. The purpose of training is to communicate the organization's needs to the staff and assist them in meeting those needs. This is a continuous process, beginning formally the first day on the job, but extending for the duration of the employee's association with the facility. Each employee will have his or her own learning curve (Argenti, 1994).

Steps in Establishing Training Needs

Staff members responsible for establishing the assisted living facility's training program normally analyze three elements in planning for this: (1) the organization, (2) the tasks, and (3) the person carrying out the work (Chruden & Sherman, 1980).

Organizational analysis consists of examining the facility's goals, resources, and internal and external environments to determine where training efforts need to be focused. A number of in-service topics may be set for the various work areas over the course of each year. These can form the initial framework for training needs.

Task analysis involves the review of job descriptions and activities essential for performing each job. The emphasis of training programs can then be placed on certain tasks that are judged to be inadequately carried out or simply in need of reinforcement because of their importance to the facility, such as fire drills and disaster preparedness.

A person or employee skill analysis can be made to arrive at the skills, knowledge, and attitudes required in each position. Person analysis involves interpreting each position in terms of the personal attributes or behaviors necessary for performing the job.

Once the goal of a training program has been determined, the following steps can be taken: (1) formulate instructional objectives, (2) develop instructional experiences to achieve theses objectives, (3) establish performance criteria to be met, and (4) obtain evaluations of the training effort (Chruden & Sherman, 1980).

On-the-job training is conducted by a staff member assigned to a new or continuing employee to help him or her acquire the abilities needed in a position in the facility. Ideally, on-the-job training permits the trainee to be an additional or extra worker for the first few days, allowing observation and progressive involvement in performing the tasks and behaviors required.

In-service training refers to employee education offered throughout the work career of the employee. Normally, in-service education consists of small seminars for groups of staff. All types of educational techniques are used, including flip charts, films, lectures, videos, role playing, and case discussions. (Ruhl & Atkinson, 1986). In many busy facilities three or more in-service training programs occur every week.

Assisted living facilities may become a training site for numerous educational programs. Most facilities participate as training sites for health care schools, physical therapy programs, pharmacy programs, and activities, social services, and hospitality training programs for nearby colleges.

Evaluating Training

Evaluating training efforts can be difficult. While it is true that tests can be devised to measure memorization, the assisted living facility is seeking to assess something more complex: changes in employee behavior. To quantify behavioral changes, it is useful to state learning objectives as behavioral objectives.

Behavioral objectives can be measured by observing whether staff, in carrying out their duties, exhibit the behaviors sought as the objective of the training. Usually the goal is to have an employee acquire a skill or change an attitude (Wehrenberg, 1983). Using performance-centered behavioral objectives can assist evaluation.

For example, performance-centered objectives in a health care aide training program might be (1) to be able to demonstrate proper procedures for helping a resident who needs assistance transferring from bed to chair and (2) to consistently greet any residents encountered in the hallways using a pleasant tone of voice.

Both of these are performance-centered objectives. Proper techniques for assisting a resident transfer from bed to chair can be physically demonstrated by the aide in training, and the aide's demeanor toward residents encountered in the hallways can be monitored by the trainer or other staff members.

2.7 Retaining Employees

2.7.1 What the Facility Needs from the Employee

We have argued that the facility needs employees who have a passion for their job and will consistently make decisions in conformity with its policies. This is possible to the extent that each staff member can be characterized as having the following:

- a high degree of interest in the job—a willingness to make every effort
- a genuine dedication to the well-being of the residents and their quality of care and quality of life—passion for the work
- a strong positive self-image, permitting employees to see beyond their own needs and to be concerned with those of the residents
- skills, both technical and interpersonal, in communication and human relationships
- the capacity and willingness to make decisions in accordance with the best interest of the facility, every act contributing toward providing the highest quality of life for the residents, their significant others, the facility staff, and the community
- the ability to be self-starting, reliable, creative, and able to exercise positive, appropriate leadership
- career commitment to the facility

Obviously, this is the description of an ideal employee. Few staff members will be able to embody all of these qualities. If, however, these characteristics can be constantly encouraged and developed among the employees, the quality of life enjoyed by the residents and staff should be high.

2.7.2 What Employees Need from the Facility

What employees require of the facility can be divided into five areas: (1) social approval; (2) self-esteem; (3) economic security; (4) "hygiene factors," that is one's use of power, accomplishment, service, and exercise of leadership; and perhaps most important, (5) a sense of working for an organization with a vision that allows the employee to participate in a larger meaning, giving him or her pride and purpose in the work.

The degree to which any one individual might seek satisfaction from employment will vary, both among the entire staff and within the person as his or her personal situation changes over time.

SOCIAL APPROVAL

Most people rely on a network of approval and satisfying social interrelationships. Whether or not they express it openly, many of them enjoy engagement in activities sanctioned by significant others—persons to whom an individual looks for favorable regard of behavior patterns, ideas, and values. Family, members of the community, and/or one's social group are typical examples of significant others.

If the community, or significant others in the community from whom approval is sought, disapproves of the employee working at the facility, he or she may not have positive feelings about the job itself or feel that being a "good" employee is worth the effort. Social approval, then, is necessary for helping employees to develop a sense of pride in and commitment to the job.

SELF-ESTEEM

Adequate self-esteem is essential in order to function. Individuals need a positive self-image; they need to feel good about themselves, about what they are doing. Each person has a need for status. Most people want to be part of an organization that has a sense of purpose to which they can dedicate their energies.

ECONOMIC SECURITY

Economic security involves the financial benefits provided by the facility. Without sufficient income for maintenance, health insurance, recreation, and funds to meet future retirement expenses, an employee may remain insecure.

HYGIENE FACTORS

Hygiene factors are those such as salary, company policies, and basic working conditions. In theory, when hygiene factors are adequate, they do not bring about appreciable levels of employee satisfaction. Hygiene factors, then, are the minimum work conditions (Argenti, 1994).

PARTICIPATION IN A VISION

Employees want to work for an organization that stimulates their dreams and aspirations and touches their hearts. They enjoy collaborating with highly motivated people who are accomplishing work that matters, that has purpose and meaning—something beyond just striving to being the largest or the best known or the highest income. The staff need the administrator to take a personal interest in them—to recognize them as essential members of the team (Riter, 1993).

ADDITIONAL NEEDS

Some employees expect even more of the work situation. Their intrinsic needs arise out of the essential nature of their personality. Wielding power and having authority in certain situations are intrinsic needs. Satisfaction from the process of completing tasks, of achievement, is another such need, as is leadership. Giving service can be a fulfilling behavior.

2.7.3 Strategies for Meeting the Facility's and Employee's Needs

Retaining high-performing employees over an extended period of time is economically desirable for the facility. The financial costs of training each new staff member can be high, especially if the employee participates extensively in in-service training programs offered by the facility and takes advantage of any additional on-the-job training for skills improvement.

In the assisted living facility setting, employee continuity is critical for the residents themselves, providing an important element of stability and continuity in their lives. More than in most work settings, employees in assisted living facilities tend to form personal relationships with the residents, often being regarded as significant friends by residents who have lost family and many cherished others.

A motivated, contented staff, capable of contributing significantly to the quality of resident life, consists of employees who are enjoying a high level of job satisfaction and are thus enabled to provide a high level of resident care.

An administrator in a large California long-term-care facility says he is successful because he primarily concentrates his energy on the staff. Only highly motivated, happy staff, he believes, give loving care to residents. His enthusiasm and evident concern enable staff members to treat residents and other employees in the same manner.

A PHILOSOPHY OF HUMAN RESOURCE MANAGEMENT

What motivates employees? Every day the administrators of the 5,000 assisted living facilities in the United States make decisions based on their assumptions of what motivates their staff. These conclusions reflect each administrator's beliefs about human resource management. We will explore one general theory about employee motivation.

Theory X and Theory Y

In 1960 Douglas M. McGregor, a management theorist, published *The Human Side of Enterprise,* in which he outlined what he called Theory X and Theory Y. McGregor wrote that the behavior of administrators is strongly influenced by their beliefs. He asserted that most business managers are Theory X types, who believe that the employee naturally dislikes work, prefers to receive extensive direction from superiors, wishes to avoid taking responsibilities in the organization, has little ambition, and is motivated more by a need for security than any other factor. This approach requires that managers use fear or punishment to motivate employees, all of whom will be closely watched if work is to be accomplished.

McGregor insisted that Theory X is not valid and that managers should be guided by what he called Theory Y. Theory Y is based on the following assumptions:

1. Using energy to work is as natural as using energy to play or rest. The administrator can control working conditions that lead to work being viewed as a source of satisfaction and therefore voluntarily performed, or to work being seen as a source of punishment and therefore avoided.
2. If individuals are committed to the organization's goals, they will exercise self-direction and self-control without need for threat of punishment or external behavior controls.
3. Rewards for achieving organizational objectives bring employee commitment; employees can achieve personal self-satisfaction in achieving organizational goals..
4. The average employee, when properly motivated, will accept and also seek responsibility.
5. Most employees have the capability of exercising imagination, ingenuity, and creativity in helping the organization to achieve its goals.
6. Most jobs underutilize the capabilities of employees.

McGregor's theory caused considerable discussion in management circles. One researcher (Allen, 1973) doubted that most managers were Theory X types. To test this, he surveyed 259 managers in 93 companies and found that managers did not completely accept either Theory X or Theory Y. In their opinion, reality is more complicated than either theory. Not surprisingly, a few years later Theory Z was developed.

Theory Z

Several writers (Argenti, 1991; Thierauf, Klekamp, & Geeding, 1973; White, 1984) proposed that, on balance, Theory Y is correct, but what motivates employees changes over time and is dependent on changing societal values. They argued that administrators will constantly come up with new strategies for motivating employees. In their view, a straightforward productivity-reward system is overly simplistic. A satisfactory quality of life, both for the individual and for the group, while more complex and abstract, is the appropriate focus.

PERSONALITY TESTS

Some facilities utilize a variety of tests to evaluate applicants and/or employees. The most widely known is the Myers-Briggs Type Indicator personality test. The test consists of 100 questions that ask respondents how they feel or act in a variety of situations. Results are used to place respondents into four categories: (1) introverted or extroverted,

(2) sensing or intuitive, (3) thinking or feeling, and (4) perceiving or judging. These characterizations are then used to place a person into one of 16 personality types. Someone whose test results show him or her to be extroverted-intuitive-thinking-perceiving is classified as a conceptualizer. This and other tests are sometimes used to categorize respondents as left brain or right brain, the theory being that left-brained people are systematic, thorough, and balanced, whereas right-brained individuals are more intuitive, quick, and less complex in their approach to decision making. While this may be edifying to the human resources personnel, most employees do not like to be put into categories, however well intentioned the testers may be.

MEETING THE EMPLOYEES' NEED FOR SOCIAL APPROVAL

Individuals have a need to be part of an enterprise that is regarded by significant others as successful. Hence, approval of the assisted living facility by significant others is important to assisted living facility employees.

In the community the word-of-mouth reputation of the facility is important. Persons and groups regarded as experts in the field (the local hospital, nursing homes, the home health agency, hospice, the local physicians, and the case managers at the local health maintenance organizations, independent practitioner organizations, professional provider organizations, and similar groups) can be important, or significant, others, whose approval is sought by the staff. Newspaper, radio, and television reports about the workplace shape employee feelings.

MEETING THE EMPLOYEE'S NEED FOR SELF-ESTEEM

Why does one health care aide strive harder than another? Why does one activities director look for additional responsibilities at the same time that another seeks to avoid taking on any? Why do wage incentives stimulate some individuals and not others? Why does a career advancement track within the facility stimulate some employees while others ignore the opportunities offered?

What motivates employees varies. Motivation is a difficult concept to define. It has been described as the factor that energizes employee behavior, directing or channeling such behavior, and sustaining it (Steers & Porter, 1979).

An individual's needs, desires, and expectations change. When one need or desire is achieved at a satisfactory level, the salience or strength of others is modified. For a nurse who has just been licensed to practice, acceptance by other health care personnel may be a priority until this recognition is achieved (Lorsch & Takagi, 1986). At that point other needs, such as maximizing income, may take precedence.

Understanding Motives

The complexity of motives has been described by Dunnette and Kirchner (1965), who attempted to apply motivational psychology to the work situation. They point out the following:

1. Identifying motives is complex. Some employees will work hard to obtain more money, but why? A strongly felt need for additional money may reflect a desire for the increased status more money brings, meeting a felt need for a sense of economic security, providing a symbol of power, or indicating simply a willingness to work harder until the car is paid off, at which point time off from work may replace the desire for more money as a primary motivation.

2. Motives are always mixed. Each individual experiences a wide range of motives that strengthen and weaken as his or her circumstances change, and some needs are met while others are frustrated.

3. The same incentive (e.g., increased health insurance benefits) may generate different responses. Individuals also differ in the ease with which their needs are satisfied.

4. Some motives may recede when satisfied (e.g., hunger and thirst). Others, such as a desire for increased status or more salary, may become intensified when, for example, more status or more income is achieved

The process of giving employees increased roles in the decision-making processes of the facility is known as *job enrichment.* For example, the administrator can assign to help motivate employees who are looking for responsibility and increased job satisfaction, resident aides complete responsibility for the care of a set of residents, rather than structuring tasks so that certain caregivers do only certain things (dispense medications, help residents get to the dining room, etc.). *Job depth* refers to the extent to which an employee has power to influence decisions. When the resident care coordinator consults the aides on a floor as to whether they are prepared to receive a proposed admission, these aides have increased job depth.

A. H. Maslow's hierarchy-of-need theory is perhaps the most often cited human need model in the literature (see Figure 2.2 Maslow theorized that needs become salient (i.e., powerfully motivating) at each successively higher level mainly after the needs at each lower level are satisfactorily met. That is, the needs for survival and basic security, will dominate the individual's motivations until they are met.

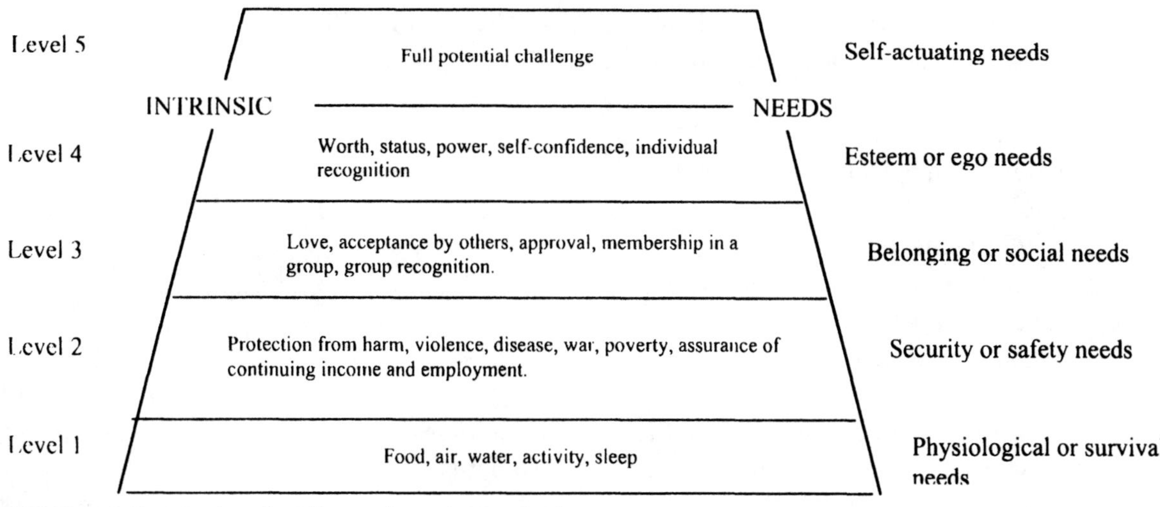

FIGURE 2.2 Maslow's Hierarchy-of-Need Theory.

Once lower level needs are met to a satisfactory degree, the individual's motivations can become more dominated by social, self-esteem, and self-actuating needs (levels 3, 4, and 5). Maslow's model is widely used. In our view, it seems to be a functional and useful explanation of some of the more basic dynamics of employee motivations.

One author (Lawler, 1973) pointed out that while the lower level needs may decrease in strength when achieved, the higher level needs, especially the need for self-actualization, tend to continue to grow stronger as they are being met. Examples of these types of needs or motivations include wielding power, accomplishing goals, and exercising leadership.

A word of caution: Each individual has a unique, ever-changing need pattern. In our view, what motivates an individual depends on life experiences and, scientists are more and more suggesting, each individual's genetic and chemical makeup.

Childhood experiences such as economic deprivation, for example, may cause an employee to be anxious about financial security, no matter how much income is being earned. The social and economic class with which an employee identifies affects his or her perceptions of his or her needs. Being raised as a male or a female can influence the needs individuals will manifest on the job. In all cases, needs are individualistic.

Personality Types: A and B

Attempts have been made to identify basic personality types. One theory categorizes people as Type A or B. Type A individuals are characterized as hard-driving, achievement-oriented people who strive to succeed to the highest level, whatever the area of activity. Type B personalities are characterized as having only moderate achievement needs and as being less competitive and more satisfied with moderation.

Type A employees come to the facility with a high internalized motivation level. They are overachievers in comparison with Type B persons.

Motivation Exercise

Supervisors' ideas about what motivates the staff and employees' ideas about what is motivating often differ significantly. The following is a list of concepts the reader can ask of a set of supervisors and employees in his or her facility. Which, among the following, do they consider the most important aspects of their jobs?

- to be treated fairly
- consistency from management
- job security
- interesting work
- full appreciation for work done
- good wages
- good working conditions
- feeling "in" on things
- promotion and growth within the facility/company
- sympathetic understanding of personal problems
- tactful discipline
- management loyalty to workers.

Ask participants to rank each of the above from most important (1) to least important (10). Chances are, you'll find that supervisors and staff will have very different rankings.

RETAINING STAFF

In the following section, we discuss nine areas available to an administrator seeking to retain staff by meeting employees' needs for approval:

- leadership by vision
- training programs
- career paths
- performance feedback and goal setting
- recognition
- power
- respect for creative potential
- teamwork
- pleasure in the job

Leadership by Vision

Most facilities set goals. Exhorting employees to meet those goals, such as making the month's budget, is, in the end, limiting. Goals limit unless goals are part of a vision. Organizations such as assisted living facilities need a vision to fire up employees, to engage their spirits, and to set long-term directions for their efforts. Each work area manager needs a vision of what his or her work area can achieve, a vision to provide meaning to each employee's efforts. Kriegel (1991) argues that a vision or dream is a goal with wings. A dream or vision is an ideal state; a goal is a more real state. The dream supplies enthusiasm, vigor, and direction for the facility's efforts. Goals are short-term targets to be achieved, such as ensuring that all the paperwork for admissions is completed in a timely manner and new residents' care plans are accomplished on a timely basis. Employees want to feel that they are doing more than contributing to the profit ratio. They want to be part of a movement, a compelling vision, something that takes hold of their imagination. Employees want to be part of a facility that has a vision, a dream about the quality of life of each resident *and* staff member.

Training Programs

Training programs increase employee skills and simultaneously communicate to them that those skills are valued by the management.

The training programs themselves serve numerous functions. They demonstrate management's interest in the staff and provide an additional arena for exchange among employees, as well as an increased opportunity for feedback to the administration about the degree of skills and understanding of facility goals among employees. As these dynamics occur, the level of employee satisfaction can improve. With the new skills or insights the employee experiences an increased feeling of being in tune with the performance expectations of the organization.

Professional Standards of Quality. Since most assisted living facilities residents use outside services, sometimes arranged by the residents, sometimes by the facility staff, the following concept of level of facility responsibility is useful for the administrator to observe.

Goal: that persons providing services are qualified to do so, that the facility's plan of care is implemented, and that those services provided meet professional standards of quality. The intent is to ensure that services being provided meet professional standards of quality (in accordance with the definition provided below) and are provided by appropriately qualified persons.

Professional standards of quality means services that are provided according to accepted standards of practice. Standards may apply to care provided by a particular discipline or in a specific situation or setting. Standards regarding quality care practices may be published by a professional organization, licensing board, accreditation body, or other regulatory agency. Recommended practices to achieve desired resident outcomes may also be found in the literature. Possible reference sources for standards of practice include

- current manuals or textbooks on activities, nursing, social work, physical therapy, etc.
- standards published by professional organizations such as the National Association of Activity Professionals, the American Nurses' Association, the National Association of Social Work, the American Dietetic Association, and the American Medical Association.
- practice guidelines published by the Agency for HealthCare Policy and Research
- current professional journal articles

Training of Nurse's Aides. One of the most debated topics in assisted living facility staffing is whether to hire only certified nursing assistants. Often facilities employ both certified aides and others whom the facility trains. A variety of staffing arrangements may be devised. A facility, for example, may employ noncertified resident assistants to give simple care measures, such as making beds or other activities that are unlikely to affect a resident negatively if insufficient training has been received.

Most resident–staff contacts will require that the staff have a minimum level of training. Such seemingly simple staff activities as assisting a resident from a bed to the bathroom when the resident is ill require the use of proper techniques to ensure resident (and staff) safety. The certified nursing assistant (CNA) has the necessary training. As a simple risk management measure, if the facility employs only CNAs, the likelihood of accidents is reduced.

Even if the facility policy is to hire only CNAs, the facility may employ a person who is not a certified nurse's aide for up to 4 months as long as that person is currently undergoing nurse's aide training and performs only those tasks for which that person has received instruction. If the facility chooses to employ only CNAs, the following requirements should be observed.

Definitions. *Licensed health professional* means a physician; physician's assistant; nurse practitioner; physical, speech, or occupational therapist; physical or occupational therapy assistant; registered professional nurse; licensed practical nurse; or licensed or certified social worker.

Nurse's aide means any individual providing nursing or nursing-related services who is not a licensed health professional, a registered dietitian, or someone who volunteers to provide such services without pay.

Volunteers are not nurse's aides and do not come under the nurse's aide training provisions. Unpaid students in education programs who use facilities as practice sites under the direct supervision of a faculty member are considered volunteers.

Private duty nurse's aides who are not employed or utilized by the facility on a contract, per diem, leased, or other basis do not come under the nurse's aide training provisions. Generally, persons designated personal care assistants do not come under the nurse's aide provisions. However, as a matter of having minimally trained staff, permanently employing only those persons who have nurse's aide training and are in the state registry may make sense, especially in the more health care–oriented level 3 assisted living facilities.

General rule. Generally, a facility should not use any individual working in the facility as a nurse's aide for more than 4 months, on a full-time basis, unless that individual is competent to provide nursing and nursing related services and that individual has completed a training and competency evaluation program, or a competency evaluation program approved by the state.

Nonpermanent employee. A facility should not use on a temporary, per diem, leased, or other basis any individual who does not meet these nurse aide requirements.

Facilities may use, as nurse's aides, any individuals who have successfully completed either a nurse's aide training and competency evaluation program or a competency evaluation program. If an individual has not completed a program at the time of employment, however, a facility may only use that individual as a nurse's aide if the individual is in a nurse's aide training and competency evaluation program (not a competency evaluation program alone) and that individual is a permanent employee in his or her first 4 months of employment in the facility.

Permanent employee. A *permanent employee* is defined as any employee that is expected to continue working on an ongoing basis.

Nurse aide training. Nurse's aide training includes at least 16 hours of training in the following subjects before any direct contact with residents is allowed:

- communication and interpersonal skills
- infection control
- safety and emergency procedures, including the Heimlich maneuver
- promoting residents' independence
- respecting residents' rights

Other areas of training should include

- basic nursing skills
- personal care skills
- understanding of mental health and social services of residents
- care of cognitively impaired residents;
- basic restorative services
- resident's rights

Registry Verification. Before allowing an employee to serve as a nurse's aide, a facility should receive registry verification that the individual has met competency evaluation requirements.

Required Training. If, since an employee's most recent completion of a training and competency evaluation program, there has been a continuous period of 24 consecutive months, during which the employee did not provided any nursing or nursing-related services for monetary compensation, the employee should complete a new training and competency evaluation program or a new competency evaluation program.

Regular In-service Education. The facility should complete a performance review of every nurse's aide at least once every 12 months and should provide regular in-service education based on the outcome of these reviews. The in-service training should be sufficient to ensure the continuing competence of nurse's aides but should be no less than 12 hours per year; the adequacy of the in-service education program is measured not only by the documentation of hours of completed in-service education but also by the demonstrated competencies of the nurse's aide staff in consistently applying the interventions necessary to meet residents' needs.

Career Paths. Offering a career path means providing upward mobility within the organization. Creating career mobility is more difficult in a freestanding assisted living facility than within a chain that owns and operates 30 facilities.

Making career paths available within the facility communicates to each employee that the organization wants to meet his or her desires to succeed and progress in job level and income. For the health care aide, a career path might include facility support through released time and/or tuition assistance. This makes more feasible enrollment at a local technical institute to become a licensed practical nurse or a registered nurse.

In a larger assisted living facility, a nurse employed by the facility might receive support to participate in a program to become a geriatric nurse practitioner. The kitchen worker might be assisted in attending classes that lead to qualifying as a dietetic service supervisor.

The labor market can be an influencing factor. If the facility is freestanding, in a rural area with a limited number of persons in the potential pool of health care aides or kitchen workers, career assistance may lead to an undesirable depletion of the worker pool.

On balance, providing career paths that create upward mobility appears to increase worker satisfaction and improve employee retention rates. Not all of the aides will aspire to become licensed caregivers, since they are not all similarly motivated. However, the availability of a career program can improve workers' attitudes. Those who choose not to participate have the satisfaction of knowing the option is available. In general, the mere presence of options is important to employees.

Performance Feedback and Goal Setting

Employees receive informal feedback on their job performance on a daily basis. Formal reaction and the formal process of goal setting for an individual employee occurs under more structured circumstances. This is known as the performance evaluation, which normally includes establishing goals for the employee to achieve until the next scheduled review. This is discussed in more detail in section 2.8.

To Err Is to Learn. The facility administrator's attitude toward errors and failures is critical to success. As Kriegel (1991) observed, failure is a good place to start. Failure itself is not a crime. The problem, really, is failure to learn from failure.

Mistakes are inevitable. If the administrator shows that he or she understands this, employees will respond with more openness about their mistakes. Cover-up of mistakes by employees takes lots of energy and usually leads to more lies to shore up the initial one. The mistake concealer is a problem for the facility. The employee who comes into the work area manager's office and says, "I screwed up," is an employee with whom there is good communication, and an opportunity to learn has been created. In short, management needs a positive attitude toward mistakes. Employees prefer to work in an open, honest atmosphere in which management helps them to learn from their mistakes.

Recognition

Most employees seek recognition for their work. Much of their behavior can be interpreted using the *expectancy theory,* which was pioneered by Victor Broom in the 1960s (Argenti, 1994). Expectancy theory holds that the level of motivation to perform (make an effort at work) is a mathematical function of the expectation individuals have about future outcomes multiplied by the value the employee places on these outcomes. Vroom (1964) defines expectancy as a "momentary belief concerning the likelihood that a particular act will be followed by a particular outcome" (Vroom, p. 170).

Believing that working long hours and asserting yourself on the job will lead to promotion upon the departure of the current manager is an example of an expectancy. It serves as a guideline for the employee in seeking promotion. The employee expects the behavior to be rewarded. Recognizing expectations can help an administrator understand how employees are motivated.

If, in this case, the employee's long hours and assertiveness lead to promotion upon departure of the manager, the expectation is reinforced. According to the *reinforcement theory,* behaviors depend on reward. When reward follows performance, performance improves. Conversely, when reward does not follow performance, performance deteriorates. If the employee in this situation had not been promoted, performance might have deteriorated.

In reinforcement theory the outcome reinforces the employee's response either positively, leading to repetition of the behavior, or negatively, leading to reduction of its use. Influencing employee behavior through reinforcement is called *operant conditioning,* literally influencing working behavior by conditioning the employee's response by rewarding (or punishing) the behavior.

When employees perform in a desired manner and are given praise and recognition for that behavior, the manager is engaging in what may be called *behavior modification.* Behavior modification involves using operant conditioning, usually rewards, praise, and positive recognition, when an employee performs as desired.

One theorist (Rotondi, 1976) suggested the following as a pattern for modifying employee behavior:

- Maintain a consistent work environment.
- Consciously identify the desired behaviors of employees.
- Decide on the rewards to be used.
- Clearly communicate to the employees both the desired behaviors and the rewards.
- Reward desired behaviors immediately.
- Scale rewards to the behavioral achievement attained (i.e., vary the rewards and minimize the use of punishments).

Power-Control

The assisted living facility administrator needs to define policies that govern decision making. However, this has both positive and negative aspects. The positive aspect is that the staff is given guidance and an appropriate framework within which to make decisions for the organization. The negative aspect is that deciding beforehand, through policy making, can substantially deprive the employee of a feeling of personal involvement in decision making for the organization.

Feelings of Powerlessness. The behavioral scientist Christopher Argyris (1972) observed a tendency for organizations to overlook a desire that he believed most employees have: to function in a mature, adult manner. In the literature this is referred to as the *immaturity-maturity theory,* which holds that, in most organizational designs, employees are treated as immature, thus frustrating their need to function as responsible adults.

Argyris believed that the typical organization tends to ignore individual potentials for competence, for taking responsibility, for constructive intentions, and for productivity. He felt that in typical lower level jobs, staff members are treated as immature. This, he argued, alienates and frustrates these workers, leading them to feel justified in rejecting responsible behavior and tempting them to defy the organization by allowing the quality of their work to deteriorate.

The same problem exists among managers who work within organizational structures that create environments hostile to trust, candor, and risk taking. In such situations, the attitudes actually encouraged are conformity and defensiveness, which tend to be expressed by producing detailed substantiation for unimportant problems and invalid information for critical issues. Argyris asserted that this leads to ineffective problem solving, poor decisions, and weak commitment to any decisions that are made.

Argyris pointed to the downside of a coherent set of policies to cover all decision making in the facility: Little significant role in decision making is left to the individual employee. This may lead to a high level of frustration among those affected.

A common reaction to frustration can be selecting an acceptable substitute goal that is attainable or engaging in behavior that is maladaptive (Chruden & Sherman, 1980). An employee barred from making any meaningful decisions at the facility may cease trying and may concentrate energies instead on a leadership role in an outside voluntary organization. Or the employee may relieve his or her frustration through aggressive or abusive behavior toward other employees or the residents.

Combating Powerlessness: Employees as "Owners." A solution to this problem is to attempt to make everybody an "owner." Giving all employees a sense of ownership in the facility means treating each employee as a member of the team. This can be accomplished by allowing them some control in their work and giving them information about what the facility is attempting to accomplish. Tom Peters and Nancy Austin call this approach "all people as 'businesspeople'" (Peters & Austin, 1985).

Ownership implies that all employees exercise some real portion of control in the facility. Of course, each employee does exercise some fraction of control over the workplace. It is up to the individual staff member, for instance, to decide whether to give care pleasantly or in a disrespectful manner.

When the organization treats every employee like an owner, the employees will feel fully engaged in the facility's goals. A sense of ownership is accompanied by a feeling of control over what happens. This is sometimes accomplished by job enlargement, increasing the number of tasks an employee performs so that he or she finds increased satisfaction through involvement in a process from start to finish. Peters and Austin (1985) cited the following examples from the experimental laboratory and from the field.

An industrial psychologist gave the subjects in a study some difficult puzzles to work and some boring proofreading to do. While the subjects were attempting to accomplish these tasks, the psychologist played a loud tape recording of one person speaking Spanish, of two speaking Armenian, and of a copy machine in use.

Half of the subjects were given a button to push to stop the noise; the other half had no control over the noise. Those with buttons to push solved five times as many puzzles and had one fourth fewer errors in proofreading, although never once did any subject with control push the button. Those who perceived that they had control over their situation clearly outperformed those who felt they had little or no control. In numerous repetitions the same results were obtained.

In the field, the same results were achieved: Workers who were given buttons to push achieved superior results for the company. The Ford Motor Company plant in Edison, New Jersey, gave every worker on the assembly line a button to push that shut down the assembly line. The Ford workers shut down the assembly line 30 times the first day and an average of 10 times a day thereafter. After the first day the shutdown lasted an average of 10 seconds.

What happened at the plant? Production remained steady. The number of defects dropped from 17 per car to less than 1. The number of cars requiring rework after coming off the line dropped by 97%. A backlog of union grievances plummeted. Why? Because the line workers felt they had some meaningful control in their jobs, a sense of ownership in the plant. Employees with a sense of ownership will try to do what is best for the organization. The health care aide with this perception is more capable of meeting his or her social needs, such as self-esteem, self-acceptance, and status.

How can health care aides be given ownership in the facility? One administrator accomplished this by consulting the aides before admitting a resident to their wing. When the aides told the administrator that the load was too great at one particular juncture, the administrator delayed the proposed admission.

These aides had a sense of control over their work situation. They worked harder than before and exercised their control judiciously to make sure the quality of resident care was not compromised by overly rapid admitting. These aides had a button to push. They never pushed it without a good reason.

Health Care Aide Ownership. Why should health care aides be involved in running the facility? The reason can be seen in the successes the fostering of ownership has had in other industries. Ford Motor Company, for example, has a practice of soliciting input from all hourly workers. The assembly line workers are asked to comment on the manufacturability of parts and are members of advance design teams. In one period hourly workers offered 1,155 suggestions for changes in design or production for three small trucks, more than 700 of these suggestions were later adopted (Peters & Austin, 1985, p. 26).

The assisted living facility administrator has three immediate constituencies: the staff, the residents, and the residents' significant others. In Part Five we will argue that one of the administrator's tasks is to create and enforce as many opportunities as possible for residents to feel in control of their lives. Here we maintain that one of the administrator's major tasks is to create and enforce as many opportunities as possible for staff to feel in control of their work. Not an easy task to accomplish for either group. The forces fostering institutionalization appear to move toward removing control from the residents. Similarly, government regulations and the accompanying need for conformity in the workplace inexorably move toward removing control over work from the staff members. Kruzich (1995) conducted a study on staff self-perceived influence on decision making (the study involved 498 staff members in 51 long-term care facilities). Nurse assistant involvement in shift reports, frequency of unit staff meetings, and administrators' decision-making autonomy from the governing board were found associated with increased levels of health care aide involvement in decision making.

Respect for the Creative Potential

The "business" of every assisted living facility is providing resident services. We mentioned in Part One that in *A Passion for Excellence,* Peters and Austin (1985) insisted that there are only two ways to create and sustain superior resident care: first, by taking exceptional care of residents by providing superior services and quality of care; second, by constantly innovating.

According to the authors, this is not accomplished by the genius of the administrator or by mystical strategic moves. Excellence in resident care comes from "a bedrock of listening, trust, and respect for the dignity and the creative potential of each person in the organization" (p. 20).

High resident care depends on whether the administrator has been able to enable the employees—the housekeepers, kitchen staff, laundry workers, maintenance persons, accountant, secretary, and health care staff—to function as a team that has bought into the facility.

Accepting Suggestions. Most individuals and organizations tend to resist change. There is a tendency on the part of administrators to ignore employee's suggestions for new ways to accomplish the facility's goals. "It's not within the budget," "It'll never work," "We've already tried that," and "We don't do it that way around here" are common responses to new suggestions.

According to Kriegel (1991), conventional wisdom holds that everything happens in cycles. The belief is that things will cycle back—back to normal, back to the good old days. Criticism of new ideas leads to sticking with the tried-and-true approach. Kreigel argued that the new reality is that change will be followed with change, that the waves will not flatten out. Rather, waves will continue to get bigger and come at the facility faster. Administrators, then, should be open to employees' suggestions and to change.

Membership on a Teams

We have mentioned the team concept several times and will return to it in the discussion of resident care planning in Part Five.

Industries repeatedly have discovered that small groups produce higher quality, more personalized service, and more innovations than do larger entities (Peters & Austin, 1985). American companies, including General Motors and Hewlett-Packard, now limit the size of plants to between 200 and 500 employees. Japanese companies generally organize their largest industrial plants into small teams of 10 to 40 workers.

A Natural Head Start. Team membership is a valuable tool in efforts to retain employees because it helps meet each employee's need for social involvement, communication with other employees, and meaningful personal involvement in the real work of the facility.

The work of an assisted living facility cannot be successfully accomplished without all work areas functioning as a team. Achieving and maintaining this necessary teamwork is one of the assisted living facility's constant challenges.

Trying Easy. Under the pressure of increased regulatory efforts and expected squeezing of funds an assisted living facility may develop a "faster is better mentality," what Kriegel (referred to as the gottas: "I gotta make cleaning rounds quickly," "I gotta finish all the paperwork," "I gotta cut costs," and so on. Kriegel (1991) cited the Charlie Chaplin film *Modern Times,* in which Chaplin is happily decorating cakes on an assembly line, adding a rose here, fancy frosting there. Suddenly the assembly line speeds up, and in his haste the icing gets sprayed everywhere the cakes begin flying.

Creativity and innovation are losers to speed. In one health care setting, Caudill and Patrick (1992) developed a 56-item questionnaire that was answered by 996 health care assistants. The researchers found that weekly and permanent resident assignments were favored over rotating responsibilities and that aides responsible for larger numbers of residents and higher turnover rates. Caudill and Patrick (1992) found that turnover rates were high as 60% in long-term care settings.

Pleasure in the Job

Work ought to be fun. Several Silicon Valley companies have led the way toward implementing this concept. At these companies dress is California informal, life is laid back, and having fun is important. Aristotle observed that pleasure in the job puts perfection in the work. If caregivers who love health care can be hired, if care assistants who love taking care of older people can be hired, if maintenance persons who love to tinker and repair and maintain can be hired, the facility will be a more pleasant place.

The Importance of Having Fun. Because of the nature of the work, it may be more important to create a relaxed atmosphere in an assisted living facility than in other work settings. As Kriegel (1991) observed, coal miners used to take canaries into the shafts with them to act as early warning systems of the presence of dangerous fumes. Laughter and good humor are the canaries of the work shift—when laughter dies, it is an early warning that life is slipping from the facility. The ice cream manufacturer Ben and Jerry's has appointed "joy gangs," whose responsibilities are to create more joy. These "gangs" must figure out activities and events that encourage the employees to stay relaxed.

This isn't an easy task in the assisted living facility environment, which makes it all the more important to try. To avoid burnout and high turnover rates, the facility, led by the activities director, with the input of staff, needs to emphasize pleasure in the job well done. Conventional wisdom says play to win. Kriegel (1991) emphasizes "play, to win" (p. 256). Actually, winning will take place, not at the end of the game, but every day along the way. Work must contain some fun each day if employees and residents are to experience quality living.

2.8 Evaluating Employees

JOB PERFORMANCE EVALUATION: A LINE MANAGER FUNCTION

Job performance evaluation is a task assigned only to line managers. Such responsibility distinguishes staff from line management functions. Staff, having no line authority, should not be assigned line responsibility for personnel matters—hiring, evaluating, promoting, reprimanding,, suspending or discharging employees—because to do so violates the concept of each employee reporting to but one manager.

PURPOSE OF JOB PERFORMANCE EVALUATION

The frequent change of staff, including work area managers, in the average assisted living facility means that the organization's "memory" can be short. For an employee seeking to build a career at a facility, if there are no records, his or her progress over an extended period is more subject to the impressions of work area managers who may pass through.

As a practical matter, all of us are judged as we go about our daily work. The organization needs some method of creating a track record, both to reward the good employee and to identify employees who function at the margin of competence and for whom considerable documentation will need to be in place when the time comes for dismissal.

A basic purpose of the job performance evaluation is to focus the energies of the employee on the performance expected (Smith, 1984). Whereas on-the-job and in-service training are part of the directing role of middle-level managers, job performance evaluation is a function of controlling personnel performance quality. The goal of the performance evaluation is, of course, to nurture the performance needed for the success of the facility and, so far as practical, to reward good work.

The Equal Employment Opportunity Commission and, more recently, the Americans with Disabilities Act have done much to stimulate employers to keep accurate evaluation records of employees' work. Court hearings have also contributed to the desirability of carefully documenting worker performance (Chruden & Sherman, 1980).

Performance Evaluation: Three Basic Objectives

Three basic objectives of performance evaluations are (1) to give employees feedback about their work performance, (2) to provide a basis (plan) for directing future employee efforts toward organizational goals, and (3) to provide a basis on which managers can decide on promotions, compensation, and future job assignments (Locher & Teel, 1977).

The performance evaluation can force communication to occur that might not otherwise concerning the manager's feelings about the employee's work. Setting up a performance evaluation system may simply be a needed formalizing of the manager's impressions of the daily work of the employee. Most industries use the performance evaluation. A study by the Bureau of National Affairs revealed that among the industries studied, 84% had regular procedures for evaluating office personnel and 58% for evaluating line workers (*Employee Performance,* 1975, pp. 1–3). The majority of evaluations were given on an annual basis.

On balance, the absence of any written system for evaluation of long-term performance exposes the individual more nearly to the whim of managers who head the employee's work area.

OUTLINE OF THE PERFORMANCE EVALUATION PROCESS

First, the manager defines the functions, tasks, demands, and expectation of the job and translates them into performance criteria (Baker & Morgan, 1984; Bianco, 1984; Smith, 1984). To implement this, forms and procedures, including standardized methods of rating employees to be used by supervisors in conducting evaluations, need to be developed.

Ideally, 2 weeks before an evaluation date, the manager completes the form, sending a copy to the employee, together with notification of time and place of the evaluation. This gives the employee time to prepare for the meeting.

At the evaluation the manager reviews the completed form and may modify sections, if appropriate. Performance goals for the next time period are reviewed, modified if employee and manager concur, and, if possible, mutually agreed upon.

At the end of the session both employee and manager should sign the evaluation. Provision is normally made for any addendum the employee may wish to write or for the employee to indicate disagreement with the findings. In the event of such a difference of opinion, appeal procedures should be available.

THE PERFORMANCE EVALUATION PROCESS: PROBLEMS ENCOUNTERED

Whatever the importance to the facility, and however rational the evaluation process may seem, resistance to its effective utilization often arises, making the program difficult to implement (Snell & Wexley, 1985).

Often evaluations are given at the time the employee hopes for an annual raise, focusing primary attention on past performance rather than future performance goals. Managers are not normally rewarded when they take time to give thorough evaluations. Most managers are uncomfortable with face-to-face judgmental roles. Employees are highly sensitive to negative evaluations, leading managers to avoid conflict. Employees want the appraising manager to (1) have had adequate opportunity to observe the employee's work thoroughly understand the employee's job, and (3) have clearly stated standards by which to judge the employee's efforts (Smith, 1984). The manager ought to be able to judge the work from an informed viewpoint. Health care aides, for example, prefer someone trained in health care, who presumably understands the nature of their job, to write their evaluation.

Performance evaluations sometimes fail. One major health care facility, the former Hillhaven Corporation, has identified the following as contributing causes to failure: (1) a lack of previously agreed upon objectives, (2) the poor skill of the manager, (3) a lack of a defined evaluation process, and (4) managerial behavior that does not contribute to the self-esteem/self-image of the employee. Employees, the corporation points out, do not normally outperform their self-image: If their self-image is high, high performance can be anticipated; conversely, if their self-esteem is low, low performance will result. Performance evaluations should not be the first time employees hear about problems. A point to remember: Evaluate performance, not the person. One can be candid and specific about performance without attacking the individual.

METHODS OF RATING EMPLOYEES

Rating Scales

Rating scales list a number of characteristics, traits, and/or requirements of the employee's position on a line or scale (Sears, 1984). The evaluator checks off the degree to which the employee is believed to meet a requirement. For example, a scale recording degree of initiative might appear as:

Initiative

Lacks initiative Meets requirements Highly resourceful

Work Quality

Needs to improve Meets standards Exceeds standards

Global Ratings

Often the manager will be asked to provide a global rating for the employee. This normally is a summary score based on the components of the evaluation. Generally, each employer establishes a numeric or alphabetic scale for the facility.

For example, 1 might represent the highest and 5 the lowest rating. Inevitably, the scale comes to resemble the grading system everyone has known in elementary and secondary school: Whatever the symbols used, the person comes to understand that he or she is an A, B, C, or D performer—or an F, in which case a termination notice might be pending. However much or little the manager may write or discuss with the employee, the employee's real concern is "Am I a top performer, and if not, why not?" because the employee knows that the top performers get first crack at whatever rewards the system has to give, whether promotions, bonuses, salary increases, or high status.

Errors Made by Managers Using Rating Scales

Rating scales, too, have their problems. At least three types of errors occur.

The Leniency Error. To avoid conflict, some supervisors give consistently high ratings. The lenient supervisor's ratings are difficult to compare with those of a stricter and more demanding supervisor.

The Error of Central Tendency. Other supervisors consistently give only moderate scores to employees, regardless of whether their performance is poor or outstanding, placing their better employees at a competitive disadvantage.

The Halo Effect. The halo effect occurs when a supervisor who values one particular type of job behavior (e.g., punctuality) permits the presence or absence of this one trait to color ratings for other traits. A habitually late employee might be excellent in resident care but be rated low in most categories because the supervisor is irritated by the persistent tardiness.

Rating by Essay. The use of essays describing employee progress is less common than rating scales. It is especially difficult to compare employees when the essay method permits supervisors simply to write whatever evaluative comments occur to them. A brief essay at the end of a rating scale can be valuable, however.

Possible Outcomes from Evaluations. Evaluations are primarily intended to give feedback to the employee about performance to date and projected activities. Results can be transfer, promotion or demotion, layoff, or discharge.

Transfer. A transfer is the placement of an employee to another position that is approximately equivalent to the present position.

Promotion. A promotion is placement of an employee at a higher level within the facility or group of facilities (e.g., promotion to a job at the regional or corporate level). There are at least two recognized bases for promotions: merit and seniority. Seniority is concerned with length of service and tends to be automatic. The merit system relies on performance evaluations of supervisors for placement of a worker at a higher level. Under the seniority system a nurse's aide who serves the required number of months or years at level 1 is automatically promoted to level 2. Under the merit system a nurse's aide may or many not be promoted from level 1 to level 2, depending on evaluation decisions of the supervisor.

Demotion. Demotion is the change of assignment of an employee to a lower level in the organization, usually with less pay, fewer responsibilities, and reduced status. "Demotions" are often accomplished by the use of transfers. A formerly more productive employee may be transferred to another position, with pay and status remaining intact. Another alternative to demotion is promotion to a position with little responsibility or power.

Layoff. Layoffs are normally temporary dismissals and are potentially demoralizing to the remaining employees as well as to those laid off. Unambiguous layoff policies can reduce anxiety among the remaining employees. However, such policies also tie the hands of management, who might, for example, seek to retain a recent but especially valued employee. Layoffs are carefully scrutinized by employees for fairness and equity in their implementation.

Discharge. When companies downsize, some basis for deciding who is dismissed is exercised. Discharging those employees with the lowest evaluation ratings first is a frequently used approach.

COP VS. COACH

One reason why some experts advise against performance evaluation reviews is that it places the manager more nearly in the role of cop than coach. The performance evaluation usually focuses on areas for improvement, the negative side of the employee's work. The focus is on what the employee is not doing right rather than on his or her strengths. The work area manager is the employee's coach. The coach's job is to bring out the best in the individual. When managers cite an employee's weaknesses in the performance evaluation, the employee feels more busted than trusted. It is the employee's strengths, not weaknesses, that will carry the employee through to success. As Kreigel (1991) observes, one can get by improving upon weaknesses; one can become great by building on strengths.

Evaluation Do's and Don'ts Learned by One Corporation

The following useful ideas about evaluations are made by one large major long-term-care corporation:

- Evaluation information should be given only to those who have a definite need and legal right.

- Evaluations should be conducted in private.
- It is unfair to an employee not to be frank with him or her in an evaluation interview and discuss areas of needed improvement.
- The evaluation form should accurately reflect the employee's performance.
- Effective evaluation interviews that produce results take time.
- Evaluations should be made only on those things that are relevant to the job.
- A supervisor will find it difficult to follow up on an "I'll try harder!" solution from the employee.
- If policy permits, the employee has a moral and ethical right to see his or her evaluation form.
- Overrating all employees is a mistake in the long run.
- Recent events, both positive and negative, can unduly bias a performance evaluation interview.

2.9 Paying Employees

The assisted living facility is labor intensive. Careful management of wages and benefits is one of the major sources of cost control available to the assisted living facility administrator.

MONEY = VALUE

The wages paid to the employees normally determine their standard of living. Wages also affect each employee's status both in the facility and in the community. Wages are perceived as a statement by the facility about the relative worth of the skills of each employee.

The most flexible benefit a facility can give to its employees is the paycheck. Health insurance, sick leave, and the like are important, but the benefit most highly valued by the employee is the dollar value of the paycheck, which provides maximum control over the product of his or her work effort.

For the typical assisted living facility employee, the wage rate is salient, and even a difference of a few cents per hour can spell satisfaction or dissatisfaction with wages for an individual making comparisons with a similarly qualified coworker.

COMPENSATION

Compensation is generally considered the reward given employees in exchange for their work effort. How willing an employee may be to work hard and assist the facility toward its goals can depend on how justly the employee feels his or her wages and benefits fit his or her work effort (Belcher, 1974).

Equity Theory

According to equity theory, employees seek an exchange in which their wages and benefits are equal to their work effort, especially when compared to wages and benefits paid to similarly situated coworkers (Whitehill, 1976). If the individual feels equitably paid, less tension may exist. If, however, the individual suspects that others with similar skills and investment of effort receive more, a tension exists that most employees will seek to resolve.

Typical worker responses to perceived inequities are to ask for a pay raise, reduce effort, file a grievance, or, in some cases, seek employment elsewhere. Alternatively, the employee may encourage those perceived as similarly situated but benefiting more not to work so hard. Reactions to perceived inequities can take many forms (Ivancevich et al., 1977).

WAGE POLICES

Developing and administering compensation policies are important administrative duties. Policies should cover such areas as the following (Chruden & Sherman, 1980):

- the rate of pay, set below, at, or above the prevailing community practice
- the discretion supervisors can exercise in differentiating an individual's pay from the set scale
- the amount of spread between pay rates for employees with seniority and pay rates for new employees
- periods between raises and the weight given to seniority and merit in determining a new pay rate

Hourly Wages or Salaries?

Most facilities distinguish between hourly and salaried employees. Hourly employees generally are required to punch in and out on a time clock and are paid only for hours worked, as verified on the time card. Salaried workers, in contrast, are paid a set wage regardless of the hours worked, which may or may not be required to be recorded on a time clock. Usually, work area managers in the assisted living facility are paid a set salary. However, some work area managers (e.g., the head of dietary) who encounter numerous occasions for long days may negotiate to work on an hourly basis or be paid overtime after a negotiated number of hours have been worked in each pay period.

HOW MUCH TO PAY: THE WAGE MIX

Determining wage rates and benefits is a complex task affected by a number of factors called the wage mix. The wage mix consists of

- the labor market
- prevailing wage rates
- cost of living increases
- collective bargaining
- individual bargaining
- key job comparisons
- wage classes

The Labor Market

Once government requirements for minimum wage rates are met and the influence of unions is taken into account, supply and demand dramatically affect the wage rate. During the early decades of the 20th century physicians were able to restrict their numbers. This resulted in favorable influences on their incomes, which now average well over $100,000 per year. Similarly, the nurse shortage of the early 1990s resulted in dramatic increases in nurses' wages.

Prevailing Wage Rates

According to one government study, more than half of businesses surveyed indicated that the prevailing wage scale for comparable jobs in their communities was the most influential factor in determining wages actually paid.

This tends to be true for assisted living facilities, which generally are viewed as paying somewhat lower salaries to employee categories such as aides than do local hospitals. In general, the local hospital's and nursing homes' wage rate sets the prevailing wage rate against which the other health care providers set their own pay scales. ("Long Term Care Employee Shortage," 1986).

Wage surveys for the community or region are taken by many organizations. They may be carried out by a single facility or through agreements with others to share this information (Brennan, 1984a). In many communities assisted living facilities share wage information with each other and other health providers.

Cost of Living Increases

During periods of inflation a cost of living adjustment may be made in wage rates. The purpose of the cost of living increase is to help workers to maintain their purchasing power. These increases, often embodied in escalator clauses of labor contracts, provide for wage adjustments based on some index, usually the consumer price index (CPI). The CPI is a government-defined measure of the cost of living compared to a base point, usually of a few years earlier, which is designated as 100. Any increase or decrease in the cost of living is then expressed as a percentage of the base figure of 100.

Collective Bargaining

Where employees are unionized (discussed in Part Four), assisted living facilities are subject to union influences, regardless of wage rates paid.

Individual Bargaining

Individuals with especially desirable skills may be able to negotiate a higher wage than others in similar positions. When a highly qualified maintenance director or resident care coordinator, for example, is sought, the facility may bargain with a candidate and offer him or her a premium.

Key Job Comparisons

In the assisted living facility the wages paid in the health care area tend to become the benchmark against which the earnings of other staff members are compared and established.

Wage Classes and Rates

To approach equity and achieve some flexibility for supervisors who evaluate employees, wage classes or grades and wage rates are normally established (Brennan, 1984a). All jobs within a class are paid at the same rate or within the same rate range. A rate range is the variation permitted within a class or grade.

2.10 Disciplining Employees

The following are some of the more common staff disciplinary problems faced by assisted living facilities:

- excessive or unexcused absences or tardiness
- leaving the facility or work area without permission
- violation of rules about smoking, intoxication, narcotics, gambling, fighting, firearms
- failure to follow safety procedures
- failure to accept direction
- failure to report accidents
- failure to take resident safety and welfare into account
- verbal, physical, or other abuse of residents
- theft, punching another employee's time card, falsifying records
- insubordinate behavior or abusive language
- failure to report an illness
- solicitation or acceptance of gratuities from residents or their families
- immoral, indecent, or disorderly conduct

RULES AND CONSEQUENCES

Each facility should carefully state and consistently enforce policies regarding disciplinary actions. The employees must be made fully aware, before any infraction occurs, of both the facility's rules and the disciplinary action that may result (Cameron, 1984; Hill, 1984). Although policies and rules may have been clearly formulated, these statements remain confusing unless they are continually reinforced by positive (motivating) and negative (disciplining) actions (Discenza & Smith, 1985). Unless the facility can document that it had a just cause for firing an employee, there is a significant chance that the employee will be able to collect unemployment benefits.

Grievance Procedures

Grievance procedures are an important safety valve for policies regarding disciplinary actions. Employees need to know that there are equitable procedures through which their reactions and views can be expressed when they feel they have been dealt with unfairly.

Progressive Discipline

For most offenses, progressive discipline—beginning with verbal warnings, followed by written warnings for any subsequent violations—makes the most sense. Progressive discipline may prevent repetition of the offending behavior after only a verbal warning, thus bringing about an early solution to the problem.

Employees who are dismissed have the right to present their case to the local Employment Security Commission, and many do. It is necessary for the employer to keep a well-documented record of having made every reasonable effort to persuade the employee to conform to facility policy before dismissal (Tobin, 1976). The administration needs to be able to demonstrate that disciplinary actions taken were based on rational judgments about the offending behavior, not on personal vindictiveness or excessive emotional reactions of supervisors to employee behavior.

Each facility needs to define clearly its own policies governing suspension and discharge procedures. Normally, several managers, including the administrator, participate in a decision to suspend or discharge an employee.

One major long-term-care chain (the former Hillhaven Corporation) recommends the following be assured regarding employee discipline:

- that the requirement reasonably relates to the operation of the facility and that the requirement has been properly communicated
- that management has investigated the matter fairly, objectively, and in a timely manner
- that the requirements and penalties are and have been administered fairly and objectively, without any form of discrimination
- that the situation is dealt with and a penalty determined in a manner consistent with past practice for similar situations
- that the penalty is appropriate to the seriousness of the infraction
- that misconduct (e.g., resident abuse, theft, or substance abuse) is reported to the appropriate agency for investigation according to state or federal regulations
- that where discharge is the penalty, employees have warning or knowledge of the probable consequences of their actions

Discharging Employees

The process of terminating employees, especially executives, can be eased by helping those individuals find alternative employment. This is called disemployment, outplacement, or dehiring (Chruden & Sherman, 1980). The managers themselves may help an employee to find another position or hire an employment firm to do so.

References

Allen, L. A. (1973). M for management: Theory Y updated. *Personnel Journal, 52*(12), 1061–1067.

Argenti, P. A. (1994). *The portable MBA desk reference.* New York: Wiley.

Argyris, C. (1972). A few words in advance. In A. J. Marrow (Ed.), *The failure of success.* New York: AMACOM.

Assisted Living. (1997). Fairfax, VA: Assisted Living Federation of America.

Assisted Living. (1998). Fairfax, VA: Assisted Living Federation of America.

Assisted Living Business Week. (1998). Vol 2, Nos. 2, 5, 7, 11 . 7–54.

Baker, H. K., & Morgan, P. I. (1984). Two goals in every performance appraisal. *Personnel Journal, 63*(9), 74–78.

Belcher, D. W. (1974). *Compensation administration.* Englewood Cliffs, NJ: Prentice-Hall.

Bianco, V. (1984). In praise of performance. *Personnel Journal, 63*(6), 40–50.

Boling, T. E., et al. (1983). *Nursing home management.* Springfield, IL: Charles C Thomas.

Brennan, E. J. (1984a). Everything you need to know about salary ranges. *Personnel Journal, 63*(3), 10–16.

_____. (1984b). Restraint of the free labor market. *Personnel Journal, 63*(5), 22–25.

Bryan, L. A. (1984). Making the manager a better trainer. *Supervisory Management, 29*(4), 2–8.

Buttaro, P. J. (1980). *Home study program in principles of administration of long term health care facilities.* Aberdeen, SD: Health Care Facility Consultants Publishers.

Cameron, D. (1984). The when, why, and how of discipline. *Personnel Journal, 63*(7), 37–39.

Carter, M. F., & Shapiro, K. P. (1983). Develop a proactive approach to employee benefits planning. *Personnel Journal, 62*(7), 562–566.

Caudill, M. E., & Patrick, M. C. (1992). Turnover among nursing assistants. *Journal of Long Term Care Administration,* pp. 29–32.

Chruden, H. J., & Sherman, A. W., Jr. (1980). *Personnel management* (6th ed.). Cincinnati: South-Western Publishing.

Cole, A., Jr. (1983). Flexible benefits are a key to better employee relations. *Personnel Journal, 63*(1), 49–53.

Davis, W. E. (1985). *Introduction to health care administration.* Bossier City, LA: Publicare Press.

Delaney, W. A. (1984). The misuse of bonuses. *Supervisory Management, 29*(1), 28–31.

Discenza, R., & Smith, H. L. (1985). Is employee discipline obsolete? *Personnel Administrator, 30*(6), 175–186.

Dunnette, M. D., & Kirchner, W. K. (1965). *Psychology applied to industry.* New York: Appleton-Century-Crofts.

Employee performance: Evaluation and control. (1975). Washington, DC: Bureau of National Affairs (Personnel Policies Forum Survey No. 108).

Equal Employment Opportunity Commission, Civil Service Commission, Department of Labor, & Department of Justice. (1978). Adoption by four agencies of uniform guidelines on employee selection procedures. *Federal Register, 43*(166), 38290–38315.

Focus on retirement. (1998, March 9). *The Wall Street Journal,* p. 22.

Givnta, J. (1984). For good job training, you need a good beginning. *Supervisory Management, 29*(6), 19–21.

Gomez-Mejia, L. R., Page, R. C., & Tornow, W. W. (1985). Improving the effectiveness of performance appraisal. *Personnel Administrator, 30*(1), 74–82.

Gordon, E. K., & Stryker, R. C. (1983). *Creative long term care administration.* Springfield, IL: Charles C Thomas.

Grant, D. A., & Kenmore, J. C. (1993). How to conduct security checks on prospective employees. *Nursing Homes,* pp. 12–14.

Green, E. (1977, October 17). Heart disease: New ways to reduce the risk. *Business Week,* pp. 135–142.

Haslinger, J. A. (1985). Flexible compensation: Getting a return on benefit dollars. *Personnel Administrator, 30*(6), 39–46, 224.

Hershizer, B. (1984). An MBO approach to discipline. *Supervisory Management, 29*(3), 2–7.

Herzlinger, R. E., & Calkins, D. (1984). How companies tackle health care costs: Part 3. *Harvard Business Review, 64*(1), 70–80.

Hill, N. C. (1984). The need for positive reinforcement in corrective counseling. *Supervisory Management, 29*(1), 10–14.

Hoff, R. D. (1983). The impact of cafeteria benefits on the human resource information system. *Personnel Journal, 62*(4), 282–283.

Ivancevich, J. M., Szjlagyi, A., & Wallace, M. (1977). *Organizational behavior and performance.* Santa Monica, CA: Goodyear Publishing.

Jauch, L. R. (1976). Systematizing the selecting decision. *Personnel Journal, 55*(11), 564–567.

Kessler, F. (1985, July 22). Executive perks under fire. *Fortune, 112*(2), 26–31.

Kriegel, R. J. (1991). *If it ain't broke.* New York: Warner.

Kruzick, J. M. (1995). Empowering organization contexts. *Gerontologist, 35,* 207–216.

Lawler, E. E., III. (1973). *Motivation in work organizations.* Monterey, CA: Brooks/Cole.

Locher, A. H., & Teel, K. S. (1977). Performance appraisal—A survey of current practices. *Personnel Journal, 56*(5), 245–247, 254–255.

Locke, E. A. (1968). Toward a theory of task motivation and incentives. *Organizational Behavior and Human Performance, 3*(2), 157–189.

Long term care employee shortage taking shape nationwide. (1986). *Today's Nursing Home, 7*(10), 2–3.

Lorsch, J. W., & Takagi, H. (1986). Keeping managers off the shelves. *Harvard Business Review, 64*(4), 60–65.

Matheny, P. R. (1984). How to hire a winner. *Supervisory Management, 29*(5), 12–15.

McGregor, D. M. (1960). *The human side of enterprise.* New York: McGraw-Hill.

McMillan, J., & Hickok, S. D. (1984). Taking stock of the options. *Personnel Journal, 63*(4), 32–37.

Meehl, P. E. (1954). *Clinical vs. statistical prediction.* Minneapolis: University of Minnesota Press.

Meyer, M. C. (1977). Six stages of demotivation. *International Management, 32*(4), 14–17.

Miller, D. B. (Ed.). (1982). *Long term care administrator's desk manual.* Greenvale, NY: Panel Publishers.

Now we know why they're so friendly. (1985, July 22). *Fortune,* p. 120.

Olian, J. D., Carroll, S. J., Jr., & Schneier, C. (1985). It's time to start using your pension system to improve the bottom line. *Personnel Administrators, 30*(4), 77–83, 152.

Owen, D. E. (1984). Profile analysis: Matching positions and personnel. *Supervisory Management, 29*(11), 14–20.

Peters, T., & Austin, N. (1985, May 13). A passion for excellence, *Fortune,* 20–32.

Printz, R. A., & Waldman, D. A. (1985). The merit of merit pay. *Personnel Administrator, 30*(1), 84–90.

Riter, R. N. (1993). Some practical advice for the new nursing home administrator. *Journal of Long Term Care Administration,* pp. 40–41.

Rodman, T. A. (1984). Make the praise equal the raise. *Personnel Journal, 63*(11), 73–78.

Rogers, W. W. (1980). *General administration in the nursing home* (3rd ed.). Boston: CBI Publishing.

Rothberg, D. S. (1986). Part-time professionals: The flexible work force. *Personnel Administrator, 31*(8), 29–32.

Rotondi, T., Jr. (1976). Behavior modification on the job. *Supervisory Management, 21*(2), 22–28.

Ruhl, M. J., & Atkinson, K. (1986). Interactive video training: One step beyond. *Personnel Administrator, 51*(5), 360–363.

Scott, R. (1972). Job expectancy—An important factor in labor turnover. *Personnel Journal, 51*(5), 360–363.

Scott, S. (1983). Finding the right person. *Personnel Journal, 62*(11), 894–902.

Sears, D. L. (1984). Situational performance appraisals. *Supervisory Management, 29*(5), 6–10.

Smith, K. E. (1984). Performance appraisal: A positive management tool. *College Review, 1*(2).

Snell, S. A., & Wexley, K. N. (1985). Performance diagnosis: Identifying the causes of poor performance. *Personnel Administrator, 30*(4), 117–127.

Steers, R. M., & Porter, L. W. (1979). *Motivation and work behavior* (2nd ed.). New York: McGraw-Hill.

Thierauf, R. J., Klekamp, & Geeding, (1977). *Management principles and practices.* New York: Wiley.

Tobin, J. E. (1976). How arbitrators decide to reject or uphold an employee discharge. *Supervisory Management, 21*(6), 20–23.

US Senate Special Committee on Aging, *Assisted Living Workgroup's final report,* April 29, 2003.

Vroom, V. H. (1964). *Work and motivation.* New York: Wiley.

Wehrenberg, S. B. (1983). How to decide on the best training approach. *Personnel Journal, 62*(2), 117–118.

White, E. (1984). Trust—A prerequisite for motivation. *Supervisory Management, 29*(2), 22–25.
Whitehill, A. M., Jr. (1976). Maintenance factors. *Personnel Journal, 55*(10), 516–519.

PART THREE

FINANCING AND BUSINESS OPERATIONS

3.0 Overview: Position of the Assisted Living Industry

No matter how skilled an assisted living administrator may be at communicating and managing human resources, if the administrator does not manage financial resources equally as well, he or she will enjoy only a brief career in this field.

TABLE 3.1 Senior Housing Construction: Total Properties by Type: 1997-2003

	1997	1998	1999	2000	2001	2002	2003
Senior Apartments	31	38	41	32	52	44	77
Independent Living	77	89	103	93	65	43	51
Assisted Living	294	460	403	164	89	43	71
Continuing Care (CCRCs)	33	27	44	31	24	20	23

Source: *American Seniors Housing Association, Seniors Housing Construction Report,* 2003, p. 14.

The Era / Error of Positive EBITDAR

As seen in the table above, the years 1997, 1998 and 1999 were years of heavy construction. In those years before the stock market's technology crash in 2000-2001 investment capital flowed freely into the assisted living industry. The industry marketed itself using a formula called EBITDAR which is net income plus depreciation and amortization plus deferred taxes. This formula, it turned out, was not a sustainable business model formula by which to analyze the financials of the assisted living industry.

The assisted living sector is influenced by a myriad of forces. Macroeconomic changes such as the stock market decline and the subsequent reduction in available of investment money affect the industry. During the years 1997 through 1999 supply outstripped demand: more assisted living units were built than the market could absorb. As the performance of individual projects declined the availability of debt and equity sources declined.

The dramatic influx of public money and the involvement of Wall Street as sources of new equity through stock and bond offerings led to dramatic building programs which, in a number of geographical areas, resulted in more units being built than could be absorbed. This can be illustrated by the assisted living industry expense ratios over the years 1994 through 2002. The expense ratio is the projected expenses for the first stabilized operating year (i.e., full occupancy), including management and capital reserves, divided by the projected revenues (Table 3.2).

The percentages in Table 3.2 suggest that, as the years have passed, the operating expenses have steadily risen as a proportion of revenues. This is likely due to a number of factors, but the increasing acuity of the assisted living resident is a major contributor to the increasing costs of providing services to persons who enter assisted living facilities. In sum, more debt per unit built was often assumed than the actual occupancy levels, or ability to charge high enough monthly rents to pay for the pervasive higher-acuity-than-expected resident population, would sustain.

TABLE 3.2 Expense Ratios of Assisted Living Facilities 1994 - 2002

1994	1995	1996	1997	1998	1999	2000	2001	2002
62%	69%	63%	66%	73%	74%	72%	75%	79%

Source: *American Seniors Housing Association, Seniors Housing Investment & Transaction Report,* 2003, p. 4.

TABLE 3.3 Sales Data for Assisted Living Facilities, 1994 – 2002 Median Price per Unit

1994	1995	1996	1997	1998	1999	2000	2001	2002
$39,000	$60,000	$65,000	$63,000	$80,000	$75,000	$90,000	$72,000	$78,000

Source: *Seniors Housing Investment & Transaction Report,* 2003, p. 4

The median price rose to $90,000, then dropped to $72,000 as a number of chains went into bankruptcy and distressed sales were made (Table 3-3).

By the year 2002 debt sources such as Wall Street offerings and bond offerings were drying up. In that year the very limited debt sources available were mostly from Fannie Mae, Freddie Mac (semi-public mortgage lenders) and the federal Housing and Urban Development (HUD) authority. The former debt sources such as local and regional banks, life insurance companies and pension funds were showing little interest in lending money to the assisted living industry.

Over the years 1994 – 2002 a number of consolidations were taking place within the industry as larger chains bought smaller chains.

Distressed Sales

During the years 1999 through 2002, 74 distressed sales occurred in the seniors housing industry with nearly 70% of all distressed sales being assisted living facilities. Distressed sales included those not generating positive cash flow at the time of sale; those sold out of bankruptcy; those sold by operators in dire need of cash.

Regional Comparison of Per Unit Distressed Sales Compared to Stable Facility Sales

The probable discount of the sale of a distressed facility compared to a stable facility was:

New England:	5%
South Atlantic:	35%
North Central:	7%
South Central	6%

Source: Seniors Housing Investment & Transaction Report, 2003, p. 24

Actual Losses

The actual losses appear to be greater than the above figures. Since most of the units sold in distressed sales were built at a cost of $120,000 to $150,000 per unit during the years 1998 through 2003, distressed properties were actually selling at $ .50 to $.60 per $1.00 of actual hard cost to build these units.

Shareholder Losses

The above figures do not take into account the literal billions of dollars of market value and venture capital invested which has been lost as chains declared bankruptcy and investors lost all their money or received pennies on the dollars invested.

Off-Balance Sheet Financing

A number of assisted living owners used financing which, until July, 2003, did not have to be reported in their financial statements because until July, 2003 companies only had to include those entities in which they had a controlling voting interest. Thus loan which increased the debt load more than represented in financial reports did not have to be reported. Currently the Financial Accounting Standards Board requires that transactions must be reported whenever a company stands to absorb a majority of the expected losses or benefit from the bulk of expected returns.

Getting a Perspective

It is important to understand business cycles and the normal operation of the free market. Assisted living construction has been largely unregulated. Builders were free to overbuild as dramatically as they wished. The overbuilding was made possible by the abundant availability of venture capital and other sources of investment to a relatively new industry: assisted living units. Investors had no history with which to compare the rate of building and the likelihood of the market absorbing the units constructed.

Overbuilding is not a characteristic of just the assisted living industry. During the same years 1996 through 2003 the apartment industry and the office building industry were busy expanding just as far beyond the capacity of the market, and all the new construction could not be absorbed quickly enough to produce the revenue necessary to pay the mortgages or bondholders. By 2003, there was as large a glut of apartments and empty office space as assisted living units.

The construction industry has historically overbuilt whenever interest rates come down, i.e., when inexpensive money is available. Overbuilding with the inevitable slow absorption of new construction is the way the free market has functioned in the U.S. for several decades. The assisted living industry had a lot of company.

3.0.1 Evaluating the Financial Strength of the Assisted Living Provider

A group of assisted living industry financial managers developed the following criteria for evaluating the financial soundness of an assisted living facility provider:

1. Cost and access to capital
2. Acquisition and development skills
3. Portable building model and product line
4. Health care industry knowledge skills
5. Efficiency
6. Higher acuity services
7. Effective community relations and marketing
8. Managed care

SIZE OF THE FACILITY

Size affects efficiency. In general, a facility with 60 to 100 residents is more efficient that one with only 20 or 30 units. In 2002, the median size of assisted living facilities was 80 (American Seniors Housing Association, *The State of Seniors Housing*, 2002). See Tables 3.4 and 3.5.

TABLE 3.4 Size Distribution of Assisted Living Residences by Number of Beds

1-40		**22.5%**
41-80		**29.4%**
81-120		**34.3%**
121 +		**13.7%**

Source: American Seniors Housing Association, *The State of Seniors Housing*, 2002, p. 19.

Table 3.5 Median Square Footage and Distribution for Assisted Living Communities

Common Area	14,000
Net Rentable Area	20,000
Gross Building Area	33,000
% Common Area	41.2
% Net Rentable	58.8

Source: American Seniors Housing Association, *The State of Seniors Housing,* 2002, p. 19.

General Assisted Living Industry Data

The median acreage of an assisted living community was 3 acres. The average number of years open is four years. Seventy three percent of assisted living communities have been built since 1996. Approximately 97% of assisted living communities are for profit, 3% not for profit. Management of these communities was 63% self managed, 17% by an affiliate of owner, and 20% managed by a third party (American Seniors Housing Association, 2002, pp. 19-24). Payment plans by assisted living facilities is nearly all (98%+) rental. Less than 2% charge entrance fees. The average length of stay was 15 months in regular units and 4 months in Alzheimer units in 2002. On average, most facilities increased their fees by about 5% each year.

COST AND ACCESS TO CAPITAL

The REITs

Real estate investment trusts (REITs) were the major funding source for assisted living providers during the years 1994 through 1999. REITs are an investment vehicle in which a number of investors pool their money to make investments in real estate. Special tax rules apply to REITs, such as requiring that 90% of all income be distributed to the investors each year. Typically, assisted living investors use REITs to obtain cash to purchase or build facilities. Often the sale/leaseback approach is used, in which the assisted living provider "sells" the project to the REIT, then leases the buildings back for a specified period of time, usually a number of years. REIT money shrank when earnings shrank.

REIT Leases

REIT leases are formulated in a variety of ways, sometimes providing for ultimate ownership by the assisted living facility investor, sometimes by the REIT. The REIT form of financing is attractive because it requires the least amount of up-front equity from the assisted living provider and has off-balance sheet characteristics. Off-balance sheet items are those items that are not required to be reported in financial statements that nevertheless have an impact on the operations of the provider. This may benefit the new assisted living provider, because operating leases do not have to be reported on the provider's financial statements as a long-term liability. Capital leases (i.e., leases in which the lessee acquired substantial property rights) must, in contrast, be reported. Providers that depend on the REIT financing are often at a disadvantage compared to providers who are self-funding or use bank lines of credit for financing.

Providers that are self-funding or use bank lines typically have lower financing costs and are thus able to compete more effectively in the market. Providers using their own cash or bank lines will have stronger balance sheets and will be better able to make further acquisitions.

ACQUISITION AND DEVELOPMENT SKILLS

Because the assisted living industry is in its infancy, most providers expect to grow by acquiring additional facilities or by building new facilities. This occurred during the years 1995 through 2003. Knowing what to pay for new acquisitions and having the management expertise to manage the newly acquired or built facilities will directly affect the performance of the provider. As providers expand into new regions of the country, they must have on board or acquire the expertise necessary to cope with the varying zoning, health care licensing, and related requirements that differ from state to state. Most providers purchased facilities during the heady days of the expanding stock market of the late 1990s. When this future failed to materialize, many went bankrupt.

Failure to manage new acquisitions or newly built facilities will result in cost overruns and greater than anticipated start-up costs, which may lead to financial instability. Further, the expected pressures for greater and greater cost effectiveness in managing the costs of each facility will be navigated only by providers with a high level of management expertise.

PORTABLE BUILDING MODEL AND PRODUCT LINE

Most providers are exhibiting a desire to expand regionally, if not nationally. To successfully accomplish this, they should have a thought-through product (e.g., facilities of *x* number of beds or units, each with an Alzheimer's wing, which is transferable to several sections of the country and which can be marketed to two or more economic groups).

The point is often made that "demographics don't buy, people do." Each region of the country has its own flavor, its own lifestyle and architectural preferences. Providers that do not take regional variations into account may end up with low occupancies in neighborhoods in which all the demographics are right, but the facility profile is out of sync. The ability to market to several income ranges with a variable product line improves the likelihood of long-term success.

HEALTH CARE INDUSTRY KNOWLEDGE SKILLS

To the extent assisted living facilities help residents to age in place, these facilities will be increasingly involved in providing health-related care. The health care field is a rapidly and constantly changing arena and will remain so for some time. Knowledge of how health care works, including the trends in service delivery and reimbursement mechanisms, will be necessary in order for the assisted living facility provider to survive.

Assisted living providers may enter joint ventures with nursing home providers, managed care organizations, hospitals, and home health care agencies. Knowledge of how these other health care organizations function, their politics and reimbursement trends, is information necessary to the survival of the assisted living facility of the future.

HIGHER ACUITY SERVICES

The financial experts who developed this list believed that implementing the concept of aging in place (remaining in a facility even as one's health deteriorates) is essential to the assisted living industry. They anticipate that successful assisted living facilities will offer an increasingly broader array of health care services. Those that do, they feel, will experience higher-margin revenues and a reduction in both resident turnover and, hence, marketing costs. That is the up side. On the down side, facilities offering an array of health care services must staff at higher staff to resident ratios. As assisted living facilities begin to approach the lower levels of health care traditionally offered by nursing homes, the proportion of revenue devoted to personnel costs has risen dramatically.

EFFECTIVE COMMUNITY RELATIONS AND MARKETING

Full census is the key to operating success. To achieve initial lease-up and quick turnover, a facility must be well connected in its community. Networking with hospital discharge personnel, nursing homes, home health care agencies, independent living facilities, and other providers is a necessary key to facility survival. To the extent the facility understands that good community relations are important, the census is likely to remain high.

Typically, it takes a year for a new facility to reach full capacity. Therefore, any favorable press, even before ground is broken for the facility, will positively affect the start-up and its associated high costs.

MANAGED CARE

While the final shape of health care delivery is not yet clear, the role that managed care and third-party payer organizations will play in assisted living's future is expected to be dramatic. Private managed care providers such as health maintenance organizations and preferred provider organizations, along with public providers such as Medicaid, may pay for resident care in the assisted living setting. This has two major implications: (1) The facility must fully understand its own costs and (2) the facility must implement a resident care record system that enables it to measure and report resident care outcomes to third-party payers. This means that health care record keeping in the assisted living facility must be compatible with record keeping used by the other providers in the health care industry. As residents age in place and require more and more extensive health care related services, third-party demands for sophisticated assisted living record keeping will need to approach that of health maintenance organizations and nursing homes.

All of this looks promising, but the road to financial solvency for the assisted living industry will become narrower as cost-conscious third-party payers such as managed care providers, Medicaid, and others use assisted living facilities, reducing the percent of individually private-paying residents.

3.0.2 Cost of Assisted Living Services

Assisted living facilities, in the mid-1990s cost perhaps 35% less than nursing homes and perhaps 15% less than home health care (Martin, 1997). However, as the acuity level of assisted living facilities rises, costs also are rising to more nearly approximate the cost of skilled nursing care. This occurs because it is necessary to staff at a higher level and to provide more amenities to safely care for and retain the residents. As the price difference decreases, the assisted living facility must market itself as a better and safe alternative to the nursing facility, i.e., a better quality of life at (typically) a lower monthly cost.

As can be seen in Table 3.6 California and Texas experienced the highest rates of construction between 1997 and 2003. This was 52% of all construction in the U.S

TYPES OF DEVELOPMENT: JOINT VENTURE OR STRATEGIC PARTNERSHIPS

Participants in joint ventures or strategic partnerships enjoy a number of advantages. The costs of development are shared by combining developers who have real estate and industry expertise with the referral network of the partner. Financially solvent partners, such as hospitals, medical groups, skilled nursing facilities, and privately owned health care organizations, can provide either necessary capital or increased access to construction financing at low interest rates due to the credit rating and borrowing power of the joint venture partner. Such an arrangement can provide both ownership to the operator and a positive rate of return on investment for the partner. Partial ownership of assisted living facilities by hospitals, medical groups, or nursing facilities creates a new synergy and an improved network for referrals.

TABLE 3.6 Geographical Location of New Construction

Between the years 1997 and 2003 the top 10 states by number of properties built were:

California	289
Texas	204
Florida	172
North Carolina	108
New Jersey	103
Pennsylvania	100
Arizona	100
New York	90
Michigan	85
Illinois	81

(Source: American Seniors Housing Association, *Seniors Housing Construction Report*, 2003.)

TYPES OF DEVELOPMENT: FRANCHISING

Franchising is often used to enter a unique market or to overcome capital limitations. It has been successful in the fast food industry and the hotel and inn keeping industry. In 1997 three publicly traded assisted living facility groups used the franchise approach. While issues of risk management do exist for fast food chains and motels, the use of franchisees in the health care field is even more complicated. Quality control of each facility is more difficult under the franchise model than other models of corporate control.

ECONOMIC PROFILE OF A STABILIZED ASSISTED LIVING FACILITY

What is the occupancy rate? How many residents does a facility have to have to break even or make money? The answer varies dramatically depending of the debt load of the facility (the more debt the larger the number of occupants needed to break even) and many additional factors such as ability to charge enough to make money, or the ability to attract mostly light care residents, and similar factors. But on the whole, the break even point is typically about 85% occupied, often higher.

According to the National Investment Center for the Seniors Housing and Care Industries (NIC) the average occupancy rate reported by the NIC for the fourth quarter of 2002 was 85%, falling to 83.5% in the first quarter of 2003 (*Provider*, September, 2003, p. 19).

3.0.3 Financing Industry Growth

From 1994 to 1996 the assisted living industry enjoyed a large infusion of invested dollars from equity offerings, convertible debt offerings, and REIT financing. Beginning in about 1998 sources of cash began to dry up as assisted living facility chains sought bankruptcy protections.

OTHER METHODS OF FINANCING ASSISTED LIVING CONSTRUCTION

HUD Section 232

Favorable financing terms are available through the 1992 Housing Act and the U.S. Department of Housing and Urban Development (HUD) 232 Act, with low interest rate mortgages, minimal equity requirements for up to 90% of cost of the real estate on which the units are built, and a long-term repayment period. Only 68% of the total development costs may be financed, however.

As of 1997 only 15 assisted living facilities (1,273 units) had been financed through HUD, since there are location requirements and extensive government regulations involved. A recent fast track program is allowing applicants to proceed faster.

Tax Exempt Bonds/Mortgages from States

Under this approach, the assisted living facility operator must be a nonprofit entity (qualifying for the 501(c)3 designation under the Internal Revenue Service rules) or a governmental body, such as a county or city government. After meeting conditions required by the governmental entity granting the tax-exempt status (usually a city, county, or state government), the assisted living facility operator may sell the bonds (usually to the public). The advantage to the bond purchaser is a tax exemption on the interest paid on the bonds.

Conventional Lenders

Typically banks or savings and loan associations, these lenders require 10% to 30% equity, working capital reserve to pay for at least one year of start-up deficits, debt coverage ratios exceeding 1.2 times on stabilized facilities, cash collateral or debt service reserves, monthly reporting, funded replacement reserves up to $400 per unit per year to guarantee continuous facility maintenance, and professional liability and other insurance coverage.

Private Funds

Housing programs, venture capital firms, and pension funds have also been sources of financing sought by the assisted living industry.

SSI Candidates

Supplemental Security Income (SSI) is a federal program to provide dollars to shore up the difference between social security income received and the federal poverty level. These dollars are paid directly to individuals, who then may use these dollars to obtain room and board.

State and Local Subsidies

Because some residents, even with social security and SSI, are unable to meet their financial needs, states and local governments may provide additional dollars to enable them to remain financially capable of paying for their care needs. In general, however, this combined income level remains below the average cost of most assisted living facility monthly fees.

Certificate of Need Laws

As of 1997, three states had adopted a version of laws applied to hospitals and nursing homes that require obtaining a certificate of need (CON) from a governmental agency before a building permit can be issued. By 2003 several additional states were contemplating requiring certificates of need.

3.0.4 Pricing Assisted Living Services

The average prices for assisted living facilities can ranged from $70 per day for a private room to $150+ per day for two bedrooms. Industry prices ranged above $200 per day for high-end facilities.

A variety of pricing strategies have evolved in the assisted living industry. The major approaches to pricing are

- home health
- service levels
- actual care
- point system

HOME HEALTH

In this model staff at the assisted living facility help with IADLs and call in home health care agency or similar personnel to help residents perform ADLs. This model allows for health care levels to be easily increased as needed; the disadvantage is that the facility may be left with only the rental fees as income.

SERVICE LEVELS

This model focuses on the amount of time spent providing services per day. A base is established, such as 30 to 90 minutes of care per day, beyond which the resident pays additional monthly fees as the time devoted to that resident rises. The advantage of this model is the ability to closely match individual resident care hours per resident day to monthly charges. The disadvantages are resident and family resistance to frequent modifications to fees and expensive time-keeping efforts on the staff's part to monitor minutes spent each day with each resident.

ACTUAL CARE

A basic price plan is established (often 45 minutes per day), and minutes above 45 minutes per day are billed monthly, much like billing for minutes used for long-distance phone calls. If a daily log of total minutes actually used by each resident is compared to a weekly average of the 315 minutes (7 x 45), the resident may not be billed for extra minutes. The variations to this plan are numerous. Disadvantages, however, are serious. The possibility of accurately keeping track of the minutes spent with each resident may be too expensive in terms of staff record keeping and nearly impossible to do with sufficient precision to please the residents and their families.

POINT SYSTEM

In this system the provider numerically scores the assistance needs of each resident using the IADLs and ADLs as the assistance categories. Scores are aggregated and averaged. Each level of the final score may indicate an increase of the monthly fee by $200 to $300. This is the most frequently used pricing approach because it provides enough precision to allow the facility to cost out care levels on dimensions that can be recognized objectively by both staff and residents. Increments are relatively easy to measure: Either Mr. Brown needs assistance with bathing or not.

For example, the following point system could be used determining whether charges are to be made for bathing and dressing.

Assistance level	Points
Independent	1
Requires assistance only in transferring into and out of the bath but is able to bathe self	2
Requires assistance in bathing and dressing but performs most of the work	3
Requires considerable assistance with bathing and dressing	4
Completely dependent upon staff for bathing and dressing	5

In evaluating a resident's ADLs, the facility can use the following definitions:

1 Point. Independent—No help or staff oversight; or staff help/oversight provided only 1 or 2 times during prior 7 days.
2 Points. Supervision—Oversight, encouragement, or cueing provided 3 or more times during the last 7 days, or supervision plus physical assistance provided only 1 or 2 times during the last 7 days.
3 Points. Limited assistance—Resident highly involved in activity, received physical help in guided maneuvering of limbs, and/or other non-weight-bearing assistance 3 or more times; or more help provided only 1 or 2 times over 7–day period.
4 Points. Extensive assistance—While resident performed part of activity, over prior 7-day period, help of the following type was provided 3 or more times:
 a. Weight-bearing support
 b. Full staff performance during part (but not all) of week.
5 Points. Total dependence—Full staff performance of activity over entire 7–day period.

3.1 The Administrator's Role as Financial Manager

An administrator's duties encompass nearly every aspect of managing the facility, from assisting in the recruitment of professional staff to ensuring the efficient operation of the laundry department. Not surprisingly, the administrator is also finally responsible for the income and expenses of the facility. It is, in reality, the administrator who is the one person held accountable for the entire financial operation of the facility.

SELECTING AND EVALUATING FINANCIAL PERSONNEL

The *bookkeeper* primarily records the daily cash transactions of the facility, keeping track of all money going out or coming in. The *accountant* uses the information compiled by the bookkeeper to generate reports on the financial standing of the facility. The bookkeepers and accountants record the financial transactions, but the administrator is chief financial officer of the facility, not the bookkeepers, accountants, or even the *business manager.*

The administrator must ensure that the business office process runs smoothly—that the bookkeeper is qualified for the job and has access to the information needed for recording all the facility's financial transactions. Thus the administrator must have some knowledge of bookkeeping in order to know whether this important task is carried out as it should be.

The administrator may also have to select an accountant, either as an employee or as a consultant for the facility. If the administrator manages one of a chain of assisted living facilities, the accountant will probably be an employee of the corporation. The administrator should therefore have some understanding of accounting to be able to assess the accountant's performance.

More important, however, the administrator must be able to interpret the financial reports generated by the accountant and the corporate office. The administrator's primary role as financial manager is to use the financial information to make informed decisions about the facility. The administrator needs to know how these reports are prepared.

CORPORATE PURPOSES

Corporations often use individual facilities for various purposes, including to balance the cash flow and tax affairs of the corporation through the network of facilities. A single facility may be carried on the books as having a high debt load, whereas another, similarly situated, may be considered as having a low debt load. The administrator must grasp the nuances of these matters to be able to compare his or her after-debt service figures and taxes with those of a sister facility carried at a different debt load. They may vary, yet the level of success of staff performance may be comparable.

MAINTAINING ENOUGH INCOME

In addition to bookkeeping and accounting, we will take a close look at costs. There are many different types of costs, and we will explore how viewing costs in different ways can provide the administrator with information not included in the financial reports prepared by the accountants.

As the facility's ultimate financial manager, the administrator must ensure the availability of funds for conducting business: to purchase supplies and pay salaries and to meet the regular payments on any borrowed funds. Without these purchases and payments, the facility cannot operate. When money is not available to meet expenses, the facility cannot continue to operate for very long and may be obliged to close its doors.

SETTING RATES

How does the administrator guarantee that the facility will receive sufficient funds? The administrator needs to know how to set rates for the services offered and how to produce the number of residents who will require these services. Appropriate rates for resident care services must reflect their true costs, so the administrator must be able to measure these costs.

Besides being available in sufficient amount, funds must be received on a timely basis. The good financial manager understands the billings and collections procedures that keep money owed to the facility coming in regularly enough to meet financial obligations.

PLANNING AND BUDGETING

Financial management is important to planning and budgeting. To make a financial plan, or a budget, the administrator must be able to predict both the costs of running the facility and the money it can expect to earn in the coming year. Knowledge of the facility's past financial performance and insight into the reason for earlier budget shortfalls or successes are essential for preparing a realistic and useful budget. The administrator who is not familiar with the cost and earnings of all the departments cannot expect to guide the organization on a reliable path in the future.

RESPONSIBILITY TO OTHERS

Finally, by virtue of his or her position as director, the administrator is responsible for the effective operation of the assisted living facility—to its residents and their significant others, to the employees, to the owners or stockholders, and to the governing body of the facility. When signs of ineffective financial management become apparent, it is to the administrator that each of these parties turns for an explanation.

Because nearly every decision made will have financial implications, an understanding of financial management is incumbent on the administrator, the person ultimately responsible for the performance of the facility, even of chain-operated facilities.

However good the relationship of the manager with staff or however capable he or she may be in other aspects of administration, if finances are poorly or improperly handled, the administrator is likely to be judged ineffectual by the board or the facility owners. One New York physician recounted an interview with the head of a large long-term care facility to which he was applying for the role of medical director. To impress her, he presented a long list of desirable (but expensive) actions he would take if appointed medical director. Aghast at the potential costs of the proposals, the head of the facility arose and observed, "Doctor, no margin, no mission."

The Search for a Sustainable Business Model for the Assisted Living Industry

Understanding a sustainable business model for the assisted living industry is vastly complex. Even so, it is not much different from the sets of calculations and speculations each of us must make in, for example, the purchase of a home. We must weigh how much debt we can sustain (what monthly mortgage payment can I sustain?). We must think about what our income is likely to be over the coming years. We must think about all the contingencies that might occur such as: will I keep my job, will I be healthy, and the like. Building and operating an assisted living facility is no different. A sustainable business model must be found. The chains that have gone into bankruptcy failed to provide for continuing successful operations if the scenario they hope occurs does not occur, e.g., the residents are sicker (more expensive to care for) than we had hoped, or if interest rates go up or down dramatically, and the like.

At the end of the first quarter of 2003, the total amount of outstanding project financing debt of the assisted living industry was 5.1 billion dollars of which 2 billion dollars was permanent financing and 2.8 billion short term debt (i.e., loan types that are bridge, acquisition, turn-around, that have less than a 10 year term [National Investment Center for the Seniors housing and Care Industries, September, 2003]).

In the end, successful operation of an assisted living facility is no different than our own personal finances. We need to have a continuing positive cash flow, i.e., some money left over after all our expenses are paid, and a debt load that we can manage even if there are downturns in our finances. Truth be known, it is not that difficult when we insist on assuring that we will be solvent over the coming years, even if we have to go to Plan B or Plan C. Surprising as it may seem, too few corporations have realistic Plan Bs or Plan Cs.

3.2 Generally Accepted Accounting Principles —the GAAPs

The accounting system defines the manner in which financial records must be kept, and it is used by nearly every type of organization, including assisted living facilities. Financial records refers primarily to the books and financial statements of the facility. Books are a set of records that list, in a prescribed manner, each monetary transaction (all money earned or spent) of the facility.

Maintaining the books constitutes bookkeeping. The books are used to prepare the financial statement. The financial statements are simply a summary of all the transactions recorded in the books, and they reflect the soundness of the organization's financial status.

The books and financial statements are prepared according to a series of rules known as the generally accepted accounting principles (GAAPs). These are consistent standards of accounting that allow the financial records to be understood by the various parties who have an interest in the financial position of the facility and also permit the financial statements of different facilities or other organizations to be more easily compared. A discussion of selected GAAPs follows.

ENTITY CONCEPT

Entity is a basic concept of accounting, under which the assisted living facility is regarded as a whole, entirely separate from the affairs of the owners, managers, or other employees. This means that if the owner, for instance, withdraws from or adds to the funds of the facility, this transfer must be recorded in the books to reflect the effect on its finances.

CONSISTENCY CONCEPT

Another basis rule of accounting is the consistency concept. This concept requires that the accounting reports for a facility be prepared in the same way from year to year, in order to compare accurately the reports between two or more different time periods. This does not require that the organization prepare reports in a manner that is not suitable to the needs of management, but suggests that the method of reporting be carefully selected and that changes occur infrequently, if at all. Clearly, financial statements that are prepared in a different format every year will make comparisons difficult.

CONCEPT OF FULL DISCLOSURE

Related to consistency is the concept of full disclosure, which means that all financial information—all money spent, earned, invested, or owed by the facility—must be shown in the financial records to represent accurately the facility's financial standing. The concept of full disclosure has important legal implications, for failure to disclose all financial information may affect the amount of taxes the facility owes or the level of reimbursement it should receive from third-party payers.

TIME PERIOD CONCEPT

Also known as the accounting period, the time period is the interval covered by the financial reports, usually 1 year. The accounting period should be consistent from one year to the next; that is, the fiscal year (the 12-month period designated for financial record keeping) should begin on the same date every year. Accounting records are frequently prepared more often than once a year, usually monthly, to provide management with current information. These shorter time periods should also remain consistent. Typically, monthly financial reports are prepared and distributed to the management, quarterly (every 3 months) and annual reports are prepared and distributed to both managers and ownership.

OBJECTIVE EVIDENCE CONCEPT

The objective evidence concept requires accounting records to be prepared with documentable records that are kept by the facility. Every transaction should be accompanied by a documented record, that is, by a piece of paper that confirms it. These pieces of paper (or equivalent electronic information) are the objective evidence of the transaction; they include receipts for bills that have been paid, bills (or invoices) for money owed by the facility, bank statements indicating interest earned periodically, and cash receipts for money received by the facility each day or designated period. These are called the *source documents* of the transactions. Objective evidence is necessary so that estimates need not be used.

Instead of estimating the cost of supplies purchased during a month, for instance, all invoices are filed in an orderly fashion and used as objective source documents in determining the cost of supplies for the month. Estimates should be used as infrequently as possible, as this introduces an element of error and inconsistency in the accounting reports. When estimates are necessary, the process used in arriving at the estimated figure should be noted in the financial statement.

3.3 Two Approaches to Accounting

There are two systems of accounting: cash and accrual. The difference between the two is primarily the time period in which expenses and revenue are recorded in the books.

Revenue, or the money coming into the facility, can be recorded for the period when, for example, the money from resident care is earned or when the cash payment is actually received by the facility.

Expenses, which will be defined in more depth later, cover the money spent by the facility and can also be recorded in two ways. An expense can be recorded when payment is made for items purchased. In accounting terminology, money paid out is called an *expenditure.* An expense can also be recorded when the items purchased are actually used by the facility.

The difference in the time of recording is the difference between the two systems of accounting and results in two very different ways of preparing the financial records.

CASH ACCOUNTING

In cash accounting, expenses are recorded when the cash is actually disbursed, and revenues are recorded when the money from, for example, resident services is received by the facility. Thus the cash system of accounting simply records expenditures and receipts (the actual flow of cash out of and into the facility) as they occur. Organizations using the cash system of accounting, therefore, do not include in their accounting records "noncash expenses" such as depreciation because depreciation, the cost of wear and tear on equipment, for example, is a cost of providing services to residents that does not involve a cash expenditure.

Cash accounting also does not recognize those expenses that are prepaid, such as insurance paid up for months or years ahead. If the premium for a 3-year insurance policy is paid in the first year that the facility is covered by the policy, an insurance expense would be recorded in the month it is paid and would be listed only as an insurance expenditure for that 1-month period. The fact that it was a prepaid expense and would last over several accounting periods is not acknowledged. Also, money that is owed to the facility for services already provided would not be recorded as accounts receivable, but would be counted as revenue only after the facility received payment. The chief advantage of cash accounting is simplicity; it is similar to an individual's personal checking account.

Cash accounting, however, has several disadvantages, one being that expenses and revenues for a single time period are not attributed to that same period. For example, supplies might be paid for in August but actually used up over the next 4 months. The cost of providing medical services in September would not include the cost of the supplies, as that expense would have been recorded in August. Thus the total cost and revenues, and therefore the real profit or loss for those months, could not be measured accurately.

As already mentioned, the cash accounting system does not recognize the very real cost of depreciation of the facility's building, or plant, major equipment, or other capital items. It also does not recognize money that is owed to creditors by the facility (known as *accounts payable,* a deferred expense) or money that is owed to the facility by residents for services provided (*accounts receivable,* a deferred revenue).

Finally, since the only means of recording expenses and revenues is when cash changes hands, the accounting records are subject to mismanagement by those involved in the accounting process. For these reasons, the cash system is infrequently used. Perhaps 99% of all health care facilities use the accrual accounting approach.

ACCRUAL ACCOUNTING APPROACH

Under the accrual system of accounting, revenues are recorded when they are earned and expenses when they are incurred, regardless of the time the cash transactions take place. The previous definition of expense can now be more precisely stated as a cost that is used up, or "expensed."

Using the example of the supplies, the cost of the supplies purchased in August is expensed over the next several months. The accounting records for September would show a supplies expense equal to the cost of the supplies used in September, and so on. This should help the reader understand why understanding the accounting and record-keeping procedures discussed in the next sections is necessary. The accrual system requires that every expense incurred by the assisted living facility be attributed to the period, usually the month, in which it is incurred and all revenues to the month in which services are rendered.

This complexity is the main disadvantage of the accrual basis of accounting, but it has numerous advantages. Most important, it allows the facility to measure the revenues earned after expenses have been paid, or losses incurred, by matching revenues and expenses for each time period. It also includes depreciation, accounts payable, accounts receivable, and prepaid expenses in the accounting records, providing a more accurate picture of the facility's actual financial position. It is less subject to tampering, as expenses and revenues are usually backed by several forms of objective evidence. The following discussion of accounting and record keeping will be based on accrual accounting.

3.4 The Two Main Steps in the Accounting Process: Recording the Transactions and Preparing Financial Statements

RECORDING TRANSACTIONS IN JOURNALS AND THE GENERAL LEDGER

The accounting process involves two main steps: keeping the books and preparing the financial statement. *Bookkeeping* is a system of recording all revenues and expenses, and matching those revenues to expenses during the same time period. This process is necessary for the preparation of the *financial statements,* which are a summary of the assisted living facility's financial well-being within a specified time period.

The accounting process is fairly universal and will be described here in chronological order, from the chart of accounts to the preparation of the financial statements.

Chart of Accounts

The chart of accounts is simply a list of every account in the facility. The accounts are organized into five main groups:

- assets — things owned by the facility
- liabilities — things owed by the facility, or its obligations
- capital — money invested in the facility, also known as the facility's net worth
- revenues — earnings from operations or other sources
- expenses — costs of salaries, supplies, etc., that have been used up, usually through the provision of services
- fund account — any funds that have been established for restricted or unrestricted uses

Table 3.7 presents the chart of accounts for Lakeside Assisted Living. As can be seen from the table, each account has a number. The first digit indicates the category into which the account falls; the second digit usually is a subcategory. For example, health care salaries are an expense (category 5) in the health care area and have an account number (5201), with 1 indicating salaries. Note that the salary expense account number for every other department also ends with 1. This system of classifying accounts is useful, as it identifies every account of the facility and thus is a means of control; expenses, for example, are automatically applied to a specific source so that random or unauthorized expenses cannot accumulate unnoticed. The numbered system also saves time by recording a number rather than a long title on many documents. It is especially convenient for a computerized bookkeeping system.

The Journals

Any transaction that takes place will affect some account. The journals are the first place that transactions are recorded; they are the books of original entry. Each facility will have its own system of journals, but generally there are six types:

- *Cash receipts journal*—records all cash received for services provided (e.g., sales refreshment machines)
- *Billings journal*—lists all bills sent for services rendered
- *Accounts payable journal* (purchase journal)—records all purchases made that will be paid within the next few months
- *Cash disbursements journal*—records all payments made for services and supplies used for resident care and for all other operations of the facility
- *Payroll journal*—summarizes all payroll checks distributed during the pay period
- *General journal*—a record of nonrepetitive entries

The journals are characterized by another concept of accounting: double-entry bookkeeping. For each transaction, two entries are made in the appropriate journal; a debit and a credit.

A *debit* in accounting simply means the left side of the journal account; *credit* refers to the right side. When all debits and credits are totaled at the end of each month, they should

TABLE 3.7 Chart of Accounts, Lakeside Assisted Living

Assets		Liabilities	
Current Assets		*Current Liabilities*	
1101	Cash – petty	2102	Accounts payable – supplies
1103	Cash – payroll account	2104	Notes payable – short term
1106	Cash – operating fund	2107	Mortgage payable – short term
1112	Investments – money market fund	2109	Debts payable – current
1114	Investments – CDs	2111	Employee benefits payable
1117	Investments – depreciation fund	2113	Employee heath insurance payable
1122	Accounts receivable – Medicare Part B	2115	Salaries payable
1123	Accounts receivable – Medicaid/DSS	2201	Taxes
1124	Accounts receivable – Private pay	2204	Taxes payable – state
1126	Accounts receivable – other (e.g., insurance, HMO, VA, workers' comp.)	2205	Taxes payable – municipal
1163	Unexpired liability insurance	2221	Interest payable
Non-Current Assets		*Noncurrent liabilities*	
1302	Land	2303	Notes payable – long term
1305	Land improvements	2313	Mortgage payable – long term
1402	Building – main	2323	Bonds payable
1414	Building "B"	2401	Pensions payable
1426	Building – garage/storage		
1430	Building improvements	*Capital*	
1502	Furniture – main	3001	Owner's equity
1512	Equipment – main	3101	Net income (loss)
1514	Equipment – Builidng "B"	*Revenue (Health Care)*	
1516	Equipment – office	4001	Medicare Part B
1518	Equipment – kitchen	4003	Medicaid/Department of Social Services
1519	Equipment – laundry	4005	Private (e.g., insurance, HMO, VA, workers' compensation)
1521	Transportation		
1524	Equipment – land maintenance	*Ancillary*	
		4212	Physical Therapy
Contra Assets, Accumulated Depreciation		4212	Occupational Therapy
1602	Accum. Depr. – main building	4216	Social services/activities
1604	Accum. Depr. – Building "B"	4218	Speech therapy (contract)
1606	Accum. Depr. – garage/storage		
1630	Accum. Depr. – building improvements	*Uncompensated Care*	
1642	Accum. Depr. – furniture, maint'nce	4311	Contract Discount – Medicare B
1644	Accum. Depr. – furniture, Welsh Hall	4313	Contract Discount - Medicaid
1651	Accum. Depr. – equipment, main building	4315	Contract Discount - other
1654	Accum. Depr. – equipment, Welsh Hall	4332	Donated care
1666	Accum. Depr. – office equipment	4341	Bad debts
1668	Accum. Depr. – kitchen	4315	Resident refunds

TABLE 3.7 Continued

1669	Accum. Depr. - laundry
1671	Accum. Depr. - transportation
1674	Accum. Depr. – land improvements
1680	Accum. Depr. – bld'g improvem'ts
Expenses	
Administration	
5001	Salaries – administration
5002	Salaries – clerical
5003	Consultation fee
5006	Health insurance
5011	Payroll tax
5013	Taxes – income
5015	Taxes – property
5022	Insurance – liability
5026	Retirement fund
5032	Supplies
5034	Telephone/Internet
5035	Travel
5037	Postage
5039	Licenses and dues
5042	Repairs
Plant Operation	
5101	Salaries
5106	Health Insurance
5111	Payroll tax
5122	Utility – electricity
5124	Utility – gas
5126	Utility – water
5128	Utility – sewage
5132	Supplies
5142	Repairs
Healthcare Workers	
5201	Salaries – nurses
5202	Salaries – aides
5206	Health Insurance
5211	Pharmacy
5224	Laboratory
5232	Supplies
5237	Uniforms
5242	Repairs
Dietary	
5301	Salary – director, food services
5302	Salary – kitchen staff
5306	Health insurance
5311	Payroll tax
5332	Supplies
5342	Repairs
Laundry	
5401	Salaries
5406	Health insurance
5411	Payroll tax
5432	Supplies
5442	Repairs
5461	Contract Services
Housekeeping	
5501	Salaries
5506	Health insurance
5511	Payroll tax
5532	Supplies
5542	Repairs
Rehabilitation (Physical Therapy)	
5601	Salaries (or contract)
5606	Health insurance
5611	Payroll tax
5632	Supplies
5642	Repairs
Occupational Therapy	
5661	Salaries (or contract)
5666	Health insurance
5671	Payroll tax
5682	Supplies
5692	Repairs
Social Services/Admissions	
5701	Salaries (or contract)
5706	Health insurance
5711	Payroll tax
5732	Supplies
5742	Repairs
Activities	
5801	Salaries – beautician
5802	Salaries – crafts
5806	Health insurance
5811	Payroll tax
5832	Supplies – beauty
5833	Supplies – crafts
5835	Transportation
5837	Special events
5842	Repairs
Capital Expenses	
5904	Interest – mortgage
5907	Interest – long-term debt
5914	Debt service – mortgage
5917	Debt service – long-term debt
5934	Depreciation – plant
5936	Depreciation – equipment

be equal. Thus, for every debit entered, one or more credits are entered that equal the debit, and vice versa. Table 3.8 indicates which transactions are recorded as debits and which as credits. Journal entries are set in the shape of a T, and thus are often called T-accounts. Data from the journal entries are the source documents, the objective evidence referred to at the beginning of this section.

To illustrate the process of journalizing, the example of the billings journal is used. When a bill is sent to a resident or to that person's payer, the bill represents revenues earned by the facility that it expects to receive. This account receivable is an asset because it is cash to which the facility is entitled. Thus, a bill to Mr. Jones for $1,000 would be recorded in the debit column as an increase in assets. On the credit side, $1,000 would be recorded as in increase in revenue. This journal entry is illustrated in Figure 3.1. The source document for this entry would be a copy of the invoice sent to Mr. Jones.

When the billings to all service recipients for the month are entered in the journal in this manner, the sum of debits should equal the sum of credits at the end of the month. Notice that the billings journal is used only for the billing of a service; the service recipient's payment of the bill will be recorded in the cash receipts journal. The complete transaction would be recorded as follows.

TABLE 3.8 Transactions Recorded as Debits and Credits

Debt		Credit	
(+)	Increase in assets	(-)	Decrease in assets
(+)	Decrease in liability	(-)	Decrease in liability
(-)	Decrease in capital	(+)	Increase in capital
(-)	Decrease in revenues	(+)	Increase in revenues
(-)	Increase in expenses	(+)	Decrease in expenses

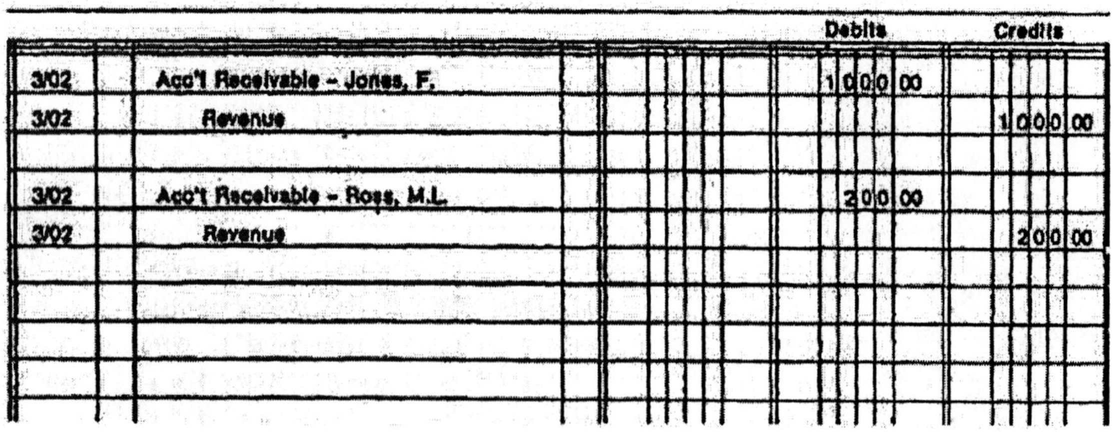

		Debits	Credits
3/02	Acc't Receivable - Jones, F.	1000 00	
3/02	Revenue		1000 00
3/02	Acc't Receivable - Ross, M.L.	200 00	
3/02	Revenue		200 00

FIGURE 3.1 Lakeside Assisted Living billings journal.

Billings Journal

Debit ______ Credit ______

3/02 Acc./Rec. $1,000.00
(account receivable)

3/02 Revenue $1,000.00

Cash Receipts Journal

Debit ______ Credit ______

4/22 Cash $1,000.00
(account receivable)

4/22 Acc./Rec. $1,000.00

The credit in the cash receipts journal would not be due to an increase in revenue, but to a decrease in accounts receivable. As mentioned, under the accrual system of accounting, revenue is recognized when the services are provided, rather than when the cash is received.

Role of the General Journal. The *general journal* records transactions that do not properly fit into any of the other journals. Note that the first five journals all record cash transactions; the general journal is used to make adjustments in the books to conform to the accrual system of accounting.

As with supplies, the supplies purchased in August, for example, will be only partially consumed in that month, but the cash disbursements journal would record the cash expenditure for the supplies purchased in August. Under the accrual method of accounting, only the costs of supplies used in August would be included in the August financial reports, so the total cost of providing services can be compared with the revenues earned in the same period. Therefore, an entry must be made in the general ledger (see below) to adjust the supplies expenditure in the cash disbursements journal to the cost of supplies used up in August. This is known as an adjusting entry.

If an expenditure of $300 for supplies is made in August and the inventory records compiled at the end of August revealed that $75 remained in inventory, the adjusting entry in the general journal would be as follows.

General Journal

Debit ______ Credit ______

8/29 Med. Supp. $225.00
(an increase in expenses)

8/29 Inventory $225.00
(decrease in expense)

8/29 Inventory $75.00
(increase in asset)

8/29 Med. Supp. $75.00
(decrease in expenses)

In addition to adjustments for inventory, entries for depreciation and prepaid expenses are also recorded in the general journal to reflect the cost of using the plant or equipment over the time period, as well as the amount of prepaid expenses used up.

Finally, the general journal can be used to correct errors made in the other journals. The general journal accounts are usually repeated from month to month and therefore should be standardized. This prevents omission of nonapparent, but very real, costs.

The General Ledger

At the end of each month, when all adjusting entries have been made in the journal accounts, the financial information in all journals is *posted* (written or entered) to the general ledger.

The *general ledger* can be thought of as a summary of all debits and credits contained in the journals for the time period. It usually has a page for each account in the chart of accounts.

The purpose of the ledger is twofold. First, it keeps a continuous balance of the amount in any account for each month. It also enables a "trial balance" to be done. Before the financial statements can be prepared, the total of all debit columns in all journals must equal the total amount from all of the credit columns. By accumulating all journal entries in one book (the ledger), debits and credits can be easily added up and compared. When total debits equal total credits, the books are said to "balance," and thus a trial balance has been calculated. If total debits do not equal total credits, then there is an error in one or more of the journal entries.

Under the double-entry concept of accounting, each debit recorded in a journal must be matched by a credit of an equal amount. The trial balance, therefore, indicates whether or not an error has been made in recording transactions.

With so many accounts, there is ample opportunity for error. Thus accuracy in preparing the journal and ledger entries will save a great deal of time spent in a search for possible mistakes. The relationship between the journals and general ledger is shown in Figure 3.2 and Figure 3.3.

The general ledger should be arranged in the order that the accounts will appear in the financial statements. Once the trial balance and gain/loss statements are prepared, the ledger is closed. This process will be discussed in the following description of the financial statements.

PREPARING THE FINANCIAL STATEMENTS: THE INCOME STATEMENT AND THE BALANCE SHEET

The financial statements are the summary of all transactions made during a particular time period and their effect on the finances of the facility. The GAAPs require that the financial statements include four reports:

- Income statement, or profit/loss statement
- Balance sheet, or statement of financial position
- Statement of changes in financial position
- Notes to the financial statements

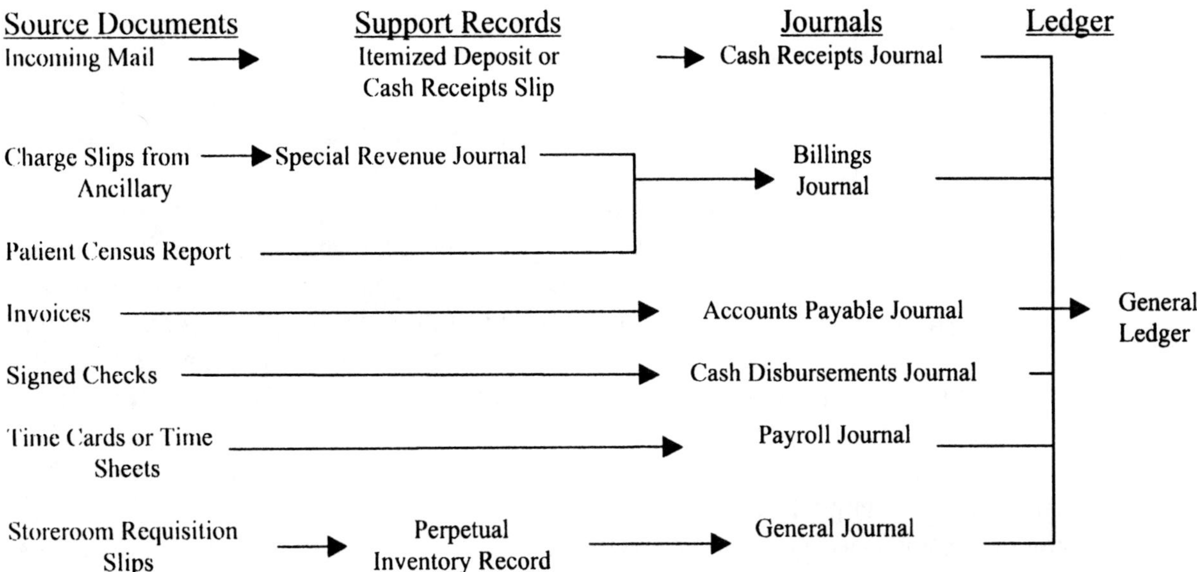

FIGURE 3.2 Source documents, support records, journals, and general ledger.

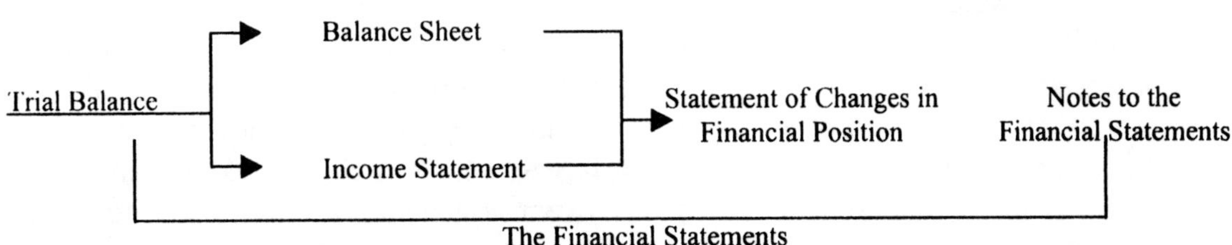

FIGURE 3.3 The financial statements.

The income statement and balance sheet are prepared directly from the general ledger and will be described below. The statement of changes in financial position and the notes to the financial statements are prepared from the income statement and balance sheet, and they will be discussed in less detail.

Profit and Loss: The Income Statement

The income statement shows whether revenues were sufficient to cover expenses, whether the facility made or lost money during the specified time period.

In accounting, income does not refer to the funds coming into the facility but to revenues minus expenses, or the profit or loss experienced by the facility (or income compared to expenses in not-for-profit operations). While net income indicates that the facility made money, or had some revenues in excess of expenses, a net loss indicates the facility lost money in the time period covered by the income statement. A net loss, or any negative figure on the financial statements, is usually shown in parentheses.

The income statement in Table 3.9 shows a net income of $833 for the month of July and $35,625 for the year until then. Revenues are listed first on the income statement, usually starting with the largest source of revenues. From the general ledger, all of the revenues earned from providing room and board and other services are calculated as routine services, separated by the level of care or type of service.

When all revenues earned from providing services, or *operating revenues,* from the general ledger have been computed, any deductions from revenue are subtracted from the gross operating revenues. Deductions from operating revenues might include money owed to the facility that cannot be collected (known as bad debts or charity care), or they might be due to contractual discounts.

In the process of setting rates at which they will reimburse the facility for care, third-party payers sometimes pay the assisted living facility somewhat less than the facility's full charges. This discount from the regular price of providing care is known as a *contractual discount.* This discounted rate is the price at which the facility has agreed to provide care when it admits the insured resident. Contractual discounts are therefore deducted from operating revenues instead of included as an expense. Today, most hospitals are forced by competition to offer contractual discounts to large groups such as HMOs. Health care facilities are similarly affected by competition and the desire to admit residents from such large third-party payers.

Total deductions are subtracted from the gross operating revenue to get the *net operating revenue.* Net operating revenues for the Lakeside Assisted Living for July are $334,693. *Nonoperating revenues* (income from sources other than direct resident care) are listed next. In July the Lakeside Assisted Living earned a total of $5,218 in nonoperating revenue ($900 in interest from funds invested in a local bank and $4,318 from a certificate of deposit). Miscellaneous sources of revenue are also included directly from the appropriate page in the general ledger. Miscellaneous revenues for Lakeside Assisted Living are from residents' meals, the beauty shop, and concession income.

Expenses are listed next, starting with the largest item, which is usually salaries. All salaries are listed by department. The salary expense generally includes any employee benefits and payroll taxes paid by the facility.

Supplies, which are separated by department in the ledger according to the chart of accounts, are combined into one expense item in Lakeside Assisted Living's income statement. A capital expense of $200 was incurred in July by the purchase of equipment. *Capital equipment* is assets that will be used by the facility to provide services for more than 1 year and will not be sold in the course of operations. In addition to equipment, capital items also include such assets as the building, units, and furniture. If we were to look at the general ledger under the chart of accounts number for capital equipment expenses, we would discover that the $200 was used to purchase office equipment for Lakeside.

Further down on the income statement there is an expense called capital costs. A *capital cost* is an expense related to the use of capital items. At some earlier time Lakeside Assisted Living had borrowed money for new dining and lounge furniture and money to purchase the building, both at an annual interest rate of 14%. For the month of July the total interest expense was $27,816. Interest expenses, then, are one cost of using capital.

A mortgage payment expense of $24,029 for July is a second source of capital costs. Another cost of using capital is depreciation; the cost of wear and tear on Lakeside Assisted Living's depreciable assets was estimated to be $39,627 for 1 month. (See section on depreciation for estimation of this expense.)

TABLE 3.9 Lakeside Assisted Living Income Statement

Revenues	July 20	Year to date (YTD)
Operating revenues		
Health care	357,603	2,207,814
Total health care	357,603	2,207,814
Ancillary		
Physical therapy	9,974	61,839
Occupational therapy	9,890	59,340
Social services	2,866	16,909
Total ancillary	22,730	138,088
Gross operating revenue	380,333	2,345,902
Less deductions	45,640	281,508
Net operating revenue	334,693	2,064,394
Non-operating revenue		
Miscellaneous		
Meals	430	2,494
Concession	1,358	8,691
Beauty shop	790	4,891
Total miscellaneous	2,578	16,004
Interest	2,640	15,312
Non-operating revenue	5,218	31,316
Total Revenues	339,911	2,095,710
Expenses		
Operating expenses		
Salaries		
Health care personnel	135,192	833,151
Dietary	15,582	93,492
Administration	9,551	54,441
Laundry	3,409	20,454
Maintenance	5,287	32,145
Physical therapy	9,652	60,808
Occupational therapy	3,450	20,735
Social services—admissions	2,146	13,305
Total salaries	184,269	1,128,531
Supplies	31,393	189,928
Activity	2,065	12,390
Capital equipment	200	1,600
Utilities	8,764	52,548
Telephone	163	1,043
Insurance	4,000	24,018
Taxes (real estate)	3,313	19,878
Capital costs		
Interest	27,816	166,896
Mortgage payment	24,029	144,174
Depreciation	39,627	237,762
Total capital costs	91,472	548,832
Total expenses	339,078	2,060,085
Net income (loss)	833	35,625
Income tax	375	16,031
Profit after tax	458	19,594

To compute the *net income,* or profit or loss, the total expenses are subtracted from total revenues. This gives the net income before taxes. Subtracting the monthly percentage for income tax shows that Lakeside Assisted Living's profit after taxes is $458 for July. Although depreciation is a real cost of providing services, it does not represent an actual cash outflow, and depreciation may be added to the after-tax profit to give the actual cash standing of the facility.

The income statement, then, shows the operating performance of the facility for a specified period of time, and it is usually prepared on a monthly and annual basis.

Closing the Books

Because revenues and expenses must be measured for finite periods of time, these accounts must be brought to a sum of zero so that they can be recorded over again for a new time period. Bringing the expense and revenue accounts to zero defines "closing the books."

To close the General Ledger:

1. For all revenue and expense accounts with a credit balance, add a debit equal to the credit to bring the account to zero.
2. For all revenue and expense accounts with a debit balance, add a credit equal to the debit to bring the account to zero.

According to the double-entry accounting system, compensation must be made for these new debits and credits in some other account.

1. Add up all the newly added debits
2. Add up all the newly added credits.
3. Subtract the debits from the credits
4. Enter the difference in the retained earning account, as follows:
   - If the difference is a profit, enter it as a credit.
   - If the difference is a loss, enter it as a debit.

Thus all revenue and expense accounts have been brought to zero, and the books are balanced and ready for a new time period.

Statement of Financial Condition: The Balance Sheet

Unlike the income statement, which summarized operating performance over a period of time, the balance sheet records the financial position of the assisted living facility at one point in time. Whereas the income statement shows the ending balance of the revenue and expense accounts, the balance sheet summarizes the assets, liabilities, and capital accounts of the facility. This document is called a balance sheet because the asset accounts must balance with the liability and capital accounts. This relationship can be expressed as an equation, called the accounting equation:

$$\text{Assets} = \text{liabilities} + \text{capital}$$

The balance sheet for the Lakeside Assisted Living for the year is shown in Table 3.10. Assets are listed on the left in order of liquidity.

Current assets refers to those possessions of the facility that will be, or theoretically can be, turned into cash within 12 months. Prepaid insurance is considered an asset

Table 3.10 Lakeside Assisted Living Balance Sheet

	July 31, 20XX	July, 31 20XX
Assets		
Current assets		
Cash	60,700	2,834
Accounts receivable		
(Less bad debts of $9032)	53,517	61,397
Securities	225,275	10,500
Inventory	62,006	54,880
Prepaid insurance	2,400	3,600
Total current assets	403,898	133,211
Non-current assets		
Equipment	1,983,000	1,981,200
Plant	5,767,004	5,767,004
Less Accumulated Depreciation	2,772,192	2,362,300
Plant and Equipment	4,977,812	5,385,904
Property	2,650,000	2,650,000
Total fixed assets	7,627,812	8,035,904
Total assets	8,031,710	8,169,115
Liabilities		
Current liabilities		
Accounts payable	2,852	24,606
Notes payable	33,625	355,271
Benefits payable	34,843	630,388
Current portion of		
Mortgage	3,460,202	3,690,883
Long term debt	75,000	75,000
Total current liabilities	367,000	1,277,498
Non-current liabilities		
Mortgage payable	3,460,202	3,690,883
Debts payable	675,000	750,000
Total noncurrent liabilities	4,135,202	4,440,883
Total liabilities	4,502,202	5,718,381
Net Worth		
Retained Earnings		
Year to date	65,625	25,507
Total	370,956	335,331
Owner's equity	3,122,927	2,087,897
Total net worth	3,529,508	2,450,735
Total liabilities and capital	8,031,710	8,169,115

because the coverage is something owned by the facility. The income statement records the proportion of the prepaid insurance that was used in the month of July ($4,000), and the balance sheet shows the amount of insurance that remains.

Noncurrent assets, of course, refers to those assets that will not be liquidated within the year; they usually include plant (the building), property, and equipment. These are also called *fixed assets* and are recorded as their cost at the time of purchase, rather than their current market value.

The *historic cost* concept is another basic tenet of accounting and relates to the ongoing concern concept: because capital assets will not be liquidated any time soon, their current market value is of little relevance. The value of these assets to the facility, however, must include the depreciation on plant and equipment over the years, and so this accumulated depreciation is subtracted from the historic cost of the depreciable assets. Although land usually appreciates in value over time, it does not do so simply through the operations of the facility and is therefore recorded at historic cost, with no depreciation from its value.

Depreciation, therefore, is an expense associated with the use of an asset, so depreciation is included both as an expense on the income statement and as a contra asset (literally, "against an asset") on the balance sheet. Note that employees are not included as an asset. This is because assets are those things owned by the facility; an organization cannot own its employees.

Liabilities are the obligations of the facility. Current liabilities are those obligations that must be met within the next 12 months, such as bills from suppliers of foodstuffs and medical or office supplies, as well as short-term bank loans.

On this particular date, Lakeside Assisted Living owes its suppliers $2,852. If this debt were paid tomorrow and a balance sheet made up for that day, Lakeside Assisted Living would have no accounts payable on its balance sheet. Notes payable refers to loans that must be repaid within 12 months. Lakeside Assisted Living owes $33,625 to a local bank for interest on its borrowed funds, as well as a portion of a long-term debt due within the year. The noncurrent liabilities sections shows which debts these are. Lakeside Assisted Living has a payment due on its debt for new furniture, and a portion of its mortgage payment is due also.

Capital accounts, or *net worth,* are recorded below the liabilities. This section is also called owners' equity, shareholders' equity, fund balance, or retained earnings, depending on the origin of the funds that make up this section. It includes funds that the owners have put into the facility, whether the owners are one person, a partnership (two or more unincorporated owners), a corporation, or a charitable organization. Net worth also usually includes retained earnings, or the net income that has been put back into the facility over the years.

If the facility incurs a net loss, this amount is subtracted from the net worth. The Lakeside Assisted Living net worth includes the retained earnings of the year to date and the retained earnings from its earlier years of operation. It also shows that the owners have invested $3,122,927 in the facility over the years. If this amount was from stockholders, it would be called shareholders' equity; if from a charitable organization, it would be a fund balance.

The most important thing to remember about the net worth is that it is not a pool of cash. The funds recorded as net worth are monies that have been put into the facility at some time; it is merely a record of these funds, not cash available for operations or investment.

To summarize, the balance sheet shows the financial position of the facility for only one point in time. Its relation with the income statement is the retained earnings, which usually include the net income in the net worth.

Thus the basic accounting equation can be expanded to

assets = (liabilities + owners' equity) + (revenues – expenses)

Two Additional Financial Statements

The statement of changes in financial position, also simply called the statement of changes, shows the major transactions that occurred over the period covered by two balance sheets, or the way that working capital was used during that period. Working capital simply refers to the current assets and current liabilities from the balance sheet. The amount of working capital available is

current assets – current liabilities

The statement of changes shows the transactions that caused the amount of working capital to change over a specified time period. It is therefore a very useful document for those interested in knowing how the facility acquires and uses its funds.

Sources of funds are generally an excess of revenues over expenses of operations, interest income, and contributions to the facility (or owners' equity). Noncash items, such as depreciation or money designated for repayment of debts, are added as a source of funds, because this is still cash (a current asset) owned by the facility.

Uses of funds would include nonoperating expenses such as repayment of a portion of a debt or additions to property. The uses of funds are subtracted from the sources of funds to give the change in working capital over the time period. This difference should equal the change in working capital calculated from the balance sheets at the beginning and end of the time period covered.

The *notes to financial statements* are included to explain the accountant's interpretation or calculation of figures, or variation in the books due to a change in their organization, which may not be readily understood by those reviewing the financial statements. The financial statements are not considered complete without these notes.

Staff Functions in the Accounting Process

The number of staff persons in the business office and their degree of specialization will vary with the size, complexity, and ownership of the facility. In general, however, those responsible for the accounting functions will be the bookkeeper, the accountant or comptroller, and the administrator.

The bookkeeper maintains the journals and ledger and performs the trial balance. An accountant or comptroller may also check the trial balance, but his or her primary task is the preparation of the financial statement.

For all practical purposes, it is legally mandatory that an assisted living facility have its books officially audited, that is, audited by a person who is a certified public accountant

(CPA). It is almost impossible to do business without having the facility's books audited by a CPA, who, in effect, serves as the public's representative.

Administrators of a chain-owned facility generally will send the data from the books to a regional or corporate office, where the financial statements, as well as a variety of other schedules, will be compiled and returned.

3.5 Putting Financial Statements to Work: Working Capital, Ratio Analysis, and Vertical Analysis

The net income is an important and readily identifiable item of interest on the financial statements. What other information can be gleaned from these reports? There are several the administrator can use. Three tools are discussed below.

WORKING CAPITAL

Current assets minus current liabilities equals the working capital available. This can also be considered the funds available to the facility.

Suppose the administrator of Lakeside Assisted Living wants to learn if enough funds are available to purchase $60,000 worth of capital equipment for the health care area. Where can this information be found?

The net income for the month of July—and the entire year—has been reinvested in the facility, as indicated by the net worth section of the balance sheet; these funds may or may not still be available. Although the net worth shows the funds that have been invested in the facility, it is not a pool of cash. Recall that the net worth is merely a record of the funds that have been invested in the facility over time and that most of the funds shown here are therefore not available for spending or investing.

The administrator might also check the cash accounts of Lakeside Assisted Living to see if the cash for purchasing the items is available. But this is not suitable either, for if the Lakeside Assisted Living owes $367,000 to various creditors, as indicated by the current liabilities section on the balance sheet, any available cash may be needed to meet these obligations.

In order to get an idea of the funds available to purchase the needed equipment, the administrator must look at the amount of working capital available. Current assets remaining after current liabilities have been subtracted yields the amount of money that the administrator has at his or her discretion.

The administrator finds that there is only $36,898 in working capital available to purchase equipment for the health care area and that the facility probably should not purchase new equipment at this time. Because current assets include relatively nonliquid accounts, such as inventory and prepaid insurance, the working capital may be calculated by excluding these accounts from the total current assets.

RATIO ANALYSIS

Another common approach to analyzing financial statements is to perform a ratio analysis. Financial managers generally express the information in financial statements as a series of ratios.

There are an infinite number of ratios that may be derived from financial statements, but the discussion here will be confined to several of the more common measures of financial performance. References for Part Three include several excellent texts that explore financial statement analysis in greater detail.

Usefulness of Ratios

Ratios are useful in several ways. First, financial ratios are no more than fractions using the numbers in the financial statement and are therefore fairly simple to calculate quickly and easily.

Ratio analysis allows the administrator to identify trends in many measures of financial performance of the facility by comparing the same ratio for several periods. Ratio analysis of the financial statements can also be used to compare the financial performance of several facilities. It is one of the most useful tools the administrator has.

That the amount of working capital available is calculated by subtracting current liabilities from current assets has already been mentioned. A positive amount of working capital indicates that the facility is able to meet its current obligations with its current assets.

If all resident revenues were collected before or immediately after they were earned, the facility would have no need of excess working capital. But because third-party payers pay health care facilities for services sometimes well after services were rendered, the facility must maintain a certain level of working capital to meet expenses during the "lag time" before the payments are received. (If the facility is part of a chain or group of facilities, the same problem is faced by the corporate managers, who have the same gaps between services rendered and payments received, but on a larger scale.) Even health care facilities that have predominantly privately paying residents must plan for collections of resident bills to extend over a period of weeks to months. How much working capital should the facility maintain to cover its lag time? One way to get an idea of an appropriate amount is to perform a current or acid-test ratio.

Current Ratio

The formula for calculating current ratio is

current ratio = current assets/current liabilities

Lakeside Assisted Living has

$403,898/$367,000 = 1.1

A current ratio greater than 1 shows that Lakeside Assisted Living is able to meet its current obligations, with a surplus of working capital. Does this mean that a current ratio of 2.5 is even better? Not necessarily; a high current ratio may show that the facility has too much money tied up in current assets and that it may make better use of some of these funds by investing them in an interest-bearing bank account or its equivalent.

Interpreting Ratios

Interpretation of an appropriate current ratio exemplifies a point of caution with the use of any ratio. One ratio itself reveals very little about the performance of the facility. Ratios must be compared either over time or with the rest of the industry. A current ratio of 1.1 may be fine if the ratio for Lakeside Assisted Living in the past has been as follows:

Year 1	Year 2	Year 3	Year 4
.80	.85	.90	1.0

A ratio of 1.1 could also indicate a decline in working capital if past ratios have been much higher than 1.1. Industry comparisons are also important. If the average current ratio for the assisted living facility industry, preferably in the same region, is 1.0, then Lakeside Assisted Living may be managing its working capital well. If, however, the industry average is .9, then Lakeside Assisted Living might rethink the amount of funds it is keeping available. Thus interpretation of all ratios is relative to both past performance and industry averages. The administrator of Lakeside Assisted Living will find out what the appropriate current ratio is and adjust his or her own working capital to maintain that ratio.

The Quick Ratio

Another commonly used ratio is the quick ratio. This ratio is similar to the current ratio, but is a more rigorous and representative measure of current assets, as only cash and accounts receivable, and sometimes marketable securities, are used to cover current liabilities.

quick ratio = (cash + accounts receivable + marketable securities)/current liabilities

($60,700 + $53,519 + $225,275)/$367,000 = 0.93

The quick ratio reveals that Lakeside Assisted Living is not quite able to cover its current obligations with its most available assets, but is quite close to the industry average.

Average Collection Period Ratio

The average collection period ratio, shows the average lag time of accounts receivable. Although the administrator of the assisted living facility will have relatively little influence in expediting the collection of funds paid by third parties, he or she should attempt to collect privately paid monies from residents as soon as possible in order to decrease working capital needs. This is therefore an important ratio (net operating revenues taken from Table 3.10).

average collection period = 365 x accounts receivable/net operating revenues

365 x $53,517/$334,693 = 58 days

Accounts Payable Average Payment Period Ratio

A related ratio is the accounts payable average payment period, which shows the average number of days used to pay creditors. Too many days in the payable period may develop into a poor credit relationship with suppliers, and too few days may indicate that funds should be invested for a longer time before creditors are paid (supplies expense taken from Table 3.10).

average payment period = 365 x accounts payable/supplies expense

365 x $2,852/$31,393 = 33 days

Because payment for bills generally is sought by the 30th day at the latest, Lakeside Assisted Living seems to be performing well in its efforts to make timely payments to suppliers. If the average payment period were much shorter, Lakeside Assisted Living might consider waiting for 30 days to pay some of its creditors and investing these funds in an interest-earning account. If a discount is offered for payment within 10 days or some short specified period, early payment of accounts payable might be more cost effective.

For both accounts payable and accounts receivable considerations, the opportunity cost (loss of use otherwise available for these funds) must be considered. In times of low interest rates, when cost for the use of money is low, the opportunity cost is less than in times of high interest rates (i.e., when using money is more costly).

Net Operating Margin Ratio

The net operating margin is the proportion of revenues earned to the amount of expenses used to earn those revenues. A low operating margin may indicate that rates for services should be raised or expenses reduced.

operating revenues – operating expenses net operating margin =

---

operating revenues

($334,693 – $339,078)/$334,693 = –0.013

Lakeside Assisted Living's negative operating margin shows that operating revenues do not cover operating expenses and that the administrator should consider increasing charges for services, if the market will allow it, or reducing operating costs, in order to increase the facility's operating margin. Another approach to this ratio is operating income as a percentage of revenues. This ratio is best compared with industry averages for an indication of performance.

Debt-to-Equity Ratio

The debt-to-equity ratio is a measure of the long-run liquidity of the facility, or the ability of the facility to meet its long-term debts. A "small" proportion of debt to equity indicates that the facility could incur more long-term debt, other things being equal, if needed; whereas a high debt-to-equity ratio (when compared to the industry) probably shows that the facility may have more debt than may be advisable, all other things being equal. This ratio is of particular interest to would-be creditors.

debt/equity = long-term debt/total equity

$4,135,202/$3,529,508 = 1.17

These are some of the more commonly used ratios. There are, of course, many other parameters of financial performance that will be of interest to the administrator.

VERTICAL ANALYSIS

A third method of analyzing the financial statements is to perform a vertical analysis. A vertical analysis converts each item on the income statement, balance sheet, or other financial report to a percentage of some total item on the same document.

A vertical analysis of the Lakeside Assisted Living income statement, using the year-to-date values, is shown in Table 3.11. Like the ratios above, these ratios are useful when compared over time or with other facilities. For example, an unusually high ratio of supplies to total expenses in July may indicate that supplies are being wasted or pilfered, provided there has not been a change in the type of services that would warrant a greater use of supplies. On the other hand, although the percentage for July may be higher than for any month that year, if supplies as a proportion of total expenses are consistently higher in July than any other month, then the administrator knows that this is a pattern that may or may not be a matter of cause of concern.

The administrator can accumulate valuable information from the financial statements by performing both ratio and vertical analyses. By comparing these ratios over time and with other facilities, trends and patterns in the operation of the facility can be identified, which is perhaps one of the most important functions of financial statement analysis. Awareness of such patterns enables the administrator to pinpoint problem areas in the facility and make more knowledgeable financial decisions.

TABLE 3.11 Lakeside Assisted Living Income Statement: Vertical Analysis

Revenues	July	Year to date	Vertical Analysis %	% YTD
Operating revenues				
Health care	357,603	2,207,814		
Total Health care	357,603	2,207,814	100	94
Ancillary				
Physical therapy	9,974	61,839	45	
Occupational therapy	9,890	59,340	43	
Social services	2,866	16,909	12	
Total ancillary	22,730	138,088	100	6
Gross operating revenue	380,333	2,345,902		100
Less deductions	45,640	281,508	12	
Net operating revenue	334,693	2,064,394		88
Nonoperating revenue				
Miscellaneous				
Meals	430	2,494	16	
Concession	1,358	8,691	54	
Beauty shop	790	4,891	30	
Total miscellaneous	2,578	16,004	100	51
Interest	2,640	15,312		49
Nonoperating revenue	5,218	31,316		100
Total revenues	339,911	2,095,710		
Expenses				
Operating expenses				
Salaries				
Nursing	135,192	833,151	68	
Dietary	15,582	93,492	8	
Administration	9,551	54,441	4	
Laundry	3,409	20,454	2	
Housekeeping	13,435	81,282	7	
Maintenance	5,287	32,145	3	
Physical therapy	9,652	60,808	5	
Occupational therapy	3,450	20,735	2	
Social secv	2,146	13,305	1	
Total salaries	197,705	1,209,812	100	59.0
Supplies	31,393	189,928	9.2	
Activity	2,065	12,390	0.6	
Capital equipment	200	1,600	0.1	
Utilities	8,764	52,548	2.6	
Telephone/internet	163	1,043	0.1	
Insurance	4,000	24,018	1.2	
Taxes (real estate)	3,313	19,878	1.0	
Capital costs				
Interest	27,816	166,896	30	8.1
Mortgage payment	24,029	144,174	26	7.0
Depreciation	39,627	237,762	43	11.5
Total capital costs	91,472	548,832	100	
Total expenses	339,078	2,060,085		100
Income tax (@45%)	375	16,031		
Profit after tax	458	19,594		

3.6 Additional Accounting Procedures That Help the Administrator Maintain Control Over the Facility

Although accounting processes are similar in every institution, the procedures for managing finances will vary from facility to facility, and so will the best methods of control.

In financial management, control refers to the development and maintenance of systematic ways to identify problems when they occur to permit the administrator to intervene appropriately. To maintain control, the administrator and the staff normally develop policies for all office procedures. Identification of possible financial problems as soon as they arise enables the staff to deal effectively with them through the use of recognized policies.

There are several tools available to assist the administrator in controlling financial operations. Procedures should be arranged so that no single person has complete responsibility for any area of the facility's finances. A system of checks and balances can be established so that part of one person's task is completed or reviewed by another. Furthermore, each employee can be required to take vacation time so that no one has uninterrupted control of certain office tasks. It is important to have procedures in place that reduce temptation to a minimum. Even the best procedures set up by the most sophisticated corporations have not been able to prevent an occasional embezzlement of funds at facilities. Eternal vigilance is necessary in such money matters.

ACCOUNTS RECEIVABLE: BILLING FOR SERVICES RENDERED BY THE FACILITY

The facility cannot receive monies for services rendered until the residents have been billed for them. Delays in billing create an opportunity cost: the loss of use or availability of funds when cash owed to the facility is not yet in its possession.

Financial Review of Applicants

At the time of admission the payment source should be established. If the client is not paying with his or her own funds, written agreement to pay must be obtained from the person who controls the resident's funds. In addition, present and potential Medicare and Medicaid needs should be determined. These agencies will normally pay for care only after an authorization number has been established for a recipient.

Just as the facility must remove temptations from its employees to embezzle facility funds, so also must the facility constantly seek to minimize temptations for residents' monies managers to withhold moneys legitimately due the facility. Experience has taught that social security and similar checks that have been pledged to pay for a resident's care are best sent directly to the facility rather than to the resident or to a family member who may feel more pressing financial needs than payment of the facility charges.

Resident Ledger Card

When the resident's source of payment has been confirmed, a resident ledger card is made up for each person admitted, listing the name, room number, source of payment, and daily (or routine) service charges. The charges and the billing and collections procedures must be explained to each resident and/or sponsor.

Preparation of Invoices

In every case, charge slips for each service not bundled into the daily rate must be collected from each service center on a periodic basis (daily or weekly). Because these charges are distinct from routine room-related services, a special revenues journal may be created to record them.

Routine Charges

Each facility or chain will determine how to package its charges to residents. Once the ancillary charges for the billing period have been determined, they are added to each resident's routine charges. The routine charge is the charge for "room and board" services, which usually include basic health care, room, and meals. Facilities will package their charges in various ways, depending on a number of considerations. Some offer a broad continuum of services from which residents may choose.

Daily Census Form

The routine charge may be determined on a daily, weekly, or monthly basis and is calculated with the aid of the daily census form. This is a summary of the facility's occupancy that lists, for each day, admissions, discharges, and transfers by level of care, if more than one is offered by the facility.

Resident Census Report

A resident census report is drawn up by the bookkeeper (usually for the month) by compiling the information from the resident census forms (see Figure 3.4). The resident census report is in turn used to calculate the total routine charges for each resident or service recipient (e.g., outside physical therapy charges). Routine and ancillary services are finally calculated for each resident and service recipient and entered on each resident's or service recipient's accounts receivable ledger card (see Figure 3.5) and in the billings journal. To expedite the billing process, the billings journal should be divided by payer type (e.g., private pay, Medicaid, perhaps a hospital reserve bed contract, HMO, PPO, IPO, workers' compensation fund, or similar third-party payer). The billing process and services covered vary with each payer. Each bill should itemize any ancillary charges (when permitted by the payer) to expedite the processing of invoices by third-party payers. Increasingly, billing may be done by electronic submission using computers and modems. Some state Medicaid programs require electronic submission. This normally means that the facility receives payment on a more timely basis.

Billing Medicaid, Other Third Parties, and Private Payers

For the most part, billing private patients is relatively straightforward if facility personnel have followed requirements for the billing system. However, billing is an increasingly complex process because of the variety of payment agreements health care facilities are negotiating with third parties. Medicaid residents' care costs are normally billed and paid for monthly, usually with one composite bill for all Medicaid residents submitted to the state or its designated payer. Payers sometimes pay promptly, but also sometimes send for many clarifications on bills, the purpose of which is to delay the final payment to the facility in order to ease cash flow problems being experienced by the third-party payers. It is a complicated game in some states.

More and more third-party payers are negotiating contracts with health care facilities that also vary in method of payment. Often a third-party payer, a health maintenance organization, for example, will negotiate a separate payment schedule for each member sent to an assisted living facility. Other third-party payers may negotiate a flat rate for all members it refers to a particular assisted living facility, regardless of acuity level. For some residents the monthly fee negotiated by their third-party payer will be all-inclusive; others will be on an itemized service use basis. It is in these circumstances that both the facility administration and the third-party payer administration are jockeying for a position that, whatever the payment arrangement, covers their actual costs.

Intense pressures on third-party payers to hold down costs are being passed on to the assisted living facility.

Accounting for Deductions from Revenue

Besides contractual discounts, charity care and bad debts are also sources of deductions from revenue. Charity care is provided to a resident when the service is not reimbursable and cannot be paid for privately. Bad debts, on the other hand, are resident accounts that are past due but are still subject to collection.

Contractual discounts are often the largest source of deductions from revenue in health care facilities. Because most deductions cannot be confirmed until payment has been received, they are accounted for in the billings journal when known rather than estimated. The payment from public insurers will be accompanied by a medical assistance remittance and status report. This report lists the resident's name and claim number, the service dates, the description of services rendered, the total amount billed to the program, and the allowed and nonallowed charges, with an explanation code stating why the service was not reimbursed. The T account for deductions from revenue would be:

Billings Journal

	Debits	Credits
2/27	Cont. Disc. $450.00	
2/27		Acc. Rec. $450.00

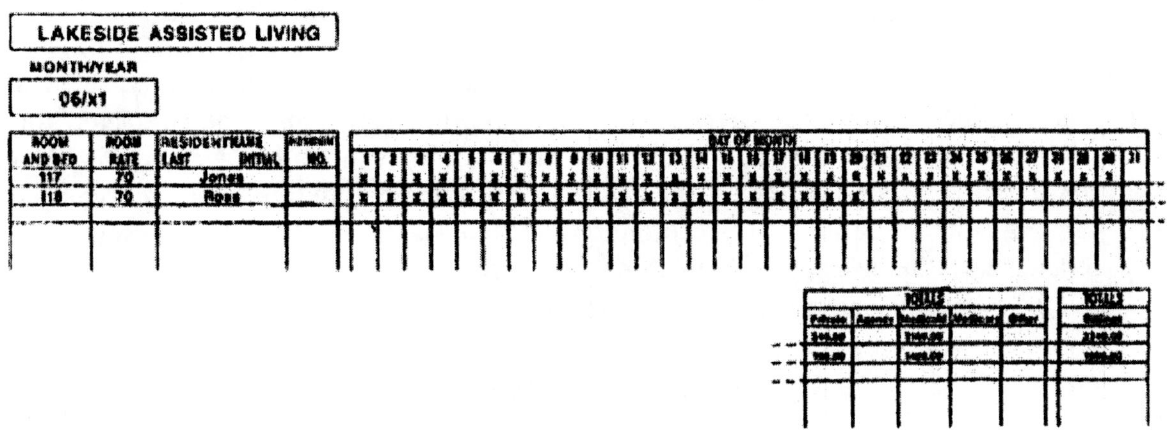

LAKESIDE ASSISTED LIVING

MONTH/YEAR

06/x1

ROOM AND BED	ROOM RATE	RESIDENT NAME LAST INITIAL	RESIDENT NO.	1	2	3	4	5	6	7	8	9	10	11	12	13	14	15	16	17	18	19	20	21	22	23	24	25	26	27	28	29	30	31
117	70	Jones		x	x	x	x	x	x	x	x	x	x	x	x	x	x	x	x	x	x	x	x	x	x	x	x	x	x	x	x	x	x	
118	70	Ross		x	x	x	x	x	x	x	x	x	x	x	x	x	x	x	x	x	x	x	x											

TOTALS					TOTALS
Private	Agency	Medicaid	Medicare	Other	[illegible]
[illegible]		[illegible]			[illegible]
[illegible]		[illegible]			[illegible]

FIGURE 3.4 Resident Census Report

ADDITIONAL CURRENT ENTRIES - COMPLETE SECTION A AND B

ACCOUNTS RECEIVABLE
INVOICE SUPPLEMENT

ADJUSTMENTS TO PRIOR MONTHS - COMPLETE SECTION A AND C

SECTION A

FACILITY NO.	FACILITY NAME				
PATIENT NUMBER	INVOICE NUMBER	YR/MO	NUMBER	INVOICE DATE	RESIDENT NAME
	[illegible]	[illegible]	1	[illegible]	Ross, M. L.

STATUS CODES
1 = PRIVATE
2 = AGENCY
3 = MEDICARE
4 = VETERAN
5 = OTHER

SECTION B

AREA
C = CERTIFIED
R = RESIDENTIAL

LEVEL
UNCLASSIFIED
SKILLED
I = RESIDENTIAL
V = VOLUNTARY

PAYMENTS

TRAN CODE	DATE MO/DAY	OPEN ITEM	DESCRIPTION	PRIVATE	AGENCY	MEDICARE	VETERAN	OTHER
	/							
	/							
	/							
	/							
			TOTAL					

RESIDENCY

TRAN CODE	DATE MO/DAY	ROOM-BED	NO. DAYS	RATE	AREA	LEVEL	PRIVATE	AGENCY	MEDICARE	VETERAN	OTHER	STATUS	
	6/20	118	30	70.00	5	8	275.00		2100.00				
	/												
	/												
	/												
						TOTAL	275.00		2100.00				

ANCILLARY

TRAN CODE	DESCRIPTION			PRIVATE	AGENCY	MEDICARE	VETERAN	OTHER	STATUS	
	PHYSICAL THERAPY					240.00				
			TOTAL			240.00				

SECTION C

EXPLANATION OF ADJUSTMENTS

ADJUSTMENTS

TRAN CODE	TRAN CODE	OPEN ITEM	NO. OF DAYS	RATE	AREA	LEVEL	PRIVATE	AGENCY	MEDICARE	VETERAN	OTHER	STATUS	NONCOLLECT
85													
85													
85													
85													
85													
85													
85													
85													
85													
85													
85													
85													
85													
85													
85													
85													
85													
85													
						TOTAL							

FIGURE 3.5 Resident card

Submitting and Resubmitting Claims

The amount of the deduction is also included on the resident's accounts receivable ledger card. If the deduction is invalid, the fiscal intermediary should be contacted for an explanation of the deduction. The claim can then be resubmitted accompanied by the information needed to justify the request for payment. Intermediaries are constantly issuing bulletins defining and redefining what covered charges include and exclude. In an era of razor-thin net operating margins, appropriate billing can have a significant impact on the result. So can inappropriate billing, however.

Medicare in the Assisted Living Facility's Future?

Currently, assisted living facilities cannot bill Medicare directly. Medicare can be billed directly by the home health care agencies, nursing homes, and hospitals that provide services to assisted living facility residents. It seems likely that more and more assisted living facilities will be able to bill Medicaid directly and, in the not-too-distant future, may be able to bill Medicare directly for some aspects of resident care.

Any funds due from Medicaid are recorded in the cash receipts journal, as follows:

Cash Receipts Journal

	Debits ________	Credits _______
11/23	Due from Medicaid $375.00	
11/23		Cont. Disc. $375.00

Sometimes services that are not allowable by an insurer (e.g., occupational therapy or some types of dental care) will be provided to residents who cannot pay for them. These services are considered charity care and are written off as essentially nonbillable. A special account should exist in the chart of accounts for this type of care, separate from other types of uncollectibles. Each facility needs policies to govern the circumstances and extent of charity care that will be given.

COLLECTING MONEY OWED TO THE FACILITY

An appropriate collections policy will depend on the facility's past experience with its payers. For bills delinquent by 1 month, a letter may be sent as a reminder. A telephone call to the payer (logged into a written record) may be made after an appropriate interval. The collections policy must indicate if and under what circumstances a collections agency or other procedure will be used.

Account Write-Off Recommendation

Problem collections are most effectively handled with an attitude of diplomacy and firmness, and an effort should be made to accommodate the payer if there is a valid reason for delinquent payment. If a resident's accounts are eventually determined to be uncollectible, some type of account write-off recommendation form (see Figure 3.6) is

Facility ______________________ # ______________________ Date ______________

Resident Name ______________________ # ______________ P__ A__ M__ VA__ Other __ Balance $______

Admission Date ______________ Discharge Date ______________ Expired: Yes ☐ No ☐

Readmission Date ______________________ Discharge Date ______________________

Readmission Date ______________________ Discharge Date ______________________

Name and address of responsible party ____

____

Home phone ______________________ Business phone ______________________

Date and amount of last payment ____

Brief History of account: (attach copy of form H-0611) ______________________________

____

____

____

Should account be assigned to a collection agency? Yes ☐ No ☐

Facility opinion by ______________________________ Date ______________

*Regional concurrence by ______________________________ Date ______________

**Corporate concurrence by ______________________________ Date ______________

If Medicare—include all intermediary correspondence.

Is coinsurance involved? Yes ☐ No ☐ If yes, please provide dates and amounts: ______________

____

____

____

______________________________ / ______________
Administrator Date

______________________________ / ______________
Regional Controller Date

______________________________ / ______________
District Director/Director of Operations Date

*For all accounts over $250.00
**For all accounts over $500.00.

Figure 3.6 Recommendation for write-off of uncollectible account.

filled out, with one copy retained in the resident's file and another going to the accountant, so that the total of uncollectible accounts can be recorded in financial statements.

Health care facilities, like hospitals and other health care providers, are victims of the cost-shifting phenomena in the United States. Because of public relations and other considerations, it is exceedingly difficult for facilities to discharge residents whose bills are uncollectible but who have no place else to go.

HANDLING CASH

Cash is easily mismanaged. It is easily concealed. The typical facility will keep only a small amount of cash on the premises, often not more than $500, as most transactions will take place through business office accounts.

Cash Handling Procedures

All cash must be handled by at least two employees, both of whom are bonded. One person should be responsible for receiving the cash, e.g., opening the mail or taking a check in person. This should not be the same person who is responsible for making bank deposits. Checks should be stamped "For Deposit Only" in the name of the facility immediately upon receipt and a daily remittance list prepared for all cash received. One copy of this list should be retained by this employee, and another should go to the person making the bank deposits.

Cash receipt slips should then be prepared, with one copy going to the payer and another to the accountant or the accountant's file. The bookkeeper should record the cash received in the cash receipts journal and also on the resident's own sheet in the resident accounts receivable ledger (see Figure 3.7).

Cash should be deposited in the bank daily to prevent it from being mislaid and to earn the maximum amount of interest on available funds. At the end of each month entries in the cash receipts journal are posted into the general ledger and these figures checked against the cash receipts entries in the resident accounts receivable ledger.

ACCOUNTS PAYABLE: THE FACILITY'S BILLS

Accounts payable are monies owed to creditors for purchases made by the facility. A health care facility's creditors usually furnish foodstuffs, linens, supplies, pharmaceuticals, laboratory tests, and office, housekeeping, and maintenance supplies, for example. A file should be set up for each regular vendor or supplier, as well as a miscellaneous vendor file for all unusual or incidental purchases.

When a purchase order is made out and sent to the supplier, a copy of the purchase order should be placed in the appropriate file. When the order is received, all supplies should be delivered to a storeroom with the exception of foodstuffs. A receiving slip will accompany the shipment; this should be checked against the items as they are being received and against the purchase order to make sure all items purchased were delivered (and, incidentally, that supplies that were *not ordered* are not delivered and signed for). Any back-ordered items on the receiving slip should be noted. The approved receiving slip is then placed with the purchase order in the vendor file.

Invoices from creditors are usually sent to the facility at the beginning of each month. The receiving slip and purchase order should be checked against the invoice to confirm that the unit price is the same as when the shipment was ordered and that all supplies charged in the bill were actually received.

All invoices should be approved by the administrator according to most owner policies, but practically speaking the administrator designates appropriate individuals to share in this task. These invoices are then recorded in the accounts payable journal by department. For example, supplies and pharmaceuticals may be attributed to health care, foodstuffs to dietary, linens to housekeeping, and so on. Invoices are placed in an invoice file.

FACILITY NO. ________ PAGE ____ of ____

DATE OF DEPOSIT 09/12/19X1 FACILITY NAME

LAST NAME	INITIAL	CASH	MISCELLANEOUS	PRIVATE	AGENCY	MEDICARE	VETERAN	OTHER	POSTED TO INVOICE NO.
Jones, F.A.						2375 00			3012-756-01
TOTALS FOR EA. COLUMN			Ⓐ						
			ACCOUNT	1211	1212	1213	1210	1217	

MISCELLANEOUS RECEIPTS SUMMARY		
ITEM	ACCOUNT	AMOUNT
EMPLOYEE MEALS - FOOD SALES	4220	
VENDING MACHINE INCOME	4860	
TOTAL A MUST EQUAL TOTAL B		Ⓑ

REDEPOSITED ITEMS RECEIVED FROM	AMOUNT

TOTAL OF THIS DEPOSIT $________ ACCOUNT 1120

FIGURE 3.7 Accounts receivable receipts ledger.

At the end of the month the accounts in the payables journal are added up, and this sum should equal the total of all invoices in the invoice file. Bills are usually payable within 30 days. Creditors should be paid on the latest possible date, unless a discount is offered for early payment. This does not mean that accounts payable should be chronically delinquent while available funds remain in the bank; it is important to maintain a good credit relationship with suppliers. Suppliers, often middlepersons, are dependent on reasonably prompt payment of invoices for their own business operations.

At the beginning of the month the invoices in the invoice file should be used to pay all bills due in that month. Checks should be signed by two designated employees, and all payments should be recorded in the cash disbursements journal at the time checks are written. Invoices should be marked "paid" and placed in the vendor file, along with the receipt of payment statement when it is received. These source documents are retained until the end of the year for the accountant's records.

INVENTORY: CONTROLLING SUPPLIES AND EQUIPMENT

A system of inventory control is needed to measure the amount and type of supplies used by each department. Under accrual accounting one must be able to measure all expenses incurred in order to match them with the revenues earned in a specified time period. Consistent records of the cost of supplies consumed enable price comparisons to be made over time between departments or services. These records are also valuable in the budgeting process.

A system of inventory control discourages waste and pilferage of supplies and provides a means of keeping supplies at optimal levels. Overstock, especially of time-dated supplies, has an opportunity cost: the cost of monies unnecessarily tied up in inventory and a possible cost of obsolescence. Excess inventory also increases the opportunity for pilferage. On the other hand, frequent shortages of needed supplies can impinge on the quality of care and result in frustration among staff or require that costly rush orders be used to meet supply needs. In the early 1990s a management approach to this continuing problem called "just-in-time" inventory was initiated. One well-known example was the Harley Davidson Motor Cycle Company, which moved to just in time inventory with notable success. By the late 1990s management viewed just-in-time inventory as much a liability as an asset. (The real problem at the Harley plants, it turned out, was not the timing of the arrival of inventory, but the quality and appropriateness of the inventory whenever it arrived.)

Ideally, the focal point of inventory control is a locked central storeroom (see Figure 3.8). All supplies should be delivered to a central storeroom as soon as they are received. A limited number of employees should have access to central stores, usually one employee on each shift, although access to supplies must be balanced so that supplies may be obtained when needed but are not subject to unwarranted use. Smaller facilities may find a central storeroom impractical, in which case decentralized storerooms can become the responsibility of personnel in the individual department.

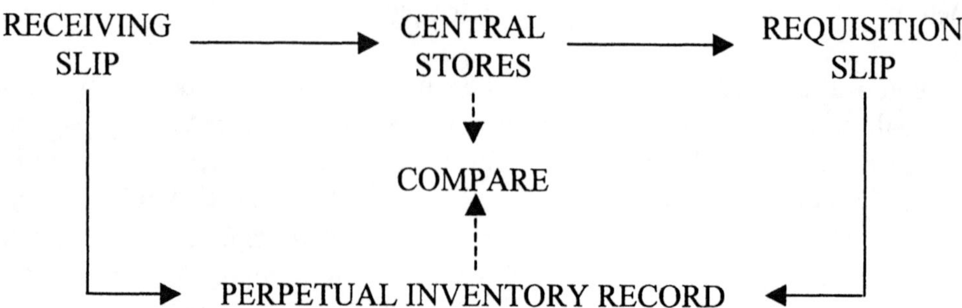

FIGURE 3.8 Perpetual inventory record.

Perpetual Inventory

A perpetual inventory system is recommended to maintain a precise count of inventory on hand, that is, an accurate count of supplies used and those remaining in the storeroom. At the beginning of each fiscal year, probably more often, all inventory in central stores (or the decentralized storerooms) should be physically confirmed. This is the beginning inventory for the time period.

Additions to inventory are noted from the receiving slips included in each shipment of supplies. The beginning inventory and the inventory received by the storerooms make up the total available inventory. When supplies are removed from a storeroom, a requisition slip identifying the supplies and date issued, by department, must be filled out. Supplies issued by storerooms may be taken as the supplies actually used in providing services. This, of course, does not account for those supplies remaining in each department or sublocation that have not yet been used.

For this reason, department heads should be encouraged to keep initial levels of supplies in their departments. Requisition slips should be initialed by a department head or other designated person. Requisition slips not only provide a check on the unjustified removal of supplies from the storerooms but are the objective measure of the supplies consumed during a particular period.

The receiving slips and requisition slips are the source documents for keeping the perpetual inventory record (see Table 3.12). At the end of each year, or other time period, the inventory in the storerooms should be counted and compared with the ending inventory from the perpetual inventory record. If the physical count of the storerooms and the inventory record do not match, this may indicate pilferage, misuse of requisition slips, or inaccuracies in the record-keeping system.

It is advisable for the business office to maintain a list of all inventory items used by the facility, the number of items in one unit, and the current price per unit. This log acts as a reference for determining the cost of the inventory used by each department and for establishing the total volume of supplies remaining in the storeroom(s).

LIFO/FIFO

To account for the effects of inflation or deflation on the price of inventory, the GAAP recognizes two methods of inventory costing—last in, first out (LIFO) and first in, first out (FIFO). The LIFO method assumes that inventory added last to stores is used first, thus making (in the case of inflation) the value of the goods remaining in inventory lower than that of the goods used to provide services. The FIFO method assumes the opposite: that the older and less expensive supplies (in the case of deflation) are used for services, and the higher-priced goods remain in inventory longer. The difference in the effect of these two methods is shown in Table 3.13. Either method of inventory cost may be adopted, but the one selected should be used consistently and should be mentioned in the notes to financial statements.

Table 3.12 Lakeside Assisted Living Perpetual Inventory Record

Item #400 Syringes, disposable	# Units	Cost/unit	Cost
July			
Beginning inventory	4	$7.00	$28.00
Goods received	5	$7.00	$35.00
Total goods available	9	$7.00	$63.00
Ending inventory	3	$7.00	$21.00
Goods used	6	$7.00	$42.00
August			
Beginning inventory		$7.00	$21.00
Goods received	6	$7.00	$42.00
Total goods available	9	$7.00	$63.00
Ending inventory	4	$7.00	$28.00
Goods used	5	$7.00	$35.00

Table 3.13 Inventory

Item #400 Syringes, disposable	# Units	Cost/unit	Cost			
August						
Beginning inventory	9	$7.00	$21.00			
Goods received	6	$7.00	$42.00			
Total goods available	9	$7.00	$63.00			
Ending inventory	4	$7.00	$28.00			
Goods used	5	$7.00	$35.00			
September	Last in, first out			First in, first out		
Beginning inventory	4	$7.00	$28.00	4	$7.00	$28.00
Goods received	5	$8.00	$40.00	5	$8.00	$40.00
Total goods available	9	4 @ 7.00	$68.00	9	4 @ 7.00	68.00
		5@ 8.00			5@ 8.00	
Ending Inventory	5	4 @ 7.00 1 @ 8.00	$36.00	5	$8.00	$40.00
Goods Used	4	$8.00	$32.00	4	$7.00	$28.00

PAYROLL

Payroll is another source of cash outflow. As mentioned in Part Two, it is the largest expense in the assisted living facility, accounting for approximately 35% to 55% of total costs, depending on whether the facility is providing level 1, level 2 or level 3 type care. It also makes up about 85% of the facility's controllable costs. A controllable cost is one over which the administrator has influence. Because it is the primary expense of the facility, accurate accounting records are essential.

PAYROLL JOURNAL

The payroll journal lists all paychecks disbursed in the time period, by department. At the end of the pay period the hours worked are entered in the payroll journal, as derived from the time cards or sheets and the salaried employee's staffing plan. Overtime hours are compensated at a higher rate, as indicated in Part Two, and are listed in a column separate from the regular rate. Gross pay is calculated by multiplying hours worked by the hourly rate:

(Pay Rate x Regular Hours) + (Overtime Rate x Overtime Hours) = Gross Pay

Payroll Deductions

Payroll deductions must be subtracted from gross pay to arrive at the employee's net pay. They include federal, state, and sometimes municipal taxes, as well as various other deductions that must be made.

The amount of federal, state, and local tax deducted is a percentage based on the employee's income. The percentages are supplied by the various government agencies. The Federal Insurance Contribution Act (FICA) deduction is the employee's contribution to the Social Security fund, described in Part Four.

A certain proportion of the employee's paycheck is withheld, matched by the employer, and remitted on a quarterly basis to the Internal Revenue Service (IRS), which collects taxes for the federal government. Because this payroll tax is part of the cost of providing services, it must be attributed to the time period in which the employee was earning the wages. The cumulative amount of payroll tax is entered in the Payables Journal for each month as a credit to the taxes payable and a debit to cash.

Other deductions from the employee's pay may include meals and uniform expense. If the employee health plan requires some contribution by them, this would also be noted in the payroll journal as a deduction. Deductions for each employee are calculated and subtracted from gross pay to give the net pay. A separate column should exist for bonuses or other adjustments to net pay. At the end of each month, salary totals for each department are posted to the general ledger. A page from a typical payroll journal is shown in Figure 3.9.

The employees who divide their time between two or more departments should be listed in the department where the majority of hours are spent, with a portion of their earnings and taxes allocated to the second department. Some reimbursement programs may require record keeping for the hours each day spent by an employee attributable to each designated resident, such as to a managed care resident.

FIGURE 3.9 Page from payroll journal.

Separate Payroll Bank Account

The facility should maintain a separate bank account solely for payroll. The person preparing the payroll does not write his or her own paycheck. All paychecks should have two signatures or be approved by the administrator before being disbursed. The paycheck number and the date of issue are recorded in the payroll journal to identify checks that are misplaced or to stop payment on checks that are not cashed within a reasonable period of time. Checks are best distributed to each employee in person.

Preparation and maintenance of the payroll is largely a bookkeeping function, although larger facilities may have a separate department devoted to this task. In recent years a number of electronic payroll services have been offered by banks and other financial service groups. A telephone call to the bank or data transmission by modem accomplishes transmission of information to the financial service or corporate office, which in turn delivers the checks to the facility at a specified time.

PROTECTING THE RESIDENTS' FUNDS

Legal Responsibilities

Health care facilities are frequently asked by residents to safeguard their assets. Any agreement to take responsibility for these assets must be conformed through a legal contract signed by both the facility and the resident or the sponsor. This contract establishes a trust relationship between the resident and the facility, and sound procedures for managing these assets must be adhered to so that the relationship is not violated.

Administrators vary in what they will protect for residents. Some may keep jewelry and similar items in safekeeping. In general, experience suggests that cash be the primary or only resident asset the facility will take responsibility to safeguard. Valuables other than cash are best managed by a legal representative of the resident.

Separate Accounting

As a check on resident cash, a separate book should be kept to record the information, as shown in Figure 3.10. A copy of a receipt signed by the resident or sponsor is kept in an envelope accompanying this book.

Facility Requirements When Managing Resident Funds

There is no requirement that assisted living facilities manage or help residents manage their finances. However, a number of facilities offer financial assistance as one of the several services available to residents. The information below summarizes the federally established principles and procedures for handling resident funds. While the assisted living facility is not bound to these principles and procedures, they provide a good checklist against which to set facility policies.

Management of personal funds. Upon written authorization of a resident, the facility may hold, safeguard, manage, and account for the personal funds of the resident deposited with the facility.

Page ____ of ____

Facility ______________ # ________ Month ending 06/30/X1

Name	Beginning Balance	Deposits	Disbursements	Ending Balance
Jones, F.A.	$210.00	$90.00	$25.00	$275.00

FIGURE 3.10 Resident trust funds trial balance.

Deposit of funds. *Funds in excess of $50:* The facility may deposit any resident's personal funds in excess of $50 in an interest-bearing account (or accounts) that is separate from any of the facility's operating accounts and that credits all interest earned on resident's funds to that account (in pooled accounts, there may be a separate accounting for each resident's share).

Funds less than $50: The facility may maintain a resident's personal funds that do not exceed $50 in a non-interest-bearing account, interest-bearing account, or petty cash fund.

If pooled accounts are used, interest may be prorated per individual on the basis of actual earnings or end-of-quarter balance. Residents should have access to petty cash on an ongoing basis and be able to arrange for access to larger funds.

"Hold, safeguard, manage, and account for" means that the facility may act as fiduciary of the resident's funds and report at least quarterly on the status of these funds in a clear and understandable manner. Managing the resident's financial affairs includes money that an individual gives to the facility for the sake of providing a resident with a noncovered service (such as a permanent wave).

"Interest bearing" means a rate of return equal to or above the passbook savings rate at local banking institutions in the area.

Proper bookkeeping techniques would include an individual ledger card, ledger sheet or equivalent established for each resident on which only those transactions involving his or her personal funds are recorded and maintained. The record should have information on when transactions occurred and what they were, as well as maintain the ongoing balance for every resident. Anytime there is a transaction the resident should be given a receipt and the facility retains a copy.

"Quarterly statements" are to be provided in writing to the resident or the resident's representative within 30 days after the end of the quarter.

If the facility accepts Medicaid, the following policies may apply.

Notice of certain balances. The facility may notify each resident that receives Medicaid benefits

1. When the amount in the resident's account reaches $200 less than the SSI resource limit for one person.
2. That, if the amount in the account, in addition to the value of the resident's other nonexempt resources, reaches the SSI resource limit for one person, the resident may lose eligibility for Medicaid or SSI.

Conveyance of Resident's Funds Upon Death Within 30 Days

Upon the death of a resident with a personal fund deposited with the facility, the facility may convey within 30 days the resident's funds, and a final accounting of those funds, to the individual or probate jurisdiction administering the resident's estate.

Surety bond or equivalent to protect resident funds

The facility may purchase a surety bond, or otherwise provide assurance to guarantee the security of all personal funds of residents deposited with the facility. Unlike other types of insurance, the surety bond protects the oblige (the resident or the State), not the principal (the facility), from loss. The surety bond differs from a fidelity bond, which covers no acts or errors of negligence, incompetence, or dishonesty.

The surety bond is the commitment of the facility in an objective manner to ensure that the facility may hold, safeguard, manage, and account for the funds residents have entrusted to the facility. The facility assumes the responsibility to compensate the oblige for the amount of the loss up to the entire amount of the surety bond. The facility cannot be named as a beneficiary.

Self-insurance is not an acceptable alternative to a surety bond. Likewise, funds deposited in bank accounts protected by the Federal Deposit Insurance Corporation, or similar entity, also are not acceptable alternatives.

Limitation or Charges to Personal Funds

The facility may not impose a charge against the personal funds of a resident for any item or services for which payment is made under Medicaid (except for applicable deductible and coinsurance amounts).

Services Included in Medicaid Payment

During the course of a covered Medicaid stay, facilities may *not* charge a resident for the following categories of items and services:

- Nursing services as required
- Dietary services
- An activities program
- Room/bed maintenance services

- Routine personal hygiene items and services as required to meet the needs of residents, including, but not limited to, hair hygiene supplies, comb, brush, bath soap, disinfecting soaps, or specialized cleansing agents when indicated to treat special skin problems or to fight infection, razor, shaving cream, toothbrush, toothpaste, denture adhesive, denture cleaner, dental floss, moisturizing lotion, tissues, cotton balls, cotton swabs, deodorant, incontinence care and supplies, sanitary napkins and related supplies, towels, washcloths, hospital gowns, over-the-counter drugs, hair and nail hygiene services, bathing, and basic personal laundry.

"Hair hygiene supplies" refers to comb, brush, shampoos, trims, and simple haircuts provided by facility staff as part of routine grooming care. Haircuts, permanent waves, hair coloring, and relaxing performed by barbers and beauticians not employed by a facility are chargeable.

"Nail hygiene services" refers to routine trimming, cleaning, filing, but not polishing of undamaged nails, and on an individual basis, care for ingrown or damaged nails.

"Basic personal laundry" does not include dry cleaning, mending, washing by hand, or other specialty services that need not be provided. A resident may be charged for these specialty services if he or she requests and receives them.

Items and Services That May be Charged to Residents' Funds

Listed below are general categories and examples of items and services that the facility may charge to residents' funds if they are requested by a resident, if the facility informs the resident that there may be a charge, and if payment is not made by Medicaid:

- Telephone
- Television/radio for personal use
- Personal comfort items, including smoking materials, notions and novelties, and confections
- Cosmetic and grooming items and services in excess of those for which payment is made under Medicaid or Medicare
- Personal clothing
- Personal reading matter
- Gifts purchased on behalf of a resident
- Flowers and plants
- Social events and entertainment offered outside the scope of the activities program
- Noncovered special care services such as privately hired nurses or aides
- Private room, except when therapeutically required (e.g., isolation for infection control)
- Specially prepared or alternative food requested instead of the food generally prepared by the facility

Matters such as inventory and payroll should not occupy too much of the administrator's time. However, it is important that all of these details be properly managed by the staff, and experience seems to show that when the administrator understands the fine points of financing and occasionally reviews these matters knowledgeably with them, the staff tend to pay attention to details also. The result is that the administrator is thus freed to deal with broader policy while procedures such as payroll and managing residents' accounts function smoothly.

3.7 The Concept of Depreciation

Depreciation has been mentioned to some extent already. Capital assets are those used to provide services during more than one time period; in the course of operations they lose value as a result of use, wear and tear, or obsolescence.

To account for this loss of value to capital assets in the accrual system of accounting, the cost of the asset is spread over the time period that it is used. This must be done because the total cost of acquiring the asset could not properly be attributed to the month in which it was purchased, when it is actually an expense of providing services for several years to come.

IDENTIFYING DEPRECIABLE ASSETS

Assets that can be capitalized or depreciated differ from other assets of the facility in that they are used in operations for more than one time period and will not be converted into cash within the year. Many facilities set a minimum value for depreciable assets, usually somewhere about $200. A calculator, for example, may be used in the business office for many years, but its acquisition cost may be so low that the depreciation expense over its useful life would be negligible. The asset must be tangible and by definition must be owned by the facility. Thus leased equipment cannot normally be depreciated. (Some leases, in which the lessor agrees not to take depreciation, can under some circumstances be depreciated.)

All new assets meeting these criteria are considered depreciable assets. Any alterations of the present fixed asset that affect either its value or its useful life, such as renovation, are depreciable expenses. Repair of damages or regular maintenance of the asset cannot be considered part of the depreciable expense.

DETERMINING DEPRECIATION EXPENSE

There are several methods of calculating depreciation expense, but all methods are based on the historical cost of the asset, its useful life (sometimes preset by tax or other regulations), and its salvage value, if any.

Historical Cost

The historical cost of the asset is the cost of acquiring the asset that is depreciated over several time periods. In addition to the purchase price, the cost of taxes, shipping delivery, installation, and so forth can be included along with any other one-time costs associated with acquiring the asset.

Useful Life

The useful life of the asset is the number of years the item can be expected to be used by the facility. This must be an estimation. However, the IRS has useful life estimates for most assets that are mandated in reporting taxes or, in most instances, in calculating depreciation reports for Medicare, Medicaid, and some other third-party payers.

Salvage Value

A capital asset may have some value at the end of its useful life. A van, which normally has an IRS determined useful life of 5 years, might be such an asset.

STRAIGHT-LINE DEPRECIATION

There are several methods for figuring the depreciation expense, once the historical cost, useful life, and salvage value are determined. Straight-line depreciation is a depreciation method in which the historical cost of an asset is spread evenly over its useful life so that the depreciation expense is the same in every time period that it functions.

historical cost / useful life = annual depreciation expense

If Lakeside Assisted Living purchases new physical therapy equipment worth $20,000 with an estimated useful life of 5 years, the annual depreciation expense for the equipment would be:

$20,000/5 = $4,000 per year depreciation

After the first year the value of the physical therapy equipment on the books would be:

$20,000 – $4,000 = $16,000

Hence, the $16,000 is called the *book value* of this asset.

Straight-line depreciation has the advantage of simplicity.

ACCELERATED DEPRECIATION

This method attributes most of the depreciation expense to the first years of the asset's life, thus enabling the facility to write it off more quickly, thereby gaining a tax advantage through earlier tax recognition of the investment. Among the several types of accelerated depreciation are the sum-of-the-years digits and double declining balance.

PURPOSES OF DEPRECIATION

We have already mentioned that depreciation must be calculated to adhere to the accrual system of accounting. To ignore the very real cost of depreciation is to underestimate the expense of providing services and to overestimate the value of the assets of the facility. For this reason, depreciation is included on the income statement as an operating expense and is subtracted from the historical cost of fixed assets on the balance sheet to reflect its impact on the financial position of the facility.

Asset Replacement

Probably the most important reason for recognizing depreciation is for asset replacement. Because the asset will eventually have to be replaced, the present asset should be expensed over its useful life to accumulate the funds needed for its replacement. Chances are, however, that an asset purchased 10 years earlier will be more expensive than the original. This is not always the case. Some assets remain about the same for replacement, whereas others actually may decrease in replacement costs. Computers, for example, have become less and less expensive to provide the same computing capacities because of advances in technology and competition among computer makers.

Few facilities actually "fund" depreciation, that is, put cash in an interest-bearing account reserved for replacing equipment. Such a fund would appear in the capital or new worth section of the balance sheet as "funded depreciation."

ENTERING DEPRECIATION INTO THE ACCOUNTING RECORDS

A portion of the depreciation expense may easily be attributed to each time period by dividing the annual depreciation expense by the number of accounting periods in the year. Since depreciation is entered in the general journal at the end of each month, the Lakeside Assisted Living's new physical therapy equipment depreciation expense after the first month of purchase under straight-line depreciation would be as follows:

General Journal

	Debit	Credit
1/29 Depreciation Expense	$333.33	
1/29 Allowance for Depreciation		$333.33

Categorization of Fixed Assets

The chart of accounts should have an account for each type of fixed asset owned by the facility. These assets can be categorized generally as

- land and improvements
- buildings

- fixed equipment
- major movable equipment
- minor movable equipment

or in more specific categories that are more useful to the facility.

In addition, depreciation schedules should be maintained for each category of assets (see Table 3.14) and for each type of depreciation, if accelerated and straight-line are both used.

If two different schedules are used to depreciate the same assets—one for reimbursement and one for other purposes—there will be a difference in depreciation expenses for each asset every year. Since the total amount of depreciation taken for each asset should be the same (total depreciation will equal the historical cost less salvage value), this difference between the two depreciation expenses is a timing difference. Depreciation in this case may be regarded as a charge that must be deferred to another time period or as revenue that is accrued if depreciation will be recognized in a later accounting period.

Table 3.14 Lakeside Assisted Living Depreciation Schedule

Item	Cost	Date purchased	Life	Method depreciated	Year	Depreciation per year Annual	Cumulative
Plant: Main	$5,767,004.00	6/10XX	30	Strt. Line	19XX	$192,233.47	$192,233.47
Welsh Hall					19XX	$192,233.47	384,466.94
Hall and Garage					19XX	$192,233.47	576,700.41
					19XX	$192,233.47	768,933.88
					Etc.		
Kitchen Equipment	$398,600.00	6/10XX	15	Strt. Line	19XX	$26,573.33	$26,573.33
					19XX	$26,573.33	53,146.66
					19XX	$26,573.33	79,719.99
					19XX	$26,573.33	106,293.32
					Etc.		

3.8 Using "Costs" in Managerial Decisions

EFFICIENCY

Efficiency, as discussed in Part One, may be defined as input over output, or the amount of input used for a certain level of output. Costs, as a component of input, are generally easier to control than are revenues or other measures of output. Revenues are subject to limitation by competition from providers of similar services and government regulation through insurance and medical assistance programs. Knowledge of costs and the ability to control and reduce them permit liquidity of limited funds, making them available for other uses.

3.8.1 Two Types of Costs: Variable and Fixed

VARIABLE COSTS

All costs can be regarded as variable, fixed, or semivariable. Variable costs are those that fluctuate directly and proportionately with changes in volume. That is, if volume is increased or decreased by a certain percentage, variable costs will rise or fall, respectively, by the same percentage. The cost of disposable supplies in the health care area will vary directly with the number of similar care type and level residents served. The cost of food in dietary or the cost of postage for resident billing will also vary with resident volume.

FIXED COSTS

Fixed costs, on the other hand, do not relate to changes in volume. The cost of resident care coordinator's salary will not change with fluctuations in the number of residents. This does not mean that the director's salary cannot change at all, but it will result from an administrative decision rather than responding to resident volume. Clearly, if volume varies enough, many "fixed" costs will not remain the same. If resident volume increases substantially, a new administrative position in the health care area may have to be created to accommodate the additional resident load. Fixed costs, then, are said to be fixed only over a relevant range of volume.

AN ADDITIONAL TYPE: SEMIVARIABLE COSTS

Semivariable costs do not fit neatly into either a variable or a fixed category, as they vary disproportionately with volume. Examples of semivariable costs might be total health care aides' salaries, which depend more on resident volume and resident level of care needs than does the resident care coordinator's salary, which does not fluctuate directly with these variables.

Utility costs that are based on ranges of usage rather than actual usage may also be considered semi-variable costs. It is helpful to think of semi-variable costs as having a much narrower relevant range than fixed costs. Semi-variable costs are often broken down into fixed and variable components for use in calculations, and so our discussion here will be limited to fixed and variable costs for the sake of simplicity.

TOTAL VARIABLE COSTS

While total variable costs (TVC) change with volume, variable costs per unit do not. If disposable pads are $1 each, the cost per pad per resident will be $1, whether 100 or 150 residents receive pads purchased at one cost in one batch. Total fixed costs (TFC), however, do vary per unit with changes in volume. If the resident care coordinator's salary is $44,000 (exclusive of benefits, etc.) and he or she oversees the care of 100 residents, the coordinator's salary cost per resident would be $440 (exclusive of benefits, etc.). If that same resident care coordinator oversees 150 residents, the cost drops to $293 per resident. Familiarity with the costs of the facility maximizes the administrator's ability to control its finances.

The behavior of variable and fixed costs is summarized in Table 3.15. As can be seen, fixed costs decrease with an increase in volume. Because the assisted living facility generally has a high proportion of fixed costs, maintaining a high volume of service is of paramount concern to administrators.

A closer study of the concept of fixed and variable costs reveals how it can be used to aid in decision making. Because all costs can be considered fixed or variable, (even semi-variable costs),

$$\text{total fixed costs} + \text{total variable costs} = \text{total costs}$$

Because total variable costs are a function of the variable cost per unit and the number of units, the above equation can be expanded to

$$\text{total fixed costs} + (\text{variable cost per unit x volume units}) = \text{total costs}$$

$$\text{total fixed costs} + \left(\frac{\text{variable costs}}{\text{units}} \text{ x volume units}\right) = \text{total costs}$$

$$\frac{\text{break-even volume}}{\text{in units}} = \frac{\text{fixed cost}}{\text{rate} - \text{variable cost}}$$

Thus, if three of these values are known, the remaining value can be calculated.

The administrator of Lakeside Assisted Living wants to find the average variable cost of supplies used per resident during the month. The general ledger shows that the total costs of the health care area for 1 month are $12,000. The administrator has determined that fixed cost accounts in that department amount to $9,000 and that supplies are its only variable cost.

The resident census report for the month shows that there have been 3,000 resident days or an average of 100 residents over 30 days. To calculate the variable cost per resident in the health care area:

$$\frac{(\text{total costs} - \text{total fixed costs})}{\text{Volume units}} = \frac{\text{variable costs}}{\text{Units}}$$

$$(\$12{,}000 - \$9{,}000)/100 \text{ residents} = \$30 \text{ per resident}$$

Thus the variable cost of providing health care services in this particular month was $30 per resident.

Table 3-15 Behavior of Fixed and Variable Costs

	Resident Care Coordinator		Disposable medical supplies	
Patients	(TFC)	FC/unit	TVC	VC/Unit
100	$44,000.00	440	100	$1.00
125	$44,000.00	352	125	$1.00
150	$44,000.00	293	150	$1.00
	(No change)	(Change)	(Change)	(No change)

VOLUME OF SERVICE UNITS

These equations can be used to determine the volume of service units required to break even. Since total costs (TC) equal total revenues (TR) at the break-even point, total revenue (TR) can be substituted for total costs (TC) in the above equations to give the costs or volume needed to break even.

If the total costs of the physical therapy department are $6,500 per month, and the total fixed costs are $5,200, and the variable cost per resident visit to physical therapy is $8, how many resident visits are needed per month to break even in this department?

total costs = total revenue

$6,500 = $5,200 + ($8 x volume unit)
volume units ($6,500 – $5,200)/$8

Volume units = 162.5 visits per month

We have assumed that the physical therapists are employees of the facility and that their salaries comprise a significant portion of the fixed costs of the department. If physical therapy is provided on a contractual basis, the therapists' salaries would become a variable cost if they were paid for each visit.

At this point, the reader may wish to revisit the tables in Part Two that depict the budgets for the 60-unit assisted living facility (Jordan Lake, Table 2.1A) and the 100-unit assisted living facility (Kerr Lake, Table 2.1B). The 100-unit facility, Kerr Lake, enjoys a number of economies of scale, making it considerably more profitable. Increased profitability for the facility results primarily from the effects of fixed and semivariable costs. An item-by-item comparison of the two tables will reveal which costs are variable, which fixed, and which semivariable. Later, the reader may wish to figure the return on investment, return on owners' equity, and similar comparisons using the formulas given below. A comparison of the Jordan Lake and Kerr Lake assisted living facilities' profitability reveal the powerful effects of fixed and semivariable costs. In order to obtain a satisfactory return on investment, the smaller facility will likely have to be able to successfully obtain higher monthly resident rates.

3.8.2 Additional Types of Costs: Indirect Costs and Direct Costs

Costs may also be categorized as direct and indirect. In order to discuss them, however, we must first define revenue and cost centers.

REVENUE CENTERS

Revenue centers are units of the facility, usually departments, that generate revenue, usually through resident care. Revenue centers in the assisted living facility will normally be health care, possibly physical therapy, occupational therapy, pharmacy, laboratory, and medical support. It may also be any other department or center earning revenue, such as a cafeteria that serves a large number of guest meals or a profitable day care program. If pharmaceuticals or supplies are included as part of the routine care and are not separately charged, they would not be revenue centers.

As facilities add service areas such as home health and hospice care, these become additional revenue centers. If the facility earns a significant amount of revenue from interest on investments, interest may also be considered a revenue center.

COST CENTERS

Cost centers are units of the facility identified with certain costs. Revenue centers are almost always cost centers because the revenue-earning departments also have costs directly associated with them. Interest as a revenue center has little or no costs associated with it. All other departments, such as administration, maintenance, housekeeping, and usually dietary and laundry, are cost centers. Depreciation, interest, insurance, telephone, utility, and transportation expenses may also be considered cost centers. These are all identifiable costs of the facility, and the concept of cost centers will become clearer as we proceed.

DIRECT COSTS

Direct costs are those directly attributable to a revenue center or directly providing resident care. In the assisted living facility direct costs are often called *resident care costs.* Direct costs of the health care area would include all health care salaries, payroll taxes, benefits, supplies, expenses associated with capital equipment used only in the department, and any other costs associated directly with this department.

INDIRECT COSTS

Indirect costs are those that cannot be directly associated with a revenue-producing center, yet support the functions of the resident care centers (or other care centers, such as an adult day care center). Indirect costs of the health care area would be administration, payroll, utility, housekeeping, maintenance, dietary, laundry, plant depreciation, tax, and interest expenses that keep these departments running. For this reason, indirect costs are also known as *support service costs.*

Support Service Costs

These indirect costs must be allocated to all the revenue-producing departments that are also cost centers in order to be included in the charge for services in each revenue center and to reflect the total cost of providing that service. To find the total costs of the revenue-producing department, then, the support costs must be spread over all revenue-producing departments in some systematic way. This process is known as *cost finding,* as it yields the total costs of the resident care centers (and other centers such as adult day care).

The concept of cost finding is illustrated in Figure 3.11. The total costs of both the support and service (or revenue-earning centers) are shown. To find the total cost of providing resident services A and B, some portion of the support centers must be allocated to the revenue centers. Support Center No. 1 divides its support equally between resident service centers A and B, so 50% of Support Center No. 1's costs are attributed to each resident service center.

Support Center No. 2 provides more services to Resident Service Center B, and this is reflected in the proportion of Support Center No. 2's costs that go to Resident Service Center B. When the costs of both support centers are allocated, the total cost of providing services A and B are known.

VALUES OF COST FINDING

Cost finding yields a representative picture of the entire expense of providing each service. This information is used in deciding whether a particular service should be discontinued or supported. For example, unless all direct and indirect costs of providing a service, such as adult day care, are calculated, it is difficult to determine the cost-effectiveness of offering such a service. Cost allocation is a subjective process in that there is an almost infinite number of ways to perform cost allocation properly.

FIGURE 3.11 Cost allocation between two support and two revenue centers.

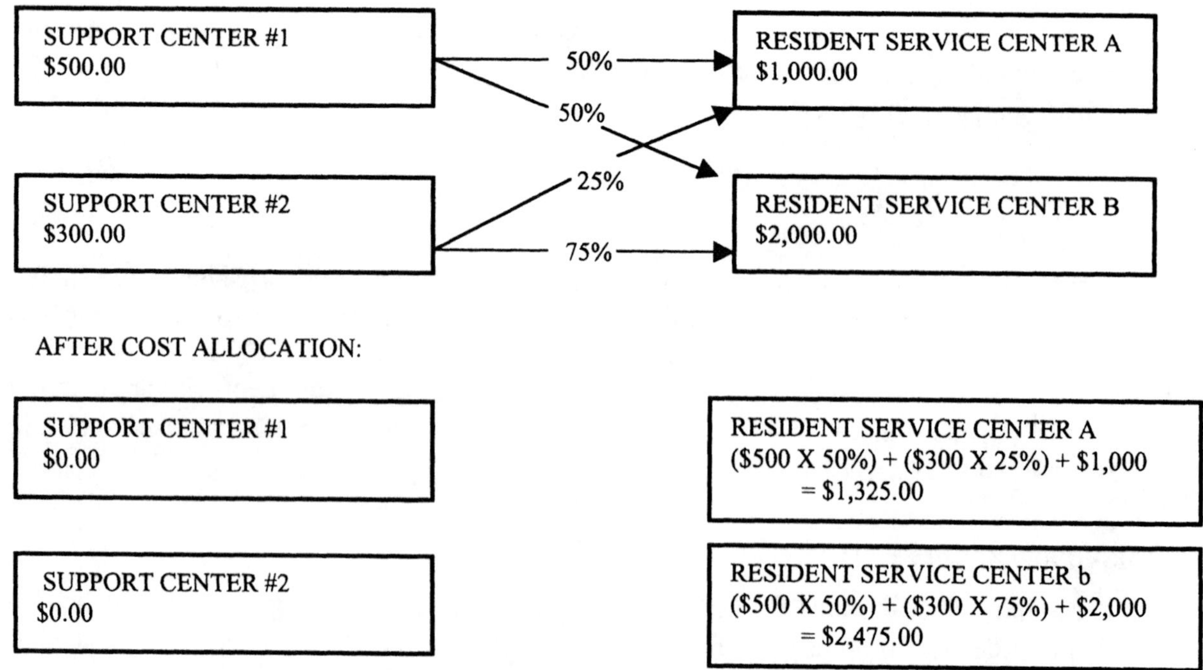

ALLOCATING INDIRECT COSTS

There are several methods for allocating indirect costs, among them the step-down and reciprocal methods. Providers that are reimbursed on a cost basis must usually use the step-down method unless another method is approved. We will discuss the step-down method in some detail here and briefly explain the reciprocal method at the end of this section.

The step-down method derives its name from the shape of the completed worksheet and involves the systematic allocation of all cost centers over all other cost centers that use the "services" of the cost center expenses being allocated. Support costs are spread not only over revenue centers but also over other support cost centers.

Once a support cost is divided among the other cost centers, no more costs can be allocated to that department. Therefore, the order in which support costs are allocated affects the final cost of the revenue centers. As a rule, cost centers that are used by most of the other cost centers are allocated first.

The basis of allocation also affects the outcome of the cost-finding process. In allocating housekeeping costs to the departments that use housekeeping services, the basis for allocation might be the number of employees in the department, the square footage of the departments, or some other criterion. Likewise, administrative costs might be allocated on the basis of number of employees, total salary of employees, volume of services provided, or total revenues earned in each department. These alternatives are examples only; clearly, the basis for allocation varies.

Third-party reimbursement will indicate the basis for allocation that should be used for residents for whom they reimburse, but in any case the method the facility uses should remain consistent to enable comparison of the resulting costs in different time periods.

The Step-Down Process

Cost allocation is best illustrated through a step-by-step example of the step-down process. The one provided in Table 3.16 is necessarily simplified; cost allocations for most health care organizations are usually performed by computer because of the volume and complexities involved in larger, more departmentalized, or multiprogram facilities.

Other Methods of Cost Finding

Two other approaches to cost finding are the reciprocal and cost-apportionment methods. The reciprocal is similar to the step-down method, except that it recognizes reciprocal services provided between cost centers, such as administration and maintenance. Because of the calculations involved and the extent of these services in most organizations, reciprocal allocation is performed by computer.

RATE SETTING

One of the primary uses of the cost-finding process is to develop a basis for setting rates for the services provided by the revenue centers. Once the costs of the revenue centers are known, the average cost per unit of service can be calculated by dividing the total cost of the revenue center by the expected service volume.

TABLE 3.16 Step-down Worksheets: Preliminary Worksheet

Cost Centers	Capital (sq. ft)	Plant (sq. ft)	Admin (1) (FTE) (-1)	Main (sq. ft)	Laundry lbs dry	House-Keeping (sq. ft)	Dietary (meals)	Social Services (visits)	P.T. (visits)	O.T. (visits)	Nursing	Total
Support and Revenue Centers												
Admin	3.0%	3.0%										
Maintenance	1.5%	1.5%	0.5%									
Laundry	9.0%	9.0%	3.0%	9.4%								
Housekeeping	8.0%	8.0%	7.4%	8.4%	5.0%							
Dietary	10.0%	10.0%	7.3%	10.5%	15.0%	12.8%						
Social Services	0.5%	0.5%	0.1%	0.5%		0.6%						
Physical Therapy	7.0%	7.0%	2.5%	7.3%	2.5%	8.9%						
Occupational Therapy	2.0%	2.0%	.04%	2.1%	2.5%	2.6%						
Nursing	59.0%	59.0%	78.8%	61.7%	75.0%	75.2%						
TOTAL	100.0%	100.0%	100.0%	100.0%	100.0%	100.0%	100.0%	100.0%	100.0%	100.0%	100.0%	100.0%

1. –FTE = full time equivalent employees
2. Total maintenance costs include all utility costs

The unit of service must first be determined. In the physical therapy department a unit of service is normally calculated as a 15-minute segment for which charges are made.

The average cost per unit of service offers a basis for rate setting, because rates should approximate the cost of providing the service. But other factors, such as demand for services, competitive rates, expected inflation rates, contractual discounts, and frequency of uncollectibles, must be considered in achieving realistic rates.

3.9 Budgets and Budgeting

CONSIDERATIONS IN BUDGETING

The budgeting process in the assisted living facility is a period of planning. The physical budget is more than a record of anticipated expenses for the next fiscal year. It represents a careful examination of internal and external changes that management believes will affect the operation of the facility and the strategy to deal with these changes for some time to come. Thus the budget is a reflection of the administrator's short- and long-term goals for the facility. Most organizations also have a 3- to 5-year budget plan following the next fiscal year as a guide to long-range planning.

The budget is a tool to be used throughout the year, rather than a document filed away to remain only in the memory of the budget participants. The budget can be changed as conditions change. It provides a meaningful comparison between actual and projected expenditures and revenues.

Most facility administrators use the budget in a monthly review with department managers on how the year is unfolding and what changes need to be undertaken.

3.9.1 Two Methods of Budget Preparation

Budgeting is done in any number of ways, and each individual facility or multifacility operation will develop its own particular style. In general, two methods of budget preparation are used: the top-down and the participatory method.

TOP-DOWN APPROACH TO BUDGETING

With the top-down approach, the administrator prepares the annual budget with little or no guidance from department heads. This method is most suitable for smaller facilities with few departments, where the administrator is familiar with all the costs of the facility. Top-down is also often the approach used by chains, in which case the local administrator is given a "suggested" budget with the corporation's goals already built into it. The top-down method is quick but has the disadvantages of possibly stifling innovation or of imposing an unpopular or unrealistic budget on department head or chain facility administrators.

THE PARTICIPATORY APPROACH

The participatory method of budgeting requires input from staff members on several levels of the organization. The administrator provides guidelines for the preparation of departmental budgets, prepared by the department heads and other key personnel. These budgets are then reviewed by the administrator, adjusted as necessary, and combined into one organizational budget.

Participatory budgeting is more appropriate for larger facilities. Although it is time-consuming, it furnishes an opportunity for communication between the administrator and department heads and results in input into the budget from those who are most knowledgeable about the daily operation of the individual departments.

Participatory budgeting will be used to describe the budgeting process in this section, as it is considerably more involved than the top-down approach. However, the process described is equally applicable to the latter.

Participatory budgeting augments the role each participant plays in the operations of the facility. Department heads and others become more aware not only of the costs of their areas and the resources available to the facility but also of the needs of the other departments. Budgeting also brings greater recognition of their own roles to the participating staff, and although the budget process is often time-consuming and frustrating, the staff is rewarded by the knowledge that their experience and ideas are valued.

Finally, the budget communicates information about the facility to external parties that have an interest in its status, such as the board of directors or stockholders, third-party payers, planning agencies, accreditation teams, rate review commissions, and unions. The administrator must often be able to justify proposed expenses and revenues to them.

3.9.2 Five Steps in the Budgeting Process

There are any number of ways to prepare the budget, whether by the administrator alone or with the input of key personnel. The optimal method will depend on, among other considerations, the size of the facility, whether it is free standing or a unit in a small or large chain, and the administrator's time constraints.

In designing the budgeting process the administrator first decides what information is desired and how detailed it must be, then maps out the logistics of the activity. The administrator determines who the participants will be. In the case of top-down budgeting, the administrator and perhaps other administrative personnel, such as the bookkeeper, comptroller, or business manager, will be involved. Participatory budgeting usually includes the administrator, the accountant or the comptroller, the bookkeeper, and other staff as appropriate. The budget timetable must also be defined. At least 2 to 5 months before the beginning of the next fiscal year should be allowed for the entire process.

STEP 1: ASSESSING THE ENVIRONMENT

The initial step in the budgeting process is the assessment of the external and internal environments. The budget cannot be prepared in a vacuum. The political, economic, and social environments outside the assisted living facility walls, as mentioned in Part One, are not static. Although the administrator does not have control over these aspects of the external environment, ignorance of the trends affecting the assisted living facility industry, and failure to anticipate their effects on the operations of the facility, leave the administrator less able to deal effectively with changes. Such trends may occur as one or more of the following:

- increased or decreased competition
- new types of competition (e.g., local hospital opening assisted living units or increasing capacity to treat at home by local home health agencies or emergence of additional hospice care agencies)
- altered reimbursement policies
- amended licensing laws
- revised quality review regulations
- swings in the economy
- inflation, deflation, or stagnation
- changes in prevailing wage rates
- reduction or enlargement of the potential service population
- changes in availability of key personnel
- changes in disease patterns among residents
- changing system pressures from hospital discharge patterns due to diagnostic related group pressures
- changing third-party payer situation, with new patterns of providing and paying for care emerging
- increasing acuity level among the resident population

Some, if not most, of these fluctuations in the external environment may affect the plans and operations of the facility.

STEP 2: PROGRAMMING

After the external environments and their anticipated effects on the facility have been evaluated, the facility's objectives for the coming year are determined. This process is sometimes known as programming; in effect, it results in a program for the facility to follow. Through this "programming" the administrator can alter internal operations over which he or she has control to respond to the external (and internal) influences on the facility.

How might an administrator use programming to cope with external events? In periods of rising inflation the cost of living goes up. This usually results in a demand for higher wages. If the administrator is aware of this trend, an objective might be to index the salaries, that is, raise them by a certain percentage to approximate the increased costs of living by a certain time during the following year. An increase in salary expense can then be included in the budget, thereby preventing a situation in which funds are not set aside for this purpose. Such an oversight could result in recruiting problems, high staff turnover, or a strain on operating funds when a salary increase is finally provided.

Similarly, if a competitor is opening a facility quite close by, a contingency fund could be set aside in the following year's budget to raise salaries to meet the new competitor's salary scale, should this become necessary.

Other considerations for programming are changes in service volume, services offered, payer mix, personnel needs, and capital needs. The cumulative effect of expected external and internal events should determine the objectives of the facility for the next years, which in turn form the basis of assumptions made in the budgeting process.

The completed budgeting process should result in four types of budgets: the operating budget, the cash budget, the capital budget, and the pro forma financial statements.

STEP 3: DEVELOPING THE OPERATING BUDGET

The operating budget has two parts: the expense budget and the revenue budget.

The Expense Budget

The expense budget, the type with which we are most familiar, lists the anticipated expenses of the facility for the coming year and is prepared largely by the department heads. The budget timetable should indicate when the final departmental expense budgets are due. Budgeting expenses on a per resident day (PRD) basis can be the most accurate.

The heads of all service units should indicate the expected resident service volume, while support departments (such as dietary) should be able to estimate the number of meals that will be served. Budgeting offers an opportunity for communication among departments. After all, dietary must learn the expected resident volume in the different areas of the facility to be able to calculate the number of meals to be served and types of diets likely to be needed (e.g., diabetic diets).

Additionally, department heads should review staff positions and note any recommended changes in the staffing pattern. In larger facilities recommendations for salary changes may be the responsibility of the personnel director and may be based on competitive salaries in the community or union agreements if employees are so organized.

Department heads should also check equipment in their departments for repair or replacement needs. Included in this assessment would be estimates of the costs of repair or replacement, supported by professional estimates, manufacturer price sheets, and the like. If equipment needs are extensive, it may be worthwhile for department heads to develop a plant and equipment budget for their departments, which will facilitate preparation of the capital budget.

The costs of supplies and other expenses are often a significant portion of departmental costs. Any change in the volume of supplies needed and the cost per unit should be noted in the budget. Catch-all or miscellaneous categories should be kept to a minimum, as there can be little control over unidentified costs.

Anticipated expenses should be broken down by months or another customary accounting period used in the facility. Monthly expense budgets also facilitate preparation of the cash budget.

Determining Expenses. In determining expenses several strategies can be used. One tactic is to increase all of the current year's expenses by a certain percentage. Although this method is quick, it defeats the purpose of budgeting and the effort involved in environmental assessment and programming.

It is more productive for the department head to identify monthly and yearly trends in costs and utilization to help reduce expenses. For example, occupancy might be consistently below average during the winter holidays but regularly above average in late January and February. Identification of such trends is useful in budgeting for monthly costs on volume levels. It is also often helpful to identify the source of variances in the current year's budget and allow for them in the preparation of the new budget.

In setting up the expense budget a checklist can be used to make sure all expense items in departments are included. A good source for this checklist is the chart of accounts, which should list all expense accounts by department.

All budget participants ought to know how and by whom the final budget levels are decided. Finally, the organizational expense budget is separated by months, and the individual department budgets were retained for comparison of actual with budgeted performance in each department throughout the year.

The Revenue Budget

The second section of the operating budget is the revenue budget, which projects the monthly income for the next fiscal year. The revenue budget need not be prepared on a departmental basis; fewer departments are involved in determining revenues than in determining expenses, and nonoperating revenues are generally under the control of the administrator. Also, service revenues are based on the prices charged for services, which are determined by administrative decision. Hence, the revenue budget is usually prepared at the administrative level.

Operating Revenue Estimates. To estimate operating revenues, all revenue centers are listed, with the number of residents appearing by type of payer. Total resident service revenues are calculated by multiplying the expected service volume in each revenue center by the charge per unit of service. As mentioned in the section on cost finding, rates for services may be determined in several ways. For publicly insured persons, the allowable rate per unit of service may be somewhat less than charges; the reimbursable rate should be used in projecting revenues for these persons.

For privately paying residents, charges can be based on the cost plus profit for providing the service, using the results of the cost-finding process and break-even analysis. Rates may also be based on competitive charges for similar services in the community or on the price that the market will bear.

Nonoperating Revenues. Nonoperating revenues, such as interest income, borrowed funds, and charitable donations, are dependent on any number of factors but are relatively predictable on a monthly basis. These revenues are added to the monthly operating revenues to arrive at the total expected revenues.

Total revenues can then be compared with total budgeted expenses. If revenues seem inadequate to meet expenses, the administrator can check the validity of the predicted service volumes. If service levels seem reasonable, the administrator can seek to increase resident service volume, reduce budget expenses, or raise rates.

Using the Operating Budget: Variance Analysis

As a managerial tool, the operating budget is used throughout the fiscal year to measure performance by a technique called *variance analysis,* which is a comparison of actual versus budgeted monetary and volume values at the end of each month.

Actual expenses that deviate significantly from the budgeted amounts can be investigated to identify the source of the variance (as mentioned in Part One). Such variances may be anything from an inadvertent miscalculation of costs or resident volume to serious mismanagement by a particular department. Typical sources of overage are items such as more pool labor being used than anticipated or a number of employees working unanticipated or unauthorized overtime. Once the source of variances is known, the budget can be adjusted accordingly or the cause of the variance can be dealt with. Budget variance analysis provides the administrator with an important means of control over the finances of the facility.

STEP 4: THE CASH BUDGET

The next step in the budgeting process is preparation of the cash budget. As its name implies, it is prepared on the cash basis of accounting, although it is based on the revenues and expenses from the operating budget. Note that the operating budget is prepared on the accrual basis of accounting: Projected revenues are based on the income earned in the time period, not on the amount of cash received for services during the month.

The cash budget is an estimate of the cash inflows and outflows for the next 12 months, enabling the administrator to identify months with possible cash shortages and overages.

This information can be used to defer nonurgent expenditures to a month with high cash inflows or retain overages in a month to cover anticipated cash shortages in the next. A cash budget is useful for anticipating effects of such events as three pay periods occurring in one month, or anticipated large third-party payments at known intervals. Facilities having corporate ownership may have little need of a cash budget inasmuch as the corporate funds can cover any temporary shortages in cash flow needs of the facility. Some administrators rely on the cash budget for daily operations and sometimes prepare weekly or even daily cash budgets a month in advance.

Determining Cash Inflows and Outflows

To develop the cash budget, cash inflows and outflows must be determined. Because the facility has less control over cash inflows, especially those received from third-party payers, projecting them is somewhat complicated. First, all payer sources must be identified. These will usually be private payers, third-party, Medicaid, insurance companies, HMOs or IPOs or similar organizations, the Veterans Administration, and all other known or anticipated sources of income for services expected to be rendered. The lag time between the billing of services and receipt of payment is determined. Most private payers do so within 30 days of billing, but time lags for third-party and Medicaid may vary considerably. This can be used to measure the percentage of revenues that will be received from each payer in each month.

When cash inflows from resident services are known, monthly cash receipts from nonoperating sources are computed to give total cash receipts for each month.

Cash outflows are somewhat easier to estimate, as most cash disbursements, such as salaries and supplies, are made at prespecified intervals. Using the expense budget and the facility 's experience with suppliers and other creditors, the amount of cash disbursements can be determined for each month. An insurance policy that is paid on a triennial basis may be due in February, for example.

As with the operating budget, the cash budget is updated as conditions or needs change throughout the year, whatever the reason. The cash budget can be a useful planning tool.

STEP 5: THE CAPITAL BUDGET

The capital budget is a summarization of all anticipated capital (items with a life of more than 12 months) expenditures in the budget year. Although many capital purchases and projects may be needed, all might not be readily affordable in the course of a single year. The capital budget is the result of the decision concerning capital projects that will be undertaken, and, most important, how they will be financed. If a competitor is to open a large all-new facility nearby, for example, a contingency capital item might be funds for renovations of a portion of the facility to compete should census drop precipitously.

Pro Forma Financial Statements

The budget process concludes with the development of the pro forma financial statements. The pro forma statements are the preliminary financial statements based on budgeted amounts. The pro forma income statement, for instance, is derived from the operating budget and shows the net income (or loss) expected under the budgeted expenses and revenues.

The budgeting process can be costly in terms of time for the administrator and all other budget participants. However, it involves a thorough investigation of the facility's finances through such tools as cost finding, break-even analysis, rate setting, programming, and cash flow analysis. Through these processes, budgeting familiarizes the administrator with the costs of running the facility and maximizes his or her ability to manage successfully.

3.10 Finance

Thus far in Part Three we have focused on the internal business and financial matters of the assisted living facility. We now turn to examine the broader business and financial context within which the assisted living facility manages its affairs.

In this section we will

- glance briefly at the sources of law and the court systems
- review a number of legal terms
- discuss the issue of risk management for an assisted living facility
- examine a number of business and financial concepts and terms, insurance terms and terms associated with wills and estates

3.10.1 Sources of Law

The daily business of the assisted living facility is conducted within the context of the United States legal system.

Constitution. The Constitution is the written agreement establishing the fundamental law of the United States of America, setting forth the conditions, mutual obligations, and rights of the federal and state governments and laying basic principles of government. The Bill of Rights guarantees specific individual rights.

Statutes. Statutes are the law under which we live. In the United States they are the acts passed by the federal and state legislatures. Lesser governmental bodies, such as the county commission, adopt ordinances; administrative agencies function by means of regulations.

Common Law. Common law is the accumulation of opinion handed down by judges. It is an outgrowth of court decisions over hundreds of years. Our common law originated in

England, where judges followed unwritten principles of "common sense" in addition to statutory laws. Common law principles change over time with the changing values and needs of society.

Regulations. To implement statutes (laws) passed by legislative bodies, the executive branch of government (the president and the various federal agencies he or she oversees) through these administrative agencies writes regulations. These regulations are the official interpretations of the intent of each statute. As a consequence, regulations become, in effect, part of the law. One may challenge a regulation on the grounds that the "official interpretation" is unconstitutional or inconsistent with the legislative intent of the statute the regulation implements.

The federal requirements for nursing facilities is an example of regulations. These were written by the executive branch of the federal government during the process of spelling out the details of how the legislation will be interpreted and implemented. The federal requirements for health care facilities were written by the employees of the Health Care Finance Administration, which administers Medicare and Medicaid. The federal requirements are published in the *Federal Register* as, for example, the OBRA regulations (the Health Care Facility Reform Amendments of 1987) have the effect of law when federal inspectors visit a skilled nursing facility and issue deficiencies based on both the written regulations and a set of "interpretive guidelines." These interpretive guidelines, although not law or regulation per se, are very real; they are the "guidelines" used by federal certification inspectors to record deficiencies and levy fines on nursing homes. No similar regulations exist, as yet, for the assisted living industry.

These requirements (not the interpretive guidelines), along with other federal administrative agency regulations, are published in the Code of Federal Regulations (CFR).

The assisted living industry hopes to avoid such federal regulations by keeping its affairs in order, thus negating the need for heavy-handed regulations.

The president of the United States has the prerogative of issuing executive orders under various statutes. Executive orders also have the effect of law.

Code. A code is a compilation of statutes and regulations. The statutes, together with the regulations written by the administrative body assigned to implement each statute, are systematically collected and placed into codes of law. The United States Code (USC) often is an example.

3.10.2 The Court Systems

Federal Courts. The United States Constitution authorizes the creation of the Supreme Court and any additional courts Congress chooses to establish. Currently, entry into the federal court system is at the level of federal district courts (general courts of original jurisdiction). Jurisdiction is the power to hear and decide a case. Situated between these and the federal Supreme Court are 12 courts of appeal, which together cover the 50 states and hear cases in the event a party is dissatisfied with the judgment of the federal district court based on what the dissatisfied party views as an error.

The federal government also operates other courts, such as a Court of Claims, the Court of Customs and Patent Appeals, the Tax Court, and federal bankruptcy courts.

State Courts. The court systems vary from state to state. The lowest level of the state system is the magistrate court, which deals with misdemeanor cases, traffic violations, and small claims (about $1,000 or under). Above the magistrate courts are the state circuit courts, or district courts, where more serious cases are tried.

Circuit or district courts have original jurisdiction over both civil and criminal cases. Most states have state courts of appeal, which normally do not have original jurisdiction and therefore limit themselves to appeals from lower courts in the state. Finally, each state has a state supreme court. This is the court of final appeal in all matters except those that involve a federal issue appealable to the United States Supreme Court.

3.10.3 Legal Terminology

Accuse. To directly charge a person with committing an offense that is recognized as being against a law. The accused person becomes the defendant and must answer the complaint or accusation through the legal process.

Acquit. To set a person or corporation free of accusation(s). Acquittal is a decision (verdict) of not guilty and is rendered either by a jury or a judge (in nonjury trials). Under the principle of double jeopardy, a person or corporation cannot be tried again for the same accusation after a verdict of not guilty.

Actionable. Conduct giving rise to a cause for legal action. For example, actionable negligence occurs only when a person unreasonably fails to perform a legal duty, resulting in damage or injury to another person. If there is no resulting damage, there may not be actionable negligence even though the person made a mistake.

Adjudication. Decision or disposition of a case by the announcement of a judgment or decision by the court or other body.

Admission. The acknowledgment of certain facts by a party in a civil or criminal case. An admission does not necessarily constitute a confession of guilt. For example, the defendant may admit that he or she was driving the automobile but deny running the red light. The term *confession* is generally restricted to an acknowledgment of guilt.

Affidavit. A written statement given under oath before an officer having authority to administer oaths. A notary public is such a public officer and is authorized to signify by his or her signature that he or she witnessed the execution (signing) of certain documents, such as affidavits, deeds, and wills.

Aggrieved party. One whose legal rights have been invaded or who has suffered a loss or injury. "Aggrieved party" is frequently used in connection with proceedings by administrative agencies. For example, a person contesting the revocation of his or her professional license in an administrative proceeding is an aggrieved party.

Amicus Curiae. Literally, a friend (*amicus*) of the court (*curiae*). An *amicus curiae* brief is a written document that provides the court with information that might otherwise escape attention. A long-term care ombudsman might, for example, appear in a court case on behalf of a resident. The "friend of the court" has no absolute right to appear in the proceeding, so must obtain the court's permission prior to intervening.

Appeal. The request by a party to a lawsuit for a higher court to review a lower court's decision when he or she believes the lower court committed error.

Appearance. The coming into court of a person on being summoned to do so. Appearance without receiving a summons is a voluntary appearance. Appearance in court after papers have been served is an involuntary appearance.

Arbitrator. An impartial person chosen by the parties to an argument to decide the issue between them. Arbitration is used to avoid unnecessary and costly court actions.

Arraignment. An early step in a criminal proceeding at which the defendant is formally charged with an offense.

Assault. See Torts.

Battery. See Torts.

Burden of Proof, or Burden of Persuasion. The obligation of the person bringing an action to prove facts in dispute. In criminal cases the state must prove its case beyond a reasonable doubt. In civil cases the burden of proof is met by a "preponderance" of the evidence.

Criminal law. Pertains to a crime, any act the government has deemed to be injurious to the public and actionable in a criminal proceeding. The criminal acts may be felonies (serious crimes such as murder, arson, rape, and armed robbery) or misdemeanors (less serious crimes such as minor traffic violations). A criminal violation may result in either a jail sentence, a fine, or both.

To picture the interaction of civil and criminal law, assume an employee intentionally runs over a resident in the facility parking lot. The employee may be sued by the resident for money damages in a civil action and may also be brought to trial on criminal charges by the district attorney for the same act. (The assisted living facility probably will be sued civilly by the resident too, particularly if the employee has very little money.)

Consent, informed. Consent given after full information regarding the matter has been provided to the person consenting. In the assisted living facility context, residents must understand the nature and risks of certain treatments before the facility can claim exemption from responsibility for resulting complications.

A diabetic resident for example, may volunteer to participate in an experimental diet program. Unless the resident fully understands the risks involved, the facility may be held liable for subsequent complications. The facility should require the resident to sign a properly prepared consent form.

Consent to one treatment or procedure is not necessarily consent to another treatment or procedure, even if such treatment or procedure is beneficial. If a resident consented to a tonsillectomy but the surgeon also removed the appendix, the surgeon may have committed a battery.

Counterclaim. A counterdemand by a defendant against a plaintiff (accuser), not merely responding to the accuser, but asserting an independent cause of action against the accuser. For example, if the resident in the knitting needle illustration (see Torts) sued the orderly for damages for assault or battery, the aide might counterclaim with a demand for damages for assault or battery.

Damages. Money awarded by a court (or jury) to a person who has been wronged by the action of another. The meaning of the terms used to describe the various types of damages available differs from state to state and depends on the type of case. Generally, actual damages, consequential damages, and incidental damages are designed to compensate the person wronged.

Nominal damages are an award of a small sum of money in recognition of the invasion of some legal right of the plaintiff, which results in no actual injury, or pecuniary loss to the plaintiff. Punitive damages are designed to punish the defendant for particularly bad conduct and to deter the defendant from such conduct in the future. Punitive damages are also sometimes called *exemplary damages*. Double and treble damages are a type of punitive damages sometimes provided for by particular statutes.

Defendant. In criminal cases, the accused. In civil cases, the one who is sued and who must "defend" against a claim of wrongdoing brought by another.

Defamation. The communication to a third person of that which is injurious to the reputation or good name of the victim. Oral defamation is slander. Written defamation is libel.

Libel is written publication that exposes someone to public scorn, hatred, contempt, or ridicule, especially if related to an individual's profession or livelihood.

Slander, because it is spoken, is more difficult to establish. The action for slander has been restricted because of the right of free speech and to avoid overloading the courts with trivial cases. Only if slanderous statements lead to actual damages (e.g., loss of employment) can they be actionable, unless the words imply crime, unchastity, or relate to a person's profession or business.

In the cases of both libel and slander, there must be communication to a third party (e.g., showing a third party written words or speaking slanderous words in the presence of a third party).

Deposition. A statement given under oath, reduced to writing, and authenticated by a notary public. A deposition gives the attorneys for both sides an opportunity to find out what the person deposed (deponent) knows about the relevant event.

Directed verdict. A verdict given by a jury at the direction of a judge. If, for example, a plaintiff fails to make a reasonable case, or a defendant fails to make a necessary defense, the judge may direct the jury to render a specified verdict.

Discovery. Pretrial devices used by the parties' lawyers to gather information or knowledge about the case. Discovery devices include depositions, interrogatories to parties, and requests for documents and articles. The purpose of discovery devices is to facilitate pretrial settlements and to reduce surprises at trials in order that cases might be decided on their merit (rather than by ambush).

False imprisonment. See Torts.

Fraud. Intentional deception that results in injury to another.

Indictment. A formal, written accusation by a public prosecutor, submitted to a grand jury and charging a crime. The grand jury is a body authorized to investigate crimes and accuse (i.e., indict) persons within its jurisdiction when it decides a trial ought to be undertaken.

Injunction. A judicial direction to a party to do or to refrain from doing some act. Injunctions guard against future acts but do not remedy past acts. When the court issues an injunction, the party to whom it is issued is said to be "enjoined."

Litigants. The parties to a lawsuit (i.e., the plaintiff and defendant).

Malice. The intentional doing of a wrongful act, without just cause or excuse, with the intent to inflict injury. Under some circumstances the law will imply evil intent. Therefore, malice (in law) does not necessarily mean personal hate or ill will. The law will imply malice to an act done with reckless disregard for another's safety, even though the actor did not dislike the party he or she injured. For example, the law may imply malice to the act of one who shoots a rifle into a crowd of strangers.

Motion. An application to the court asking for an action favorable to one's side.

Negligence. The failure to exercise the degree of care a reasonable person would exercise under the same circumstances, which results in injury to another. Negligent conduct falls below the standard established by society (a jury) for the protection of others from an unreasonable risk of harm. Negligence may arise from either an overt act or from a failure to act.

The term *negligence* is used in several different ways:

1. *Comparative negligence.* In some states an individual can recover damages even though he or she was negligent. For example, a resident slips and injures himself or herself partly as a result of the unreasonably slippery floors in the facility and partly because the resident had chosen very slippery shoes. The facility is negligent because it failed to warn the resident that the floors were unusually slippery. But the resident was also negligent because he or she wore shoes that had slippery soles. In states that have comparative negligence, the jury determines how much of the resident's injury should be blamed on the facility's negligence and how much the resident is to blame. The jury then apportions the damages (money) accordingly.
2. *Contributory negligence.* Contributory negligence is similar to comparative negligence in that the victim is partly responsible for his or her own injury. However, in states where the doctrine of contributory negligence applies, all recovery by the victim is barred. Contributory negligence is a favorite of defendants because they can win the case by convincing the jury that the victim was just the least bit to blame for his or her own injury.
3. *Negligence per se.* Conduct treated as negligence without proof. It is usually necessary to show failure to exercise a reasonable degree of care. Negligence per se is found where the act complained of is in violation of a safety statute. Negligence per se also includes acts that are so clearly harmful to others that it is plain to any reasonable person that negligence must have occurred.
4. *Criminal negligence.* Recklessness or carelessness resulting in injury or death punishable as a crime. Criminal negligence implies reckless disregard or indifference to the safety or rights of others.

Prosecutor. A public official, either elected or appointed, who conducts cases on behalf of the government against persons accused of crimes.

Risk, Assumption of. The principle that a person may not recover for an injury he or she received when he or she voluntarily exposed himself or herself to a known danger.

Res ipsa loquitur. A Latin phrase that literally means "the thing speaks for itself." The defendant's negligence is inferred from the mere fact that the event happened and that the instrumentality causing the injury was under the exclusive control of the defendant. *Res ipsa loquitur* could apply to an otherwise unexplained gas furnace explosion in an assisted living facility.

Res judicata. Latin for "a thing decided." Once a court of competent jurisdiction has decided a matter, that decision continues to bind those parties in any future litigation on the same issue.

Retainer. A fee paid an attorney in advance for services on a case. In exchange, the attorney must refuse employment as the client's adversary in the case.

Search warrant. A written order from a judge permitting certain law enforcement officers to conduct a search for and seize specified things or persons. Warrants are issued on sworn testimony or affidavits supporting probable cause. Law enforcement officers may not search or seize items or persons not within the scope of the search warrant.

Stare decisis. A Latin phrase meaning "to stand by that which was decided earlier." The doctrine of stare decisis means that once a court has laid down a principle of law as applicable to a certain set of facts, it will adhere to that principle in all future cases in which the facts are substantially the same. *Stare decisis* gives the law a measure of predictability. However, a court will reverse itself occasionally where considerations of public policy demand it. For example, nonprofit health care institutions were once immune from lawsuits. Public policy has demanded that such immunity no longer apply.

Subpoena. A written order issued by a court to require the appearance of a person in court. A person failing to appear may be held in contempt of court.

Subpoena duces tecum. A written court order for a person to bring to a judicial proceeding certain objects or documents in his or her possession. The court, for example, may require an assisted living facility administrator to bring resident records to a court proceeding.

Summons. A written instrument notifying a defendant that a lawsuit has commenced against him or her. Failure to appear may result in a default judgment, wherein the defendant has a judgment entered against him or her for failure to appear.

Tort. A wrong. Literally, tort means "twisted." A tort exists when (1) a legal duty is owed by a defendant to a plaintiff, (2) that duty is breached, and (3) the plaintiff is harmed as a direct result of the breach of duty.

For example, the duty to provide care to residents is imposed on the assisted living facility by virtue of holding itself out as a licensed care provider. If the facility breaches its duty to provide care for a resident and the resident is harmed as a direct result of the breach of duty, a tort has occurred. The general term *tort* includes several specific types of bad or wrongful conduct. Assault, battery, false imprisonment, and negligence are among the types of conduct labeled by the law as torts.

An assault is an attempt to inflict bodily harm on another person that creates well-founded fear of imminent peril. An assault does not require actual touching. It can be the basis for a civil action (actions outside criminal practice) and/or a criminal action (violation of criminal laws). In the civil action for assault, the person assaulted brings the action seeking to be awarded money. In the criminal action for assault, the district attorney brings assault charges for the purpose of punishment.

The tort of assault is closely linked to, and often confused with, the tort of battery. Battery is the unlawful touching of or application of force to another human being without his or her consent. For battery to occur there must be an intent to touch, actual touching, and a lack of consent. If the touching is knowingly consented to, it is not battery.

Assault has been defined as a "failed battery," because an assault must cause apprehension of immediate harmful contact, without actual contact. For example, if the doctor ordered pills and the health care personnel approaches the resident with a 4–inch-long needle, causing apprehension in the resident of immediate contact, it is an assault. When the health care personnel actually uses the needle (the touching), it becomes a battery (unless the resident has consented).

To illustrate the differences between assault and battery, consider the following. An aide bumps into a female resident's breast. If it is purely accidental, no battery has occurred. If the aide intended to bump into the resident's breast, it may be battery. The angry resident retaliates by throwing a knitting needle at the aide. If the knitting needle misses but the aide is apprehensive about immediate harmful contact, the resident has committed an assault. If the knitting needle hits the aide, it is battery (even if the aide was not apprehensive of the contact). The aide then throws a towel at the resident. If it hits the resident, it is battery. If it misses the resident but the resident apprehends immediate harmful contact, it is assault.

False imprisonment is another tort occasionally related to assault and battery; it is the confining of another human being within fixed boundaries against his or her will. Numerous circumstances within the health care setting can give rise to false imprisonment. If a competent resident refuses bed (side) rails but the health care personnel raises the bed (side) rails anyway, false imprisonment has occurred.

If a physician leaves orders to restrain a competent resident to remain inside the facility but that resident refuses, keeping the resident inside the facility will constitute false imprisonment. (Keeping the resident inside the facility may also be battery.)

Tort-feasor. The person who commits a tort.

Warrant, Arrest. A written order for the arrest of a person from a judge having authority in that jurisdiction.

Witness. A person who gives sworn testimony in a court proceeding.

3.10.4 Risks Assumed by the Operation of an Assisted Living Facility

The act of obtaining a license to operate a long-term care facility automatically brings a set of risks to the facility. Some of these are defined below.

EMPLOYER'S LIABILITY ACTS

Various states have statutes that set forth the extent to which employers are liable to their employees for injuries to them. Generally, the employer is held responsible only for injuries to employees occurring in the course of their work. Workers' compensation acts and the federal Employer's Liability Act are examples. Employer's liability acts usually pay for physician and hospital costs. These statutes removed the earlier claims by employers that the employee knew the hazards of a job and accepted them when agreeing to work for the facility.

Often these statutes also hold the employer responsible for negligent acts of fellow employees within the zone of employment. The zone of employment is the physical area within which employers are liable (legally responsible) under workers' compensation acts. This usually includes the parking areas, entryways, and other areas under the control of the employer.

STRICT LIABILITY

An employer held strictly liable is subject to liability without fault (i.e., without the employee having to show employer fault).

VICARIOUS OR IMPUTED LIABILITY (*RESPONDEAT SUPERIOR*)

The employer is held responsible for the acts of employees within the scope of their employment. For example, if a health care aide carelessly drops a resident from a wheelchair, causing injuries to the resident, the employer is normally held liable for the injuries. *Respondeat superior* is a Latin term literally meaning "let the master answer for the acts of his or her servants," or "let the employer answer for the acts of his or her employees."

SCOPE OF EMPLOYMENT

The range of employee activities held by the courts to be the legal responsibility of the employer is called the scope of employment. Basically, it includes any acts performed in the process of carrying out one's duties. Ascertaining the scope of employment is important when determining the employer's liability for the acts of his or her employees.

The health care aide who, in the process of hurrying down the hall to aid another resident, knocks down and injures a resident on crutches, is likely to be found to be acting as a servant within the scope of employment, resulting in employer liability for the accident. An employee may be found to be acting within the scope of employment even though the employee is doing his or her job contrary to the instructions of the employer.

BORROWED SERVANT

A borrowed servant is a person under the temporary employ of another person. In an assisted living facility, a health care personnel employed by the local community college as a health care instructor, but temporarily working under the direction of the assisted living facility's health care personnel, might be found to be a borrowed servant. Using the concept of respondeat superior, the assisted living facility might be found liable for the wrongful acts of the "borrowed" health care personnel.

INDEPENDENT CONTRACTOR

An independent contractor agrees with another person to perform a certain job and remains in control of the means and methods of performing the job. Because an independent contractor is not an employee, the doctrine of *respondeat superior* has no application to the independent contractor. Therefore, the assisted living facility would not be liable ordinarily for the negligence of an independent contractor.

Determining whether a person is acting as an employee, with the facility liable for the employee's negligence, or as an independent contractor, without this liability, depends on a number of factors:

- the extent to which the facility controls the details of the work
- whether the person is engaged in a distinct occupation or profession
- whether the work is usually done under the direction of the employer or by a specialist without supervision
- the skill required
- the portion of time the person is employed
- who supplies the equipment used
- whether the work is part of the regular business of the facility
- whether the facility and worker believe they have formed an employer-employee relationship
- whether or not the person is in business

Depending on the circumstances, physical therapists under contract to the assisted living facility and private duty health care personnel may (or may not) be found to be independent contractors. Because facilities would naturally prefer to have a number of its employees be viewed as independent contractors in order to reduce liability, courts do give great weight to the label the facility places on the worker. Liability for injuries sustained by a resident under treatment by a physical therapist on contract to the facility might more nearly be ascribed to the facility than an injury to a resident caused by an outside painting contractor employee.

MANAGING RISKS

How Much Risk?

How much risk is faced in an average 100-bed assisted living facility over a year? Assuming that each assisted living facility resident will have at least 20 contacts with staff members each day, over 2,000 staff/resident contacts occur daily in this typical assisted living facility. Over the course of a month, 60,000 contacts occur. Over the course of a year nearly three quarters of a million staff/resident contacts occur. Each of these contacts potentially incurs risks to the facility. Consider the following scenarios from the nursing home industry, which delivers the type of assistance with the activities of daily living increasingly being provided by assisted living facilities that assist their residents to age in place (level 2 and level 3 assisted living facilities).

Care Decisions of a Nursing Home Aide

An Alabama jury awarded $2.5 million in punitive damages to the family of an 86-year-old nursing home resident who strangled to death while restrained in a Posey vest. The health care personnel aide, not realizing that Posey vests are color coded, chose a vest to match the resident's gown, rather than body size. She then placed the vest backwards on the resident, causing the resident to choke to death. The J.T. Posey Company, a codefendant, was found not guilty of negligence because it had warned the health care facility that the vests' V neck should be placed in front (*Quality Care Advocate,* 1989). Health care personnel aides give the preponderance of hands-on care in health care facilities. Certainly this is a good argument for assisted living facilities to avoid the use of physical restraints (discussed further in Part Five).

Staff Performance Under Stress.

At a 150+ bed nursing home facility in a southern state, 9 persons died, 141 people were hospitalized, and 98 received significant injuries and treatment for smoke inhalation from a fire started by smoking materials at the foot of a resident's bed. State and local officials said the facility had undergone recent inspections and was in compliance with state fire codes. An administrator for the group of facilities said the facility was fully up to code, was well equipped to deal with fires, prohibited smoking in bedrooms, and had fire alarms, smoke and heat detectors, and fire-resistant doors. Fire, and effective or ineffective staff responses, can occur at any time.

Uncontrolled Resident Behavior

An 89-year-old resident in a Dade City, Florida, facility beat to death his roommate and another sleeping resident with his cane, then injured four others in a room-to-room rampage sparked by squabbles with roommates.

Transferring a resident, however, is not a simple matter. Consider the recommendations of the *Assisted Living Workgroup Report* to the U.S. Senate Special Committee on Aging (April, 2003, p 128).

The following reasons may be given for transfer or move-out by the resident:

- The resident desires to move
- Following a documented assessment, the facility is no longer able to care for the resident as disclosed to the resident upon move-in and when the facility has attempted to work with the resident so move out would be unnecessary
- The resident fails to pay or arrange payments after reasonable and appropriate notice
- The resident's behavior or conditions presents a direct and serious threat to the well-being or safety of the resident or other residents or staff
- An immediate transfer is acceptable if temporary and due to a disaster, etc.
- The facility ceases to exist.

What Is a Risk?

A risk can be defined as any event or process that can lead to actions that result, directly or indirectly, in economic losses of damage to the facility and/or its reputation.

Each of the events cited above is a risk to be managed. One writer in this field (Kapp, 1987) has cited several definitions of risk management that appear in the literature: "A program that attempts to provide positive avoidance of negative results. Liability control; loss prevention" (Showalter, 1987); "prediction of resident injury, avoidance of exposure to predicted and other risks, and minimization of malpractice claims loss" (Orlikoff, Fifer, & Greeley, 1981).

Troyer and Salman (1986) define risk as "exposure to the chance of injury or loss; a hazard or dangerous chance." They note that there are "many considerations other than professional liability," and define loss control broadly as an attempt to prevent "financial, human or intangible harm" (p. 24). They include personnel and intangible resources such as position in the community as risks to be managed.

Essentially, risk management is identifying and solving problems before they get out of hand, thus preventing being sued.

For a definitive discussion of the legal aspects of risk management in long-term care, see *Preventing Malpractice in Long Term Care: Strategies for Risk Management* by Marshall B. Kapp. Troyer and Salman's *Handbook of Health Care Risk Management* provides a broad statistically oriented treatment of risk management.

Resident environment free of accident hazards. Accidents are one of the most recognizable risks faced in the day-to-day life of the assisted living facility. The facility must ensure that the resident environment remains as free of accident hazards as is possible. The intent is that the facility prevent accidents by providing an environment that is as free as possible from hazards over which the facility has control. *Accident hazards* are defined as physical features in the facility's environment that can endanger a resident's safety, including but not limited to

- physical restraints
- poorly maintained resident equipment (e.g., wheelchairs or geri-chairs with nonworking brakes, and loose nuts and bolts on walkers)
- bathing facilities that do not have nonslip surfaces
- hazards (e.g., electrical appliances with frayed wires, cleaning supplies easily accessible to cognitively impaired residents, wet floors that are not obviously labeled and to which access is not blocked)
- handrails not securely fixed to the wall, difficult to grasp and/or with sharp edges/splinters
- water temperatures in hand sinks or bath tubs that can scald or harm residents

Adequate Resident Supervision and Assistive Devices to Prevent Accidents. Each resident should receive adequate supervision and assistance devices to prevent accidents. The intent is that the facility identify each resident at risk for accidents and/or falls, and adequately plan care and implement procedures to prevent accidents.

An *accident* is an unexpected, unintended event that can cause a resident bodily injury. It does not include adverse outcomes as a direct consequence of treatment or care (e.g., drug side effects or reactions).

Accident-reducing Questions the Assisted Living Administrator Can Ask:

1. Are there a number of accidents or injuries of a specific type or on any specific shift (e.g., falls, skin injuries)?
2. Are residents who smoke properly supervised and monitored?
3. Are specific identifiable residents repeatedly involved in accidents? What care planning and implementation is the facility doing to prevent accidents and falls for those residents identified as at risk? How does the facility fit, and monitor, the use of that resident's assistive devices? How are drugs that may cause postural hypotension, dizziness, or visual changes monitored?

Terms Associated with Risk Management

Civil Liability. The three primary sources in health care malpractice suits are (1) failure to obtain effective consent before intervening in the life of the resident; (2) breach or violation of a contract or promise, and (3) the rendering of substandard, poor-quality care (Kapp, 1987).

Claims-made Policy. The insurance company pays for the claims made only during the term of the policy and only for events occurring during the term of the policy (Kapp, 1987). (See Occurrence policy.)

Durable Power of Attorney. Appointment of an agent who is empowered to act on behalf of the person creating the power in case of future incompetence. (Ordinary power of attorney ends when the person creating the power becomes incompetent.)

Empty Shell Doctrine. View that the facility merely provides a workplace for health professionals and has no corporate liability for their actions. Abandoned after *Darling v. Charleston Community Memorial Hospital* (1965), in which the facility was held liable for acts of staff.

Euthanasia. A "good" or "easy" death. Active euthanasia in the assisted living facility setting is involvement of facility caregivers in nonaccidental termination of a resident's life.

Guardianship. Appointment by a probate court of a substitute decision-maker for an incompetent person.

Malpractice system (purposes of). (1) The just financial compensation of innocent, injured residents and (2) the maintenance of a high level of care by deterring undesirable provider practices (Kapp, 1987).

Occurrence policy. The insurance company pays for claims for events occurring during term of the policy regardless of when claims are filed (Kapp, 1987).

Palliative care. Alleviating suffering even where "cure" of underlying disease is no longer possible.

Resident/resident's rights—sources. (1) Judge-made (common) law based on society's values, (2) specific statutes (i.e., legislative law) resulting in rules and regulations defining resident rights.

Standard of Care. The duty to have and to use the degree of knowledge and skill that is usually possessed and used by competent, prudent health care providers in like or similar circumstances (Kapp, 1987).

Substandard Care. Four elements are required for a civil lawsuit: (1) duty owed, (2) breach or violation of that duty, (3) damage or injury, and (4) causation (Kapp, 1987).

3.10.5 Business-Related Concepts and Terms

ACCOUNTING CONCEPTS

Activity-based costing. An accounting method that assigns identifiable costs and allocates common costs to specific activity areas in the facility, sometimes known as *departmental area costing*. This allows the facility to identify the profit contribution of each activity or departmental area (Argenti, 1994). Similar to or the same as the step-down accounting method described above.

Agency. A relationship in which one person acts on behalf of and under the control of another. The acts of the agent are binding on the person or business the agent represents. The administrator is the agent of the facility; thus the facility is bound by the agreements the administrator makes on behalf of the facility.

Allowance for Bad Debts. A provision a facility makes for uncollectible accounts receivable. On the balance sheet, net receivables—the amount the facility realistically expects to collects from resident billings—is calculated by reducing the accounts receivable by the allowance for bad debt (Argenti, 1994).

American Institute of Certified Public Accountants (AICPA). A national organization of certified public accountants. This organization develops standards for its members and offers advice to such government agencies as the Securities and Exchange Commission (Argenti, 1994). Decisions of this group usually become the standard of practice.

ARR, Accounting Rate of Return. A method of measuring the potential profitability of an investment. ARR is calculated by dividing the net income by the amount (or average amount) of the investment.

Annual Report. A detailed statement of the facility's financial position at the end of its reporting year, either fiscal or calendar. Annual reports, as described above, contain the facility's income statement, balance sheet, statement of cash flows, statement of owners' or shareholders' equity, management's discussion and analysis of operations, notes to the financial statements, audit opinion, and other selected data. The Financial Accounting Standards Board (FASB), described below, also requires reporting on all other financial activities (e.g., pharmacy holdings, or any other business activities that affect the facility's financial status.

Audit. An examination of a facility's compliance with accounting standards and policies. There are four types of audit: financial, internal, management, and compliance. In the financial audit an independent certified public accountant examines the facility's financial records and gives an audit opinion. In the internal audit the internal financial officer studies the financial records to ensure they meet facility policies. The management audit examines management's efficiency. The compliance audit determines whether the facility is meeting specific rules and regulations.

Audit Opinion. A report given by an independent certified public accountant that gives the auditor's opinion as to the reasonableness of the facility's financial statement.

Big Six. A term given to the six largest CPA firms in the United States. The rankings change over time, depending on criteria used, such as billings and number of staff.

Certified Public Accountant (CPA). A title given to accountants who pass the Uniform CPA examination administered by the American Institute of Certified Public Accountants and who satisfy the experience requirements of each given state. CPAs are licensed to issue an audit opinion of a facility's financial statements (Argenti, 1994).

Change in Accounting Estimate. A revision of an accounting forecast or assumption about the facility's expected or experienced performance.

Cumulative Effect of a Change in Accounting Principle. In accounting, the income statement account showing the effect of switching from one accounting principle to another. Cumulative effect shows the difference between the retained earnings reported at the beginning of the year under the old method and the retained earnings that would have been reported at the beginning of the year had the method never been changed (Argenti, 1994).

Extraordinary Item. In accounting, an economic item that is both unusual and infrequent (such as the replacement of the emergency power generator, which might occur once every 15 years).

Financial Accounting Standards Board (FASB). The independent institution that establishes and disseminates the generally accepted accounting principles (GAAPs) and recording practices. The American Institute of Certified Public Accountants and the Securities and Exchange Commission both recognize the statements of the FASB. All practicing CPAs are required to adhere to FASB guidelines.

Generally Accepted Accounting Principles (GAAP). The policies, standards and rules followed by accountants in the preparation of financial statements and in recording and summarizing transactions (Argenti, 1994).

Materiality. In accounting, the relative importance of an accounting error or omission in a facility's financial statements. A $200 error in an earnings statement of $2 million income would be immaterial, whereas a $500,000 error would clearly be material (Argenti, 1994).

Qualified Opinion. An auditor's report of a facility's financial statement pointing to some particular limitation (e.g., inability of the CPA to obtain objective evidence of a certain transaction that might directly or adversely affect the facility's financial standing (Argenti, 1994).

Unqualified opinion. Sometimes known as a clean opinion, that the report meets all the GAAP requirements (Argenti, 1994).

ASSETS-RELATED TERMS

Attachment. A legal procedure in which a defendant's property is seized by court order pending the outcome of a claim against the defendant. The purpose is to gain control over property that may be used to satisfy payment of a judgment if the plaintiff's suit is successful.

Bad faith. Generally implies a design to mislead or deceive another. Good faith means being truthful and faithful to one's obligations in business dealings.

Brand Mark. The portion of a brand in the form of a symbol, design or distinctive coloring or lettering; also called a logo (Argenti, 1994).

Intangible Asset. An item or right that has no physical substance and provides an economic benefit. The reputation of an assisted living facility as the best caregiver in the community is a valuable intangible asset, for example.

Liquidity. The ability of current assets to meet the financial obligation of current liabilities. Having high liquidity enables a facility to take advantage of investment opportunities and to borrow capital or receive a line of credit at a more favorable rate.

Long-Term Asset. An asset with future economic benefits that are expected for a number of years. Long-term assets are reported on the balance sheet as noncurrent assets and include buildings and equipment. A new central building for an assisted living facility may have a long-term expected asset value for perhaps 40 or more years to come.

Net Present Value. In corporate finance, the present value (i.e., the value of cash to be received in the future expressed in current dollars) of an investment in excess of the initial amount invested. When a proposed project, such as building a new wing, has a positive net present value, it should perhaps proceed; when a proposed wing shows a negative net present value, it should perhaps be delayed or abandoned.

Note receivable. A contract to receive money at a future date. Notes receivable are reported on the balance sheet as either current assets (less than 1 year) or noncurrent assets (more than 1 year).

Off-balance sheet. An item not reported in financial statements that nevertheless has an impact on the operations of a facility. An example might be an estimate of the monetary value of a strong reputation for quality of a recently purchased facility. Assisted living facilities have sometimes successfully sought expansion funds by not having to report such off-balance sheet liabilities as a noncapitalized lease.

Present Value. The current value of a future payment or stream of payments. Present value is calculated by applying a discount (capitalization) rate to future payments. This is sometimes referred to as the *discounted cash flow method* or the *discounted earnings method* (Argenti, 1994). Its purpose is to estimate the fair market value of a potential investment.

COMPETITION/RISK RELATED TERMS

Bankruptcy. Inability to pay one's debts, insolvency. Also refers to the legal process of the federal Bankruptcy Code, under which the assets of the business or individuals are liquidated, creditors paid, and the debtor given a fresh start. In a Chapter 11 reorganization, the dominant form, under the Bankruptcy Code, the debtor's assets are not liquidated. Instead, the debt structure and business are rearranged, creditors are paid some or all of what they are owed under a "plan," and the business continues to function without serious interruption. Under Chapter 7, the conventional form under the 1978 Bankruptcy Reform Act, all the assets must be auctioned or sold in order to pay creditors. A court appointed trustee gathers, liquidates all assets, then distributes the proceeds to the creditors. In most cases, debts remaining after liquidation distribution are discharged. Generally, debtors at the bottom of the creditor ranking receive little or nothing. Attorneys usually refer to a Chapter 7 bankruptcy as a "straight" bankruptcy.

Better-Off Test. A method of evaluating the strategic impact of an acquisition or business venture on the facility's financial standing. The better-off test stipulates that the new venture must either gain a significant competitive advantage through its functioning or offer a significant competitive advantage to the facility (Argenti, 1994).

Cannibalization. The reduction of income in the sales of a product caused by the introduction of another similar product by the same facility or company. A facility may decide to offer newer forms of physical therapy that reduce use of currently used physical therapy methods. If the total combined income using the new method of physical therapy and the reduced use of the old method yields a higher final income, cannibalization is justified.

Caveat emptor. Latin expression for "let the buyer beware." The purchaser buys at his or her own risk. In recent years, consumer protection laws and the Uniform Commercial Code have implied certain warranties in most purchases, unless the goods are bought "as is."

Competitive Advantage. The elements within a facility's operations that give it an edge over its competitors. Building a new enlarged dementia wing might give facility A competitive advantage over its competitors. If, however, a competing facility B counters by building an even larger and more attractive state-of-the-art dementia wing, facility A is placed at a competitive disadvantage. These are calculations used in developing the corporate strategy to be followed by facility A.

Competitor Analysis. The evaluation of the intent and actions of one's competitors (Argenti, 1994). This is part of corporate strategy. The information gained in competitor analysis is used to estimate the probable future actions of competitors, such as their future goals and assumptions about the marketplace.

Cost of Entry Test. A method of evaluating the strategic impact of the acquisition or start-up of a new business venture for the facility (Argenti, 1994). This test specifies that the cost of entering the new venture must not exceed the future profits generated by that venture.

Debt-to-Assets Ratio. A measure of the relative obligations of a facility. Generally, the lower the debt ratio, the more financially sound the facility is believed to be. The ratio is calculated by

$$\frac{\text{Current Liabilities + Noncurrent Liabilities}}{\text{Total Assets}}$$

Differentiation. The emphasis a facility places on some important product benefit or set of benefits that is valued by the entire market but not offered by the competition. Numerous facilities sought to differentiate themselves by being the only facility to offer, for example, a dementia or Alzheimer's unit. These competitive advantages through differentiation are usually short lived, as competitors emulate and begin to offer the same services.

Externality. Any incidental by-product(s) (both positive and negative) associated with a particular course of action chosen by a facility (Argenti, 1994). A positive externality for a facility that chooses to admit dementia residents from local hospitals might be an increased census. A negative externality associated with this course of action would be the necessity to hire additional staff and provide additional training for present staff.

Inflation. An increase in the general price level (Argenti, 1994). Inflation can be viewed as an increase in the cost of doing business or an erosion of the value of the facility's income. Inflation rates usually force facilities to offer higher salary increases in years of higher inflation.

Management's Discussion and Analysis of Operations. A section in the facility's annual report required by the Securities and Exchange Commission that summarizes the reasons for changes in operations, liquidity, capital resources, and working capital available to the facility. The purpose is to help readers of the financial statements to understand the effects of changes in activities and accounting procedures.

Perfect competition. A market that is so competitive that all its participants have virtually no control over the price (Argenti, 1994). Characteristics of a perfect market are thought to be (1) a large number of relatively small buyers and sellers, (2) easy entry and exit from the market, (3) a standardized product, and (4) complete information about market price. Few, if any, health care markets meet these requirements.

Price Elasticity of Demand. The effect price change has on income. This is calculated by

$$\frac{\text{\% Change in Quantity Demanded (Sales)}}{\text{\% Change in Price}}$$

Each facility, in setting its rates for private paying residents, for example, must calculate the impact on census of any rate increases. Potential private-paying persons might go to a competitor if rates at facility A are raised significantly above rates at facility B, other things being equal.

Return on Investment (ROI). A measure of the earning power of a facility's assets. A high return on investments is desirable whether a for-profit or a not-for-profit operation. Return on investment is broadly thought of as net income divided by investments but may be calculated using three different figures: return on assets, return on invested capital, and return on owners' equity.

Return on Assets (ROA). Calculated by dividing the net income after any taxes by the average total assets:

$$\frac{\text{Net Income After Any Taxes}}{\text{Average Total Assets}}$$

where average total assets are calculated by adding the ending balance of total assets of the previous year and the ending balance of total assets for the current year and dividing by 2.

Return on Invested Capital (ROIC). Tells how well a facility has used the funds given to it for a long time period. Invested capital equals noncurrent liabilities plus owners' equity.

$$\frac{\text{Net Income After Any Taxes}}{\text{Noncurrent Liabilities + Owners' Equity}}$$

Return on Owners' Equity (ROE). Measures the return that a facility has earned on the funds invested in it. These funds may be invested by shareholders (public or private) or may be, for example, the funds invested by a REIT in its own facilities. The ratio is calculated by dividing net income after any taxes by investors' equity:

$$\frac{\text{Net Income After Any Taxes}}{\text{Investor's Equity}}$$

BENEFITS/PENSIONS-RELATED TERMS

Accumulated Benefit Obligation (ABO). The present value of the amount a facility would owe to its pension plan if its eligible employees retired during that accounting period (Argenti, 1994).

Charter. A document issued by a state or other sovereign government establishing a corporate entity (same as article of incorporation).

Contract. An agreement between two or more persons that creates legally enforceable rights and remedies. Contracts must have the following elements:

- competent parties (of majority age and of sound mind)—in the case of some health care facility residents, the courts decide on their competence to enter into a contract.
- consideration—something of value given in return for performance of an act or the promise to perform an act. A promise to refrain from an act, that is, giving up a legal right, may qualify as consideration
- mutuality of agreement—the parties must agree willingly. Often stated as a "meeting of the minds."
- mutuality of obligation—all parties must be bound to some reciprocal performance. A promise by one person to do something at the will of another person without any consideration (benefit) to the first person is not a contract.

An oral contract is an enforceable agreement that is not in writing or signed by the parties. Oral contracts are enforceable but are subject to limitations. Various state statutes impose monetary limits on oral contracts for the purchase of goods, and almost every agreement dealing with real estate must be in writing to be enforceable.

Normally, no punitive damages are available for breach of contract. A person or facility suing for breach of contract can recover only what would have been received had the contract been fulfilled. Generally, the nonbreaching party can recover money damages but cannot command performance of actual work. Ordinarily, attorneys' fees cannot be recovered by the successful party.

Contractor. One who agrees to do work for another and retains control over the means, method, and manner in which the work is done. Concerning building, a general contractor is one who contracts with the owner of a property to accomplish agreed-on construction. A subcontractor is one who deals only with the general contractor for performance of some portion of the work to be accomplished by the general contractor.

Defined Benefit Pension Plan. A program of pension benefits that employees will receive when they retire. Normally, benefits are based on a formula involving years of service and compensation levels as employees near retirement. Whenever a facility establishes a defined benefit pension plan it must ensure that its pension fund has enough assets to pay the promised benefits. Delivering promised health benefits has become a major liability to pension plans in recent years because of the escalation of health care costs.

Defined Contribution Pension Plan. A program designating the annual dollar amount an employer contributes to a pension plan. Under a defined benefit pension plan, specific benefits such as dollar amounts and other benefits are promised. Under a defined contribution pension plan, in contrast, the employer makes no guarantee of future benefits beyond the value of the dollar amount of the funds set aside in the pension fund each year (Argenti, 1994).

Employee Stock Ownership Plan (ESOP). An employee benefit plan that gives employees shares in the facility. These may be voting shares, but more often are a special class of nonvoting common stock. ESOP rules change with revisions to the Internal Revenue Service code. Employers are allowed a tax deduction for part or all of their donations to ESOPs. Sometimes ESOPs are used as the acquiring mechanism, via bank loans to the ESOP, to achieve management buyout of part or all of a company (Argenti, 1994). ESOPs may borrow from banks and acquire additional shares in the company.

Minimum Pension Liability. In accounting terms, an obligation recognized when the accumulated benefit obligation of a pension plan is greater than the fair market value of plan assets. This must be shown on the balance sheet as a pension liability. This became so great among American corporations in recent years that the Financial Accounting Standards Board instituted a new rule for accounting for pensions that resulted in companies taking millions of "losses" on their balance sheets to show this obligation.

Pension Funds. The money set aside by an employer to meet the obligations under the pension plan. A pension fund is administered by trustees who actually pay the retirement benefits.

401(k). An employee retirement plan, sometimes called a *salary reduction plan.* This plan allows employees to set aside up to a government- and company-specified percentage of their salary in a special retirement investment account. The IRS does not count contributions to a 401(k) plan as income. Contributions and earnings accumulate tax free until they are withdrawn. Early withdrawals (before age 59_) are subject to full taxation plus a 10% withdrawal penalty. Companies sometimes match contributions. Some long-term care chains use 401(k) plans in lieu of a defined pension plan as a cost-saving device. A drawback to the 401(k) approach is that workers, especially when changing companies, often cash in their 401(k) plan for present needs.

COST-RELATED TERMS

Acceptable Quality Level (AQL). The actual percentage, specified by administration, of goods in a lot of incoming materials that a facility will allow to be defective and still accept the lot as "good." This applies to such areas as dietary, where large deliveries of items such as baked goods or canned goods are received.

Alternative Work Schedules. A method of increasing worker flexibility by offering a number of different job-scheduling options. Job sharing by two or more employees is such an option. Health care personnel have for some years been offered plans such as the "Baylor Plan," under which personnel may work long hours over a full weekend and receive a regular "week's" pay.

Cost-Benefit Analysis. A method of determining whether the results of a particular proposed course of action are sufficient to justify the cost of undertaking it. If a facility wished to purchase a similar facility 50 miles away, a cost-benefit analysis would assist in deciding whether the purchase should be undertaken.

Default. A failure to perform an act or obligation. A common example is a default on mortgage payments due.

Deferred Expense. An expense incurred in one accounting period that will benefit future accounting periods, also called a deferred charge. Insurance prepaid, as mentioned above, is a good example.

Economic Order Quantity (EOQ). A method of determining the optimum amount of materials that needs to be ordered on a regular basis. The costs of possession (storing, pilferage, becoming too old to use) are compared with the cost of acquisition.

Just-in-Time (JIT). An approach to dealing with materials inventories that emphasizes the elimination of all waste and the continual improvement of the production process. This concept was developed in the 1970s by Toyota Motor Company in Japan to ensure that materials are replenished exactly when they are needed and not before or after. JIT is so widespread that traditional materials and supplies inventory is sometimes referred to as "just in case." In the assisted living facility, however, health care supplies for sick care (e.g., oxygen tanks) are of critical importance vis-à-vis availability when needed.

Marginal Costs. The increase or decrease in the total costs that results from the output of one more unit or one less unit; also called the *incremental cost.* In an assisted living facility, for example, adding one more resident might trigger need for an additional aide on a shift, dramatically increasing the marginal cost of adding one more resident to a wing.

Materials Requirements Planning. A system of materials or supplies management designed to reduce or eliminate the need for excessive inventories of supplies by analysis of product needs and lead times.

Methods-Time Measurement (MTM). A system for measuring individual motions called micro-motions, such as reach, grab, and position. One method of changing a resident's bed may take significantly less time than a second method, for example, or designing a facility to have no bed farther than *X* feet from a health care station might produce more care time.

Price Controls. The use of government powers to keep the price either above or below its equilibrium point. When the government tries to keep what is paid for a product above the equilibrium, it is establishing a "price floor," such as the price paid for a bushel of wheat being set to ensure that farmers continue to raise wheat. In the health care situation, however, the government has sought to keep the price of a product below its equilibrium level (i.e., a "price ceiling"). By paying only the lesser of usual, customary, or actual health care charges in Medicare, the government establishes price ceiling. This normally results in cost shifting from Medicare or Medicaid residents' costs to charges made to private-paying residents.

Queue Time. The time a job or activity has to wait before a particular facility is available. The amount of time it takes housekeeping and health care to "turn a room," to make it available for the next resident, is a queue time that affects the occupancy rate a facility can achieve.

FINANCING: FORMS, TERMS

Arm's-Length Transaction. A business transaction at market-established prices between two unrelated parties. For example, a chain establishes and operates its own pharmacy to provide drugs to its own facilities. To be reimbursable as an arm's-length transaction, that chain must sell drugs to other assisted living facility chains and disinterested other purchasers at the same price it "sells" drugs to itself.

Bonds. A debt obligation of a facility, corporation, or other body to pay a specific amount on a stated date. Facilities usually issue bonds to raise capital for building or renovation projects. Not-for-profit facilities may often be allowed to issue tax-free bonds. Issuing bonds usually involves a very detailed and expensive prospectus conforming with SEC-required information. Junk bonds are debt securities rated below investment grade by credit-rating agencies. Long bonds are 30-year United States Treasury bonds or other bonds that mature beyond 10 years. Interest charges used to measure the market in corporate bonds are reflected in basis points: 100 basis points equal one percentage point of interest.

Borrowing Base. The facility assets used as collateral to secure short-term working capital loans from banks and other lenders.

Capital. The amount on the balance sheet that represents ownership in a business; also called *equity* or *net worth* or available funds or cash, as in working capital, or financing, as in "raising capital."

Capital Asset. An asset purchased for use rather than resale, including land, buildings, equipment, goodwill, and trademarks.

Capitalize. To classify an expense as an asset because it benefits the facility for more than 1 year.

Capital Market Theory. A set of complex mathematical formulas that strive to identify how investors should choose common stocks for their portfolios under a given set of assumptions.

Commercial Paper. Short-term securities (2 to 270 days) issued by corporations, banks, and other borrowing institutions to raise short-term working capital. Investors buy commercial paper as a very short term investment. Commercial paper is unsecured debt that can be sold at a discount or bear interest.

Cost of Capital. The rate of return available in the marketplace on investments that are comparable both in terms of risk and other characteristics, such as liquidity and other qualitative factors.

Disclosure. A necessary explanation of a company's financial position and operating results. Impending lawsuits and other liabilities must be part of disclosure.

Federal Trade Commission Act of 1914. The act that established the Federal Trade Commission (FTC) and gave it responsibility for promoting "free and fair competition in interstate commerce in the interest of the public through the prevention of price-fixing agreements, boycotts, combinations in restraint of trade, unfair acts of competition, and unfair and deceptive acts and practices" (Argenti, 1994, p. 183).

Leases. There are different types of leases.

- *Capital lease*—a lease in which the lessee acquires substantial property rights.
- *Finance lease*—a long-term rental commitment by both lessor and lessee that usually runs for the entire useful life of the asset. Usually the total of the payments approximates the purchase price plus finance charges. Most leases are net leases,

under which the lessee is responsible for the maintenance of the property, taxes, insurance, and the like. In the health care facility industry most leases are known as net net net, or *triple net leases,* under which the lessee's role is strictly that of a financier whose responsibility extends solely to financing the facility, assuming no liability from the operating of the facility.

- *Leasehold improvement*—Any refurbishment made to leased property (e.g., painting, reroofing, and redoing the interior). Leasehold improvements (if a for-profit facility) must be amortized over the life of the improvement.
- *Sale/leaseback*—a transaction in which a facility sells some or all of its hard assets to a leasing company for cash, then leases them back over a period of time. This allows for raising immediate capital while retaining control over the assets. A cash-poor small chain, for example, might use this mechanism to obtain money to purchase additional facilities.

Leveraged buyout (LBO). Purchase of controlling interest in a company using debt collateralized by the target company's assets to fund most or all of the purchase price. This has allowed small assisted living facility chains to purchase much larger assisted living facility chains.

Leveraging. The advantage gained by using debt financing to create asset appreciation. This is used by most purchasers or builders of health care facilities, which, in today's market, cost upwards of $4 million for a 100–unit facility. Someone buying a condominium with a small down payment and a large mortgage is leveraging, as are persons buying an assisted living facility with a small amount of cash and a large loan.

Letter of Credit. A bank instrument stating that a bank has granted the holder the amount of credit equal to the face amount of the letter of credit (L/C). This transfers collection risk from the seller to the bank. A "standby L/C" cannot be drawn unless the payee fails to perform or pay as agreed upon by the contract.

Leverage. In accounting and finance, the amount of long-term debt that a company has in relation to its equity.

Recapitalization. The revision to a company's capital structure (Argenti, p. 329). May involve exchange of debt obligations for equity interests, or exchange of one type of debt for another. Some reasons to recapitalize are to reduce debt service that will allow additional borrowing, to clean up a balance sheet prior to a sale or merger, to increase tax deductions (by for-profit facilities) by substituting interest payments for dividends.

Mortgage. A use of the value of a purchase to borrow money for the purchase of that property by promising to repay the debt on a scheduled basis. The interest rate on most mortgages is set in reference to the prime rate (i.e., the interest rate established by money center banks as a measuring base against which to calculate customer interest charges). Banks define prime rate as the rate of interest charged to their best commercial customers.

Notes. A borrowing of money for an agreed upon purpose between a lender and borrower. A demand note is a promissory note with no set maturity date; the holder may require payment at any time. Notes spell out the principal amount of the loan and the interest rate and may identify a final date for liquidation of the note. Promissory notes with a term of 5 to 6 years are regarded as medium-term notes.

Securities and Exchange Commission (SEC). The federal agency responsible for regulating financial reporting and monitoring use of accounting principles, trading activities, and auditing practices of publicly held companies. SEC requirements are issued as Accounting Series releases and Staff Accounting bulletins.

Additional Paid in Capital. An accounting concept of the excess amount over par value that shareholders pay for a company's stock; usually treated as a donation.

STOCKS TERMS

Nearly all assisted living facility chains issue stock. Many of them are traded on the various stock exchanges.

Arbitrage. The process of simultaneously buying a stock, currency, or commodity on one market and selling it on another. The price difference between the two markets gives the arbitrageur his or her profit.

Blue Chip. A common stock with a long history of dividend payments and earnings.

Book value per share. The assets of a company available to common shareholders (i.e., what each share is worth based on the historical stockholders' equity costs maintained in a company's accounting books).

Capital Stock. The shares representing ownership of a company.

Common Stock. Certificates that represent ownership in a corporation. A variety of types of stock exist (e.g., common and preferred) and are used by most assisted living facility chains.

Common Stock Equivalent. A security that is not currently in common stock form but can be converted to common stock. Executives, for example, are often given stock options (i.e., the right to purchase stock at a stated price over a specific time period) as a benefit.

Convertible security. Stocks and bonds that can be converted into capital stock at some future date.

Debenture. An unsecured bond, normally in a subordinated position. Debentures often have convertible features or warrants attached that permit the holders to exchange their debenture or the warrants for common stock on a stated date or when specified events occur.

Garnishment. A legal process through which a plaintiff can obtain goods or money belonging to a defendant, held by a third party, that are due or will become due to the plaintiff. Garnishment is similar to attachment.

A person who receives notice to retain assets belonging to a defendant is the garnishee. Thus the health care facility may be the garnishee when a court directs the facility to pay over a portion of an employee's salary to a plaintiff to repay a portion of an employee's debt.

Grandfather clause. Provision whereby persons already engaged in a business or profession receive a license or entitlement without meeting all the conditions new entrants would have to meet.

Option. A right that is granted in exchange for an agreed-upon sum to buy or sell property (e.g., a set amount of stock during some specified time period).

Penny Stocks. Stocks of young public companies that are not listed on any stock exchange (see below) and typically sell at a very low price ranging from pennies to $10 per share (Argenti, 1994). One major nursing home facility chain did a reverse split in the mid-1990s (see below) to escape being viewed as a penny stock.

Preferred stock. A type of capital stock giving its holder preference over common stock in the distribution of earnings or rights to the assets of the company (Argenti, 1994).

Price/Earnings (P/E) Ratio. A measure of the company's investment potential, literally how much a share is worth per dollar of earnings:

$$\frac{\text{Market Price per Common Share}}{\text{Primary Earnings per Common Share}}$$

Reverse Split. A procedure whereby a company "buys back" a portion of its outstanding stock (Argenti, 1994). One major health care chain, in the mid-1990s, reduced the number of outstanding shares dramatically by giving one new share for each four old shares held, thereby increasing the value of each remaining share.

Stock Dividend. A dividend consisting of stock rather than of cash paid to shareholders.

Stock Exchanges. There are three major United States stock exchanges: the New York Stock Exchange (NYSE), and the National Association of Securities Dealers Automated Quotation System (NASDAQ), and the American Stock Exchange (ASE). The minimum listing requirements for the NYSE are (1) publicly held shares of $1 million, (2) market value of $16 million for those shares, (3) annual pretax net income of $2.5 million, (4) at least 2,000 shareholders, and (5) net assets of $18 million. In addition, the company must engage a registrar and a transfer agent in New York City.

The American Stock Exchange requires (1) 300,000 publicly held shares; (2) market value of $2.5 million for those shares; (3) annual pretax net income of $750,000; (4) 900 shareholders, of which 600 must own 100 shares or more; and (5) net assets of $4 million.

The minimum listing requirements for the NASDAQ are (1) 100,000 publicly held shares, (2) minimum of 300 shareholders, (3) net assets of $2 million, (4) net worth of $1 million, (5) two or more market makers, and (6) annual fee of $2,500 or $0.0005 per share.

These stock listing requirements are given because most assisted living facility chains strive to move up the ladder to the NYSE. One midsize nursing facility chain, for example, was forced to list initially on the ASE but worked diligently to become listed on the NYSE, which afforded it more status and net worth growth potential.

Treasury Stock. Shares of common stock that have been issued to the general public but are repurchased by the issuing company (Argenti, 1994). A health care chain might choose to repurchase some of its stock in order to increase the value of its remaining shares.

Value Line Investment Survey. An investment advisory service that tracks over 1,700 stocks in 91 industries. There are a number of such investment services available, most of them at public libraries. Considering going to work as an administrator for a particular chain? Go to the library and learn all you can about the chain's financial position. This information can help you decide whether to interview with the company, and if so, to appear well informed during the interview.

INCOME-RELATED TERMS

Annual Percentage Rate (APR). A measure of the true cost of credit. APR yields the ratio of the finance charge to the average amount of credit used during the term of a loan, or during the time money is owed to the facility in accounts receivable on which interest is charged by the facility after a specified due date.

Cash Cow. A facility or product that generates cash. The term, according to Argenti (1994), was coined by the Boston Consulting Group as an element of its growth/market share matrix.

Cash Equivalent. Any asset, such as a bond or easily sold stock, held as an investment that can easily and quickly be converted to cash.

Cash Flow. The cash receipts less the cash disbursements from a given operation or set of operations for a specific time period. If a facility has $300,000 cash income from accounts receivable for a month and operating costs of $275,000, there is a $25,000 cash flow for that month.

Contribution Margin. The amount by which sales exceed the variable costs, such as supplies and labor costs, of a service. The resulting money left over is available to cover fixed costs, such as mortgages, insurance, and the like. A contribution margin can be calculated for each income-producing area of the facility.

Lien. A claim on the property of another person as security for a debt owed. A lien does not give any title (ownership) to the property; it is a right of the person holding the lien to have a debt satisfied out of the property to which the lien applies. If a general contractor building a health care facility is not paid money due under the terms of the contract, he or she may seek to have a lien placed on the facility until the indebtedness is satisfied. Similarly, regular creditors of the assisted living facility, if not paid within a specified period of time, might seek to have a lien placed against the facility.

Perceived Value Pricing. A pricing approach based on the buyer's perception of value rather than the seller's cost. A facility with a strong reputation for quality care may choose to price daily room rates above the prevailing market rate in its community.

Profit Margin. The ratio of income to sales. There are two types of profit margin: gross profit and net profit. Gross profit margin shows the percentage return that the facility is earning over the cost of providing services. It is calculated as

$$\frac{\text{Gross Profit}}{\text{Sales}}$$

Net profit margin. (Also known as return on services rendered) shows the percentage of net income generated by each service-billed dollar in for-profit facilities. It is

$$\frac{\text{Net Income After Tax}}{\text{Sales}}$$

Rate of Return. The annual percentage of income earned on an investment. There are numerous ways to calculate rate of return. These are variously termed return on investment, return on equity, return on total assets, or return on sales. Rate of return on fixed-income securities is usually calculated as the current yield, (i.e., the annual interest or dividend payments divided by the price of the security). Some bonds, for example, may have been purchased at above or below the face value and may or may not have an additional pay out at maturity or when called before maturity. In such cases, a *yield to maturity* rate of return is calculated, which assumes the asset is held until maturity.

OWNERSHIP—TYPES, FORMS OF

Article of Incorporation. The instrument that creates a corporation under the laws of a state.

Business Combination. The process of associating two or more different companies. According to Argenti (1994), there are three forms of business combination: statutory merger, statutory consolidation, and acquisition. A statutory merger occurs when two separate companies combine in such a way that one of the companies will no longer exist: $x + y = x$. A statutory consolidation occurs when two or more separate companies combine such that both companies no longer exist and a new company is formed: $x + y = xy$. A number of hospital mergers are of this nature (e.g., Columbia-HCA—a combination of two hospital companies). An acquisition occurs when two separate companies combine in such a way that both keep their separate identities: $x + y = x + y$.

Core Competence. The particular capabilities of a company that separate it from competitors and serve as the basis for growth or diversification into new lines of business. One health care chain, Manor Care, has been particularly successful in attracting and maintaining a large share of the private-paying resident market in the communities they serve, possibly being that company's core competence.

Corporation. An association of shareholders (even one shareholder) created by statute and treated by the law as a "person." In effect, it is an artificial person with a legal existence entirely separate from the individuals who compose it. A corporation may have perpetual existence: buy, own, and dispose of property; sue and be sued; and exercise any other powers conferred on it by statute.

Normally, a stockholder's liability is limited to the assets of the corporation; thus stockholders avoid personal liability for their corporation's acts. Corporations are taxed at special rates, but usually stockholders must pay an additional tax on any profits received from the corporation (dividends).

A small corporation earning a modest profit may elect to be taxed as a partnership (see below). Stockholders, in this case, avoid personal liability for the acts of the corporation and avoid double taxation. A corporation choosing to pay federal taxes as a partnership is called an S corporation. For tax purposes, all income and losses of a corporation pass through to its shareholders.

To qualify for S status, a corporation and its shareholders must meet the following criteria: (1) be a domestic corporation and not part of an affiliated group of corporations; (2) not own 80% or more of the stock of another corporation; (3) not have more than 35 shareholders; (4) no nonresident aliens as shareholders; (5) shareholders must be individuals, estates, or some trusts, not corporations or partnerships; and (6) only one class of stock issued. Voting and nonvoting shares of stock are permitted.

Each state enacts its own corporation laws. Some states, such as Delaware, give the officers and board of directors more freedom from minority shareholder controls and thereby attract unusually large numbers of groups to incorporate under their state's laws.

De facto corporations are those that exist in fact without actual authorization by the law. Three conditions must be met: (1) a statute exists under which it could be incorporated, (2) it behaves in such a way as to appear to be functioning as a corporation, and (3) it assumes some corporate privileges.

Public corporations are created by authorization of the federal government and the states to accomplish certain purposes. They include town, counties, water and sewage districts, and radio and television stations. The United States Postal Service and the Corporation for Public Broadcasting are two such entities.

Private corporations are corporations created by private individuals for nongovernmental purposes.

Professional corporations are professional associations of one or more professionals (e.g., physicians, dentists, physical therapists, health care personnel) who form a corporation.

Courts may choose to ignore the protection provided to stockholders from personal liability, typically when it can be shown that the purported corporation is found to be the "alter ego" of a principal (person). When, for example, it can be shown that the purported corporation does not hold stockholder meetings or generally ignores the duties and activities associated with operating a corporation, and neglects other corporate formalities, the courts may ignore the stockholders' usual immunity from personal liability and assign personal liability to the stockholders for acts of the corporation. If the incorporation itself was undertaken to defraud, the courts may hold the stockholders and officers personally liable for acts of the corporation.

Decentralization. The diffusion of authority, responsibility, and decision-making power throughout different levels of a company. Beverly Enterprises, long the largest publicly owned health care chain, a few years ago chose to move its national offices from the West Coast to a central United States location and to give each region decision-making power formerly reserved to the national office. As the assisted living industry matures into a few national firms, a similar transition is likely.

Horizontal Integration. A growth strategy in which a company buys a competitor at the same level of services. Several assisted living chains have purchased others in recent years, thus increasing the amount of horizontal integration of the industry.

Joint venture. A legal form of business organization between companies whereby there is cooperation toward the achievement of common goals between entities that were, prior to the joint venture, separate. A *contractual joint venture* is a joint venture not created as a separate legal corporate entity. It is an unincorporated association set up to attain specific goals over a specified time period. An *equity joint venture* has two or more partners based on the formation of a legal corporation with limited liability and the joint management of it by the partners. Profits and losses are shared on the basis of their equity in the joint venture. There are, in addition, *hybrid joint ventures,* which take a variety of shapes.

Limited Liability Company or Limited Liability Corporation. Limited liability companies or corporations provide the flexibility of a partnership with the same kind of financial protection offered by a C corporate structure. Wyoming passed the first state law allowing this form in 1977, and over 40 states are now following suit. In 1988 the Internal Revenue Service ruled that it would treat limited liability companies as partnerships for tax purposes. The limited liability company provides liability protection for its owners, similar to that of a corporation, but allows the limited liability corporation or company to be taxed as a partnership.

Limited Liability Partnership. A new form of partnership used by professional groups, such as physicians, health care personnel, and physical therapists, to limit a partners' liability to the partnership's general contractual debts, the partner's individual malpractice, and the wrongful acts of persons acting under the partners' direct supervision. Unlike the standard partnership, there is no individual liability for the malpractice of the other partners. About half the states have adopted this form of business formation. In some states, protection extends even to the partnership's contractual debts that exceed the value of a partner's interest (Lasser, 1995).

Merger. A combination of two or more companies. The combination may be accomplished by the exchange of stock, by forming a new company to acquire the assets of the combining companies, or by a purchase.

Minority Interest. An ownership interest of less than 50%. In consolidated financial statements, minority interests are shown as a line item in the noncurrent liability section of the balance sheet (Argenti, 1994).

Partnership. A contract between two or more persons to pool resources and efforts for the purposes of conducting a business operation. Normally, partnership status requires an agreement to divide profits and assume indebtedness in some proportionate share. Unlike stockholders in a corporation, the partners do not have limited liability, unless it is a limited partnership—an entity in which one or more persons are designated general partners (who assume unlimited personal liability for the acts of the partnership) and one or more persons are designated limited partners (whose liability is limited to their investment). Limited partners do not share in the management of the partnership (Argenti, 1994).

Privately Held Company. A company whose ownership shares, unlike publicly held companies, are not publicly traded. A privately held company may be of many forms, including corporations, partnerships, proprietorships, limited partners, joint ventures, and limited liability corporations. The same accounting principles apply to privately held companies as publicly held companies. However, reporting requirements from regulatory agencies, such as the Securities and Exchange Commission, and public stock exchanges do not apply to them. Hence, in most reports on health care chains and ownership, privately held companies' financial statements are usually not shown, because they choose not to make them available to the public at large. Privately held companies do make their financial statements available to lenders, private investors, and, as required, some state agencies.

Product liability. The liability of manufacturers and sellers for products they place on the market that cause harm to a person because of defects.

Sole Proprietorship. Ownership of a business by one individual. Before incorporation became popular among physicians, most of them were the sole proprietors of their office practices.

Vertical integration. Expansion by moving forward or backward within an industry (Argenti, 1994). For example, health care chains frequently integrate backwards by owning and operating their own pharmacies. Some chains are integrating forward by owning and operating home health care agencies.

3.10.6 Insurance Terms

Actuary. A person who computes insurance costs, usually for the purpose of determining rates to be charged, an especially important function for continuing care retirement communities, which take lifetime responsibility for their residents.

Annuity. A fixed amount of money payable periodically by an insurer under the terms of an insurance contract. Normally, the annuitant (the person receiving the payments) has no rights other than entitlement to payments for a fixed period of time. Often, assisted living facility residents have insurance annuities that can be applied to their costs of care.

Beneficiary. The person named in an insurance policy to receive the proceeds or benefits under the policy.

Binder. A contract for temporary insurance until a permanent policy can be issued.

Coinsurance. A division of responsibility for losses or risks between the insurer and the insured. The insured individual might agree to pay, for example, the first $50 of any claim.

Life insurance. Insurance that may be one of several types. Whole life insurance policies can build cash value (i.e., can be turned in by the insured for cash) and normally pay dividends (i.e., interest on the cash value). Term insurance, on the other hand, has no cash value; hence, no dividends. When term insurance expires, no value is left. Whole life insurance costs more than term insurance. A variety of types of policies can now be offered as variations on these two basic forms of life insurance.

Types of insurance

- fidelity or bond coverage of key employees
- pharmacy
- vehicle and driver
- workers' compensation
- property damage—coverage against fire, flood, earthquake damage to buildings, furniture fixtures; building contents
- furnace and machinery

- business interruption
- accounts receivable—protection against loss of income from destruction of financial records
- comprehensive general liability or casualty against losses sustained by residents, visitors, others resulting from negligence not related to rendering professional services
- directors' and officers' coverage for acts done in their official capacities
- malpractice or professional liability coverage protecting against losses sustained by others, resulting from negligence related to the rendering of professional services

3.10.7 Terms Associated with Wills and Estates

Inevitably, as residents age in place, the assisted living administrator will want to be increasingly knowledgeable about wills and estates.

Administrator. A person appointed to transfer the property of one who dies intestate to those who succeed in ownership. To die intestate is to die without leaving a will. The estate (or property) of persons who die testate (with a will) is administered by an *executor* of the estate, usually named in the will.

Codicil. See Will.

Decedent. The person who has died.

Competence. The capability of a person to make a will. A person is judged capable or competent if he or she understands the nature and extent of his/her property, the identity of the property owned, and the consequences of the act of making a will.

Estate. A term that originally referred to ownership of land, but now refers broadly to all real and personal property a person owns or leaves at death.

Health Care Power of Attorney. Increasingly, state laws are allowing persons of the resident's choice to be given power of attorney control over their health care decisions. Persons exercising health care power of attorney are expected to make, as nearly as possible, the same health care decisions the grantor would have made.

Incompetence. Inability to function within limits judged normal by a court of law. A *guardian* must be appointed if a person is found to be incompetent. The guardian must handle the incompetent person's affairs until the court determines that competency has returned, in which case the guardian is discharged.

Probate. The process of proving that an instrument presented as a will is in fact the valid and duly executed will of the deceased person. Some states have special courts, called probate courts, to conduct theses procedures.

Will. A person's declaration as to how he or she wishes his or her real and personal property to be disposed of after death. A will may call for actions desired by the decedent (testator) but must dispose of some property, real or personal, to be valid. Originally *will* referred to real estate and *testament* to personal property. "Last will and testament" refers to the most recent valid will left by the decedent.

A *holographic will* is an entirely handwritten will. In some states a will may be handwritten and need not be witnessed to be valid. A *codicil* is a supplement or amendment to a will. *Codicil* literally means "to say along with." A codicil must meet the same formal requirements as the will.

Living will. Some assisted living facility residents make a *living will,* which governs the type(s) of treatment to be given the resident in the event the resident becomes comatose or in a similar condition. Several states have passed laws establishing living wills as valid legal instruments. A living will has noting to do with disposition of property.

REFERENCES

American Seniors Housing Association. (2003). *Seniors Housing Construction Report, 2003.* Washington, DC: Author.

American Seniors Housing Association. (2003). *Seniors Housing Investment & Transactions Report, 2003.* Washington, DC: Author.

American Seniors Housing Association. (2002). *The State of Seniors, 2002.* Washington, DC: Author.

Argenti, P. A. (1994). *The portable MBA desk reference.* New York: Wiley.

Assisted Living Business Week. (1998). *2*(2,5,7,11), 7–54.

Assisted Living Today. (1996). *4*(1).

Focus on Retirement. (1998, March 9). *Wall Street Journal,* p. 22.

Kapp, M. B. (1987). *Preventing malpractice in long-term care.* New York: Springer Publishing Co.

Lasser, J. K. (1995). *Monthly tax letter.* New York: J. K. Lasser's Tax Letter.

Martin, P. (1997). *The assisted living industry.* New York: Jeffries & Co.

Orlikoff, J., Fifer, W., & Greeley, H. (1981). *Malpractice prevention.* Chicago: American Hospital Association.

Provider, September, 2003.

Quality Care Advocate. (1989, September/October). Washington, DC: National Citizen's Coalition for Nursing Home Reform.

Showalter, J. (1984). *Quality Assurance and Risk Management Journal of Legal Medicine, 5,* 497.

Trager, G. T., & Salman, S. L. (1986). *Handbook of health care risk management.* Rockville, MD: Aspen.

U.S. Senate Special Committee on Aging. (2003, April 29). *Assisted Living Workgroup's Final Report.* Washington, DC: Author.

Union membership fell further in 1997. (1998, March 18). *Wall Street Journal.*

PART FOUR

THE LONG-TERM CARE CONTINUUM:

LAWS AND REGULATIONS

4.1 The Long Term Care Continuum

4.1.1 Origins

Each culture evolves modes of caring for its elderly. Various institutions such as churches have often provided assistance to the elderly. During the agricultural era the children typically provided assistance in the home, which often housed three generations. Today, due to a variety of demographic and cultural forces, care for aging adults is increasingly unavailable in the home.

Every day over 5,000 Americans celebrate their 65th birthday and join the "elderly" sector of the population. In 1900, 4% of the U.S. population were age 65 or older; in 1980, 11%. It is projected that, in 2030, 18% of the U.S. population will be 65 years of age or older (see Table 4.1).

INCREASED LIFE EXPECTANCY

Increased life expectancy accounts for much of the change in the elderly population that is of the most direct concern to the assisted living facility administrator and staff. Since 1900 life expectancy has increased from 46 years to 75+ years. Greater and greater numbers of people are reaching age 65.

Year	No. 65 or over In thousands	% of U.S. population
1950	12,397	8.1
1980	24,927	11.2
2000	31,822	12.2
2020	45,102	15.5
2030	55,024	18.3

Source: U.S. Bureau of the Census as referenced in Doly, P., Korbin, L. and Wiener, J. (1985, Spring). An Overview of Long Term Care. *Health Care Financing Review*, 6(3), 69.

TABLE 4.1 U.S. Population 65 Years of Age and Older and Percentage of Total Population: Selected Years and Projections: 1950-2030

Increased Proportions of the "Old-Old"

As a group the elderly are growing older all the time. The 64–74 cohort, now referred to as the "young-old," increased at approximately the rate of the general population during the 1980s and 1990s. Those 74–84 and 85 and older are increasing at twice the rate of the general population (Liu, Manton, & Allston, 1982). Thus, in 2000 a full quarter of the elderly were old-old (see Table 4.2 and Figure 4.1). Live to 90? According to the National Center for Health Statistics, the percentage of people age 65 expected to survive to age 90 has increased dramatically since 1940 and is expected to top 40% by 2050:

Percentage of Elderly Expected to live to age 90

1940	7%
1960	14%
1980	24%
2000	27%
2050	42% ("Focus on Retirement," 1998)

Fewer Men, More Women

As the elderly grow older, their age group becomes more and more dominated by women. In 1900 men in all age groups outnumbered women 102 to 100, but by 1975 the ratio had reversed, with fewer men than women: 69 men for every 100 women. In the 1990s this is even further reduced to 66 men for every 100 women. The preponderance of women is even more pronounced in the 75+ age group: The ratio of men to women for 1900 in this age group was 96 men for every 100 women; in 1975 this had decreased to 58 men per 100 women. Today, the ratio is 54 men for every 100 women. No wonder that most of the residents in long-term care facilities are women.

Year	All ages	65-74 years	75-84 years	85 and over
1950-1960	18.7	30	41	59
1980-1990	10	14	26	20
1990-2000	7	-3	16	29
2000-2010	6	13	-3	19

Source: U.S. Bureau of the Census as referenced In Doly, P., L. Korbin, and J. Wiener (1985, Spring). An Overview of Long Term Care. *Health Care Financing Review, 6*(3), p. 69.

TABLE 4.2 Percentage Increases in U.S. Population for Selected 10-Year Intervals by Age Group, 1950-2010.

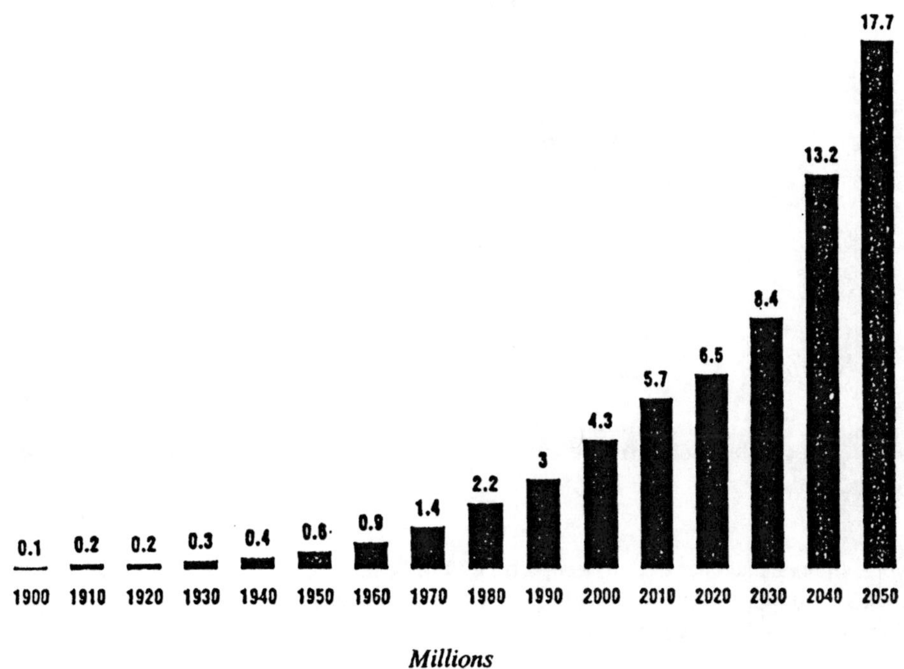

FIGURE 4.1 U.S. population group aged 85 and over from 1950 to 2050

THE NEED FOR INSTITUTIONAL CARE

In the mid-1990s a total of 1,640,000 elderly Americans were estimated to need institutional care, as were 710,000 working-age adults and 90,000 children (see Table 4.3). When community-based long-term care is added to institutional care needs, 57% of the elderly, 40% of working-age adults, and 3% of children were calculated to be in need of such care in 1995 (see Figure 4.2 and Table 4.4).

INCREASING DEPENDENCY LEVELS AMONG THE AGED

As individuals age, they become susceptible to chronic conditions. Therefore, it is no surprise that older Americans also dominate the dependent population. Of people relying on others for eating, bathing, dressing, getting to and using the bathroom, getting into or out of a bed or chair, and mobility in general activities (activities of daily or ADLs), approximately 7 in every 10 are elderly (Weissert, 1985). Persons better able to care for themselves are described using the concept of instrumental activities of daily living or IADLs (see Figure 4.3).

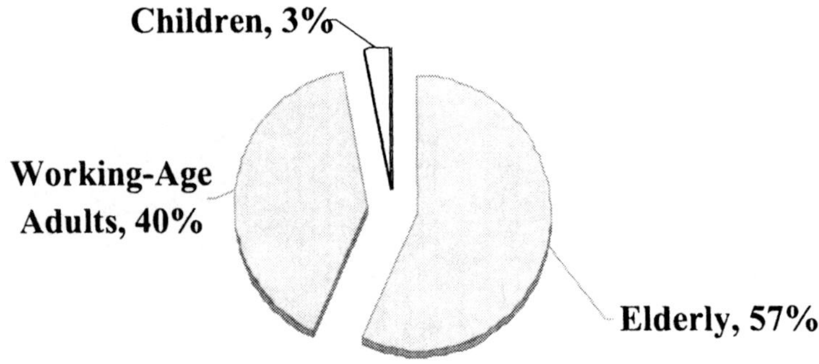

Need for institutional and community-based long-term care, 1995

Note: Includes people needing long-term care in institutions or in the community. Children are those under 18 years old, working-age adults are those 18 to 64 years old, and the elderly are those 65 years old and older.

Source: Based on our analysis of information form HHS and Institute for Health Policy Studies at the University of California, San Francisco. From: Ross, J. L. (April, 1995). long-term care: Current Issues and Future Diections. United States General Accounting Office: Report to the Chairman, Special Committee on Aging, U.S. Senate. GAO/HEHS-959109, long-term care Issues, p. 7

FIGURE 4.2 Need for institutional and community-based long-term care.

	Numbers in thousands		
Age group	In institutions	At home or in community settings	Total population
Children	90	330	420
Working-age adults	710	4,380	5,090
Elderly	1,640	5,690	7,330
Total	2,440	10,400	12,840

Note: Based on our analysis of information from HHS and the Institute for Health Policy Studies at the University of California, San Francisco.

Source: Ross, J.L. (April, 1995) Long-Term Care: Current Issues and Future Directions United States General Accounting Office: Report to the Chairman, Special Committee on Aging, U.S. Senate. GAO/HEHS-95-109, Long Term Care Issues, p.8.

TABLE 4.3 Numbers of persons needing long-term care in institutions and in community settings.

	Source of assistance				
Year	Institution[a]	Spouse[b]	Offspring[b]	Other relative[b]	Nonrelative[b]
	Number in thousands				
1980	1,187	1,442	1,438	1,213	655
1990	1,623	1,801	1,950	1,610	880
1985	1,411	1,612	1,701	1,414	771
1995	1,861	1,953	2,232	1,814	1,003
2000	2,081	2,049	2,484	1,989	1,110
2020	2,805	2,976	3,392	2,728	1,530
2040	4,354	3,900	5,172	4,028	2,298

[a]These projections refer to a full day of care in an institution.
[b]These projections refer to the number of episodes of caregiving on a given day.

Source: Preliminary data from the Department of Health and Human Services, 1982 National Long-Term Care Survey, 1977 National Nursing Home Survey, National Center for Health Statistics, and Social Security Administration projections as referenced in Doty, P., Korbin, L. and Wiener, J. "An Overview of Long Term Care" Health Care Financing Review, Spring 1985, Vol. 6, No. 3, p. 71.

TABLE 4.4 Projections of daily volume of long-term assistance by sources of assistance, 1980-2040.

ADL	Activities of Daily Living	Generally include eating, bathing, dressing, getting to and using the bathroom, getting in or out of a bed or chair, and mobility.
IADL	Instrumental Activities of Daily Living	Generally include going outside the home, keeping track of money or bills, preparing meals, doing light housework, using the telephone, and taking medicine.

Source: Ross, J.L. (April, 1995) Long-Term Care: Current Issues and Future Directions. United States General Accounting Office: Report to the Chairman, Special Committee on Aging, U.S. Senate. GAO/HEHS-95-109, Long Term Care Issues, p. 5.

FIGURE 4.3 Definitions of activities of daily living and instrumental activities of daily living.

4.1.2 The Care Continuum

OVERVIEW OF THE CARE CONTINUUM

The American long-term care system, insofar as it can be called a system, is loosely interconnected. Each agency and program is separately authorized by various pieces of legislation. No single agency or program is authorized, or indeed able, to coordinate the various efforts on behalf of the elderly. Although the Older Americans Act of 1965 calls for and authorizes coordination, in reality officials have not been empowered to bring this about.

Sources of payment for long-term care costs are given in Figure 4.4. Federal and state programs—mainly Medicaid and Medicare—account for nearly two thirds of the payments. Figure 4.5 demonstrates the dramatic rise in expenditures. In the years 1995 to 2003 the proportions paid by each program have changed only slightly.

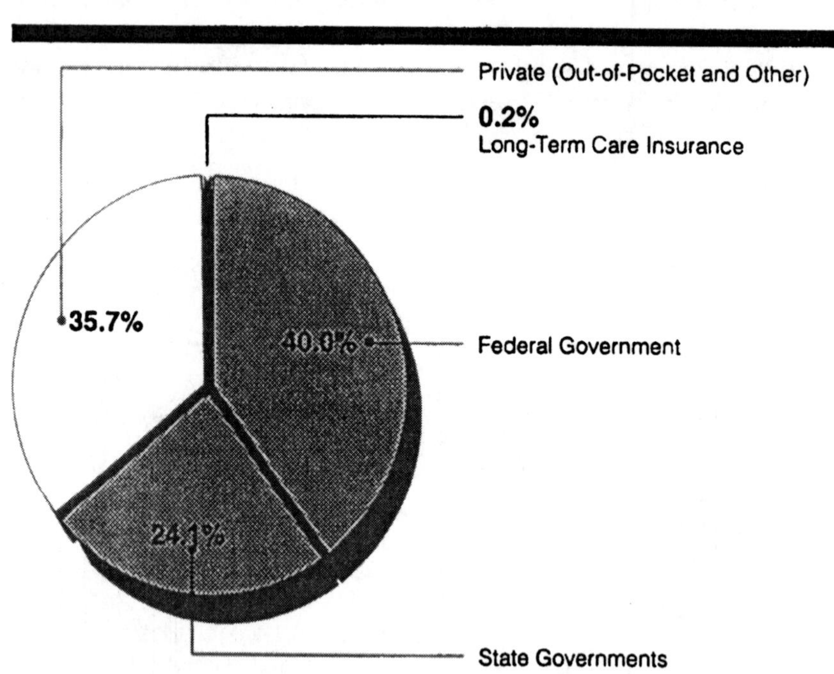

Source: Office of the Assistant Secretary for Planning and Evaluation, HHS.

Source: Ross, J.L. (April, 1995) Long-Term Care: Current Issues and Future Directions. United States General Accounting Office: Report to the Chairman, Special Committee on Aging, U.S. Senate. GA0/HEHS-95-109, Long Term Care Issues, p.9.

FIGURE 4.4 Sources of payment for long-term care costs, 1995.

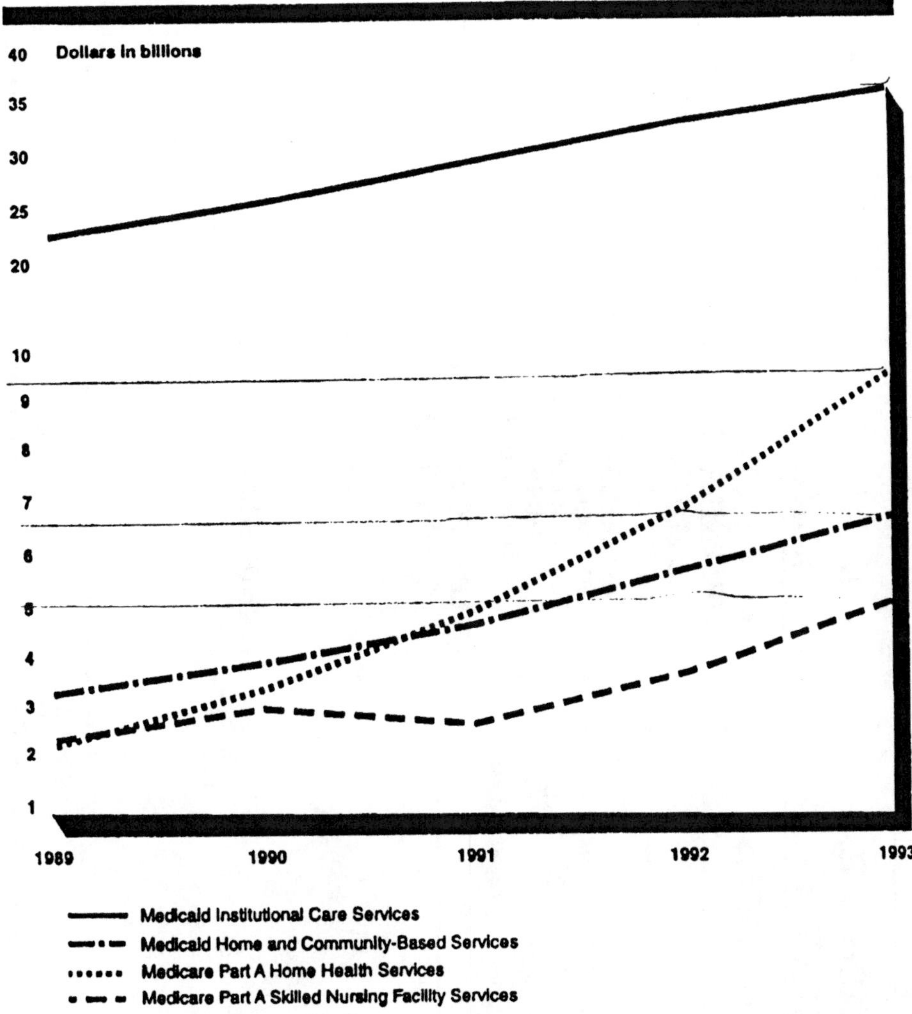

Note: Medicare Part A Home Health Services include post-hospital services and long-term care services for persons with qualifying chronic conditions. Medicare Part A Skilled Nursing Facility Services are post-hospital services but have often been counted as long-term care because they are provided primarily by nursing homes, traditional long-term care providers.

Sources: Medicare Expenditure Data from 1994 Green Book, Overview of Entitlement Programs. Medicaid Expenditure Data from Systemetrics (MEDSTAT, using data from HCFA-64).

Source: Ross, J.L. (April, 1995) Long-Term Care: Current Issues and Future Directions. United States General Accounting Office: Report to the Chairman, Special Committee on Aging, U.S. Senate. GA0/HEHS-95-109, Long Term Care Issues, p.14.

FIGURE 4.5 Medicaid and Medicare long-term care expenditures, fiscal years 1989-1993.

Figure 4.6 describes the major sources of services available to older Americans, moving from the least restrictive to the most restrictive.

An overview of the major federal programs supporting long term care services for the elderly and for persons with disabilities, fiscal year 1993, is presented in Table 4.5 which gives the programs, their objectives, fiscal year 1993 funding levels, administers of the programs, and the services offered.

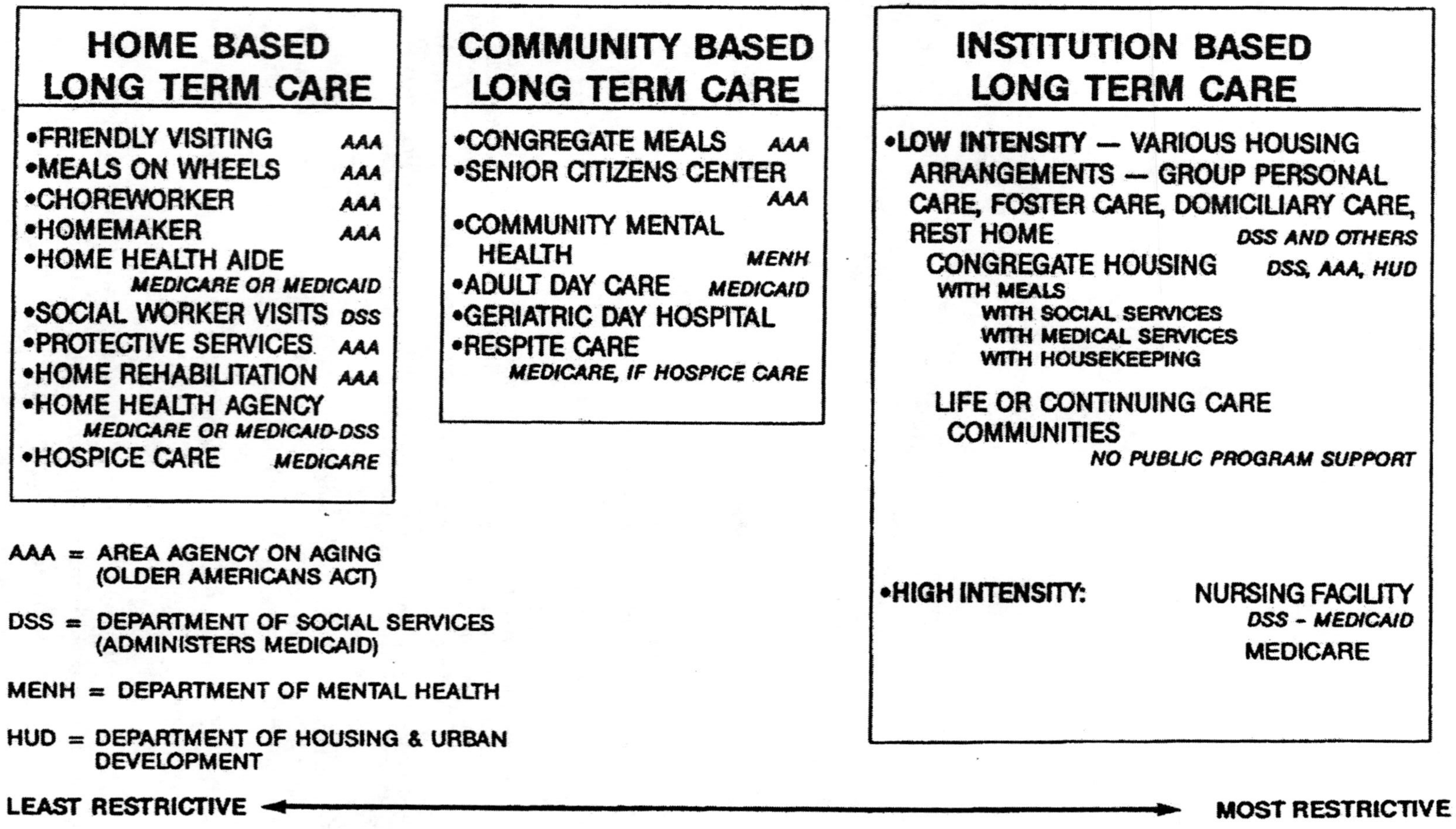

HOME BASED LONG TERM CARE

- FRIENDLY VISITING — *AAA*
- MEALS ON WHEELS — *AAA*
- CHOREWORKER — *AAA*
- HOMEMAKER — *AAA*
- HOME HEALTH AIDE — *MEDICARE OR MEDICAID*
- SOCIAL WORKER VISITS — *DSS*
- PROTECTIVE SERVICES — *AAA*
- HOME REHABILITATION — *AAA*
- HOME HEALTH AGENCY — *MEDICARE OR MEDICAID-DSS*
- HOSPICE CARE — *MEDICARE*

COMMUNITY BASED LONG TERM CARE

- CONGREGATE MEALS — *AAA*
- SENIOR CITIZENS CENTER — *AAA*
- COMMUNITY MENTAL HEALTH — *MENH*
- ADULT DAY CARE — *MEDICAID*
- GERIATRIC DAY HOSPITAL
- RESPITE CARE — *MEDICARE, IF HOSPICE CARE*

INSTITUTION BASED LONG TERM CARE

- LOW INTENSITY — VARIOUS HOUSING ARRANGEMENTS — GROUP PERSONAL CARE, FOSTER CARE, DOMICILIARY CARE, REST HOME — *DSS AND OTHERS*
  - CONGREGATE HOUSING — *DSS, AAA, HUD*
    - WITH MEALS
      - WITH SOCIAL SERVICES
      - WITH MEDICAL SERVICES
      - WITH HOUSEKEEPING
  - LIFE OR CONTINUING CARE COMMUNITIES — *NO PUBLIC PROGRAM SUPPORT*
- HIGH INTENSITY: NURSING FACILITY — *DSS - MEDICAID*; MEDICARE

AAA = AREA AGENCY ON AGING (OLDER AMERICANS ACT)

DSS = DEPARTMENT OF SOCIAL SERVICES (ADMINISTERS MEDICAID)

MENH = DEPARTMENT OF MENTAL HEALTH

HUD = DEPARTMENT OF HOUSING & URBAN DEVELOPMENT

LEAST RESTRICTIVE ←——————→ MOST RESTRICTIVE

Figure 4-6 Overview of the long term care continuum.

TABLE 4-5 Major Federal Programs Supporting Long Term Care Services for the elderly and for persons with disabilities, FY 1993

Program	Objectives	Fiscal year 1993 federal spending (billions)[a]	Administration	Long-term care services
Medicaid/Title XIX of the Social Security Act	To pay for medical assistance for certain low-income persons	Total: $77.4 Long-term care: $24.7 (estimated)	Federal: HCFA/HHS State: State Medicaid Agency	Nursing home care, home and community-based health and social services, facilities for persons with mental retardation, chronic care hospitals
Medicare/Title XVIII of the Social Security Act	To pay for acute medical care for the aged and selected disabled	Total: $138.8 Long-term care: $15.8 (estimated)	Federal: HCFA/HHS State: none	Home health visits, limited skilled nursing facility care
Older Americans Act	To foster development of a comprehensive and coordinated service system to serve the elderly	Total: $1.4 Long-term care: $.8	Federal: Administration on Aging/Office of Human Development, HHS State: State Agency on Aging	Nutrition services, home and community-based social services, protective services, and long-term care ombudsman
Rehabilitation Act	To promote and support vocational rehabilitation and independent living services for the disabled	Total: $2.2 Long-term care: $.1	Federal: Office of Special Education and Rehabilitative Services/Department of Education State: State Vocational Rehabilitation Agencies	Rehabilitation services, attendant and personal care, centers for independent living
Social Services Block Grant/Title XX of the Social Security Act	To assist families and individuals in maintaining self-sufficiency and independence	Total: $2.8 Long-term care: (not available)	Federal: Office of Human Development Services, HHS State: State Social Services or Human Resources Agency; other state agencies may administer part of Title XX funds for certain groups; for example, State Agency on Aging	Services provided at the states' discretion, may include long-term care

[a] Data represent total fiscal year 1993 obligations as reported in the Budget of the United States Government, Appendix, Fiscal Year 1995, except for estimates of Medicare and Medicaid long-term care spending. These figures are estimates for 1993 from the Assistant Secretary for Planning and Evaluation, HHS. Under the Medicaid program, states contributed an estimated $19.0 billion in support of long-term care in addition to the federal share of $24.7 billion.

Source: Ross, J.L. (April, 1995) Long-Term Care: Current Issues and Future Directions. United States General Accounting Office: Report to the Chairman, Special Committee on Aging, U.S. Senate. GA0/HEHS-95-109, Long Term Care Issues, p.10.

HOME- AND COMMUNITY-BASED LONG-TERM CARE OPTIONS

Table 4.6 provides an overview of various types of services offered under home- and community-based services in 1995. Table 4.7 illustrates the expected dramatic growth in the number of home health care agencies.

TABLE 4.6 Examples of Home and Community Based Services, 1995.

Service	Description
Case management	Assists beneficiaries in getting medical, social, educational, and other services.
Personal care	Includes bathing, dressing, ambulation, feeding, grooming, and some household services such as meal preparation and shopping.
Adult day care	Includes personal care and supervision and may include physical, occupational, and speech therapies. Also provides socialization and recreational activities adapted to compensate for any physical or mental impairments.
Respite care	Provides relief to the primary caregiver of a chronically ill or disabled beneficiary. By providing services in the beneficiary's or provider's home or in other settings, respite care allows the primary caregiver to be absent for a time.
Homemaker	Assists beneficiaries with general household activities and may include cleaning, laundry, meal planning, grocery shopping, meal preparation, transportation to medical services, and bill paying.

Source: Ross, J.L. (April, 1995) Long-Term Care: Current Issues and Future Directions. United States General Accounting Office: Report to the Chairman, Special Committee on Aging, U.S. Senate. GA0/HEHS-95-109, Long Term Care Issues, p.4.

TABLE 4.7 Estimated Number of Current Patients 65 Years and Over Receiving Home Health Care, and Number per 1,000 populatio 65 and over, by geographic region: United States, 1991, 2000 (Est.).

Geographic region	*Estimated number of current home health patients (in thousands)*[1]	*Number per 1,000 U.S. population*[2]
United States	918	28.9
Northeast	295	41.8
Midwest	201	25.6
South	321	29.3
West	101	17.1

[1]Source: unpublished home health care data from the 1991 NHPI.
[2]Based on U.S. Bureau of the Census estimates of the United States resident population ages 65 years and over, as of July 1, 1991.

United States 2,000 (est)	1.239	39

Source: 1991 data: Sirrocco, A. (1994) Nursing homes and board and care homes: data from the 1991 National health Provider Inventory. NCHS: Advance Data, 244, February 23, 1994.
Source: Allen, J.E. (2,000 data) (1996) Extrapolation on 1990s trend. Estimates a 35% increase in number of home health patients.

HOME-BASED OPTIONS

Friendly Visiting

Both the Area Agency on Aging and local volunteer groups arrange for regular visits to the elderly living alone. This offers both needed social contact and continuous monitoring of these individuals.

Meals on Wheels

Title 3c of the Older Americans Act pays for home-delivered meals. To qualify, an organization must deliver meals (usually only the noon meal) on each of 5 days or more per week and meet certain standards, including providing one third of the daily nutritional requirements. As a rule, the Area Agency on Aging contracts with groups to provide these meals. long-term care facilities frequently offer Meals on Wheels, both as a public service and as a contact mechanism with potential applicants. The dietary department of the facility automatically meets the various requirements of the program by preparing food for its residents.

Chore worker/Homemaker

Area Agency on Aging subcontractors offer the services of workers who will come into older persons' homes to perform specific tasks. A chore worker usually does window washing or other less routine tasks. A homemaker visits on a more regular basis and performs housekeeping, tasks such as dusting, dish washing, and laundry.

Home Health Aide

The home health aide, in contrast to the homemaker and chore worker, is expected to perform only health-specific tasks, such as administering medicines, changing bandages, and the like. The home health aide is paid from Medicaid or Medicare funds, not by the Area Agency on Aging. A home health care agency, discussed below, can send such an aide if the older person is receiving Medicare services in the home for a specific illness or injury. Over the past few years local Medicaid offices have increasingly been permitted to use Medicaid funds to pay for services designed to prevent or postpone institutionalizing older persons. Originally, these were called Title 19 waivers, for which states had to apply.

In 1984 the Department of Health and Human Services authorized all Medicaid programs to offer a variety of services similar to those available under the Older Americans Act if they were conducive to postponement or prevention of institutionalization. Usually, these services will be funded up to three quarters of the costs of institutionalizing the client.

Social Worker Visits

The local department of social services, under Title 20 or other authorizations, is permitted to pay for social worker visits to the homes of the elderly. This is similar to a social worker or case worker visiting any other client.

Protective Services/Home Rehabilitation Services

The Area Agency on Aging or its subcontractor is authorized to assist elderly persons to bring their homes up to minimum standards and to provide added security measures to reduce the possibility of break-ins.

Home Health Care

In the mid-1960s the federal government fueled an exponential growth in nursing facilities through its funding legislation. In the mid-1990s federal (and state) support resulted in increasing numbers of home health care agencies on the assumption, probably erroneous, that they can provide care more inexpensively than nursing facilities. As we have seen, an assisted living facility may neatly fill the niche of unmet need between home health care and institutionalization in a nursing facility.

An older person is entitled to receive home health care through any one of three programs, all under the Social Security Act: Medicare Plan A, Medicare Plan B, and Medicaid.

Services Under Medicare Plan A. Unlimited home health care visits at no cost are available to any Medicare recipient hospitalized under Plan A and evaluated to need post-hospital home health care for the final DRG (diagnostically related group) diagnosis.

Services Under Medicare Plan B. Unlimited visits, at 80% of cost, are available to persons covered by Medicare Plan B who are found to need part-time health care in their home for the treatment of an illness or injury. No prior hospitalization is required, but four conditions must be met: (1) the care must include part-time nursing care, physical therapy, or speech therapy; (2) the client must be confined to his or her home; (3) a doctor must diagnose the need and design the plan; and (4) the agency must participate in Medicare.

Medicare does not cover general household services, meal preparation, shopping, assistance in bathing or dressing, or other home assistance to meet personal, family, or domestic needs (U.S. DHHS, 1985). Thus, to keep an ailing older adult who requires various types of home assistance functioning, several agencies, with separate priorities and interests, must be coordinated by the client or by a friend or a caseworker acting in his or her behalf. During the period from 1966 (the year Congress authorized Medicare to pay for home care) to 1988 the number of home health care agencies rose from 1,000 in 1966 to 10,850 in 1988. Home health care agencies are increasingly able to care for persons as nearly disabled as at the skilled nursing facility (Simon-Rusinowitz & Hofland, 1993). A cost-effectiveness study by Greene, Lively, and Ondrich (1993) found that 41% of persons studied could be effectively cared for outside the nursing facility. There has been a steady movement toward increasing utilization of home health care (Manton, Stallard & Woodbury, 1994). In 1995 the American Academy of Medical Administrators formed a division for home health care executives, a further recognition of the maturing of this field (Shriver, 1995)

In 1982, 1.1 million Americans were receiving home health care; by 1988 the number had risen to 4.0 million. By 1993 there were 7,400 home health care agencies, of which 37% were proprietary, 43% nonprofit, and 20% government and other. A high percentage were certified by Medicare (84%) and Medicaid (83%) (Strahan, 1994). Of all patients receiving home health care, the proportion publicly paid for is even higher: 89% on Medicare, 91% on Medicaid. In short, when compared to nursing home care payment sources, a dramatically higher percentage of costs of home health care patients are paid by Medicare and Medicaid. The same is equally true of hospice patients, 90% of whom are both Medicare and Medicaid eligible. Assisted living facilities are beginning to enjoy reimbursement from such third parties. It has been estimated that between 5% and 10% of physician time is spent in home health care (Council on Scientific Affairs, 1990).

Home health care expenditures by all payers increased from $8,421,000,000 in 1988 to $29,255,000,000 in 1998 (Office of the Actuary, HCFA, September 27, 2000).

Medicaid Services. If a Medicaid recipient is found to need full-time institutional care, Medicaid can pay for nearly any of the types of in-home services available through either Medicare or the Area Agency on Aging, and increasingly through waivers for assisted living facility services.

The economic rationale of this program is to reduce public expenditures by offering services that allow people to function in their own home where they, or often their family, will be sharing the financial burden, thus reducing public costs. The care rationale to encourage them to remain at home is based on the positive psychological and emotional benefits. The assisted living facility offers an in-between level of care.

HOSPICE CARE

Hospice care is given to persons usually believed to be at the end of their lives, with perhaps 6 months or less to live, who mainly seek alleviation from pain rather than intensive technological medical treatment. Hospice care is usually provided at home. There is a trend for hospice agencies to attend such patients in assisted living facilities and nursing facilities. Hospice is also offered in freestanding hospice centers for inpatients and patient wards in hospitals designated as hospice units, as well as individual patients on other wards.

Medicare Plan A pays for hospice care if three conditions are met: (1) medical certification exists that the patient is terminally ill; (2) patient's choice is to receive care from a hospice instead of the standard Medicare benefits; (3) the program must be offered by a Medicare-certified hospice. People who choose hospice can be given Medicare Plan A hospitalization care for events unrelated to their terminal illness (e.g., a bone broken during an accidental fall).

The Health Care Financing Administration, which administers Medicare and Medicaid, defines hospice as a public agency or private organization that is primarily engaged in providing pain relief, symptom management, and supportive services to terminally ill people and their families (U.S. DHHS, 1985). Medicare pays 100% of all hospice services except for outpatient drugs and respite care.

The first national survey of hospice providers (the National Home and Hospice Care Survey) was conducted from September through December 1992. (Hospice data are given in Table 4.5 for the United States and each state.) Of 1,000 hospice agencies identified in the survey, 4% were proprietary, 94% were not-for-profit, and 2% were government and other. Seventy percent of these 1,000 hospices were certified by Medicare and 63% by Medicaid (Strahan, 1994).

During the years 1991 through 2001 hospice care giving increased substantially in the US. Dollars spent by Medicare on hospice increased from 0.4 billion dollars in 1991 to 3.6 billion in 2001. The average amount spent per beneficiary during those years increased from $4,000 to $6,000. The number of beneficiaries increased from 108,000 to 579,000. The average number of days increased only slightly from 44 days in 1991 to 50 days in 2001. Many assisted living facilities are taking advantage of hospice services for residents who choose to age in place.

COMMUNITY-BASED LONG-TERM CARE

Congregate Meals at Nutrition Sites and Senior Citizens Centers

Under Title 3c of the Older Americans Act, an effort has been made to make congregate meal sites available to as many elderly citizens as possible in both urban and rural areas. To accomplish this, the Area Agencies on Aging contract with many thousands of groups that serve such meals 5 or more days a week. Often these nutrition sites, as they are called, are rural schools or churches that are usually centrally located. Transportation is usually provided, as well as counseling, nutrition education, recreation, and referral services at the same site and time.

Senior Citizens Centers Activities and In-Center Services

The Area Agencies on Aging offer a variety of activities and services at these centers, and usually congregate meals as well.

Community Mental Health Centers

Mental health legislation over the past two decades has resulted in the establishment of an extensive network of community mental health centers to which older persons may refer themselves or be referred. However, the utilization rate of these centers has tended to be disproportionately low among the elderly.

Adult Day Care

An adult day care program is a community organization providing daytime health and/or recreational services to groups of impaired older adults in a centralized protective environment, often for long periods of time. Assisted living facilities and nursing facilities are uniquely positioned to offer adult day care programs, and some do. Payments for adult day care can come from various sources, including federal revenue-sharing programs, Title 4 of the Older Americans Act, Title 6 of the Social Security Act, and Medicaid.

People enter an adult day care program for a variety of reasons, such as the need for the primary caregiver to be at work during the day. Its primary function is to allow older persons with various kinds of disabilities to remain in the home setting longer.

Often the adult day care participant in an assisted living facility eventually becomes a resident there. This earlier exposure to the environment serves to reduce the trauma usually involved in the transition to institutional care. (This trauma is discussed in Part Five.)

Adult day care began in the mid-1970s. The National Institute of Adult Day Care was established in 1979. The average day care program cares for about 20 persons, between 9:00 a.m. and 3:00 p.m. Day care programs normally offer a structured day, including social interaction, exercise, and a hot noontime meal. Some offer case management, health assessment, nutrition education, and therapeutic diets (Weissert, 1985).

A majority of adult day care centers are located in nursing homes. The majority of participants are functionally dependent elderly white women. Most are unmarried, and about a third are mentally impaired. Compared to the nursing home resident, they tend to be younger, less dependent, and have less mental impairment. Few, if any, adult day care programs are physically located in a hospital (Weissert, 1985). Assisted living facilities are well situated to enter this market.

Geriatric day rehabilitation hospitals are a medical model of the adult day care program. Adult day care programs range from offering recreation with no health care to providing nearly full health care services similar in intensity to those of the nursing facility.

Respite Care

Respite care is a relatively new program under Medicare Plan A, where it is defined as a short-term inpatient stay that provides temporary relief to the person who regularly assists with home care (U.S. DHHS, 1985).

Under Medicare, respite care is available only to caregivers of hospice patients. Medicare will pay 95% of the costs and 100% of the costs after the patient has paid a specified number of dollars of coinsurance. Medicare limits inpatient respite care to stays of no more than 5 consecutive days.

Depending on occupancy level, nursing facilities have offered respite care over the years. Some organizational obstacles to their ability to do so are (1) the costs involved in the extensive paperwork required at each admission and discharge, regardless of whether the patient is a regular or a hospice patient, and (b) the costs associated with keeping units empty for hospice-type admissions, which by definition are of short duration and therefore incur higher administrative costs to the facility. Assisted living facilities often accept respite care residents, but such care is not normally eligible for Medicare reimbursement.

Depending on the needs of the individual and the skills available in the facility, the assisted living facility may be ideally situated to offer respite care as a market niche if funding becomes available.

INSTITUTION-BASED CARE

CONTINUING CARE RETIREMENT COMMUNITIES (CCRCS)

The original CCRCs, often called life care communities, were usually set up and managed by religious communities. In return for all their worldly possessions, participants were promised care for the rest of their life. Today the typical resident pays a one-time entrance fee plus monthly fees.

The CCRC that offers life care is, in essence, an insurance pool. The entry and monthly fees are set based on actuarial calculations to cover the expected lifetime costs of each resident. In exchange for the entry and monthly fees, residents of life care communities are guaranteed care no matter how long they live, even if one's personal funds run out. Not every resident will need expensive nursing facility care, but the fees paid by all residents cover those who do. As with an insurance annuity, those who live longer receive more benefits than those who die earlier.

Normally, the new resident initially occupies either a detached (garden) apartment or moves into an apartment building. As the need arises for more protected and/or assisted living, residents may move progressively from a detached unit, to an attached apartment, to "sheltered" care (assisted living), and, as needed, into full-time nursing care. As mentioned in Part One, CCRCs are now building and staffing regular assisted living units as a new formalized level of care on their campuses.

In the early 1990s, 527 CCRCs were serving some 230,000 residents whose average age was 82, 79% of whom were women. The average age at entrance was 77 (a second retirement for most). The average age in the nursing centers was 86. The number of CCRCs is expected to double to 1,000+ by the year 2000.

The CCRC is predominantly a middle-class elderly housing phenomenon—the rich typically have assistance brought into their homes. Entry fees usually are set to collect 25% of projected lifetime costs, the monthly service fees collecting the remaining 75%. Few if any facilities place a cap on monthly service fees: These fees must fluctuate to account for inflation and other costs. CCRC administrators prefer to admit only persons capable of independent living. The relationship between the resident and the administration is lengthy—24 hours a day, 12 to 14 years. The administrators guarantee a service package with no time constraints and no limit on cost in the full-featured CCRC.

Array of Facilities

A broad array of financial arrangements have emerged. Three types of CCRCs are identified in the literature.

Type A, or all-inclusive CCRCs (about 33% of facilities), guarantee fully paid nursing care for as long as needed at no extra cost beyond the resident's monthly fee. Many services are "bundled" or included in the monthly fee (e.g., two or more meals a day, cleaning, laundry, linen, utilities, and recreation facilities). Fees vary by geographical area and size of living unit, averaging $70,000 to well over $200,000 entry fees and $900 to well over $2,000 monthly fees.

Type B, or modified CCRCs (about 26% of facilities), usually offer nursing care at no substantial increase in monthly fees, but include fewer services. Fees, for example, may be charged for cleaning or laundry, and only one or two meals may be included. Residents in this type of community assume some of the financial risk of extended nursing care costs. Entry and monthly fees are commensurably reduced.

Type C, or fee-for-service CCRCs (about 38% of facilities), usually offer no meals or personal care service in the monthly fee. Access to nursing care, on-site (usually) or off-site, is normally guaranteed, but the resident using the service bears the full costs.

Originally, entry fees were usually nonrefundable. Competition for residents has spawned an array of approaches, varying from no refund to 100% refund upon resale of one's unit.

Eighty percent to 90% of all CCRCs are not-for-profit, most of them also having a church affiliation. However, for-profit corporations have been eager to enter the field.

Regulation

Resident contracts vary. By 2000, 31+ states had some type of regulation in effect, but little uniformity existed among them. Some states regulate through the insurance department, others through the health department, offices on aging, or even departments that supervise securities and corporations.

Successfully building and operating a CCRC is a complex business venture. The most common reason for failure is low occupancy rate, because major costs are fixed (see Part Three for a discussion of fixed and variable costs).

Quality Control

The industry has formed the Continuing Care Accrediting Commission, headquartered in Washington, D.C. In the early 1990s, 91 communities in 20 states had successfully achieved accreditation by conducting the required self-examination and opening their books to a 3-day industry inspection team.

Hospitals

There are only about 5,300 community hospitals in the United States. Hospitals are seeking alternative sources of income because their occupancy rates and average length of stay are continuing a downward trend. Between 1989 and 1993 median occupancy rates decreased from 49% to 47%, and the average length of stay decreased from 4.34 days to 3.83 days (Lutz, 1994).

NURSING HOMES

Ownership of Nursing Homes

In general, the ownership pattern has remained the same for the past 20 years:

Facility type	Ownership (%)
For-profit facilities	70
Not-for-profit	25
Government	5

Furthermore, the breakdown of types of ownership within these categories has remained relatively stable over the past 20 years:

Facility type	Ownership (%)	Total (%)
public for-profit chains	13	
private for-profit chains	10	23
private for-profit individual facilities		52
not-for-profit chains	3	

not-for-profit individual facilities	17	20
government (federal, state, local)	5	5

The sources of payment for nursing homes is about 33%. The assisted living facilities sources of payment, in stark contrast, are 90% private pay.

Nursing Home costs to all payers increased from $40,000,000,000 in 1988 to $88,000,000,000 in 1998 (Office of the Actuary. (2000). HCFA, September 27, 2000).

4.2 The Social Security Act: Medicare / Medicaid

4.2.1 The Social Security Act: Medicare

The long-term care industry is molded by the Social Security Act and owes its economic existence (approaching $100 billion per year) to this original legislation and its later amendments.

ORIGINS OF THE SOCIAL SECURITY ACT

When the Social Security Act was enacted in 1935 it was a response to a fundamental societal change in American life: the evolution from an agrarian to a highly industrialized form of society. Growing old suddenly became visible nationally during the shift from an agricultural form of society, in which the aged were normally cared for by the family in the home, to a society where the workplace was a factory. Workers in this era were controlled by economic conditions beyond their influence. Urbanization and industrialization brought increased problems to the aged, such as unemployment and economic survivorship of the dependents when the wage earner died.

The event that brought these problems to the attention of America in dramatic terms was the Great Depression of the 1930s. By 1935, 50% of the aged were indigent. Within 5 years, the proportion had grown to 66% (Clement, 1985).

EFFECTS OF THE SOCIAL SECURITY ACT

Although additional factors are involved, a comparison of the number of aged persons receiving Social Security checks and the percentage of them living at the poverty level reveals a clear association. By 1959 the proportion of aged Americans who were indigent had fallen to 35%. Although this reflected some improvement, it still constituted a major social problem. As Social security benefits during the 1950s and 1960s continued to expand, the percentage of aged living in poverty declined to 14% of older persons by 1978 (Kaplan, 1985). According to the U.S. Census Bureau, during the inflation and recession period from 1979 to 1982, the elderly receiving Social Security checks based on cost of living adjustments (COLAs), which began in 1975, were the only group studied whose poverty rate did not increase.

In 1985 the President's Council of Economic Advisors declared that older Americans were no longer disproportionately poor, that the percentage of the general population in poverty (15.2%) was slightly higher than that of the same segment of the elderly population (Kaplan, 1985). Today nearly all Americans are covered by Social Security, although on occasion a person will apply for admission to a long-term care facility who has no Medicare eligibility, a matter to which the assisted living facility administrator must be alert if the person cannot pay privately for such care. In 1950 only 1 of 4 persons received Social Security checks, but by 1977, 9 out of 10 did.

Many factors, such as the political activism of the aged, general improvements in the economy, the Older Americans Act of 1965, and related actions, have led to general improvement in the economic condition of the elderly. Even so, although direct measurement is not feasible, it appears that a significant number of older Americans have little more than their Social Security check for income—a poverty level income.

The Original Social Security Act and Its Amendments

The original Social Security Act, as passed in 1935, consisted of 11 titles enacting the program, authorizing the necessary taxes, and establishing the administrative mechanisms of the act. Numerous amendments have been added to the Social Security Act over the years. Only those more directly affecting the long-term care industry are discussed here.

In 1950 permanently and totally disabled persons, who might at some time need nursing home care, were added as beneficiaries. In that same year, federal matching money was made available to states to pay for medical care for persons on public assistance—a precursor of Medicaid, which was to come in 1965. States were required to establish licensing programs for nursing homes. Some already had done so.

By 1956 the Social Security program was known as OASDI—old age (OA), survivors (S), and disabled (D) insurance (I). It was not until 1960 that the H (for health) was added, and it became OASDHI. The next step toward the Medicaid program, so critical to the long-term care industry, came in 1960 with the Kerr-Mills Act, which amended the Social Security Act to provide Medical Assistance to the Aged (MAA). This amendment offered 50% to 84% in matching funds to states, depending on the per capita income of each state. However, during the following 5 years, only 25 states implemented this program to assist their aged.

The major amendments affecting the long-term care industry were added in 1965, with the passage of Title 18, known as Medicare, and 1 year later, Title 19, known as Medicaid. These are discussed below.

Title 20 was added in 1974, supporting, among other things, in-home services to the elderly. In 1977 antifraud amendments were passed to minimize abuse of the program. Numerous additional amendments were passed during the 1980s. The primary focus has been containment of costs, rather than expansion of services, since the mid-1970s.

In general, it appears that from 1935 to about 1975 the federal government sought to expand benefits under the Social Security Act, whereas since 1975 the thrust has been reduction in the rate of cost increases and the units of service for which payment is made.

MEDICARE

As of this printing, the following information on basic Medicare coverage was accurate. (We use the past tense in our discussion, although the information may still be current.) See also the publication *Federal Requirements and Guidelines to Surveyors* for any new changes.

Attempts have been made to modify Medicare during each session of Congress, and these attempts continue. Beginning July 1, 1998, for example, Medicare implemented a new payment system for skilled nursing care providers. This is known as the Prospective Payment System (PPS), under which Medicare reimbursement is calculated on a per diem basis that covers routine and ancillary (including therapy) care as well as capital costs. The PPS system is based on the Resource Utilization Group III (RUG-III) payment system, which is driven by the resources required to provide care, not the patient's diagnosis or the actual costs incurred by the skilled nursing facility. This marks a radical departure from the payment system described below.

Plan A

Everyone receiving Social Security was automatically covered under Plan A.

Hospital Costs. Covered hospital-related costs were paid on the following basis: During the first 60 days of hospitalization for each period of illness (defined below), the patient pays for the equivalent of the first day, and Medicare pays for the other 59. During the years of Medicare coverage the cost of this first-day coverage rose from an initial cost of under $100 to almost $1,000.

During days 61 to 90 of hospitalization, the patient paid for about 25% of the daily rate. Medicare picked up the remaining costs. Inpatient days were covered only during the first 90 days of any period of illness. Each Medicare recipient had a lifetime reserve of 60 days, which could be used after the 90th day of hospitalization. During days 91 to 150 the patient paid for about 50% of the daily rate. In addition, each Medicare recipient was eligible for up to 190 days of inpatient psychiatric care during his or her lifetime.

Prospective Payment: The Era of DRGs. Beginning with federal fiscal year 1984, the federal government began to pay hospitals for Medicare patient costs on the basis of 467 diagnostic/reimbursement categories. Each year, Medicare officials prospectively decided on the amount of reimbursement for each Medicare hospital admission based on the principal diagnosis, that is, the condition established after study to be chiefly responsible for admission of the patient.

DRG stands for diagnostically related group (of diseases). There are 9,000 disease codes listed in the *International Classification of Diseases*. Using the ninth edition's clinical modifications (called ICDM9CM), the federal government identified 467 diseases for reimbursement to hospitals for care of Medicare patients based on the principal diagnosis and the severity of the disease for which a Medicare patient was admitted.

The theory was that some patients' length of stay was shorter than average and some longer. Medicare reimbursed on the average length of stay for each disease, based on the level of severity experienced by the patient. At the end of each year, Medicare made adjustments, using up to approximately 6% of its total funds to reimburse hospitals for especially expensive cases (called outliers).

Payments varied for each of the nine geographical regions in the United States established by Medicare and by whether the hospital was rural or urban. For example, an urban hospital in New York City would be reimbursed at a higher rate than a rural Georgia hospital for treating a patient with the same principal diagnosis. The basis of each hospital's reimbursement rate was based 25% on whether it was rural or urban and 75% on the cost experience of that hospital during the first year it was in the program, called the base year. New base years were designated as time passed.

One effect for the long-term care industry was that, because payment was by disease, no matter how extended the length of stay of each patient, hospitals sought to place Medicare patients into a nursing home, home health care agency, or nursing home equivalent for what is currently called "subacute" care. This resulted in hospitals discharging Medicare patients "quicker and sicker." As has already been seen, hospitals often opened their own nursing home equivalent (i.e., Medicare-certified beds in the hospital itself) in order to start up a new stream of cash income.

Nursing Facility Costs. For each period of illness, Medicare paid 100% of "reasonable costs" during the first 20 days. During days 21 to 100 the patient copaid a required amount, set usually at well over half the daily cost. Medicare paid nothing beyond 100 days of nursing facility care during any one spell of illness.

New Nursing Home Reimbursement Methodology

During the year beginning July 1998 through June 1999, Medicare phased in a new method of reimbursing nursing facilities: the prospective payment system. The year 1995 was designated as the base year on which future years' payments are based. Under prospective-payment system reimbursement schedules, facilities are reimbursed according to the amount of care is required by each resident using a scale divided into 44 levels of care. To continue receiving Medicare payments facilities must submit information using the minimum data set forms after days 7, 14, 30, 60, and 90 of a Medicare resident's stay.

In addition to instituting the prospective payment system, in 1998 Medicare began identifying a number of diagnoses for which hospitals would be only partially reimbursed if a patient is discharged to a nursing-facility bed before the average length of stay has been achieved in the hospital. This is expected to reduce the acuity level of residents entering nursing facilities.

In 2002 the rate of reimbursement to nursing homes dropped 15% and has been slowly rising back toward its earlier level.

Home Health Care Costs. Medicare paid 100% of all home health care costs associated with any one period of illness (care provided for a diagnosed illness for which 3 or more days of hospital care was given).

It is important to realize that Medicare was intended to cover brief periods of illness. Medicare provided short-term acute care; it was never intended to cover long-term care. Medicaid is the vehicle for covering long periods of illness, but only after an individual has spend all but about $2,000 of his or her total resources (discussed in more detail below).

Home health care expenditures by Medicare increased from $1.6 billion in 1988 to $10.3 billion in 1998—an annual average growth of 17% (Office of the Actuary, HCFA, September 27, 2000).

Eligibility for Nursing Facility Care. To be eligible for inpatient nursing facility care, at least four conditions had to be met by the Medicare patient: He or she had to

- have spent 3 consecutive days in a hospital (not including the day of discharge)
- be transferred to a nursing facility because treatment for the original cause of hospitalization is required
- be admitted within 14 days of hospital discharge (leeway is generally allowed up to 30 days)
- be certified by a physician to be in need of and receiving nursing care or rehabilitation services on a daily basis

Nursing home expenditures by Medicare increased from $700 billion in 1988 to $10.4 billion in 1998 (Office of the Actuary. (2000). HCFA, September 27, 2000)

Plan B. Plan B was voluntary

The Medicare recipient had to pay a small monthly premium, which was determined every 2 years and based on the benefits paid and administration costs of Plan B. General funds from the U.S. Treasury paid half of the costs of Plan B, and the participants paid the other half.

Three major expenses were covered under Plan B:

1. medical expenses (including physician services inpatient and outpatient medical services, and supplies, physical and speech therapy, ambulance transportation, diagnostic X-ray, laboratory and other tests, dressings, splints, and medical equipment)
2. outpatient hospital treatment
3. home health care

Payments Under Plan B. After the recipient paid an annual deductible amount, Medicare Plan B paid 80% of Medicare-determined reasonable charges for medical expenses, outpatient hospital treatment, and home health care. If home health care qualified under Plan A posthospital care, 100% of home health care costs were paid under Plan A.

Excluded From Coverage. Many health care costs associated with the elderly were excluded from payment by Medicare plans A and B. Neither plan would pay for

- routine physical and related tests
- eyeglasses or eye examinations
- hearing examinations or hearing aids
- immunizations (except for pneumococcal shots)
- routine foot care
- orthopedic shoes or other supportive devices for the feet
- custodial care
- preventive care, filling, removal, or replacement of teeth

Intermediaries and Carriers. Medicare payments were actually made by private insurance organizations that had contracted with the federal government to do so. Organizations handling claims from nursing facilities, hospitals, and home health care agencies were called intermediaries. Organizations dealing with claims from doctors and other medical suppliers covered under Plan B were called carriers.

Approved Charges. Under Plan B, approved charges were those determined as follows: The carrier in each geographic area annually reviewed the charges made by physicians and suppliers during the previous year. Suppliers were persons or organizations other than physicians who furnished equipment or services, such as ambulance transportation, laboratory tests, and medical equipment (e.g., wheelchairs).

To calculate an approved charge, the carrier determined the customary charge (i.e., the one most frequently made by each physician and supplier during the previous year). Then the carrier found the prevailing charge for each service and material supplied during that year. The prevailing charge was an amount sufficient to pay for the customary charges in three out of every four bills that were submitted in the previous year for each service and supply (limited by an economic index ceiling). When a claim was received from a physician or supplier, the carrier compared the actual charge with the customary and prevailing charges for that service or supply and paid 80% of the lowest of the three. The Medicare recipient paid the remaining 20%, either out of pocket or through a limited insurance policy (called Medigap insurance), which was designed to pay the remaining 20%.

Assignment. When a physician or supplier accepted an assignment of the medical insurance payment under Plan B, he or she agreed that the total charge to the patient would be the one approved by the carrier. In this case, Medicare paid the physician or supplier directly, after subtracting any part of the annual deductible not met.

Assignment was voluntary and had to be agreed to by both the provider and the patient. It guaranteed that the physician or supplier would not charge the patient more than the 20% of approved charges not paid by the carrier.

4.2.2 Title 19: Medicaid

Medicaid and Medicare were both passed as amendments to the Social Security Act. Medicare essentially has been an insurance program for recipients of Social Security benefits. Medicaid has not been insurance. As designed, it has been, literally, medical aid for persons receiving welfare and for comparable groups of persons who were defined as medically indigent.

Whereas Medicare was a federally run program, Medicaid was a program of federal grants to the states to enable them to provide medical assistance to

- families with dependent children (AFDC)
- the aged—persons receiving Old Age Assistance (OAA)
- the blind—Aid to the Blind (AB)
- persons permanently and totally disabled (i.e., persons receiving federally aided public assistance)
- comparable groups of medically indigent persons, not currently on welfare but who fall into the preceding four categories; such persons are categorized as medically needy when medical expenses reduce their income below the Medicaid eligibility level

The federal share ranged from 50% to 83% of costs, depending on the state's per capita income. Each state determined its coverage above a basic minimum of at least some of each of the following services: inpatient hospital, outpatient hospital, other laboratory and X-ray, nursing, and medical.

In addition to these basic services, a state could include any medical care recognized under state law if it chose. No residency requirements could be established for eligibility of services. Medicaid recipients have not been subject to deductible payments, as in the case of Medicare, but states have been allowed to require some copayments for recipients for care. Some states, for example, charged copayments for prescriptions, usually 50 cents per prescription; dental visits, eye exams, and similar services involved a $1 to $2 copayment per visit (Muse & Sawyer, p. 96).

Changing Congressional Goals. Originally the federal government set July 1, 1975, as the date by which all participating states were to be offering comprehensive services to all eligible persons. As costs soared under the program, Congress scaled back this goal and in the 1980s and 1990s moved toward containing Medicaid costs rather than expanding its services. Congress has been concerned because Medicaid has no ceiling on annual expenditures. The federal government was committed to paying its share of services that the states provided Medicaid recipients.

A glance at the total expenditures for personal health care in the United States over the years demonstrates the validity of Congressional concern about escalating health costs. All payers costs increased from $497,040,000,000 in 1988 to $1,016,129,000,000 in 1998, an average annual 9.0% growth (Office of the Actuary, Centers for Medicare and Medicaid, April 1, 2002). The total costs for personal health care have risen from 10% of the Gross National Product in 1988 to 12% in 1997 (Centers for Medicare and Medicaid Services, Office of the Actuary, National Health Statistics Group, April 1, 2002).

Buy-in Agreements. To maximize the contribution of federal dollars to state programs, participating states have signed "buy-in agreements," under which the state pays for Medicare's Plan B costs for Medicaid recipients. The buy-in obligated the federal government to pay entirely for medical costs that might have been cost-shared by the states' Medicaid programs, thus reducing the total dollar costs to the states.

To further contain costs, some states have obliged county governments to use their own funds to pay for a portion (usually about 3% to 5 %) of Medicaid costs. Medicaid dollars, initially committed by county social workers, became thus more carefully supervised by the county governments.

Eligibility for Medicaid generally has been determined at the county level by a social worker, and the program is usually administered by the local Department of Social Services, which assigns recipients as part of the case load of its social worker.

As mentioned elsewhere, the elderly have benefited to a great extent under the Medicaid program; they represent approximately 15% of all recipients but have received slightly more than one third of the benefits paid out (Muse & Sawyer, p. 8). Unmarried persons are 5 times more likely than married persons and Medicaid enrollees 10 times more likely than those without Medicaid to use nursing homes (Feinleib, Cunning, & Farley, 1994).

In the 1990s both the federal and the state governments sought ways to reduce expenditures under Medicare and Medicaid. Consequently, details of the payment plans change constantly. The reader should obtain current information and check with the local Medicare and Medicaid offices for the latest coverages and payment mechanisms.

Medicaid expenditures for home health care has been increasing at an average annual rate of 17% from $1.3 billion in 1988 to $5 billion in 1998 (Office of the Actuary. (2000). HCFA, September 27, 2000). Assisted living facilities are heavy users of Medicaid and Medicare home health care dollars.

Medicaid expenditures for nursing home care increased from $18 billion in 1988 to $40 billion in 1998 (Office of the Actuary. (2000). HCFA, September 27, 2000).

4.3 Older Americans Act of 1965

The Older Americans Act can be characterized as Congress's response to noninstitutional, primarily nonhealth care needs of the elderly. Medicare and Medicaid provide for institutionalized health care needs (home health care being an exception). Title 20 of the Social Security Act is a response to the primarily noninstitutional needs of the elderly.

The Older Americans Act authorizes payment for almost any activity that may lead to an improved quality of life for persons 60 years of age and older (with some programs, e.g., "reemployment" programs, for persons 55 and older). The funds and agencies authorized and generated by the Older Americans Act play major roles in shaping the long-term care industry in the United States. For this reason, some of its more important features are explored below.

PRECURSORS OF THE OLDER AMERICANS ACT

Events that laid the foundation for the passage of the Older Americans Act in 1965 began about 1945, when the first state, Connecticut, set up a commission concerned with the needs of older individuals. By 1961 all states had established similar commissions or aging units. That same year a White House Conference on Aging was held, at which heavy pressure for a federal role in addressing the needs of the elderly was brought to bear by lobbyists. Two years later President John F. Kennedy sent a message to Congress entitled "Elderly Citizens of Our Nation." He recommended federal help for older individuals who do not need institutional care but are encountering the expected increase in difficulty of successfully performing the activities of daily living, such as bathing, dressing, and toileting. Continued lobbying for federal aid for the functional elderly led to passage of the Older Americans Act in 1965.

GRAND OBJECTIVES: TITLE 1

Title 1 states the goals of the Older Americans Act: equal opportunity of every older individual to the full and free enjoyment of

- adequate income
- the best possible physical and mental health science can offer, without regard to economic status
- affordable, suitable housing
- full restorative services for those needing institutional care
- employment
- retirement in health and dignity

- pursuit of the widest civic, cultural, educational, and recreational opportunities
- efficient community services: low-cost transportation, choices in living arrangements, coordinated social service assistance
- immediate benefit of technological developments
- freedom, independence, and the free exercise of individual initiative in planning and managing his or her own life

Other portions of the Older Americans Act authorize the Commissioner on Aging, who is the administrator of the Older Americans Act, to pay for virtually any service or activity that will foster these broadly stated goals. The goals and authorizations are sweeping; however, the economic realities of the level of funding have prevented implementing large-scale programs to achieve these goals.

OTHER TITLES

Title 2 established the Administration on Aging within the Office of Human Development Services, which is in the federal Department of Health and Human Services. A Commissioner on Aging, appointed by the president and confirmed by the Senate, is empowered to administer the Older Americans Act and report directly to the Secretary of Health and Human Services.

Title 3 authorized grants to the states to create Planning and Service Areas within which the local Area Agencies on Aging function. Title 3b is concerned with social services, Title 3c1 with congregate nutritional services for those age 60 and older as well as their spouses, and Title 3c2 with home-delivered meals. Title 4 deals with research and training. Title 5 created the Senior Community Services Employment Program (SCSEP) for those age 55 and older with limited incomes (usually 125% of the poverty level). Title 6 addresses grants to Native American tribes. Title 7, passed in 1984, authorizes a health education and training program for older individuals.

AMENDMENTS

The Older Americans Act was substantially amended in 1967 and 1969, annually from 1972 to 1975, and in 1977, 1978, 1981, 1984, and 1992. Most of the significant amendments focused on expanding and repositioning the various programs, especially those under Title 3. The amendments of 1978 are of special interest to the long-term care industry. They require state plans to include a long-term care ombudsperson program that will

- investigate and resolve complaints by or on behalf of long-term care patients
- monitor, develop, and ensure implementation of federal, state, and local laws governing long-term care facilities
- give public agencies information about problems of older individuals residing in long-term care facilities
- train volunteers and enlist and develop community citizen organizations

To accomplish these goals, the states had to initiate procedures allowing ombudspersons to have access to any long-term care facility records and patient records without disclosing the plaintiff's identity, without his or her written consent, or a court order. Furthermore, each state has had to set up a statewide complaint-recording system to spot problems over time and report them to the state agency that licenses and certifies the long-term care facilities, and to report to the federal Commissioner on Aging.

Finally, under the 1978 amendments, the states have had to ensure that the ombudspersons' files are secure, meaning accessible only to the ombudspersons themselves unless the inquiring person, such as a concerned facility administrator, has written permission from the person who lodged the complaint or has a court order. In short, the state agency is to serve as a watchdog over the long-term care facilities, and although it cannot take legal action against a facility, it is expected to go to the state licensing and certification agency, which is empowered to do so. Amendments in 1992 again addressed and expanded provisions for ombudspersons (Cherry, 1993; Sharma & Fallavollita, 1992).

Beyond the ombudsperson program itself, the state agency and the local Area Agencies on Aging have been authorized to serve as advocates for the elderly. This is interpreted to mean that they ensure that the facilities observe the laws and give good quality resident care.

COMPREHENSIVE SERVICES SYSTEM

Another major assignment to the states and their local Area Agencies on Aging is to foster the development of comprehensive and coordinated service systems for all of the elderly. This is to be accomplished primarily by establishing numerous supportive services, nutrition programs, and multipurpose senior centers.

Definition of Supportive Services

The local Area Agency on Aging has legislative approval to engage in all of the following very broad range activities:

- health services, including education, training, welfare information, recreation, homemaker, counseling, and referral to specialists
- transportation to and from supportive services
- services to encourage the elderly to use supportive services
- helping older persons to obtain housing, to repair and renovate housing to meet minimum housing standards, to adapt homes to an individual's disabilities, and to introduce modifications to prevent unlawful entry
- services to avoid institutionalization, including preinstitutional evaluation and screening, home health, homemaker, shopping, escort, reader, letter writing, and similar services
- legal services, including tax and financial counseling
- physical exercise services
- health screening
- career counseling

- ombudsperson services for long-term care complaints
- unique disabilities services
- job counseling
- other services necessary for the welfare of older individuals

In sum, the local Area Agency on Aging is empowered to engage in a wide variety of activities on behalf of older persons in the community. Generally, however, funding has been at a modest level.

Effectiveness of the Act

The extent to which the Older Americans Act has achieved its goals is debatable. Clearly, the local Area Agencies on Aging, although being given a mandate that could cost billions of dollars if implemented, operate on a shoestring budget. Whether the services under the Older Americans Act should be available to every elderly person no matter how wealthy is also in question.

One of the greatest burdens of growing old is the loneliness resulting from loss of friends and family members of the same generation. Participating in the congregate meal is, for many individuals, regardless of their income level, a primary source of social contact with other people. In this regard, the act has been effective and has affected countless seniors.

Have the Area Agencies on Aging been successful in establishing a coordinated service system for long-term care in their communities? Generally, no. They have had neither the funds nor the organizational authority to bring together and organize the long-term care providers in the communities. Despite the meager funding levels and lack of authority, however, there is a network of services in place for all older Americans who need assistance to remain outside an institution. This is a major improvement over the decades before the 1960s, when such services did not exist at all. This network and the nutritional assistance to all older Americans have become integral to the long-term care system in which assisted living facilities and nursing facilities are active participants.

Still, much need remains unmet. In a 1994 *Wall Street Journal* article, "Frayed Lifeline: Hunger Among Elderly Surges; Meal Programs Just Can't Keep Up," Michael McCarthy, a staff reporter, reviewed some unsettling data. In 1993 as many as 827,000 Americans had received Meals on Wheels and 2.5 million had received subsidized meals at community centers. Even so, the Urban Institute (a private nonprofit research group in Washington, D.C.) estimated that in 1994, 4.9 million elderly persons were either malnourished or hungry (about 16% of the population over 60). The Urban Institute found that two thirds of needy older persons are not being reached by food assistance projects. In New York 2,500 older persons were on waiting lists for home-delivered meals. About 62,000 of the elderly in that state were in the program, but officials estimated that about 10,000 more were eligible. The funding levels for the Older Americans Act have fallen behind with each succeeding year as inflation and a dramatically increasing elderly population outstrip funding. This is not surprising, since the government funds available to feed the elderly amounted to about 0.53 cent per person, according to a 1992 Government Accounting Office study. Funding has improved slightly over the intervening years.

Recent Activities under the Older Americans Act

In Fiscal Year (FY) 2001, 15 million units of assistance were provided under the Act, 433,000 older Americans were receiving case management services. By 2002 the Act administrators were testing models of what they named Naturally Occurring Retirement Communities (NORCs) where persons were aging in place in a community setting such as an apartment complex or area of town. Of their clients 35% relied almost exclusively on the Act's transportation services.

Over 4,000 nutrition services providers in FY 2001 provided 112 million congregate meals to 1.8 million older adults in states and 143 million home delivered meals were served to 1 million older Americans.

In 2000, the National Family Caregiver Support Program was established. By 2002 more than 325,000 caregivers were being supported by the Act.

In 2002, $128 million was given to states, $5.5 million to Indian Tribal and Native Hawaiian Organizations, and $7 million awarded to 39 innovation projects.

The Ombudsman program which oversees assisted living and nursing facilities investigated 260,000 complaints in FY 2002. The Ombudsman staffing nationally consisted of 1,000 paid and 14,000 volunteer staff. Legal services providers under the OAA reached 1,000 providers nationwide and provided about 1 million hours of legal assistance each year to low income or otherwise needy elderly.

Since 1998 the OAA has funded 51 Senior Medicare patrol projects in 45 states resulting in the recovery of $3 million in Medicare funds and $76 million in Medicaid funds.

During the years 1996 through 2002, the OAA budget increased an average of 8.7% yearly, totaling $1.2 billion in 2002. States, on average, added $2. to each federal $1.

The OAA 2002 budget $1.2 billion was spent in the following percentages:

Nutrition Services	46%
Home and Community Based Supportive Services	30%
Caregiver Services	11%
Program Innovations & Network Support	5%
Health Promotion and Elder Rights	3%
Native American Services	3%
Federal Administration	2%

(*Source*: Administration on Aging 2002 annual report. U.S. Department of Health and Human Services, Washington, DC.)

4.4 Labor and Management: Laws and Regulations

What rights do long-term care administrators have when employees in the facility are seeking to form a union? What rights do the employees have? What are the basic laws and regulations governing the managers dealings with employees?

This section provides a framework to help the reader begin to answer these questions.

4.4.1 Early Management–Labor Relations in the United States

During most of the earlier years of its history, the government of the United States strongly supported management in its dealings with employees. It was not until 1935 that American workers won government sanction of the right to form trade unions.

The passage of the National Labor Relations Act (better known as the Wagner Act) in 1935 was the first nationwide labor legislation to favor the growth of trade unions. This was the culmination of a long, slow process.

A BRIEF HISTORY OF THE LABOR MOVEMENT IN THE UNITED STATES

So powerful were employers in the 18th century that workers contented themselves with forming "fraternal unions" to help each other in coping with personal economic adversity, but certainly not to act collectively for improved working conditions and more pay (U.S. Department of Labor, 1976). Employers were able to prevent effective unionization. At their own discretion, they could fire any worker seeking to organize a union, refuse to negotiate with any union representative, and require each new employee to sign a "yellow dog" contract, by which the worker agreed not to join a union (Chruden & Sherman, 1980).

During the 19th century U.S. courts consistently sided with management. In 1806 a federal court ruled that workers who sought to combine to exert pressure on managers were participating in a "conspiracy in restraint of trade," which in effect meant that such grouping was to be treated as criminal activity (Ivancevich & Glueck, 1983). The first hint of rights for workers did not appear until 1842, when the Massachusetts Supreme Court ruled that unions that did not resort to illegal tactics were not guilty of criminal conspiracy. Still, employers could fire any worker at will for union activity, impose yellow dog contracts, and, when all else failed, obtain a court injunction against threatened strikes. The employers still retained nearly all of the power. Despite this, the union movement grew. By 1886 skilled workers such as machinists, bricklayers, and carpenters formed the American Federation of Labor (AFL).

It was not until 1935 that another major labor force, the Congress of Industrial Organizations (CIO), emerged and in 1955 merged with the AFL. It was a slow process because the government did not substantially back labor until the Wagner Act was passed in 1935 (Raskin, 1981).

The federal government had actually given American workers some negotiating rights earlier in the century in order to keep the nation's railroads running. The Railway Labor Act of 1926 was the first federal legislation sanctioning union organization and the right to bargain collectively with management.

The first national effort to define workers' and employers' respective rights came just 6 years later. In 1932 the Norris-LaGuardia Act, also called the Anti-Injunction Act, limited the powers of federal courts to side with management by issuing injunctions, court decrees that stopped or limited union efforts to picket, boycott, or strike. Yellow dog contracts were prohibited (Ivancevich & Glueck, 1983).

MANAGEMENT PREFERENCES

Most managers would prefer not to have to deal with organized labor. Unionization is perceived as intensifying the difficulty of the administrator's responsibilities. There is a natural tendency for what organizational theorists call the "we-they" phenomenon to occur in the relationship between labor and management. Workers often perceive their interests as different from those of managers, whose task is to operate cost-effectively, that is, to produce the best results for the least cost.

The administrator would be happy to pay nurses and nurse's aides the premium wages that will attract the most competent workers available, but pressures to keep costs down do not often permit this. As discussed in Part Two, the result is that most long-term care workers, especially the nurse's aides and the kitchen and housekeeping staffs, are paid at prevailing rates in the particular geographical area, which are usually close to the required minimum wage levels. Understandably, these workers, many of whom hold second jobs to make ends meet, seek to increase their personal incomes from the nursing facility and obtain the best working conditions on their jobs. Tensions between managers and workers are inevitably built into the situation.

4.4.2 Major Legislation Affecting Employer-Employee Relationships

THE WAGNER ACT OF 1935

The Wagner Act of 1935 is the landmark law that, for the first time in federal legislation, defined the rights of workers (Boling, Vrouman, & Sommers, 1983). The Wagner Act limited the freedom of employers to give their views on proposed unionization. The

Wagner Act also guaranteed employee bargaining rights: "Employees shall have the right to self-organization, to form, join, or assist labor organizations, to bargain collectively through representatives of their own choosing, and to engage in concerted activities, for the purpose of collective bargaining or other mutual aid or protection" (Chruden & Sherman, 1980, p. 354).

THE TAFT-HARTLEY ACT OF 1947

In the provisions of the Taft-Hartley Act unions were prohibited from the following actions (Chruden & Sherman, 1980; Ivancevich & Glueck, 1983)

1. Restraining or coercing employees in the exercise of their right to join a union or not (unless an agreement existed with management that every worker must be a union member). Union members could not physically prevent other workers from entering a facility, nor act violently toward nonunion employees, nor threaten employees for not supporting union activities.
2. Causing an employer to discriminate against an employee for anti-union activity, nor could unions force employers to hire only workers acceptable to the union.
3. Bargaining with an employer in bad faith. They could not insist on negotiating "illegal" provisions, such as the administration's prerogative to appoint supervisors.
4. Participating in secondary boycotts or jurisdictional disputes. Unions may not picket a long-term care facility, for example, in an attempt to force it to apply pressure on a subcontractor (e.g., a food service contractor) to recognize a union, nor can a union force an employer to do business only with others, such as suppliers, who are unionized; nor can one union picket for recognition when another union is already certified for a long-term care facility.
5. Charging excessive or discriminatory membership fees. They may not charge a higher initiation fee to employees who did not join the union until after a union contract was negotiated.
6. Coercing or restraining employees in the selection of the parties to bargain on management's behalf. The manager is free to hire the best labor lawyer available to represent the facility.
7. Forcing managers to hire employees when they are not needed (called featherbedding).

However, when the Wagner Act was amended by the pro-management Taft-Hartley Act, certain employees' rights were retained (Ivancevich & Glueck, 1983). Under the act, employers may not

1. Interfere with, restrain, or coerce employees in the exercise of their rights. Employers, for example, may not give wage increases timed to discourage employees from joining a union or threaten with loss of their jobs employees who vote for a union.
2. Interfere with or attempt to dominate any labor organization, or contribute financial or other support to a labor organization. For example, employers cannot take an

active part in union affairs or permit a long-term care supervisor to participate actively in a union, or show favoritism toward one union over another.

3. Discriminate in hiring or giving tenure to employees or set any terms for employment so as to encourage or discourage union membership. For example, they cannot fire an employee who urges others to join a union or demote an employee for union activity.
4. Fire or discriminate against any employee who files charges or gives testimony under the Wagner Act.
5. Refuse to bargain collectively with the duly chosen representatives of its employees. For example, the long-term care administrator must provide financial data to a union if the facility claims to be experiencing financial losses, must bargain on mandatory subjects such as hours and wages, and must meet with union representatives duly appointed by a certified bargaining unit.

An important consideration for long-term care administrators is the denial of legal protection to supervisors seeking to form their own unions, thus keeping the roles of these persons (usually department heads in long-term care facilities) clearly managerial in function and identification.

Probably the single most important provision of the Taft-Hartley Act for long-term care administrators is the restoration of the right of managers to express their views regarding unions and unionizing efforts. This means that administrators are free to express their opinions about their employees voting for a union in the workplace and judgments about unions in general. Administrators are still prohibited from threatening, coercing, or bribing employees concerning their union membership or their decision to join or not to join a union.

THE NATIONAL LABOR RELATIONS BOARD

A major aspect of the Taft-Hartley Act was its creation of the National Labor Relations Board (NLRB), which plays a dominant role in U.S. labor-management relations. It has the following responsibilities (Chruden & Sherman, 1980):

- to determine what the bargaining unit or units within an organization shall be (a unit contains those employees who are to be represented by a particular union and are covered by the agreement with it)
- to conduct representation elections by secret ballot for the purpose of determining which, if any, union shall represent the employees within a unit
- to investigate unfair labor practice charges filed by unions or employees and to prosecute any violations revealed by such investigations

The board is empowered to initiate action against illegal strikes or unfair labor practices by unions. In a typical month as many as 4,000 new cases are filed with the NLRB.

One of the more controversial features of the Taft-Hartley Act is a provision allowing the president of the United States, through the Office of the Attorney General, to seek an injunction for a period of 80 days against strikes or walkouts affecting the nation's welfare or health. Some labor leaders have called this "slave labor" (Chruden & Sherman, 1980, p. 356).

THE LANDRUM-GRIFFIN ACT OF 1959

Officially designated the Labor-Management Reporting and Disclosure Act of 1959, the Landrum-Griffin Act seeks to protect the interests of the individual union member against possible union abuses. Specifically, the act gives to each union member several rights (Ivancevich & Glueck, 1983):

- nominate candidates for union office
- vote in union elections
- attend union meetings
- examine required annual financial reports by the union to the Secretary of Labor

In addition, employers are required to report any payments or loans made to unions the officers or any members—to eliminate what are called "sweetheart contracts," under which union officials and the managers benefit, but the rank and file of union members do not.

SPECIAL DISPUTE-SETTLING RULES FOR LONG-TERM CARE AND HOSPITAL ADMINISTRATORS

The NLRB has jurisdiction over health care institutions. However, until 1974 the board was expressly forbidden by the original Taft-Hartley law to hear cases in the nonprofit sector. Because the vast majority of nursing homes and hospitals that operated in the 1950s and 1960s were nonprofit, this meant that most of the health care industry was not subject to these labor laws.

In 1973 Congress began considering having the law apply to not-for-profit long-term care facilities and hospitals. Long-term care facilities and hospitals pressed for the following benefits (American Hospital Association, 1976; Rosmann, 1975):

- special protection against strikes
- priority for rapid NLRB action on disputes
- mandatory mediation requirements
- limit on the number of bargaining units to one each for professional, technical, clinical, and maintenance and service workers

The nursing homes and hospitals were successful on the whole.

In 1974 Congress amended the Taft-Hartley Act to bring long-term care facilities and hospitals under its regulations (1974 Non-Profit Hospital Amendments, Public Law 930360; see Wilson & Neuhauser, 1982). However, special provisions were made (Pointer & Metzger, 1975):

- Long-term care facilities, hospitals, and unions must give to the other party 90 days' notice of a desire to change an exiting contract (this is 30 days more than that required of other organizations).
- The Federal Mediation and Conciliation Service (FMCS) must be given 30 days' notice if an impasse occurs in bargaining for an initial contract after the union is first recognized.
- A long-term care facility or hospital union may not picket or strike without 10 days' prior notice, in order to allow the facility to make provisions for continuity of care. (No prior notice is required of other unions.)
- The FMCS may appoint a board of inquiry to mediate the dispute if it decides a strike would imperil the welfare or health of the community. Neither the long-term care facility nor the union is obliged to accept the board's recommendations, but each must provide any witnesses or information sought by the board.

For-profit long-term care facilities benefited from the 1974 amendment to the Taft-Hartley Act because of the four special labor relations rules cited above (Miller, 1982). These benefits are equally available to the assisted living facility.

THE BARGAINING UNIT

Labor unions must seek recognition as representing the majority of persons in a specific bargaining unit of a long-term care facility. As indicated above, long-term care facilities and hospitals sought to limit the number of bargaining units in negotiations to professional, technical, clinical, and maintenance and service workers.

During most of the decade after the 1974 amendments to the Taft-Hartley Act, the NLRB ruled that in long-term care facilities and hospitals, service and maintenance workers, clerical staff, licensed practical nurses, registered nurses, and security guard units constitute appropriate bargaining units (Miller, 1982).

In August 1984 the NLRB issued a new ruling. In the case of *St. Francis Hospital* (Memphis) *v. International Brotherhood of Electrical Workers Local 474,* the NLRB ruled that a group of 39 maintenance workers did not constitute an appropriate bargaining unit. Health care workers thereafter had to represent either "all professionals" or "all nonprofessionals" rather than the particular interest groups allowed during the previous decade.

The unionization of long-term care facilities is a complicated affair. Vigorous attempts to unionize facilities have been undertaken by several unions over recent years. A study by the AFL-CIO and data from 1983–1986 showed that 15.9% of nursing home facilities were unionized. By the early 1990s, about 20% of U.S. nursing facilities were believed to have unions (*long-term care News,* 1990).

All regions of the United States have unionized nursing facilities. From "most unionized" to "least unionized" were the Mid-Atlantic, followed by the West Coast, New England, Midwest, Southeast, and South Central. The Service Employees International Union (SEIU), for example, had organized 225 of the 1,832 long-term care facilities in California by 1990.

Since 1990 the SEIU has been the most active union seeking to organize long-term care workers. In the mid-1990s the SEIU waged a campaign against a number of major nursing chains, including attacking the quality of care provided by long-term care facilities and arguing that nurses in particular are overworked, stressed out, and sick (The National Nurse Survey, 1995; Falling Short, 1995; "Caring till it hurts,". In some cases the SEIU claimed harassment (Scott, 1994); in others, it attempted to prevent mergers of nursing home chains (Shriver, 1995). Strikes have been called to draw attention to "patient care and demands for a new contract" (Moore, 1995). In 1989 the National Union of Hospital and Health Care Employees, which had about 74,000 members, merged with two other unions. About two-thirds of their members joined the SEIU and the remaining one third the American Federation of State, County, and Municipal Employees. To complicate the picture, long-term care facilities have been organized by numerous other unions, such as the United Food and Commercial Workers, the Teamsters, and the Federation of Nurses and Health Professionals, which is an offshoot of the American Federation of Teachers.

The largest proportion of long-term care facilities with unions are in the SEIU which in 2003 had a membership of over 755,000 health workers including 110,000 nurses and 20,000 physicians.

In 2003 the SEIU was the largest union of long term care facility workers: more than 130,000. In 2002, 71,000 home care workers joined the SEIU. During the summer of 2003 long-term care workers in facilities in Florida, Connecticut, Ohio and Illinois joined the SEIU (Service Employees International Union, AFL/CIO, CLC www.seiu.org September, 2003).

Normally, employees in nursing, dietary, housekeeping, and laundry are the most likely to be unionized. A growing number of employers, particularly the larger chains, attempted to prevent unionization of nurses by arguing that all nurses (RNs and LPNs) are statutory supervisors and thereby excluded from labor law protection to join a union. The employers insisted that because all nurses supervise nurse's aides, all nurses are supervisory personnel and therefore not covered by labor laws. In a setback for unionization of nursing home workers, the U.S. Supreme Court, by a 5–4 decision, agreed and ruled in May 1994 that nurses who supervise lesser-skilled employees are not protected by the National Labor Relations Act (*NLRB v. Health Care & Retirement Corporation of America;* see Burda, 1993).

PROPORTION OF WORKERS IN UNIONS: 1932-2003

In 1933 there were 3 million unionized workers in the United States. By 1947 they numbered 15 million, representing about 31% of the workforce. Union membership increased until about 1956, then declined until 1963, when it resumed at a slower pace. In 1980 about 20 million workers were in unions—approximately 20% of the total workforce and 29% of nonagricultural workers (Ivancevich & Glueck, 1983). According to a 1998 release by the U.S. Bureau of Labor Statistics, in 1997, 16.1 million workers were represented by unions. This comprised 14.1% of the workforce.

The period from 1935 to 1947 was one of dramatic growth in union membership. The power given to unions through the Wagner Act resulted in what Congress in 1947 viewed as abuses. This led to the Taft-Hartley Act, which placed limitations on unions, just as the Wagner Act had placed limitations on managers 12 years earlier.

NONUNION WORKERS

At least 75% of the total labor workforce in this country is not unionized. What of their rights?

Over the years the federal government has enacted legislation establishing and protecting the rights of workers in general. Three of these laws are the Civil Rights Act of 1964, the Equal Employment Opportunities Act of 1972, and the Americans with Disabilities Act of 1992.

CIVIL RIGHTS ACT OF 1964

Title 7 of the Civil Rights Act of 1964 prohibited employers and others from discriminating against employees on the basis of race, color, religion, sex, or national origin. It also prohibits discrimination with regard to any employment condition, including hiring, firing, promotion, transfer, and admission to training programs.

Minority groups that are specifically protected under the Civil Rights Act are African-Americans, Hispanics, Native Americans, Alaskan natives and Asian-Pacific Islanders.

CONSUMER CREDIT PROTECTION ACT OF 1968

Title 3 of this act limits the amount of an employee's earnings that may be garnished and protects employees from being discharged for any one indebtedness. In general, an employee's earnings that may be garnished is the lesser of 25% of disposable earnings or the amount by which disposable earnings are greater than 30 times the federal minimum wage. Other conditions apply. The Department of Labor's Wage Hour Division administers and enforces Title 3. Violations can require back pay, reinstatement, and fines up to $1,000 or imprisonment for not more than 1 year, or both.

THE EQUAL EMPLOYMENT OPPORTUNITIES ACT OF 1972

The Equal Employment Opportunities Act (EEOA) amended Title 7 of the Civil Rights Act. The EEOA strengthened enforcement of the original act and expanded its coverage to additional groups, such as state and local government workers and private employment of more than 15 persons.

What Is Discrimination?

Congress did not define discrimination in its legislation. Over the years the courts have established three definitions:

- During World War II, discrimination was defined as harmful actions motivated by personal animosity toward the group of which the target person was a member.
- Later this was redefined as unequal treatment. Accordingly, a practice is illegal if it applies different standards or different treatment to different groups of employees or

applicants. For example, minorities may not be kept in less desirable departments (different treatment); rejecting women with preschool-age children is not permissible (different standards). Point: The administrator may impose any standards so long as they are applied equally to all groups or individuals and do not result in any intended or unintended adverse treatment of any group.

- In *Greggs v. Duke Power Co.* (1971), the U.S. Supreme Court defined employment discrimination as unequal impact (or adverse impact). In this case, Duke Power was using employment tests and educational requirements that screened out a greater proportion of African-Americans than Caucasians (Ivancevich & Glueck, 1983).

Adverse impact is often measured (for the purposes of Title 7 cases) when the selection rate for a protected minority group is less than 80% of the selection rate for a majority group.

Although the practice in the *Duke Power* case was not motivated by prejudice against African-Americans, and the tests were all applied equally, they had the result of adverse impact, that is, unequal impact on African-Americans. The job involved was that of shoveling coal into a furnace. Duke failed to prove that passing employment tests and requiring a level of education were related to success on the job. The burden of proof is on the employer to show that a hiring standard is job related.

Discrimination Based on Sex

Few situations exist that justify discrimination based on sex. In the current U.S. cultural setting, perhaps employment of a wet nurse is justifiable, of a woman to model women's clothes, or of a woman as an attendant inside a locker room for other women. In the final analysis, the only legitimate basis for discrimination based on sex may be that the employee must use body organs specific to his or her sex to accomplish the job requirements (e.g., wet nursing).

Sexual Harassment

Sexual harassment has been defined in the EEOA guidelines as follows:

> Unwelcome sexual advances, request for sexual favors, and other verbal or physical conduct of a sexual nature constitutes sexual harassment when (1) submission to such conduct is either explicitly or implicitly a term or condition of an individual's employment, (2) submission or a rejection of such conduct by an individual is used as a basis for employment decisions affecting such individual, or (3) such conduct has a purpose or effect of reasonably interfering with an individual's work performance, or creating an intimidating, hostile, or offensive work environment.

In recent years two general categories of cases have emerged: quid pro quo and hostile work environment. In quid pro quo the harassment is not only a demand for sexual favors but also the adverse employment decision that results from the rejection of those demands. A hostile work environment case requires evidence of pervasive offensive conduct of a sexual nature (e.g., proof that obscenities and sexual gestures, remarks, or touching were commonplace). Some hostile work environment cases have involved the pictures or calendars of nude or partially nude women as part of the proof of discrimination (e.g., *Robinson v. Jacksonville Shipyards,* 1991).

The assisted living facility can be held strictly liable for the acts of department managers who are found to be sexually harassing employees. A written policy against sexual harassment containing procedures available to employees is an advisable step for facility management to take. It has been pointed out that sexual harassment laws apply equally to both females and males, to heterosexuals, homosexuals, bisexuals, and transsexuals (Argenti, 1994). Sexual harassment laws generally are aimed at superior-subordinate relationships, but apply equally to peer relationships and those between residents and employees.

THE PREGNANCY DISCRIMINATION ACT OF 1978

The 1964 Civil Rights Act was amended in 1978 to end discrimination against pregnant women. The act makes it illegal to discriminate on the basis of pregnancy, childbirth, or related medical conditions in hiring, promoting, suspending, or discharging women who are pregnant. In addition, the employer is required to pay medical and hospital costs for childbirth to the same extent it pays for other conditions.

EQUAL EMPLOYMENT OPPORTUNITY COMMISSION: ENFORCING THE EEOA

The Equal Employment Opportunity Commission (EEOC) was established by the 1964 Civil Rights Act. The commission was empowered to interpret the EEOA and resolve charges brought under it. The 1972 amendments gave the commission additional authority to bring lawsuits against employers in the federal courts. Since 1979 the EEOC has enforced the Age Discrimination in Employment Act (ADEA) of 1967, the Equal Pay Act (EPA) of 1963, Section 501 of the Rehabilitation Act of 1973, and the Americans with Disabilities Act (ADA) of 1990.

Even so, the commission still cannot directly issue enforceable orders, as do other government agencies, such as the Environmental Protection Agency. Hence, the EEOC cannot order an employer to discontinue discriminatory practices, nor can it order back pay to victims of discrimination. It must seek action through the courts.

The average backlog of cases for the EEOC runs approximately 20,000. It is not possible to handle all of them, of course. Only a small percentage of charges are eventually resolved by the EEOC or by the courts (Ivancevich & Glueck, 1983). Nevertheless, legal history is being made by the EEOC, and its presence is felt in employment practices.

EEOC Procedures

Step 1. The EEOC has the power to require employers to report employment statistics on federal forms.
Step 2. If the EEOC feels that charges are justified, it authorizes its preinvestigation division to review the complaints.
Step 3. The investigation division then interviews all parties concerned.
Step 4. If there is substance to the case, the EEOC seeks an out-of-court settlement.
Step 5. If the parties cannot be reconciled, the EEOC can sue the employer.

In cases settled by court decisions, the courts have required such actions as back pay, reinstatement of employees, immediate promotion of employees, hiring quotas, abolition of testing programs, and creation of special training programs. Some settlements have been in the millions of dollars.

Specifically, the EEOC may seek any or all of the following:

- back pay
- hiring, promotion, reinstatement, benefit restoration, front pay, and other affirmative relief (Title 7, ADA, ADEA)
- actual pecuniary loss other than backpay (Title 7, ADA)
- liquidated damages (ADEA, EPA)
- compensatory damages for future monetary losses and mental anguish (Title 7, ADA)
- punitive damages when employer acts with malice or reckless disregard for federally protected rights (Title 7, ADA)
- posting a notice to all employees advising them of their rights under the laws EEOC enforces and their right to be free from retaliation
- corrective or preventive actions taken to cure the source of the identified discrimination and minimize the chance of its recurrence
- reasonable accommodation (ADA)
- stopping the specific discriminatory practices involved in the case

LAWS AFFECTING FEDERAL CONTRACTORS AND SUBCONTRACTORS

Several laws and executive orders (orders issued by the president of the United States under authority vested in him or her) govern hiring and job practices of firms that hold federal contracts of over $50,000. Although it is unlikely that any long-term care facility would be directly affected by these regulations, many contractors doing construction work for a facility are subject to these regulations.

Executive Order 11246

This order by requires written affirmative action programs of all contractors with 50 or more employees and $50,000 or more in federal contracts.

To enforce this order, the Office of Federal Contract Compliance Programs (OFCCP) was established. This agency was later given responsibility for administering laws protecting veterans.

The Vocational Rehabilitation Act of 1973

This act requires federal government contractors to mount affirmative action programs for the handicapped. It is enforced by the OFCCP. The act also provides a measure of federal support for programs to assist in training the handicapped. By 1980 approximately half of the 15 million Americans of working age deemed to be handicapped had been able to find employment (Ivancevich & Glueck, 1983).

Vietnam Era Veterans Readjustment Act of 1974

This act requires firms with more than $10,000 in federal contracts to have affirmative action programs for employment and advancement of Vietnam veterans.

The American with Disabilities Act of 1990

Title 1 of the Americans with Disabilities Act of 1990 (ADA) prohibits facilities from discriminating against qualified individuals with disabilities in job application procedures, hiring, firing, advancement, compensation, job training, and other terms, conditions, and privileges of employment.

An individual with a disability is a person who

- has a physical or mental impairment that substantially limits one or more major life activities (e.g., walking, lifting, seeing, learning, or doing manual tasks)
- has a record of such an impairment (e.g., has been treated for a mental illness)
- is regarded as having such an impairment (e.g., a person who has extensive scars from burns)

The act applies to any qualified individual with a disability who can perform the essential functions of the position with or without reasonable accommodation. Individuals who have HIV or AIDS are considered disabled within the meaning of the ADA. Current users of illegal drugs are not protected as disabled persons. The facility may not limit, segregate, or classify a disabled job applicant or employee in any way that adversely affects his or her opportunities. Facilities may not fire or refuse to hire disabled persons for any cause that could be eliminated by a reasonable accommodation.

Reasonable Accommodation. This may include making existing facilities freely accessible to handicapped persons, supplying readers or interpreters, modifying policies, examinations, or training manuals, restructuring jobs or changing work schedules, reassigning the individual to a vacant position, or acquiring or modifying equipment for use by the disabled.

"Undue Hardship." The facility is required to make an accommodation to the known disability of a qualified applicant or employee if it would not impose an "undue hardship" on the facility. Undue hardship is defined as an action requiring significant difficulty or expense when considered in light of factors such as a facility's size, financial resources, and the nature and cost of the proposed accommodation.

Standards. The facility is not required to lower quality or production standards to make an accommodation nor to provide personal use items such as glasses or hearing aids.

Medical Examinations. The facility may not ask job applicants about the existence, nature, or severity of a disability. Applicants may be asked about their ability to perform specific job functions. A job offer may be conditioned on the results of a medical examination if the examination is required for all entering employees in similar jobs. Medical examinations of employees must be job related and consistent with the employer's business needs. Medical tests must involve only "normal" test aspects given all preemployment applicants and have no features that could be construed to be testing for or testing a disability. EEOC Notice 915.002 describes a number of scenarios and illustrations concerning preemployment medical examinations around which the facility should build its medical examination policies.

If an applicant is not hired because of post-offer medical exam results, the reason must be given and a statement made that no reasonable accommodation was available that would have enabled the applicant to perform the essential job functions or that accommodation would impose an undue hardship.

Employee/Applicant Rights. Employees and applicants are entitled to apply to the Equal Employment Opportunity Commission. If the applicant is successful, the EEOC may require that the person be placed in a position as if the discrimination had never occurred. This might entitle the applicant to hiring, promotion, reinstatement, back pay, or other remuneration, or reasonable accommodation including reassignment. The successful complainant may also be entitled to damages for future money losses, mental anguish, and inconvenience. Punitive damages may also be imposed on the facility if the EEOC feels it acted with malice or reckless indifference. The complainant may also be entitled to their attorney's fees. Charges can be filed at any field office of the EEOC.

Patient Self-Determination Act of 1990

The Patient Self-Determination Act (PSDA) of 1990 was technically an amendment to the federal Medicare and Medicaid law passed as part of the 1990 Omnibus Budget Reconciliation Act. It is usually referred to, however, as the Patient Self-Determination Act.

Requirements. The act requires that all health care facilities accepting Medicare or Medicaid funding:

- provide written information to residents at the time of admission concerning an individual's right under state law to make decisions concerning medical care, including the right to accept or refuse medical or surgical treatment and the right to formulate advance directives

- maintain written policies an procedures with respect to advance directives (e.g., living wills and health care power of attorney) and to inform residents of the policies
- document in the individual's medical record whether or not the individual has executed and advance directive
- ensure compliance with the requirements of state law respecting advance directives at facilities of the provider
- provide (individually or with others) for education for staff and the community on issues concerning advance directives

The facility may not condition the provision of care or otherwise discriminate against an individual based on whether or not the individual has executed an advance directive.

A signed copy of each resident's acknowledgment of receipt of his or her information and the opportunity to act under the provisions of the PSDA should be in his or her file. Relevant advance directives should be prominently located in the resident's medical record.

Safe Medical Devices Act of 1990

Under the Safe Medical Devices Act of 1990, long-term care facilities must report to the Food and Drug Administration and/or the manufacturer all incidents in which a medical device caused or contributed to a resident's death or serious injury or illness.

A medical device is any instrument, implement, machine, implant, or related article intended for use in diagnosing, treating, or preventing disease. (Drugs are not considered medical devices.) Examples of such items include blood glucose devices, blood pressure devices, catheters, hearing aids, infusion pumps, pacemakers, restraints, scales, thermometers, and wheelchairs (Carley, 1991). As assisted living facilities offer additional health care services, reporting requirements may apply.

Reasonable Probability. All incidents that reasonably suggest a likelihood that a medical device has caused or contributed to a resident's death, serious illness, or injury must be reported. Reports are to be made as soon as possible, but no later than 10 days.

Clinical Laboratory Improvement Act

The Clinical Laboratory Improvement Act (CLIA) requires that any medical facility that conducts named tests meet stringent CLIA requirements. Most nursing facilities and assisted living facilities do not conduct laboratory tests that do not come under the "waived" test list (e.g., the use of glucometers is waived). Changes to the list of waived tests has occurred periodically. However, all such facilities must obtain a certificate of waiver from the Food and Drug Administration. It is unclear how many assisted living facilities will be affected by this act.

The Family and Medical Leave Act of 1993

Under the Family and Medical Leave Act (FMLA), a covered employer (50 or more employees) must allow up to 12 weeks per year of unpaid leave connected with pregnancy, childbirth, and recovery, or a serious health condition affecting an employee or his or her family member.

Benefits Eligibility. The employee must have worked for at least 12 months (1,250 hours at least) prior to the leave. The 12 months need not be consecutive.

Benefits. These cover birth of a son or daughter or adoption or foster care and caring for a spouse, son, daughter, or parent with a serious health condition or a serious health condition that prevents the employee from performing his or her job functions. A serious health condition does not normally include any short-term condition that could be covered under regular sick leave policies. Absence for substance abuse without a treatment program is not within the definition of a serious health condition for the purposes of this act.

Options. The employee may ask for leave as reduced work hours or any combination of modified work schedule to accommodate covered reasons for unpaid leave under the act.

Return. Generally, the employee is entitled to return to his or her former job or its equivalent at the same pay, benefits and other equal working conditions.

The Personal Responsibility and Work Opportunity Reconciliation Act of 1996

This act requires all states to maintain a Directory of New Hires. The purposes of the law are to (1) help officials locate absent parents in order to establish or enforce child support and (2) reduce fraud and abuse in unemployment insurance and welfare programs. The New Hire Reporting Law requires that every employer report the hiring of all new employees within 20 calendar days of their start time.

4.4.3 Regulation of Compensation

Most states and the federal government have passed laws that regulate compensation for work done.

Federal jurisdiction covers only those workers engaged in producing goods for interstate and foreign commerce. Technically, the federal government does not have authority to regulate worker compensation within states.

More than 40 states have their own wage and hour laws and also regulate other conditions of employment, such as hours allowed per week before overtime must be paid.

The practical effect of having both federal and state regulations compensation is that both prevail. In reality, the federal laws are applied to most workers regardless of whether they are producing goods for interstate or foreign commerce. This breadth of application of the federal wage laws is achieved by including persons whose work is closely related to any production for interstate or foreign commerce. On a day-to-day basis, this means that long-term care facility employee compensation and other work conditions must meet both federal and state regulations.

The original goals of federal wage and hour regulations were (1) to encourage the spreading of work among as many wage earners as feasible and (2) to establish a floor for wages for any worker regardless of the job. Requiring a rate of 1_ times the regular pay rate for all overtime has helped to accomplish spreading the work. Requiring a minimum wage for all persons has accomplished the second goal.

FAIR LABOR STANDARDS ACT (FSLA) (WAGE AND HOUR ACT)

The Fair Labor Standards Act was originally passed in 1938, but like the Social Security Act of 1935, it has been amended many times. The four primary foci of the act are (1) minimum wage rates, (2) overtime, (3) child labor, and (4) equal rights.

Minimum Wage Rates

When first instituted, the minimum wage was 25 cents an hour. Over the decades it has risen nearly 15–fold.

The new minimum wage must be calculated on the actual earning wage before any additional payments are added. For example, the employee works a 46–hour week. He or she received the minimum wage for the first 40 hours and is paid at 1_ times that rate for the additional 6 hours. Generally, the employee must be paid in cash or in a "negotiable instrument payable at par" (a check) except that board, lodging, and other facilities regularly furnished to employees may be provided in lieu of cash wages or the cost deducted from cash wages.

What Is Work?

Preparatory activities integral to the employee's job may be considered work time. If an employee performs work that is prohibited, with the knowledge and/or acquiescence of management, the employee must be paid, even if the work is away from the facility, if the employer has reason to believe the work is being performed. On-call or waiting time may be considered work if the employee is "engaged" by the employer to wait for the work. Travel associated with or required by the job is compensable. Bona fide meal periods are not compensable, must be 30 minutes in duration, and must totally free the employee from performing any work. If meal periods are frequently interrupted, as happens often in a long-term care facility setting, the whole meal period may be considered compensable work time. Rest periods and coffee breaks are compensable.

The minimum wage rates are especially important to long-term care facilities because many of them pay nurse's aides and housekeeping and maintenance employees at or just above the minimum wage.

Overtime

The Fair Labor Standards Act requires overtime for all hours over 40 hours a week, to be paid at one and one half the regular rate of pay. Hospital, nursing home, and assisted living facility employees are entitled to an exception in that overtime may be calculated on the basis of a 14-day period if overtime is paid for hours worked in excess of 8 daily and in excess of 80 during the 14-day period. There must be an agreement between employees and employer to this arrangement.

Overtime must be calculated on the basis of a single work week and not be averaged over 2 or more weeks. A fluctuating work week is permitted under certain circumstances.

Whenever compensatory time is given for overtime hours worked, the employee must be given 1_ hours off for every hour of overtime worked. Employees may not accumulate more than 240 hours, however.

If bonuses are paid for some other period—a month or a quarter, for example—the base for overtime wages must be recalculated to add any additional remuneration to the base rate for that period in calculating the time-and-a-half rate for all hours worked over 80 hours in each 2-week period.

Because of their exemption from coverage by the Fair Labor Standards Act, management personnel are referred to as exempt employees. Nonmanagement employees are considered nonexempt. A number of complicated definitions apply to this area.

Congress amends this act frequently, so it is important to check with the Department of Labor to keep abreast of current and upcoming regulations and changes.

Enforcement of FSLA

Records may be subpoenaed without a warrant at off-site locations. Normally, a warrant is required for on-site inspections. Violations are subject to a penalty of up to $1,000 per violation. Injunctions may be issued regarding minimum wage, overtime, child labor, and record-keeping violations. Criminal proceedings may be brought by the Department of Justice. First offenders may be fined no more than $10,000. Second offenders may be so fined, and a maximum prison sentence of 6 months may be imposed. Wage and Hour inspectors are liable to show up unannounced. In general, the word of the employee is taken most seriously by these inspectors. If an employee said that he or she worked 2 hours a week "off the clock" for the previous year, the facility may be required to pay that employee for 2 hours of overtime per week for that past year.

Child Labor

Minors under 16 may not be employed except under a temporary permit issued by the Department of Labor. Many states have regulations concerning the employment of persons between ages 16 and 18 in certain industries, such as long-term care facilities, where the worker can be exposed to disease or other hazardous conditions. Generally, special temporary work permits must be obtained.

EQUAL PAY ACT

In 1963 the Fair Labor Standards Act was amended by the Equal Pay Act. Under that amendment,

> [n]o employer shall discriminate between employees on the basis of sex by paying wages to employees less than the rate at which he [sic] pays wages to employees of the opposite sex for equal work on jobs which require equal skill, effort and responsibility, and similar working conditions. (Quoted in Chruden & Sherman, 1980, p. 453)

Progress has been slow in this area. U.S. Department of Labor, Bureau of Labor Statistics, studies have shown that women earn slightly more than 60 cents for every dollar men earn in comparable positions.

The equal pay provision of the Fair Labor Standards Act is of special concern to long-term care operators, who may employ both male and female nurses, male and female aides, and male and female maintenance and laundry persons.

4.4.4 Workers' Compensation

Workers' compensation laws are based on the principle that employees themselves should not have to pay costs associated with injuries that occur at work. On-the-job injuries, the lawmakers have reasoned, are a cost of doing business and should be passed on to the consumer.

In New Jersey, Texas, and South Carolina, workers' compensation insurance is voluntary. In all other states it is compulsory for employers to participate in a state-sponsored or state-approved program.

Under most state laws, workers are paid a percentage of their regular wages while recovering from an injury suffered on the job. States normally set limits to benefits and specify how long they must be paid.

Hospitalization and other medical costs are also normally covered by workers' compensation insurance funds. There are usually death benefits for a worker's family. States establish commissions that handle any claims that are in dispute. Generally, the result is little cost to the injured worker and reasonably rapid assistance.

States usually take one of two basic approaches to funding workers' compensation insurance. Sometimes the state operates its own insurance system in which employers are usually obliged to participate. In other states, employers are allowed either to self-insure or to join a private insurance company program.

One characteristic of most worker accident compensation plans is that the amount the employer must pay each month is experience-based. Under this system, employers with good safety records pay less than those with large numbers of claims. In some states, benefits to an injured worker are reduced if the worker is willfully negligent in following safety procedures.

In 1993 alone, 216,400 employees in nursing, assisted living, and personal care facilities suffered work-related illnesses and injuries, an incident rate of 16.9 non-fatal injuries and illnesses per 100 full-time employees (Burda, 1993). This was 50% higher than hospitals' 10.9 rate. The nursing, assisted living, and personal care homes injury rate in 1993 was the second highest of all industries, with 100,000 or more total injuries and illnesses; the motor vehicle and equipment makers' rate (17.7) was slightly higher.

4.4.5 Unemployment Compensation

Employees who participate in the Social Security Act program are eligible for unemployment compensation when they are laid off by their employer. Nearly all long-term care employees are covered by the Social Security Act.

Unemployment compensation is available for up to 26 weeks through the state employment agency if the worker registers and is willing to accept any suitable comparable work offered through the agency.

Unemployment compensation is funded by a federal payroll tax based on the wages of each employee up to a certain maximum. The federal government turns these funds over to the states for disbursement.

A separate record is kept for each employer. Once a company has paid an amount equivalent to the required reserve, its rate of taxation is reduced. In actual practice, this means that assisted living facilities with few unemployment compensation claims against them pay at a lower tax rate than those with a large number of such claims.

Experience has shown that, although they are discharged or let go for valid reasons (unrelated to lack of work), unless the facility has extremely good documentation on the circumstances of the dismissal, employees may be successful in claiming unemployment compensation. When this happens, the costs of the unemployment compensation paid by the state are allocated to that individual facility's account.

4.4.6 Retirement

AGE DISCRIMINATION EMPLOYMENT ACT OF 1967 (AMENDED 1978)

This act protects employees from being discriminated against on the basis of age. It is intended to prevent companies from replacing older employees with younger ones, whether to achieve a younger average age among the working force or to avoid paying pension benefits. There are some exceptions, such as certain occupational groups and employers with fewer than 20 employees, but the practical effect is that no employees in the typical long-term care facility can be forced to retire against their wishes solely on the basis of age.

During the 1960s Congress investigated pensions for American workers and discovered that for a variety of reasons, up to one half of American workers covered by pension plans would never receive any benefits. The largest problem was a failure of businesses to fund their pension plans adequately. For the workers, the basic problem was loss of any pension benefits when leaving the company for almost any reason before retirement. The EEOC is the primary agency responsible for enforcing this act.

THE EMPLOYEE RETIREMENT INCOME SECURITY ACT OF 1975

In reaction, Congress passed the Employee Retirement Income Security Act (ERISA) of 1975. This act sets minimum funding levels for pension funds, requires certification every 3 years of the actuarial soundness of the plan, and requires vesting of each employee's equity in the pension fund. Employers are *not* required under ERISA or any other law to provide a private pension fund for their employees.

Among its regulations ERISA set up the Pension Benefit Guaranty Corporation, established in 1974, which is supported by premiums from employers to ensure that employees will eventually receive retirement funds. Companies that decide to withdraw from the plan must make substantial payments into the corporation before being permitted to do so. This and other elements of the act create hardships for employers who otherwise are committed to providing pension benefits for employees.

One major drawback to the ERISA legislation is that its rules are so demanding that many employers choose not to offer pension plans. Also, upon implementation of the act, many employers chose to withdraw their plans rather than try to comply with the law when it went into effect. Another unfortunate result is that many employees are electing to receive their accumulated "retirement" benefits when they leave the organization. Studies have documented that all to often these pension benefits never find their way into 401k or similar retirement mechanisms.

In place of regular company-created and -maintained pension plans, a number of employers have opted to offer employees participation in what are known as 401k and similar plans, under which employees contribute money on a tax-deferred basis for retirement purposes. The major drawback for the employee is that upon leaving the company, he or she often receives his or her 401k contributions in a lump sum. Employees can roll over these 401k funds to similar tax-deferred investments within specified days and retain them for eventual retirement purpose, but, as with regular lump sum pension proceeds given to an employee at termination, for too many employees the temptation to use the funds for current expenses is too great.

4.4.5 Workplace Safety: The Occupational Safety and Health Act of 1970

ORIGIN AND PASSAGE

For the first 7 decades of the 20th century state governments were responsible for safety in the workplace. During that period organized labor became less and less satisfied with the enforcement of state laws, the variation in laws among the states, and often the absence of any safety laws. In the half-decade before the passage of federal legislation, job-related accidents were causing up to 2.5 million disabilities and 14,000 deaths annually (U.S. Department of Labor, 1976).

After 3 years of intense lobbying by employees and the unions, Congress passed the Occupational Safety and Health Act (OSHA) in 1970 (Public Law 91–596). OSHA applies to nearly all employees and includes all of those working in long-term care facilities.

FEDERAL IMPLEMENTATION

Two federal agencies have been set up to implement OSHA. The act is administered by the Occupational Safety and Health Administration in the Department of Labor. The National Institute of Occupational Safety and Health was established to conduct research and develop standards.

A major goal of the act has been to turn workplace safety enforcement back to the states with a strengthened workplace-safety law. States have been encouraged to establish their own inspection programs and industrial safety laboratories.

In addition to meeting all standards set, OSHA imposes on employers a general duty to provide each employee a safe workplace, free from recognized hazards causing or likely to cause death or serious physical harm. For example, pending the publication of final regulations regarding the control of infections (e.g., AIDS), OSHA invoked the "general duty" obligation when inspecting long-term care facilities.

THREE OSHA IMPACT AREAS

OSHA directly affects the operations of long-term care facilities in at least three areas:

1. meeting the standards set by OSHA
2. cooperating in OSHA inspections of the facility
3. keeping the necessary records on job-related accidents and illnesses

SOURCES OF STANDARDS

OSHA standards may originate from a variety of sources. The Secretary of Labor may issue and revise standards at will. This may be done on the secretary's own initiative, on the recommendation of the National Institute of Occupational Safety and Health, or at the urging of interested parties, such as labor unions or groups of affected employees.

Adopting Standards of Other Organizations

OSHA has adopted several national consensus standards that were developed by other groups, including the National Fire Protection Association's Life Safety Code and the Standards for the Physically Handicapped of the American National Standards Institute.

DEFINITION OF "STANDARD"

OSHA safety standards are "practices, means, operations or processes, reasonably necessary to provide safe . . . employment" (Ivancevich & Glueck, 1983, p. 595). The administrator is responsible for knowing OSHA standards for his or her facility.

The original standards ran to 350 pages of small print in the *Federal Register*. Subsequently, supplementary volumes of standards have been published. Some annual volumes have been over 700 pages in length. Even so, the administrator is responsible for knowing applicable standards and is subject to both fines and imprisonment if found to be in violation of them.

SOME OSHA REQUIREMENTS

OSHA bulletins have listed the following requirements.

Employers

Every employer must furnish a workplace free from recognized hazards that are causing or are likely to cause death or serious harm to employees and shall comply with OSHA standards, displaying the OSHA poster that informs employees of their rights and responsibilities, and compiling annual figures on work-related illnesses and accidents.

Employees

Each employee shall obey all OSHA requirements. However, the facility is held responsible for worker violation of OSHA standards. The employer has the choice of dismissing such a worker, but there are no punishments for the worker who willfully ignores OSHA requirements. Willful disregard of OSHA rules is, however, grounds for termination permitted under federal law.

Any employee may lodge a complaint with OSHA. The complaint must be in writing and signed, with a description of the hazardous condition. The signed complaint is submitted to the OSHA regional director and to the employer, unsigned, if the employee wishes to remain anonymous.

Inspections

OSHA inspectors will visit at times of their own choosing, or at the invitation of any employer, union, or employee. Employees requesting an inspection need not be identified.

The employer and the employees must each designate a representative to accompany the OSHA inspector(s). If the employees do not do so, the OSHA compliance officer must consult several employees during the visit. This officer must hold an opening conference to discuss the scope and reason for the inspection and a concluding conference in which findings are presented to the employer.

Employers must not discriminate against any employee(s) who asks for an OSHA safety or health inspection. Any employee may file a complaint with the nearest OSHA office within 30 days for any such alleged discrimination.

OSHA inspectors examine the premises for compliance with regulations and the records of illnesses and injuries to employees.

Citations

Citations may be issued at the end of the inspection itself or later by mail. Any citation issued must be posted at or near the site of violation for 3 days or the duration of the violation, whichever is longer. One citation must be issued for each serious and nonserious violation found and a time limit specified for its correction.

OSHA compliance officers may categorize employer violations as

1. *imminent danger* (can close operations down)
2. *serious* (calls for a major fine)
3. *nonserious* (a violation in which a direct and immediate relationship exists between the condition and occupational health, but not such as to cause death or serious physical harm)
4. *de minimus* (small violation)—a notification is given, but no fine imposed; a violation of a standard that is not directly or immediately related to occupational safety or health

In every case, a time period is specified within which the violation must be corrected. A fine of $7,000 per day per violation may be imposed after the time limit set for abatement (correction) of the violation.

Fines

Fines, some mandatory, are imposed for the following reasons:

1. *willful or repeated violations*—up to $70,000 per violation (mandatory); may double after first conviction
2. *serious violation*—mandatory penalty up to $7,000 for each violation
3. *nonserious violation*—optional penalties up to $7,000 each
4. *failure to correct* within proposed time period—up to $7,000 per day
5. *willful violation*—minimum fine: $5,000

Employers have the right to appeal fines or citations within the OSHA structure or in the courts. Notice of contest must be filed within 15 days.

Under Title 3 the facility may assessed a civil penalty of up to $55,000 for the first violation and $110,000 for any subsequent violation (Enforcing the ADA: A Status Report from the Department of Justice, January – March, 2003).

Record Keeping

The area that most directly affects long-term care facility administrators on a daily basis is keeping standardized records of illnesses and injuries from which ratios must be calculated. This record, "Log and Summary of Occupational Injuries and Illnesses," must be kept by each facility.

Accidents and illnesses that do not have to be reported are those that require only first aid and do not result in any work time lost. Accidents and illnesses that do have to be reported are those that result in death(s), disabilities that cause the employee to miss work, and injuries that require treatment by a physician. Reporting requirements were tightened on May 2,1994. Fatal or serious multiple cases (three or more hospitalized) must be reported to the OSHA regional director orally, by telephone within 8 hours, which begins as soon as any facility representatives becomes aware of the situation. Also, such incidents must be reported if death or hospitalization occurs within 30 days of the incident. Other cases must be recorded within 6 days and reported on routine forms as requested by OSHA.

Occupational illness is a definition of special relevance to the long-term care setting. An occupational illness is any abnormal condition or disorder, other than one resulting from an occupational injury caused by exposure to environmental factors associated with employment. It includes acute and chronic illnesses or diseases that may be caused by inhalation, absorption, ingestion, or direct contact (Chruden & Sherman, 1980).

OSHA defines an occupational injury as any injury, such as a cut, fracture, sprain amputation, that results from a work accident or from an exposure involving a single accident in the work environment (Chruden & Sherman, 1980).

Each time a recordable case is entered in the log mentioned above, a "Supplementary Record of Occupational Injuries and Illnesses" must be completed, giving information on what the employee was doing, which part of the body was affected, and the identity of the employee.

OSHA Form "Summary of Occupational Injuries and Illnesses," must be submitted annually and posted where employees can easily see it (e.g., above the time clock), at least during January and February of every year.

In 2001 the incidence rate of injuries and illnesses in private industry as a whole was 5.7 cases per 100,000 full-time workers. The rate for assisted living and nursing facilities was 13.5—one of the highest for any occupation (Enforcing the ADA: A Status Report from the Department of Justice, January – March, 2003).

The Current and Emerging Situation

Completing, submitting, and posting accident and illness forms as required will remain a continuing requirement for long-term care facility administrators, but the inspection issue is another matter. After years during which few, if any, long-term care facilities were being inspected in the various states, OSHA inspectors have begun showing up to perform routine inspection of facilities. In many locales OSHA inspectors will, at the invitation of the facility, perform "dry run" inspections for an employer, advising on any violations and providing an opportunity for correction before any official inspection.

Since OSHA was enacted, fatalities in the workforce are estimated to have decreased by 10% and total injuries to have decreased by 15% (Inancevich & Glueck, 1983, p. 601).

Due to constant lifting and similar activities assisted living and nursing home facilities have traditionally had one of the higher rates of occupational illness and injuries. The incidence rate (the number of injuries and illnesses per 100 full-time workers) for assisted living and nursing facilities in 2001 was 13.5 compared to the national average of 5.7. This represents about 200,000 cases in assisted living facilities and nursing homes in the year 2001 (Bureau of Labor Statistics, U.S. Department of Labor, December, 2002).

In the Assisted Living Workgroup Report to the U.S. Senate Special Committee on Aging, (April, 2003, p. 346) the following emergency and disaster preparedness plans are recommended:

- The means by which residents or their families or representatives are notified of the evacuation plan
- The training staff will receive related to the plan; execution of the plan, how soon after hiring, how frequently reviewed
- How changes in the plan will be communicated to everyone
- Sepcific responsibilities of each staff member
- List of residents needing assistance;where list is kept
- Identification of the staff member responsible for each of the following:
- Ensuring all residents are accounted for
- Ensuring medications are taken from the building in emergencies
- Ensuring medical records are removed from the building
- Back up plan if cannot remove medications or records
- How family will be notified of evacuation

- Frequency of practice of the plan
- Evacuate the building every 6 months

Contingency Plan

- Where residents will be housed
- How to transport residents to alternate location
- How to assure adequate staff is available

4.5 Fire Safety: The *Life Safety Code*®

The National Fire Protection Association is a private, nonprofit organization with headquarters in Quincy, MA. It is not a government agency, nor does it write federal regulations. However, because the regulations for licensing nursing homes include adherence to the *Life Safety Code,*® these fire safety standards have, in effect, the force of law for nursing homes. They may or may not have the force of law for the assisted living administrator. Some states and/or localities have their own life safety laws that they enforce. In some states assisted living facilities may be inspected using this *Life Safety Code.*® In any case, the *Life Safety Code*® represents the best understanding of how to provide for resident safety in the institutional setting, such as assisted living communities.

The National Fire Protection Association has more than 150 committees, one of which, the Committee on Safety to Life, establishes and revises these standards. The committee has met since 1913 and currently has several standing subcommittees.

The code has evolved over the years, benefiting from the hindsight gained from the experience of many tragic fires. This code represents the collected wisdom on fire prevention and fire containment.

The regulations passed in the *Federal Register* in 1974 required nursing facilities to "meet such provisions of the *Life Safety Code*® of the National Fire Protection Association as are applicable to long-term care facilities" (405.1134A). These regulations have been revised regularly with new editions approximately every 3 years. The ones described in the following sections are from the 1994 *Life Safety Code*® edition.

The actual wording of the *Life Safety Code*® is not used in the following pages. The major concepts and a number of the essential features of the code presented below are summaries of the code presented for study purposes. The code itself is not directly quoted, only paraphrased. Under no circumstances, then, should the reader treat this material as a substitute for obtaining the actual *Life Safety Code*®.

The sixth edition (1994), edited by Ron Cote, P.E., offers highly useful interpretations of the *Life Safety Code*® and the National Fire Protection Association's *Health Care Facilities Handbook,*® 4th edition, (1993), edited by Burton R. Klein, P.E. Copies of the code itself may be ordered from National Fire Protection, Inc., Batterymarch Park, Quincy, MA 02269; telephone 800-344-3555.

The material here is reprinted with permission from NFPA *101,*® the sixth edition of the *Life Safety Code Handbook,* ©1994. National Fire Protection Association, Qunicy, MA 02269. This reprinted material is neither the actual wording nor the complete and official position of the NFPA on the referenced subjects which are represented only by the standard in its entirety. This material is intended to apprise persons in the long-term care field of the general nature and functions within the facility of the *Life Safety Code.*®

(Note: Assisted living is covered under chapter 21 of the *Life Safety Code,*® "Residential Board and Care Occupancies." The reader may wish to study this section. As assisted living facilities become more involved in providing health-related care, the more rigorous regulations presented below may become the expected standard.)

HEALTH CARE OCCUPANCIES (SECTION 31-4 OF THE FIRE SAFETY CODE)

Life Safety Code® and *101*® are registered trademarks of the National Fire Protection Association, Inc., Quincy, MA 02269.

A-31-4 Compromised Health

Due to the compromised health and mobility of residents a primary emphasis in placed on superior construction, quick discovery of fire, quick notification of the fire department, and early extinguishment.

31-4.1 Emphases

Emphasis must be placed on removing patients from the room of fire origin and anyone directly exposed to the fire. The current emphasis is on moving occupants themselves rather than on having movable beds (an earlier, now deleted requirement).

31-4.1.1 Fire Plan

Every administration must have written copies of a fire plan available to all supervisory personnel and an evacuation plan to areas of refuge. All employees must receive periodic in-service training and drill practice for their specific individualized duty assignments. A copy of the plan must be at the security center or telephone operator location.

31.4.1.2 Fire Drills

Drills must be conducted with actual transmission of a fire alarm signal and a simulated emergency condition (e.g., placement of an object in a room or area designated as the fire origin, which must be quickly located and transmitted by staff). All personnel in the facility, including administrators, maintenance, etc., must be trained. Quarterly drills for each shift must be conducted (9:00 p.m. to 6:00 a.m. drills may use a coded announcement rather than an audible alarm). Infirm and/or bedridden patients do not have to be physically moved to safe areas or the exterior.

A-31-4.1.2 Drills (continued)

To reduce patient anxiety doors to patient rooms in the area of planned fire origin may be closed. Drills must be on a random basis, at least once every 3 months for every employee. Empty wheelchairs may be used to simulate relocation of residents to adjacent safe smoke compartments.

31-4.1.3 Training

All employees must be trained in life safety procedures and devices.

31-4.2.1 Minimum Response

Minimum response must include all personnel, removing all patients directly involved in the fire area, quick transmission of an alarm signal, confinement of the fire by closing doors to isolate the fire, and all duties assigned in the fire safety plan.

Upon discovering a fire the discoverer must come to the aid of any person involved while calling aloud an agreed upon code phrase; any individual within hearing must activate an alarm at the nearest manual fire station (if no person is endangered, the discoverer must activate the nearest manual alarm). All personnel must immediately undertake their assigned duties. The telephone operator, who must be immediately notified of the fire location, must notify the fire department and alert all building occupants.

31-4.2.2 The Written Fire Safety Plan

The written fire safety plan must include: using alarm devices, transmitting alarms to the fire department, how to respond to alarms, how to isolate the fire, how to evacuate the fire area, preparation for building evacuation, and extinguishing the fire.

31-4.2.3 The Goal

The goal is to close as many doors as possible to prevent smoke from spreading and, to the extent feasible, to confine the fire to the room of origin. No or low loss of life occurs when staff close the doors, according to studies conducted. Closing the doors has the most significant effect on limiting the spread of fire and smoke and limiting or eliminating any loss of life.

31-4.3 Maintenance of Exits

All exits must be maintained. If locks exist on any exits sufficient staff must be available 24 hours a day to assure prompt release of any locks in fire or any emergency situation.

31-4.4 Smoking

[Many, if not most facilities are adopting a no smoking policy. For those that do not universally prohibit smoking in the building, the following requirements must be met.] Smoking is not permitted in any location with flammable liquids, combustible gases, or where oxygen is being used or any other location designated as hazardous. Such areas must post No Smoking signs. Any smoking by nonresponsible patients must be prohibited except under strict supervision. Ashtrays must be safely designed, of noncombustible material, and metal closable containers must be available.

Assisted Living Workgroup Report to the U.S. Senate Special Committee on Aging (April, 2003, p. 349) recommendation: If the assisted living residence permits smoking, it must have a written smoking policy which addresses:

- Who may and may not smoke
- When and where smoking may occur
- Appropriate signage
- Resident education
- Staff education
- How smoking policies will be published and enforced
- Documentation needed to permit resident smoking
- How and how often to screen smoking residents for ability to smoke safely
- Maintenance of ventilation and fire protection systems.

A-31-4.4

In cases where a ban on all smoking is not possible or not enforced it is important to train staff and to exercise full control over all smoking. Smoking in bed and placing smoking materials in improper waste containers lead the causes of fire in long-term care facilities.

31-4.5 Furnishings, Bedding, and Decorations

31-4.5.1 Draperies and Any Similar Hanging Material

Draperies and any similar hanging material including bed cubicle curtains must not interfere with the operations of smoke detectors and sprinklers. One option (12-3.5.3) is to hang curtains 18" below the sprinkler or detector or use a thin mesh that will not inhibit their functioning. Or (13.3.5.6) have a minimum vertical distance meeting NFPA 13 Standard for the Installation of Sprinkler Systems, which assumes occupants are basically nonambulatory with sufficient staff 24 hours each day. Draperies, furniture with upholstery, and mattresses must be tested to meet heat release standards.

31-4.4.4 Combustible Decorations

Combustible decorations are prohibited. Photographs and paintings in limited quantities are permitted.

31-4.5.5 Soiled Linen and Trash Collection Containers

Soiled linen and trash collection containers must be limited to a capacity of 32 gallons within any 64 square foot area. Mobile soiled linen and trash collection receptacles of 33 gallons and more must be mobile and in an area or room protected as a hazard area when unattended. Housekeeping staff, for example, who must leave an area for whatever reason must store mobile containers in such a hazard protected area.

31-4.6 New Engineered Smoke Control Systems

New engineered smoke control systems must meet standards of NFPA 92A, *Recommended Practice for Smoke-Control Systems,* and NFPA 92B, *Guide for Smoke Management Systems in Malls, Atria, and Large Areas.*

31-4.7 Portable Space Heating Devices

Portable Space Heating Devices are prohibited except for use in nonsleeping staff and employee areas where the heating elements do not exceed 212° Fahrenheit.

SECTION 12-1 NEW HEALTH CARE OCCUPANCIES

[Only certain sections applying directly to facilities are mentioned here. Numerous exceptions are cited in the full document to which the reader should refer when planning any new building.]

GENERAL REQUIREMENTS (SECTION 12-1)

New facilities must either meet the standards stipulated here or demonstrate equivalent safety. Alternative designs are allowed as long as they provide equivalent safety as based on Chapter 3 of NFPA 101M, *Manual on Alternative Approaches to Life Safety.*

These requirements apply to new buildings or sections used as health care occupancies.

12-1.1.2 Objective:

To limit the development and spreading of a fire to the room of fire origin and reduce the need for evacuation, except from the room of fire origin. These are achieved partially through requirements aimed at prevention of ignition, fire detection, controlling fire development, confinement of the fire effect, the fire's extinguishment, provision of evacuation facilities, and staff action.

12-1.1.3 Total Concept

It is believed that evacuation between floors in a facility is too time consuming (up to 30 minutes being required); hence the basic approach is to defend in place.

12-1.1.4.1 Additions

Additions not meeting these standards must be separated by a fire barrier having at least a 2-hour fire resistance rating and of required construction materials.

12-1.1.4.2 Communicating Openings

Communicating openings shall be limited to corridors protected by approved self-closing fire doors. These doors, when necessary, may be held open by automatic release devices. These doors are normally kept closed.

A-12-1.1.4.5 Automatic Sprinkler Protection

Automatic sprinkler protection is required of all new health care occupancies.

12-1.6.1 Construction Requirements

The primary level of exit discharge of a building is the lowest story with a floor level at or above finished grade on the exterior wall with 50% or more of its perimeter. The following (Figure 4.7) is a figure of a three-story building.

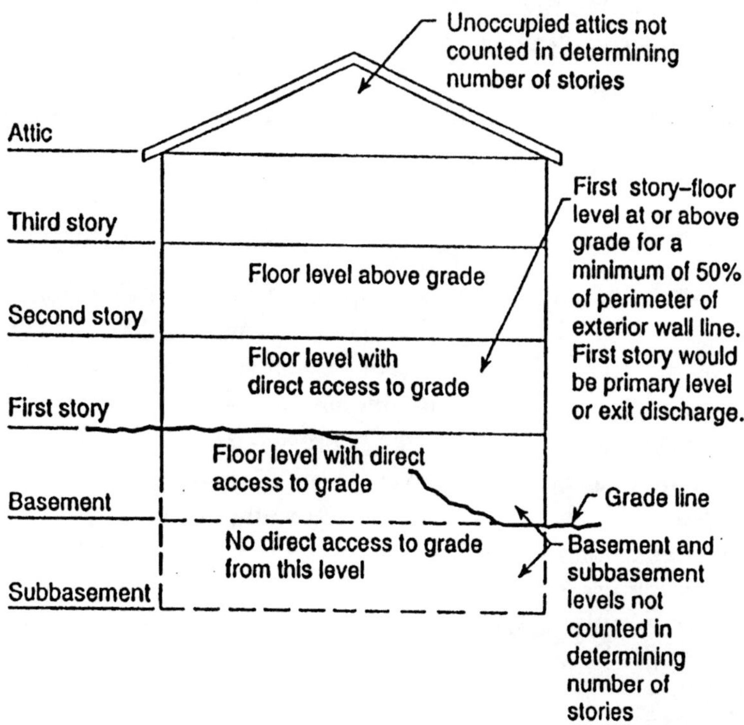

Determining number of stories for application of minimum construction requirements. Because of sloping grade, the primary level of exit discharge is not obvious. The fifty percent perimeter guideline of 12-1.6.1 clarifies that for the arrangement illustrated, the first story is the primary level of exit discharge. Number of stories includes primary level of exit discharge and all occupiable floors located above. This is an example of a three-story building.

FIGURE 4.7 Building section view illustrating grade line and story designation. Reprinted with permission from *NFPA Life Safety Code® Handbook*, 6th Ed., Ron Cote, P.E., Editor, 1994, p. 374.

12-1.6.2 Construction and Multistory Buildings

Construction types are specified for a variety of buildings. All multistory health care facilities must be constructed of noncombustible materials. In three- or more story buildings the major construction elements must be protected by a 2-hour fire resistance rating.

12-1.6.4 Openings for Pipes, Etc.

All penetrations of walls must be protected with such means as metal plates, masonry fill, or similar approved product to prevent the spread of fire and smoke.

12-1.7 Occupant Load

Means of egress must be provided for one person for each 120 square feet of gross floor area in health care sleeping areas and for one person for each 240 square feet of gross floor area in inpatient treatment areas (e.g., physical therapy). If the actual count of persons exceeds these numbers, the actual number of persons becomes the minimum occupant load for determining required egress.

12-2.2.2-7 Doors

Locks are not permitted on patient sleeping room doors. An exception is permitted for using a device that locks a door so that staff can unlock it from the corridor and the patient can exit the room without use of any key. Such an approach would prevent patients from accidentally wandering into an isolation room, but the patient in the isolation room would be able to exit the room without use of a key or tool. Also, for patients that might endanger themselves (e.g., Alzheimer's patients), a lock may be installed provided staff carry keys at all times or other provision for remotely unlocking all such doors. Doors in a required means of egress may not be equipped with a latch or lock that requires the use of a tool or key from the egress side. At maximum, only one delayed egress device may be used along the length of any egress.

5-2 Means of Egress

Interior stairs, in general, must have a minimum clear width of 44 inches except for handrails not exceeding 3½ inches at or below handrail height on each side. Riser maximum height is 7 inches, minimum height of risers is 4 inches. Minimum tread depth is 11 inches, minimum headroom is 6 feet 8 inches. Maximum height between landings is 12 feet.

Handrails

Handrails are required on both sides and must be not less than 34 inches nor more than 38 inches above the surface of the tread measured vertically to the top of the rail from the leading edge of the tread. Handrail clearance must be at least 1½ inches when smooth surfaces are used, more if rough surfaces. Handrails must be graspable firmly with a comfortable grip so the hand can slide along the rail without encountering any obstructions.

5.2.3 Smokeproof Enclosures

A smokeproof enclosure is a set of enclosed stairs designed to limit the infiltration of heat, smoke, and fire gases from a fire in any part of a building that limits entry of the products of combustion into the stairway. Such stairwells must have a 2-hour fire resistance and a door with a 1½ hour fire protection rating.

5-2.4 Horizontal Exits

A horizontal exit is a passage from one area of a building to another, separated by a fire barrier, space, or other protection, enabling each area to be a fire compartment independent of the one in which a fire exists. It can be a bridge to another building. No stairs or ramps are normally involved. At least 30 square feet per patient must be provided within the aggregated area of corridors, patient rooms, treatment rooms, lounge dining area, and other low hazard areas on each side. A single door may be permitted provided the exit serves one direction only and is at least 41½ inches wide. If separating two fire areas, two doors swinging opposite directions, each at least 41½ inches is required.

5.2.5 Ramps

The usual definition is:

- 20° to 50° = a stairway
- 7° to 20° = a stairway and landings
- under 7° = a ramp

Nearly horizontal landings are required at both ends of ramps. Ramps are to be slip resistant and have a clear width of at least 44 inches. The maximum rise for a single ramp run is 30 inches.

12-2.3.3 Aisles, Corridors, and Ramps Used for Exit

Aisles, corridors, and ramps used for exit must be at least 8 feet in width clear and unobstructed.

12-2.4 Number of Exits

At least two exits located remotely from each other must be provided for each floor and fire section of a building. At least one exit from each floor or fire section must lead directly outside, to a stair, a smokeproof enclosure, a ramp, or an exit passageway. At no time can an exit passageway require return through the compartment of origin.

12-2.5 Arrangement of Means of Egress

Every patient room must have an exit access door leading directly to an exit access corridor (some exceptions exist, e.g., a door opening directly to the outside).

12-2.6.2 Travel Distance to Exits

Travel distance between the door in any room and an exit access and an exit must not exceed 150 feet, and travel from within any patient room to same must not exceed 200 feet. Travel distance within a room to an exit must not exceed 50 feet.

12-2.7 Discharge from Exits

Each required exit ramp or stair must lead directly outside at grade or be an enclosed passage meeting all fire-resistance regulations at grade.

12-2.8 Illumination of Means of Egress

Illumination of means of egress must be continuous, with all exit floor surfaces illuminated at the level of 1 foot-candle measured at the floor of the exit access, the exit, and the exit discharge. Failure of any single light source (electric bulb) must not leave any area in darkness, hence the need for overlapping light sources, separately wired.

5-9 Emergency Lighting

Emergency lighting must have automatic transfer between normal power and an emergency source. Storage batteries are acceptable if they meet the candlelight requirements for a period of 1½ hours. Automotive type batteries are not acceptable. An on-site generator normally is required as the second source of emergency lighting.

5-10 Exit Marking

Exit signs must be readily visible from any direction of exit access. Tactile signage is required at each door into an exit stair enclosure. No point in the exit access route may be more than 100 feet. Exit signs must have letters at least 6 inches high and not less than ¾ inches wide and be of contrasting color.

Emergency Power

Most facilities have an emergency electrical generator. This generator must go on within 10 seconds of a power failure. Such a generator is not required, however, in a freestanding building in which the management precludes the provision of care for any patient who may need to be sustained by electrical life-support equipment such as a respirator or suction apparatus, and in which battery-operated systems or equipment are provided to maintain power to exit lights and means of egress, stairways, medicinal preparation areas, and the like for a minimum of 1½ hours. Battery power is also required to operate all alarm systems. Separate power supplies controlled by separate switches that are protected from fire threat are required.

12-3 Protection

12-3.1 Vertical Openings

Any stairway, ramp, elevator, hoist or chute (e.g., for laundry) between stories must be enclosed with protective construction (e.g., fire resistance of 1 hour in buildings required to have 1-hour protection, 1-hour fire resistance for buildings of not more than three stories, and 3 hours for enclosures in buildings of over three stories).

12-3.2 Protection From Hazards

Hazardous areas are spaces with contents that are flammable or combustible and represent a higher than normal hazard. Hazardous areas must be protected by fire barriers with a fire resistance rating of 1 hour or a completely automatic extinguishing system. Hazardous areas include

- mechanical equipment rooms
- laundry
- kitchens, repair shops
- handicraft shops
- employee locker areas and
- gift shop

The following must have both 1-hour fire resistance and a compete extinguishment system: soiled linen rooms, paint shops, trash collection rooms, and rooms or spaces, including repair shops, used for the storage of combustible supplies and equipment in quantities deemed hazardous by the authority having jurisdiction.

Cooking Facilities

Numerous regulations govern cooking facilities. A major focus is the requirement for a regularly serviced, fixed, automatic fire-extinguishing system for cook stoves. Small appliances such as equipment for food warming or limited cooking, such as a small microwave, are exempted from cooking regulations for commercial cooking equipment.

12-3.3 Interior Finish

A number of requirements specify the type of wall materials usable and the degree of flame spread, smoke development, and similar characteristics so as to ensure that walls do not contribute to the spread of fire. No specific requirements pertain to floor finishes.

12-3.4 Detection, Alarm, and Communications Systems

This is an extensive section with numerous provisions and exceptions. The following are some of the more salient requirements.

A manually operated fire alarm system electrically monitored is required. This means that when any component part of the fire alarm system malfunctions, a continuous trouble alert indication is sent electronically to a continuously attended location.

The fire alarm system must be designed to notify all building occupants when any alarm station is activated. The local fire department (or its equivalent) must be automatically notified whenever any fire alarm station is activated. Codes for identifying fire zones are permitted.

Emergency Control. Activating any fire alarm station must automatically activate all appropriate devices (e.g., the sprinkler system, alarms, and door releases).

New long-term care facilities must have an automatically operated smoke detection system. Smoke detectors must be located no farther apart than 30 feet and not more than 15 feet from any wall.

The automatic smoke detection and fire detection systems must both be connected electrically. Manual pull stations should be located so no employee has to leave the fire area to activate the alarm. A distinct, supervisory signal must be provided to a constantly attended location in the event of any malfunction or action that would reduce sprinkler system performance. The main health care station is often chosen for such a location.

12-3.5 Extinguishment Requirements

A **supervised automatic sprinkler system** must be installed. Quick response sprinklers must be used in the smoke compartment. Some exceptions may be made regarding sprinkler type.

Portable fire extinguishers meeting NFPA and local codes must be installed. Hand fire extinguishers are required on every floor and in every hazardous area. The travel distance to any extinguisher may be no more than 75 feet to a Class A extinguisher, 50 feet to a Class B or C extinguisher. Short persons must be able to reach the extinguisher. Every extinguisher must be in operating condition at all items Fire extinguishers must be checked quarterly and be serviced annually by a qualified examiner who must show the date that the inspection and servicing was accomplished on an attached tag.

12-3.6 Corridor Doors

Doors protecting openings in corridor partitions must be able to resist the passage of smoke but need not have a fire protection rating. Doors must have a positive latch that cannot be held in the retracted position. Roller latches are not permitted. The latch must be able to hold the door in a closed position.

12-3.7 Subdivision of Building Spaces

Smoke barriers are required

- to divide every story used by patients for sleeping or treatments into at least two smoke compartments
- to divide every story having an occupant load of 50 or more persons, regardless of use, into at least two smoke compartments
- to limit the size of each smoke compartment required above to no more than 22,500 square feet
- to limit the travel distance in the required smoke barrier to 200 feet

Doors shall be 1¾ inches thick, solid-bodied wood core or of construction of 20 minute resistance fire rating. Vision panels must be provided in swinging doors.

12-3.8 Outside Window or Door

Each patient sleeping room shall have an outside window or outside door. The maximum allowable sill height is 36 inches above the floor. The window does not have to be operable.

CONCLUDING OBSERVATIONS

The administrator who is planning new construction must meet all state and local codes as well. Many areas covered by the *Life Safety Code®* have been left uncovered. There are, for example, additional sections on utilities, heating, ventilation, air conditioning, elevators, rubbish chutes, incinerators, laundry chutes, and so on that have not been discussed.

The reader realizes, of course, that this is an introduction to only a few of the more salient aspects of the *Life Safety Code.®* The reader is strongly urged to purchase the *Life Safety Code® Handbook* for the year containing the requirements that he or she must meet.

The *Life Safety Code® Handbook* is an essential tool for administrators. It is the administrator's job to understand the code and its basic requirements in order to ensure that his or her facility is in basic conformity with regulations and to work intelligently with engineers, architects, and state building code officials in planning and pursuing any assisted living facility construction project.

4.6 Americans with Disabilities Act of 1990: Accessibility Guidelines for Facilities

On Friday, July 26, 1991, the federal Department of Justice, Office of the Attorney General, issued the following final rule Part III 28 CFR Part 36 for the purpose of achieving nondiscrimination on the basis of disability. These requirements apply to long-term care facilities that are newly built or renovated and are available from the Americans with Disabilities Act's Architectural and Transportation Barriers Compliance Board, U.S. Department of Justice, Civil Rights Division (Washington, DC), and are found in the Federal Register, Vol. 56, No. 144 / Friday, July 26, 1991, pages 35544–35691.

The following section provides an overview of these requirements, most of which are based on the standards developed and approved by the Council of American Building Officials/American National Standards Institute, Inc., entitled American National Standard Accessible and Usable Buildings and Facilities, CABO/ANSI A117.1-1992, which, along with the federal final rule cited in the paragraph above, must be obtained and utilized by any administrator planning, building, or renovating a long-term care facility. The following information, figures, and tables are reproduced here with the permission of the Council of American Building Officials, Executive Offices, 5203 Leesburg Pike, #708, Falls Church, VA 22041. As indicated in each figure and table, however, the ordering address for copies of American National Standard Accessible and Usable Buildings and Facilities is located in Country Club Hill, IL (see addresses below).* The information given here is designed to provide only an introduction to the reader of the nature and importance of the directions of these requirements. Under no circumstances may the following pages be utilized in actual planning, construction, or renovating of a long-term care facility.

STANDARDS FOR ACCESSIBLE DESIGN (APPENDIX A TO PART 36)

The following is an overview of these standards.

1. Purpose
2. General
3. Miscellaneous Instructions and Definitions
4. Accessible Elements and Spaces

4.1 Minimum Requirements
4.2 Space Allowance and Reach Ranges
4.3 Accessible Route
4.4 Protruding Objects
4.5 Ground and Floor Surfaces
4.6 Parking and Passenger Loading Zones
4.7 Curb Ramps
4.8 Ramps
4.9 Stairs
4.10 Elevators
4.11 Wheelchair Lifts
4.12 Windows
4.13 Doors
4.14 Entrances
4.15 Drinking Fountains and Water Coolers
4.16 Water Closets
4.17 Toilet Stalls
4.18 Urinals
4.19 Lavatories and Mirrors
4.20 Bathtubs
4.21 Shower Stalls
4.22 Toilet Rooms
4.23 Bathrooms, Bathing Facilities, and Shower Rooms
4.24 Sinks
4.25 Storage
4.26 Handrails, Grab Bars, and Tub and Shower Seats
4.27 Controls and Operating Mechanisms

4.28 Alarms
4.29 Detectable Warnings
4.30 Signage
4.31 Telephones
4.32 Fixed or Built-in Seating and Tables
4.33 Assembly Areas

6. Medical Care Facilities (included in 4 above)

1. Purpose

To set guidelines for accessibility for individuals with disabilities. Are to be applied during the design, construction, and alteration of facilities.

2. General

Departures from these guidelines are permitted where equivalent access is provided.

3. Miscellaneous Instructions and Definitions

Graphic conventions. These are illustrated in Table 4.8.

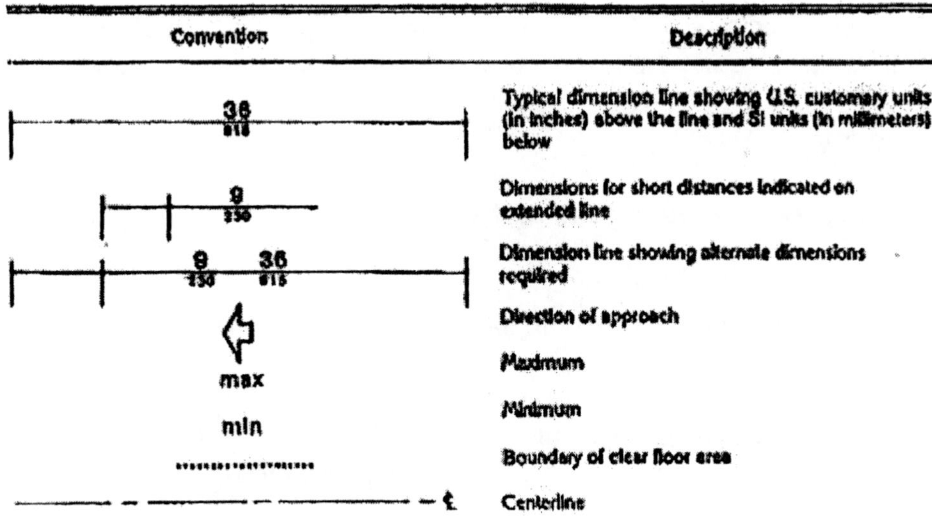

Convention	Description
36	Typical dimension line showing U.S. customary units (in inches) above the line and SI units (in millimeters) below
9	Dimensions for short distances indicated on extended line
9 36	Dimension line showing alternate dimensions required
	Direction of approach
max	Maximum
min	Minimum
....	Boundary of clear floor area
℄	Centerline

Americans with Disabilities Act of 1990, Accessibility Guidelines for Facilities. Federal Register / Vol. 56, No. 144 / Friday, July 26, 1991 / Rules and Regulations, p. 35622. Final Rule Part III CFR 28 Part 36. A copy of the final federal rule should be obtained from American with Disabilities Act's Architectural and Transportation Barriers Compliance Board, U.S. Department of Justice, Civil Rights Division (Washington, DC). A copy of American National Standard Accessible and Usable Building and Facilities, CABO/ANSI A117.1-1992 should be obtained from American National Standards Institute, 11 West 42nd St., New York, NY, 10036.

TABLE 4.8 ADA Graphic Conventions

Access Aisle. An accessible pedestrian space between elements, such as parking spaces, seating, and desks that provides clearances appropriate for use of the elements.

Accessible. Describes a site, building, facility, or portion thereof that complies with these requirements.

Accessible Element. An element specified by these requirements (e.g., telephone).

Accessible Route. A continuous unobstructed path connecting all accessible elements and spaces of a facility. Interior accessible routes may include corridors, floors, ramps, elevators, lifts, and clear floor space at fixtures. Exterior accessible route may include parking access aisles, curb ramps, crosswalks at vehicular ways, walks, ramps, and lifts.

Accessible Space. Space that complies with these requirements.

Addition. An expansion, extension, or increase in the gross floor area of a facility.

Area of Rescue Assistance. An area, which has direct access to an exit, where people who are unable to use stairs may remain temporarily in safety to await further instructions or assistance during emergency evacuation.

Assembly Area. A room or space accommodating a group of individuals for recreational, educational, or amusement purposes or for consumption of food and drink.

Clear. Unobstructed.

Clear Floor Space. The minimum unobstructed floor or ground space required to accommodate a single, stationary wheelchair and occupant.

Egress, Means of. A continuous and unobstructed way of exit travel from any point in a facility to a public way.

Element. An architectural or mechanical component of a facility, space, or site, (e.g. telephone, curb ramp, door, drinking fountain, seating, or toilet).

Signage. Displayed verbal, symbolic, tactile, and pictorial information.

Space. A definable area (e.g. room, toilet room, hall, assembly area, entrance, storage room, alcove, courtyard, or lobby).

Tactile. Describes an object that can be perceived using the sense of touch.

Walk. An exterior pathway with a prepared surface intended for pedestrian use.

4. Accessible Elements and Specifications of Section 6, Medical Facilities)

(6)(3) long-term care facilities—At least 50% of patient bedrooms and toilets, and all public use and common use areas, are required to be designed and constructed to be accessible. [Note: Given the nature of the patient mix in the typical assisted living facility, it seems illogical to build any resident rooms and toilets that are not accessible to handicapped persons.]

4.1 Minimum requirements

Accessible sites must provide at least one accessible route that complies with section 4.3 within the boundary of the site from public transportation stops, accessible parking spaces, passenger loading zones, if furnished, and public streets or sidewalks to an accessible building entrance.

Accessible routes must have at least one complying with section 4.3 connecting accessible buildings, accessible facilities, accessible elements, and accessible spaces that are on the same site.

Several other minimum requirements are stated, most of which are outlined below.

4.2 Space allowance and reach ranges.

Wheelchair passage width. 36 inches continuously, 32 inches at any one point (see Figure 4.8).

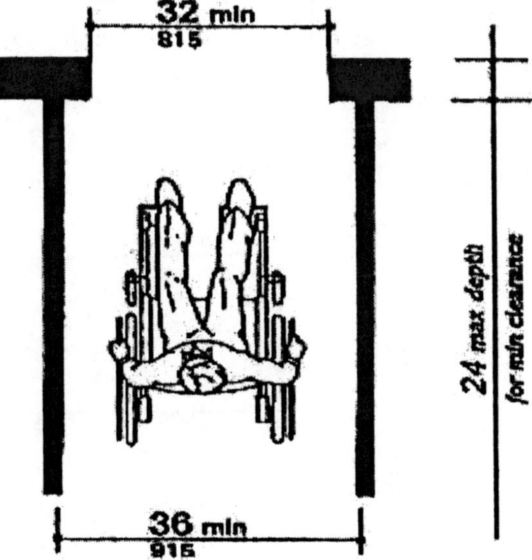

FIGURE 4.8. Minimum clear width for single wheelchair.

Americans with Disabilities Act of 1990, Accessibility Guidelines for Facilities. Federal Register / Vol. 56, No. 144 / Friday, July 26, 1991 / Rules and Regulations, p. 35622. Final Rule Part III CFR 28 Part 36. A copy of the final federal rule should be obtained from American with Disabilities Act's Architectural and Transportation Barriers Compliance Board, U.S. Department of Justice, Civil Rights Division (Washington, DC). A copy of American National Standard Accessible and Usable Building and Facilities, CABO/ANSI A117.1-1992 should be obtained from American National Standards Institute, 11 West 42nd St., New York, NY, 10036.

Width of wheelchair passing. 60 inches (see Figure 4.9).

Wheelchair Turning Space (to make 180° turn). Clear space of 60 inches or T-shaped space (see Figure 4.10).

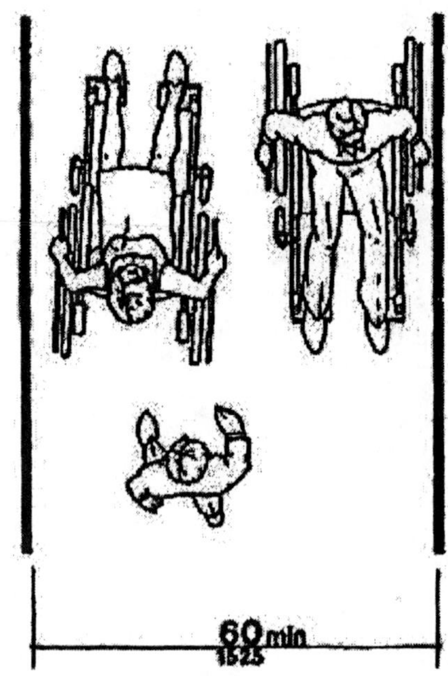

FIGURE 4.9. Minimum clear width for two wheelchairs.

Americans with Disabilities Act of 1990, Accessibility Guidelines for Facilities. Federal Register / Vol. 56, No. 144 / Friday, July 26, 1991 / Rules and Regulations, p. 35622. Final Rule Part III CFR 28 Part 36. A copy of the final federal rule should be obtained from American with Disabilities Act's Architectural and Transportation Barriers Compliance Board, U.S. Department of Justice, Civil Rights Division (Washington, DC). A copy of American National Standard Accessible and Usable Building and Facilities, CABO/ANSI A117.1-1992 should be obtained from American National Standards Institute, 11 West 42nd St., New York, NY, 10036.

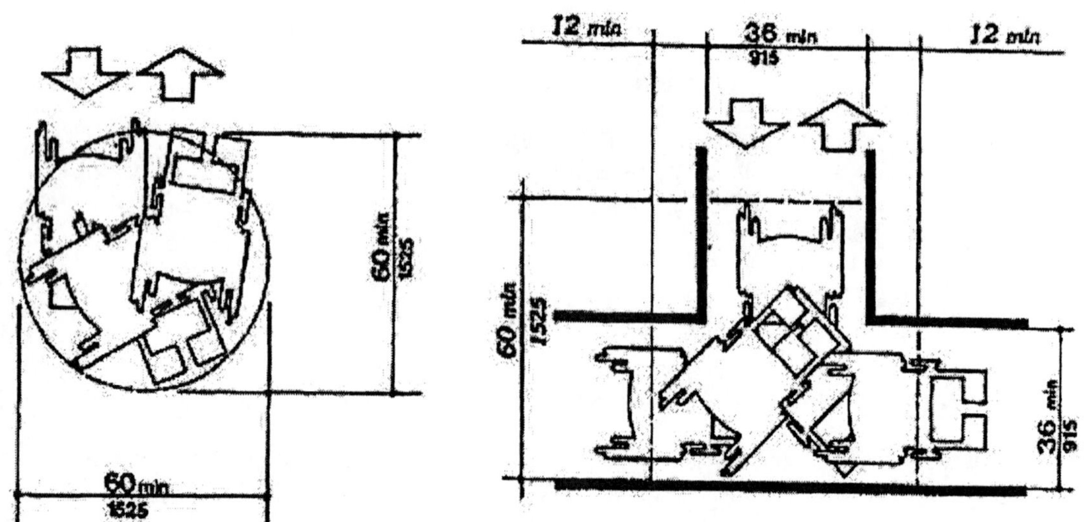

FIGURE 4.10. Wheelchair turning space.

Americans with Disabilities Act of 1990, Accessibility Guidelines for Facilities. Federal Register / Vol. 56, No. 144 / Friday, July 26, 1991 / Rules and Regulations, p. 35622. Final Rule Part III CFR 28 Part 36. A copy of the final federal rule should be obtained from American with Disabilities Act's Architectural and Transportation Barriers Compliance Board, U.S. Department of Justice, Civil Rights Division (Washington, DC). A copy of American National Standard Accessible and Usable Building and Facilities, CABO/ANSI A117.1-1992 should be obtained from American National Standards Institute, 11 West 42nd St., New York, NY, 10036.

Relationship of Maneuvering Clearances to Wheelchair Spaces. One unobstructed side adjoining an accessible route (see Figure 4.11).

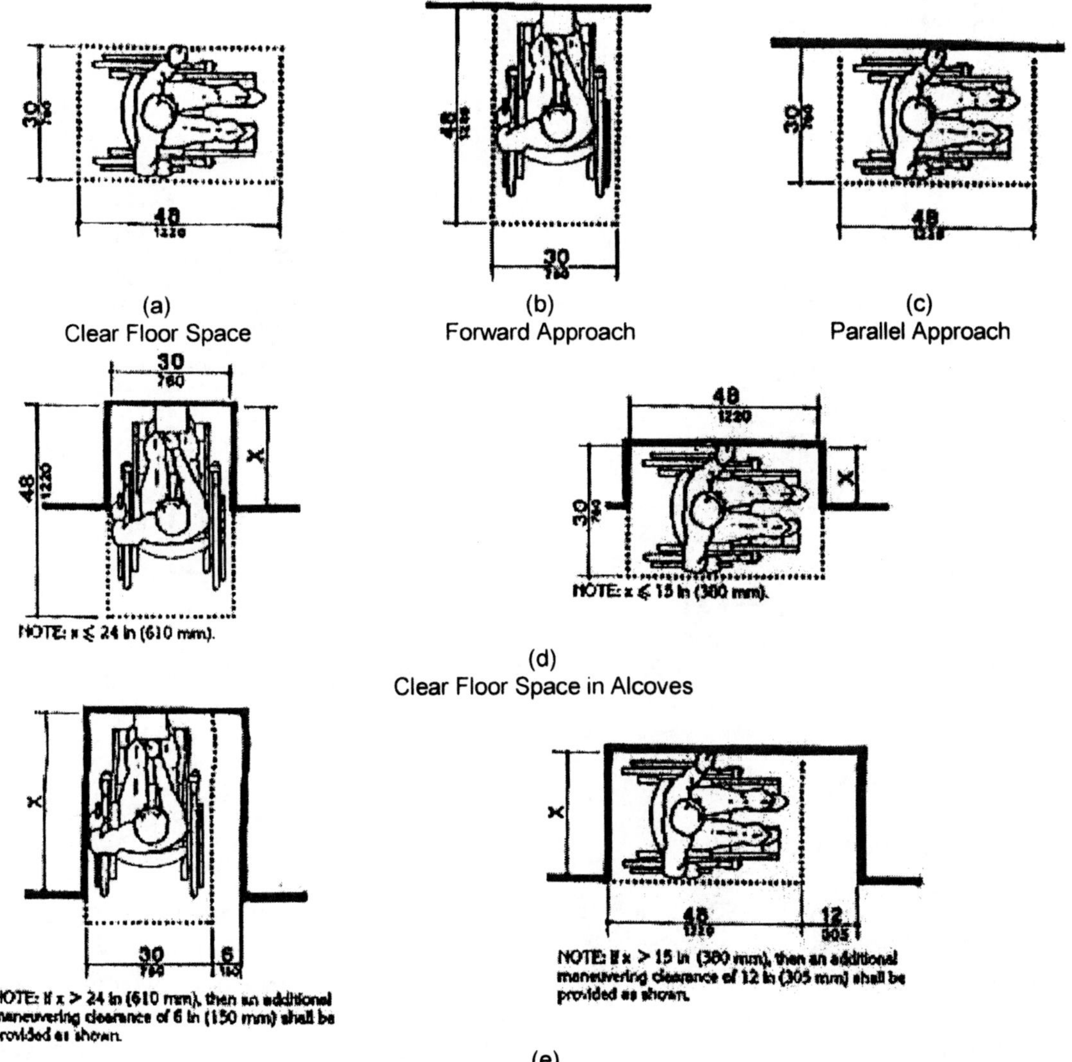

FIGURE 4.11. Minimum clear floor space for wheelchairs.

Americans with Disabilities Act of 1990, Accessibility Guidelines for Facilities. Federal Register / Vol. 56, No. 144 / Friday, July 26, 1991 / Rules and Regulations, p. 35622. Final Rule Part III CFR 28 Part 36. A copy of the final federal rule should be obtained from American with Disabilities Act's Architectural and Transportation Barriers Compliance Board, U.S. Department of Justice, Civil Rights Division (Washington, DC). A copy of American National Standard Accessible and Usable Building and Facilities, CABO/ANSI A117.1-1992 should be obtained from American National Standards Institute, 11 West 42nd St., New York, NY, 10036.

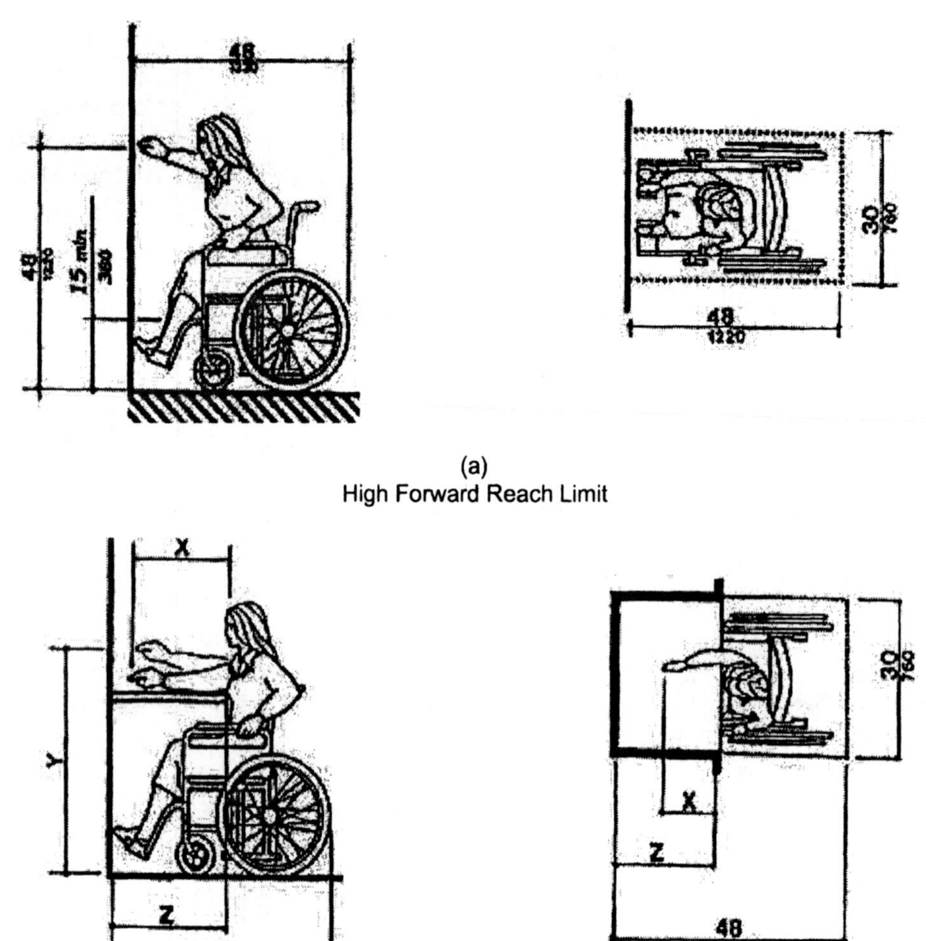

(a)
High Forward Reach Limit

Note: x shall be < 25 in (635 mm); z shall be > x. When x < 20 in (510 mm), then y shall be > 48 in (1220 mm) maximum. When x is 20 to 25 in (510 to 635 mm), then y shall be 44 in (1120 mm) maximum.

(b)
Maximum Forward Reach over an Obstruction

FIGURE 4.12. Forward reach

Americans with Disabilities Act of 1990, Accessibility Guidelines for Facilities. Federal Register / Vol. 56, No. 144 / Friday, July 26, 1991 / Rules and Regulations, p. 35622. Final Rule Part III CFR 28 Part 36. A copy of the final federal rule should be obtained from American with Disabilities Act's Architectural and Transportation Barriers Compliance Board, U.S. Department of Justice, Civil Rights Division (Washington, DC). A copy of American National Standard Accessible and Usable Building and Facilities, CABO/ANSI A117.1-1992 should be obtained from American National Standards Institute, 11 West 42nd St., New York, NY, 10036.

Side Reach. Between 9 inches and 54 inches off the floor (see Figure 4.13).

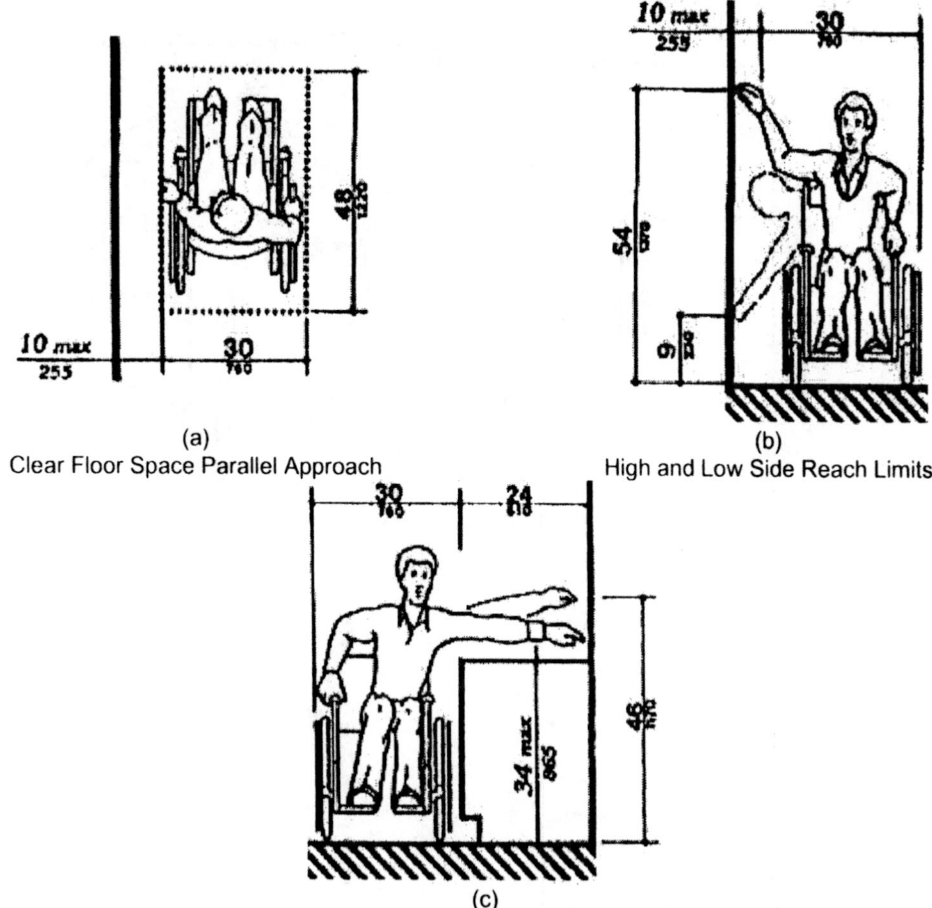

(a)
Clear Floor Space Parallel Approach

(b)
High and Low Side Reach Limits

(c)
Maximum Side Reach over Obstruction

FIGURE 4-.3. Side reach

Americans with Disabilities Act of 1990, Accessibility Guidelines for Facilities. Federal Register / Vol. 56, No. 144 / Friday, July 26, 1991 / Rules and Regulations, p. 35622. Final Rule Part III CFR 28 Part 36. A copy of the final federal rule should be obtained from American with Disabilities Act's Architectural and Transportation Barriers Compliance Board, U.S. Department of Justice, Civil Rights Division (Washington, DC). A copy of American National Standard Accessible and Usable Building and Facilities, CABO/ANSI A117.1-1992 should be obtained from American National Standards Institute, 11 West 42nd St., New York, NY, 10036.

4.3 Accessible Route

Must meet definition in section 3 above, be at least 36 inches wide (32 inches at doors), allow for turns around objects (see Figure 4.14) have passing spaces 60 inches wide at least every 200 feet, 80-inch turn room, stable, firm, and slip-resistant surface texture, and meet change of level requirements.

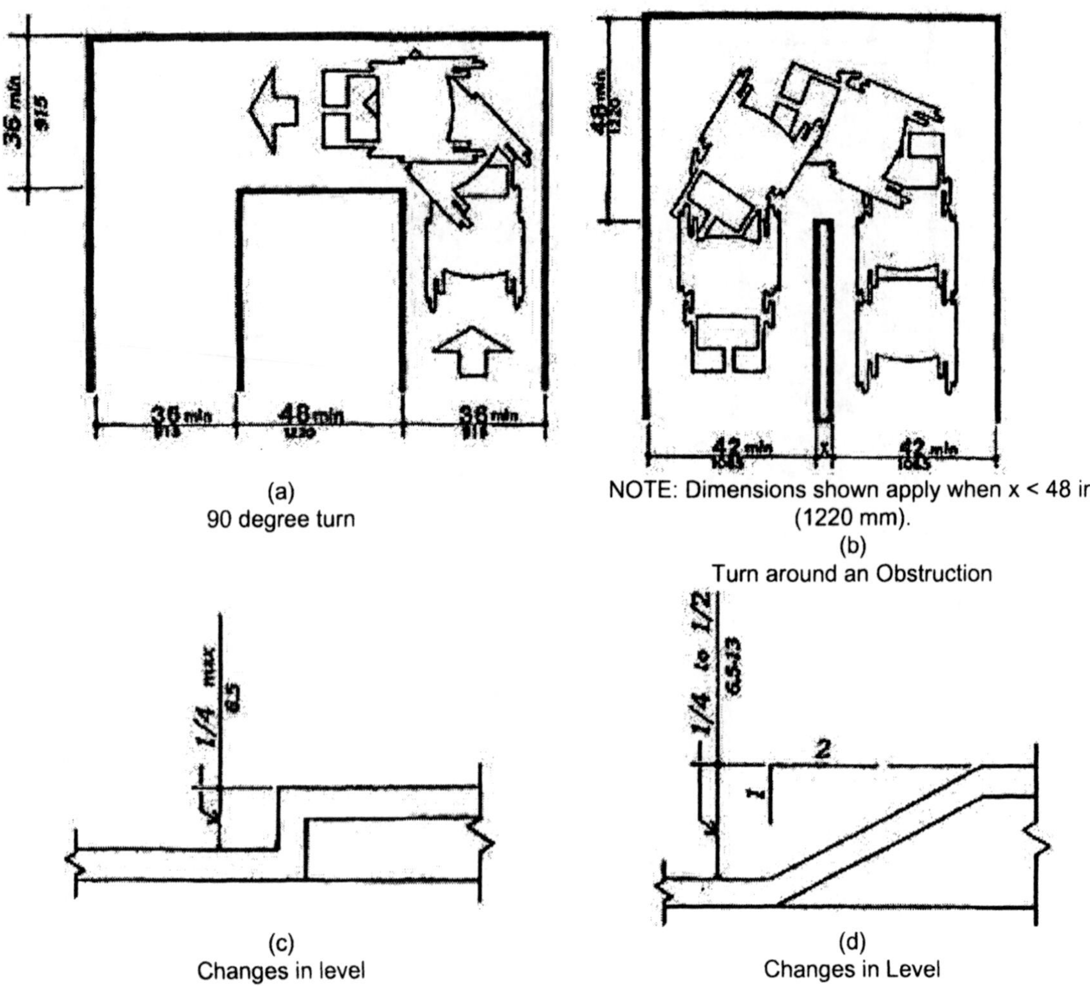

FIGURE 4.14. Accessible route.

Americans with Disabilities Act of 1990, Accessibility Guidelines for Facilities. Federal Register / Vol. 56, No. 144 / Friday, July 26, 1991 / Rules and Regulations, p. 35622. Final Rule Part III CFR 28 Part 36. A copy of the final federal rule should be obtained from American with Disabilities Act's Architectural and Transportation Barriers Compliance Board, U.S. Department of Justice, Civil Rights Division (Washington, DC). A copy of American National Standard Accessible and Usable Building and Facilities, CABO/ANSI A117.1-1992 should be obtained from American National Standards Institute, 11 West 42nd St., New York, NY, 10036.

4.4 Protruding Objects

Objects located between 27 and 80 inches above the floor must protrude no more than 4 inches into any hall or passageway or walk. Objects with their leading edge 27 inches high or less may protrude any amount from the wall. Freestanding objects mounted on posts or pylons may overhang 12 inches when mounted between 27 and 80 inches above the floor (e.g. a telephone booth). In no case may protruding objects reduce the clear width of an accessible route or maneuvering space (see Figure 4.15 and 4.15A to D).

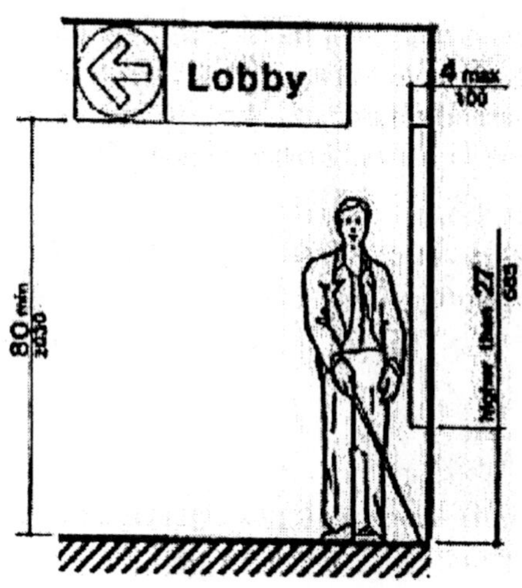

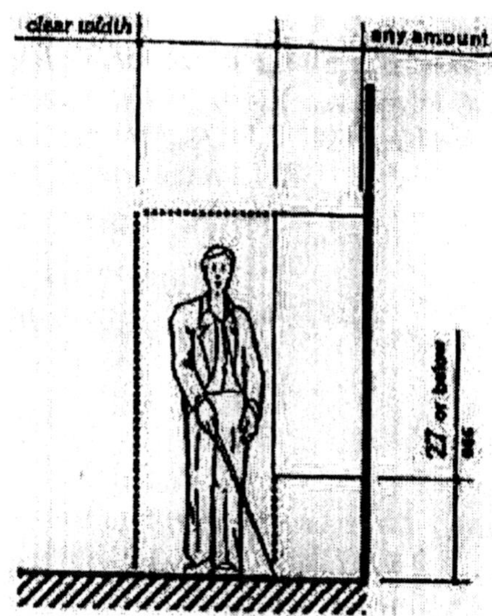

FIGURE 4.15. Protruding objects. (a) Walking parallel to a wall.

Americans with Disabilities Act of 1990, Accessibility Guidelines for Facilities. Federal Register / Vol. 56, No. 144 / Friday, July 26, 1991 / Rules and Regulations, p. 35622. Final Rule Part III CFR 28 Part 36. A copy of the final federal rule should be obtained from American with Disabilities Act's Architectural and Transportation Barriers Compliance Board, U.S. Department of Justice, Civil Rights Division (Washington, DC). A copy of American National Standard Accessible and Usable Building and Facilities, CABO/ANSI A117.1-1992 should be obtained from American National Standards Institute, 11 West 42nd St., New York, NY, 10036.

4.5 Ground and Floor Surfaces

General. Must be stable, firm, and slip-resistant.

Changes in level

- Up to _ inch may be vertical and without edge
- Between _ and _ inch: beveled edge required
- Over _ inch: ramp treatment required

Carpet. Must be securely attached, firm or no pad, with maximum pile height of _ inch, level cut, and trimmed along exposed edge that conforms to changes in level in paragraph above (see Figure 4.16).

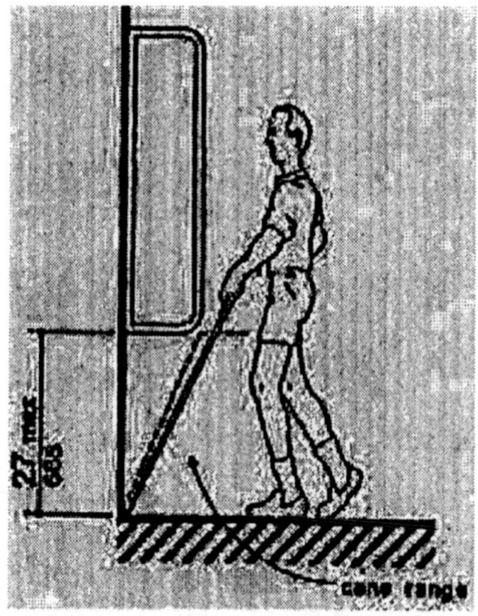

FIGURE 4.15 (b). Walking perpendicular to a wall.

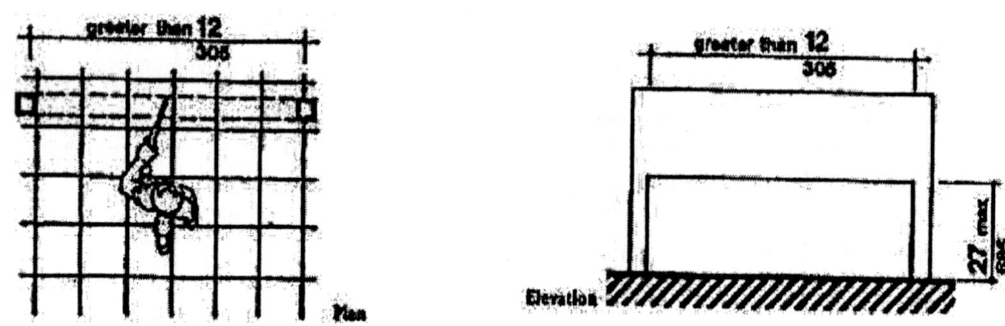

FIGURE 4.15 (c). Free standing overhanging objects.

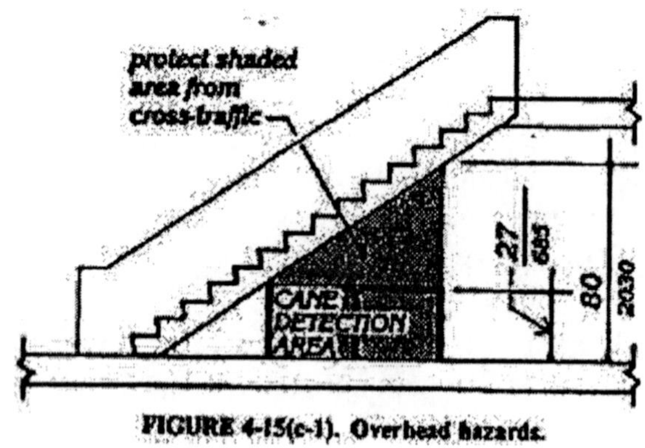

FIGURE 4-15(c-1). Overhead hazards.

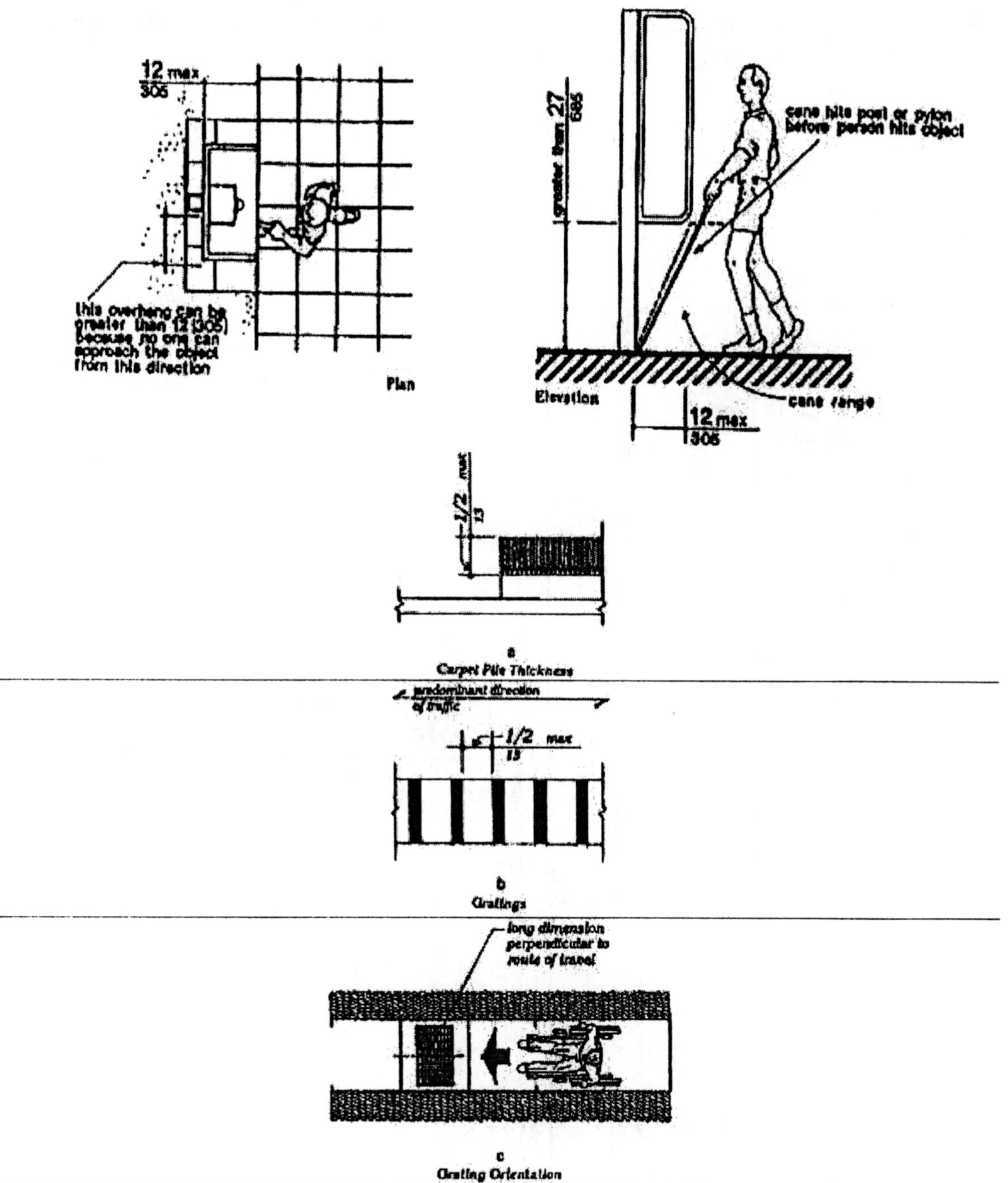

FIGURE 4.16 Protruding objects. (a) Carpet pile thickness, (b) gratings, (c) grating orientation.

Americans with Disabilities Act of 1990, Accessibility Guidelines for Facilities. Federal Register / Vol. 56, No. 144 / Friday, July 26, 1991 / Rules and Regulations, p. 35622. Final Rule Part III CFR 28 Part 36. A copy of the final federal rule should be obtained from American with Disabilities Act's Architectural and Transportation Barriers Compliance Board, U.S. Department of Justice, Civil Rights Division (Washington, DC). A copy of American National Standard Accessible and Usable Building and Facilities, CABO/ANSI A117.1-1992 should be obtained from American National Standards Institute, 11 West 42nd St., New York, NY, 10036.

Gratings. Maximum width of openings: _ inch. If in walkways, the _ inch openings must be perpendicular to dominant direction of travel .

4.6 Parking and Passenger Loading Zones

Parking spaces	Space requirements Minimum accessible spaces
1–25	1
26–50	2
51–75	3
76–100	4
101–150	5
151–200	6
201–300	7
301–400	8

Spaces shall be at least 96 inches wide with an accessible aisle at least 60 inches wide (two spaces may share one aisle). A van space must be provided and designated by signage (see Figures 4.17 and 4.18).

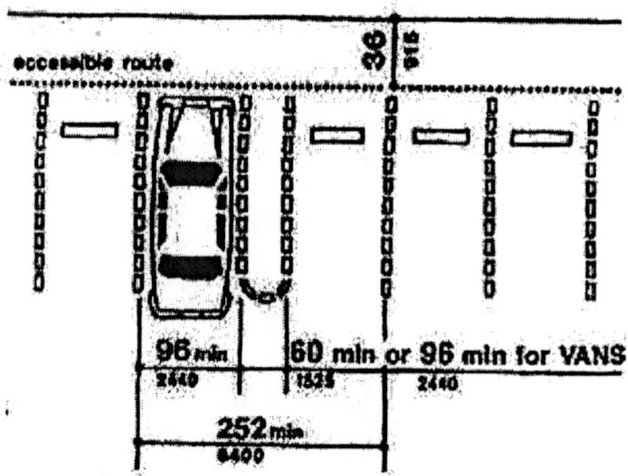

FIGURE 4.17. Dimensions of parking spaces.

Americans with Disabilities Act of 1990, Accessibility Guidelines for Facilities. Federal Register / Vol. 56, No. 144 / Friday, July 26, 1991 / Rules and Regulations, p. 35622. Final Rule Part III CFR 28 Part 36. A copy of the final federal rule should be obtained from American with Disabilities Act's Architectural and Transportation Barriers Compliance Board, U.S. Department of Justice, Civil Rights Division (Washington, DC). A copy of American National Standard Accessible and Usable Building and Facilities, CABO/ANSI A117.1-1992 should be obtained from American National Standards Institute, 11 West 42nd St., New York, NY, 10036

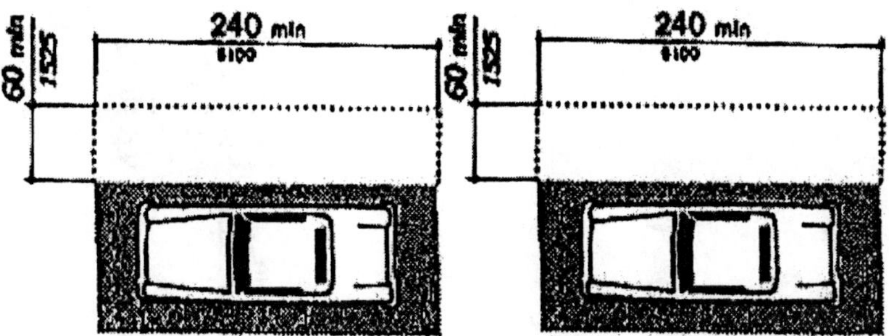

FIGURE 4.18. Access aisle at passenger loading zones.

Americans with Disabilities Act of 1990, Accessibility Guidelines for Facilities. Federal Register / Vol. 56, No. 144 / Friday, July 26, 1991 / Rules and Regulations, p. 35622. Final Rule Part III CFR 28 Part 36. A copy of the final federal rule should be obtained from American with Disabilities Act's Architectural and Transportation Barriers Compliance Board, U.S. Department of Justice, Civil Rights Division (Washington, DC). A copy of American National Standard Accessible and Usable Building and Facilities, CABO/ANSI A117.1-1992 should be obtained from American National Standards Institute, 11 West 42nd St., New York, NY, 10036

The **standard handicapped symbol** must be placed so that it is not obscured by a parked vehicle. A passenger loading zone at least 60 inches wide and 20 feet long adjacent and parallel to the vehicle pull-up space must be provided.

4.7 Curb Ramps

Location. Wherever an accessible route crosses a curb (see Figures 4.19 and 4.20).
Figure 4.20 Built-up curb ramp.

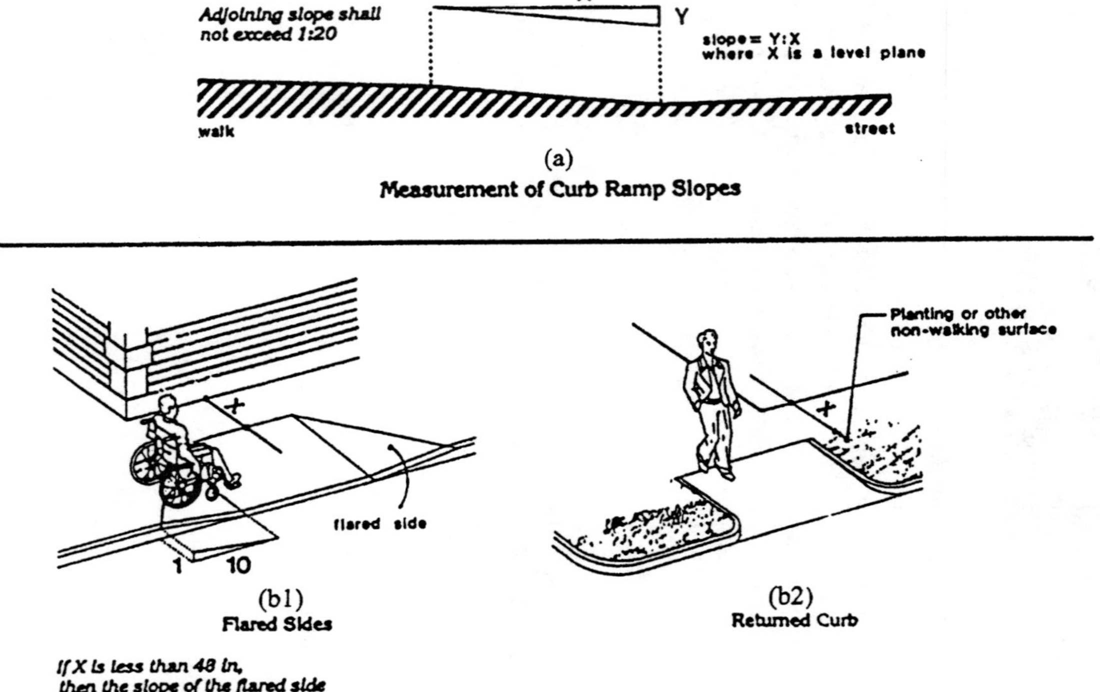

FIGURE 4-19. Measurement of curb ramp slopes (a), sides of curb ramps (b).
Americans with Disabilities Act of 1990, Accessibility Guidelines for Facilities. *Federal Register* / Vol. 56, No. 144 / Friday, July 26, 1991 / Rules and Regulations, p. 35622. Final Rule Part III CFR 28 Part 36. A copy of the final federal rule should be obtained from American with Disabilities Act's Architectural and Transportation Barriers Compliance Board, U.S. Department of Justice, Civil Rights Division (Washington, DC). A copy of *American National Standard Accessible and Usable Buildings and Facilities,* CABO/ANSI A117.1-1992 should be obtained from American National Standards Institute, 11 West 42nd St., New York, NY, 10036.

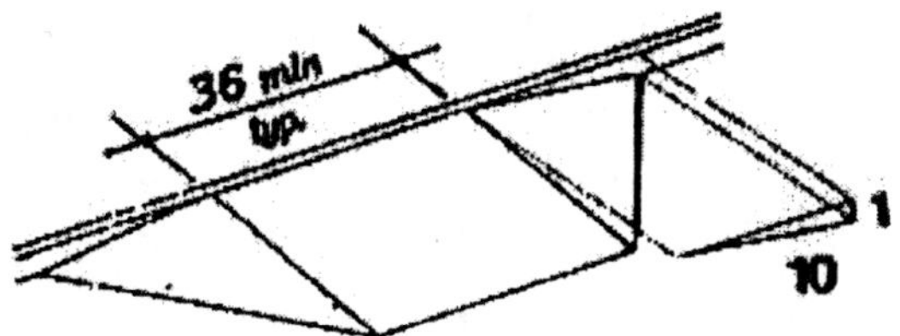

FIGURE 4.20. Built-up curb ramp.
Americans with Disabilities Act of 1990, Accessibility Guidelines for Facilities. Federal Register / Vol. 56, No. 144 / Friday, July 26, 1991 / Rules and Regulations, p. 35622. Final Rule Part III CFR 28 Part 36. A copy of the final federal rule should be obtained from American with Disabilities Act's Architectural and Transportation Barriers Compliance Board, U.S. Department of Justice, Civil Rights Division (Washington, DC). A copy of American National Standard Accessible and Usable Building and Facilities, CABO/ANSI A117.1-1992 should be obtained from American National Standards Institute, 11 West 42nd St., New York, NY, 10036

4.8 Ramps

Ramp. Any part of an accessible route with a slope greater than 1:20.

Rise and Slope. Least possible slope is to be used. Maximum slope is 1:12, maximum rise 30 inches.

Landings. Required at bottom and top of each run, as wide as widest ramp run leading to it (minimum of 60 inches). Minimum 60 inches by 60 inches if ramp changes direction at a landing.

Handrails. If there is a rise of more than 6 inches or a horizontal projection of greater than 72 inches, it must have handrails on both sides (see Figure 4.21).

Cross Slopes. Maximum of 1:50.

4.9 Stairs

Treads and Risers. On any given flight of stairs, riser heights and tread widths must be uniform. Treads must be no less than 11 inches apart, measured from one riser to another. Risers must be a maximum of 7 inches high. Open risers are never permitted on an accessible route. Nosing must project no more than 1_ inches (see Figure 4.22).

Handrails. See "Ramps" (section 4.8) above. Also, at the bottom, the handrail shall continue to slope for the distance of one tread past the bottom riser, then extend parallel to the floor or ground surface for 12 inches.
Gripping surfaces must be uninterrupted by newel posts, other construction elements, or obstructions. Top of handrail gripping surface shall be mounted between 34 and 38 inches above stair nosings. Ends of handrails shall be either rounded or returned smoothly to floor, wall or post. Handrails must not rotate within their fittings (see Figure 4.23).

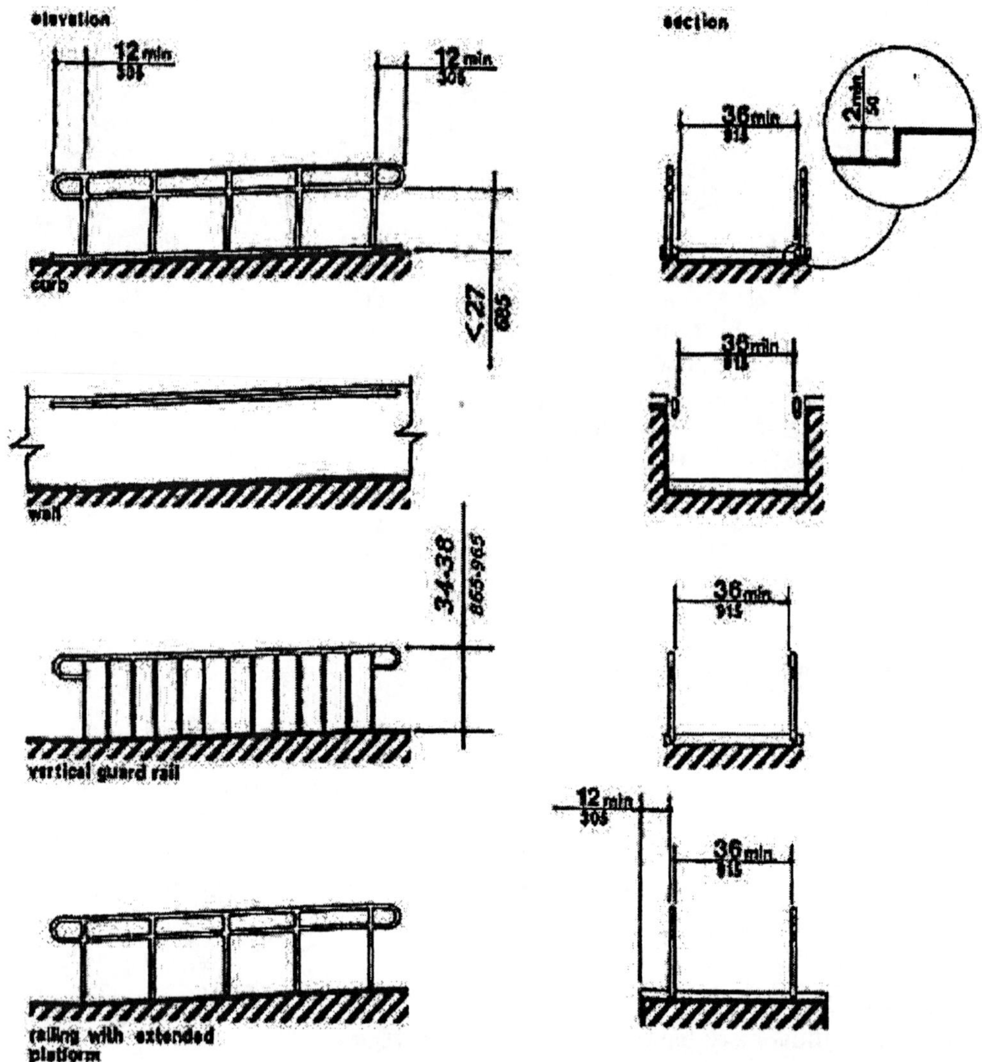

FIGURE 4.21. Examples of edge protection and handrail extensions.

Americans with Disabilities Act of 1990, Accessibility Guidelines for Facilities. Federal Register / Vol. 56, No. 144 / Friday, July 26, 1991 / Rules and Regulations, p. 35622. Final Rule Part III CFR 28 Part 36. A copy of the final federal rule should be obtained from American with Disabilities Act's Architectural and Transportation Barriers Compliance Board, U.S. Department of Justice, Civil Rights Division (Washington, DC). A copy of American National Standard Accessible and Usable Building and Facilities, CABO/ANSI A117.1-1992 should be obtained from American National Standards Institute, 11 West 42nd St., New York, NY, 10036

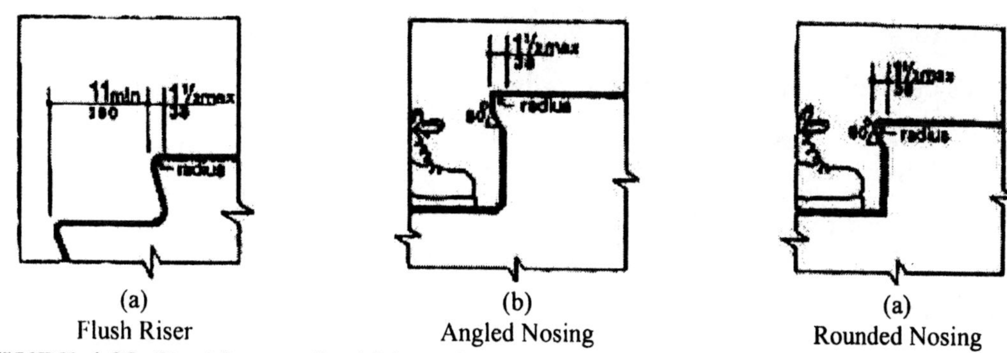

(a) Flush Riser (b) Angled Nosing (a) Rounded Nosing

FIGURE 4.22. Usable tread width and examples of accessible nosings.
Americans with Disabilities Act of 1990, Accessibility Guidelines for Facilities. See Below

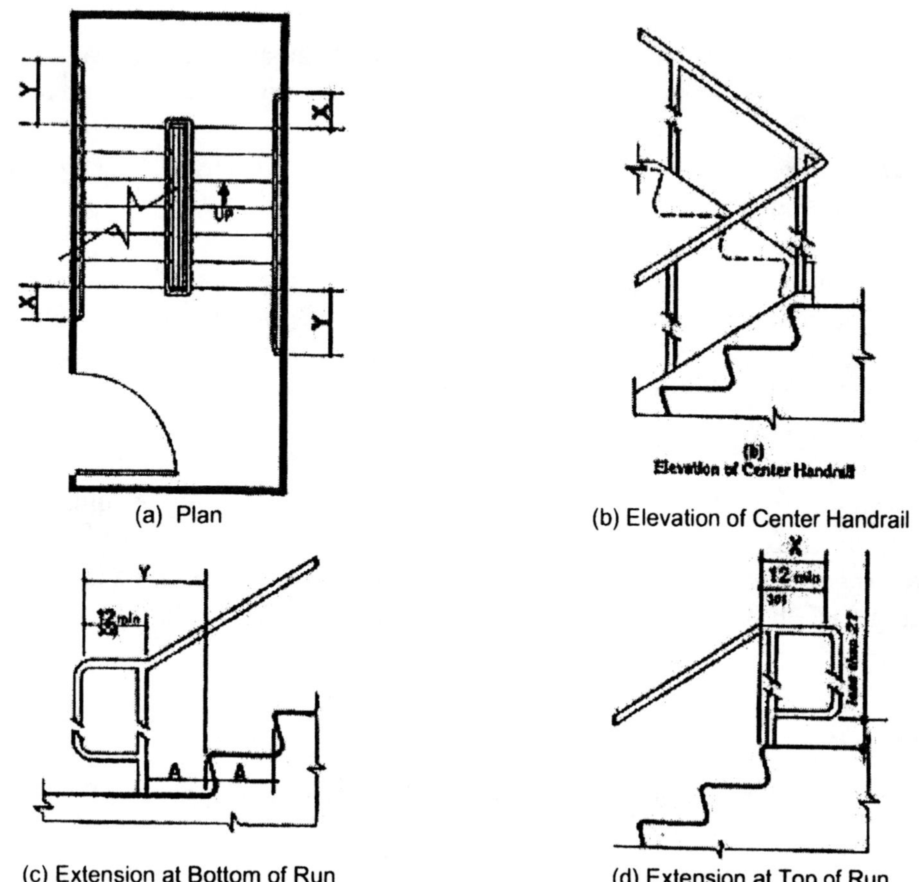

(a) Plan (b) Elevation of Center Handrail

(c) Extension at Bottom of Run (d) Extension at Top of Run

NOTE: X is the 12 in minimum handrail extension required at each top riser.
Y is the minimum handrail extension of 12 in plus the width of one tread that is required at each bottom riser.

FIGURE 4.23. Stair Handrails.
Americans with Disabilities Act of 1990, Accessibility Guidelines for Facilities. Federal Register / Vol. 56, No. 144 / Friday, July 26, 1991 / Rules and Regulations, p. 35622. Final Rule Part III CFR 28 Part 36. A copy of the final federal rule should be obtained from American with Disabilities Act's Architectural and Transportation Barriers Compliance Board, U.S. Department of Justice, Civil Rights Division (Washington, DC). A copy of American National Standard Accessible and Usable Building and Facilities, CABO/ANSI A117.1-1992 should be obtained from American National Standards Institute, 11 West 42nd St., New York, NY, 10036

4.10 Elevators

Numerous detailed requirements are set forth.

4.11 Wheelchair Lifts

Are permitted, must meet local requirements.

4.12 Windows

Reserved (i.e., no requirements set at this time).

4.13 Doors

Clear Width. Must be 32 inches at openings, which must be at an angle of 90° to accessible route. Two doors in series must have at least 48 inches between them.

Thresholds at Doorways. Shall not exceed _ of an inch in height for exterior sliding doors or _ inch for other types.

Hardware. Handles, pulls, latches, locks, and other operating devices on accessible doors must have a shape that is easy to grasp with one hand and does not require tight grasping, tight pinching, or twisting of the wrist to operate. Lever-operated mechanisms, push-type mechanisms, and shaped handles are acceptable designs, no more than 48 inches above the finished floor.

Door Opening Force. Five pounds maximum for interior and sliding or folding doors.

Automatic Doors and Power-Assisted Doors. Should be slow opening and low powered: not opening back to back faster than 3 seconds, needing no more than 15 pounds to stop movement.

4.14 Entrances

Must be part of an accessible route and all accessible spaces and elements within a facility.

4.15 Drinking Fountains and Water Coolers

Spouts. Shall be no higher than 36 inches, located at the front of the fountain, flowing parallel with the front of the unit and at least 4 inches high (to allow for a cup or glass to be inserted under the stream of water) (see Figure 4.24).

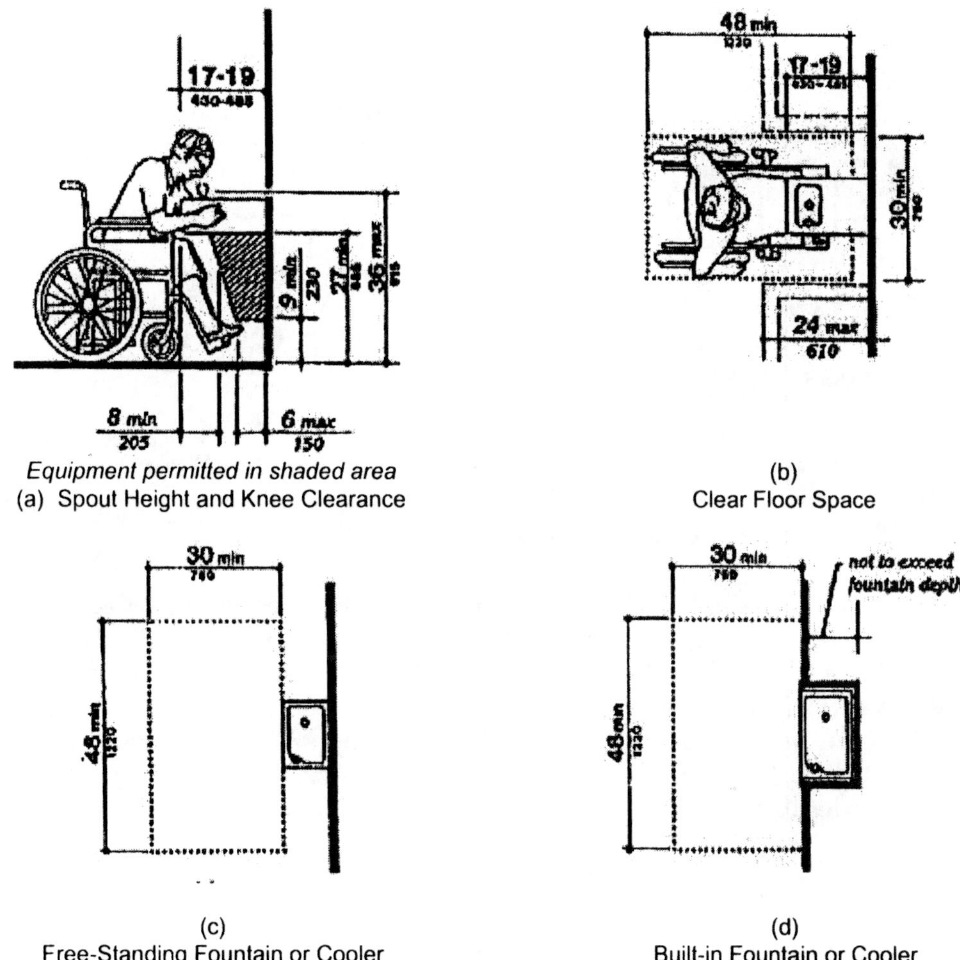

Equipment permitted in shaded area
(a) Spout Height and Knee Clearance

(b)
Clear Floor Space

(c)
Free-Standing Fountain or Cooler

(d)
Built-in Fountain or Cooler

FIGURE 4.24. Drinking fountains and water colors.

Americans with Disabilities Act of 1990, Accessibility Guidelines for Facilities. Federal Register / Vol. 56, No. 144 / Friday, July 26, 1991 / Rules and Regulations, p. 35622. Final Rule Part III CFR 28 Part 36. A copy of the final federal rule should be obtained from American with Disabilities Act's Architectural and Transportation Barriers Compliance Board, U.S. Department of Justice, Civil Rights Division (Washington, DC). A copy of American National Standard Accessible and Usable Building and Facilities, CABO/ANSI A117.1-1992 should be obtained from American National Standards Institute, 11 West 42nd St., New York, NY, 10036

Controls. Shall be located at or near the front edge of the fountain, be operable with one hand, easily grasped, needing no more than 5 pounds of pressure to operate.

4.16 Water Closets

Toilets not in stalls must meet clear floor space requirements and may have either right-handled or left-handled approach. Height of 17–19 inches to top of toilet seat, with grab bars on walls mounted 33–36 inches off floor on side and rear walls. Flush control to require no more than 5 pounds of force to operate (see Figure 4.25).

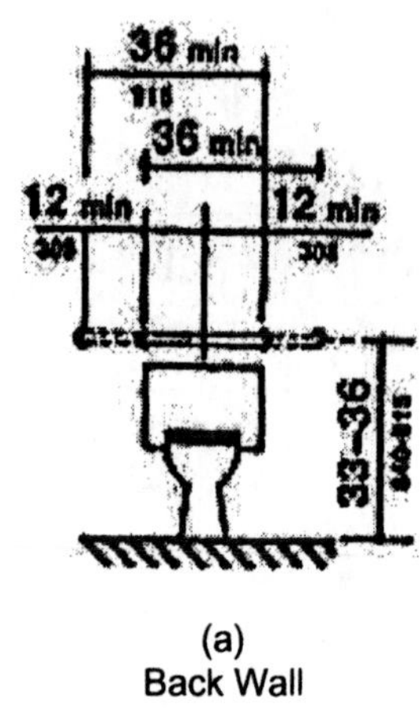

(a)
Back Wall

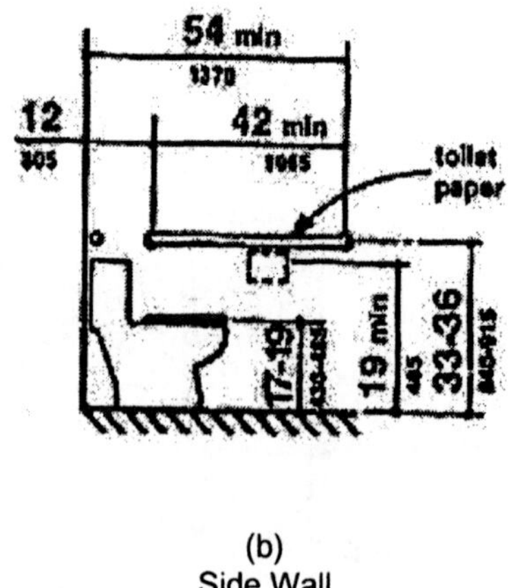

(b)
Side Wall

FIGURE 4.25. Grab bars at water closets.

Americans with Disabilities Act of 1990, Accessibility Guidelines for Facilities. Federal Register / Vol. 56, No. 144 / Friday, July 26, 1991 / Rules and Regulations, p. 35622. Final Rule Part III CFR 28 Part 36. A copy of the final federal rule should be obtained from American with Disabilities Act's Architectural and Transportation Barriers Compliance Board, U.S. Department of Justice, Civil Rights Division (Washington, DC). A copy of American National Standard Accessible and Usable Building and Facilities, CABO/ANSI A117.1-1992 should be obtained from American National Standards Institute, 11 West 42nd St., New York, NY, 10036

4.17 Toilet Stalls

Toilet stalls must meet numerous dimension requirements (see Figure 4.26). They may be a specified standard or alternative size, must include grab bars, and if less than 60 inches in depth must provide 9 inches of toe clearance.

4.18 Urinals

Urinals may be wall-hung or stall type with elongated rim a maximum of 17 inches above the finished floor; clear floor space of 30 inches by 48 inches is required; hand-operated flush lever (5 pounds of force to operate at most) not more than 44 inches off floor.

4.19 Lavatories and Mirrors

Lavatories must be mounted with the rim or counter surface no higher than 24 inches above the finished floor; provide a clearance of at least 29 inches above the floor to the bottom or the apron (see Figure 4.27).

Hot water and drain pipes under lavatory shall be wrapped and any sharp or abrasive surfaces protected.

Faucets: five pounds of pressure maximum to operate.

Mirrors. Mounted with bottom edge of reflecting surface no higher than 40 inches above the finished floor.

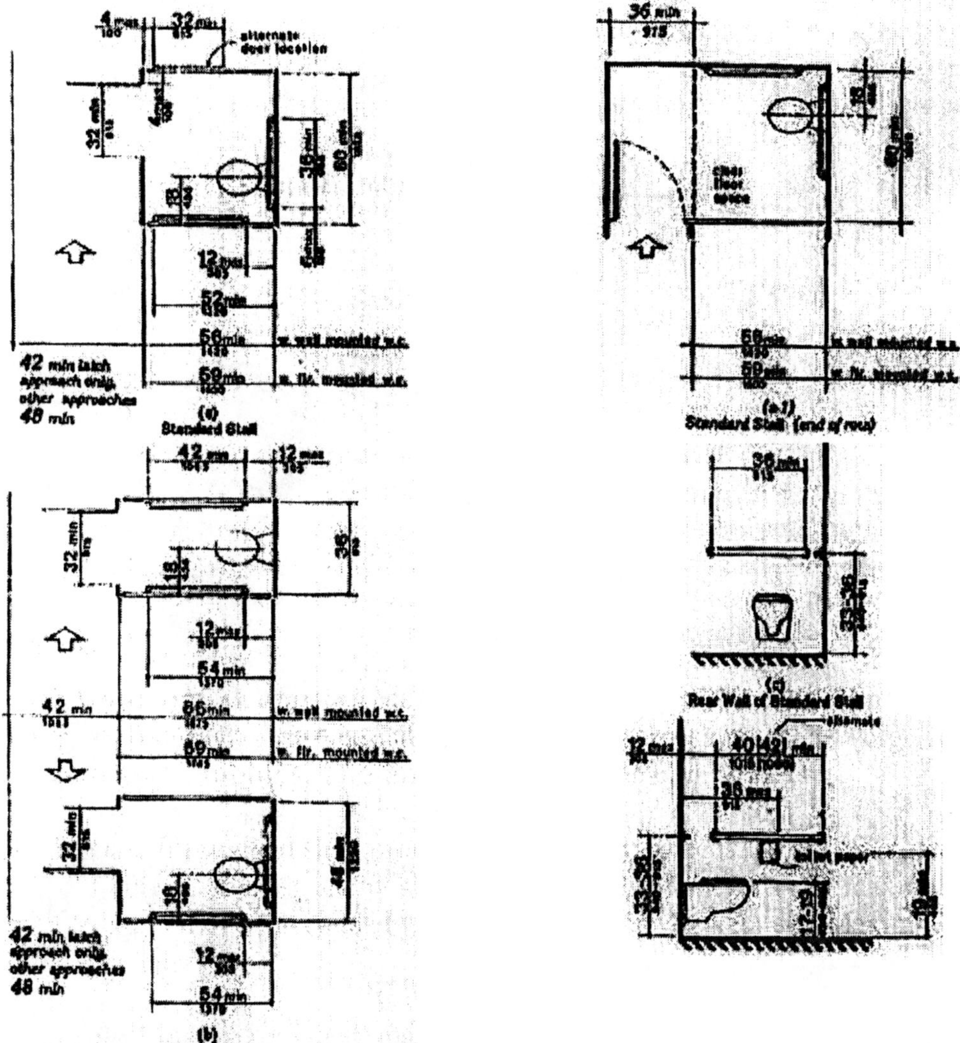

FIGURE 4.26. Toilet Stalls.

Americans with Disabilities Act of 1990, Accessibility Guidelines for Facilities. Federal Register / Vol. 56, No. 144 / Friday, July 26, 1991 / Rules and Regulations, p. 35622. Final Rule Part III CFR 28 Part 36. A copy of the final federal rule should be obtained from American with Disabilities Act's Architectural and Transportation Barriers Compliance Board, U.S. Department of Justice, Civil Rights Division (Washington, DC). A copy of American National Standard Accessible and Usable Building and Facilities, CABO/ANSI A117.1-1992 should be obtained from American National Standards Institute, 11 West 42nd St., New York, NY, 10036

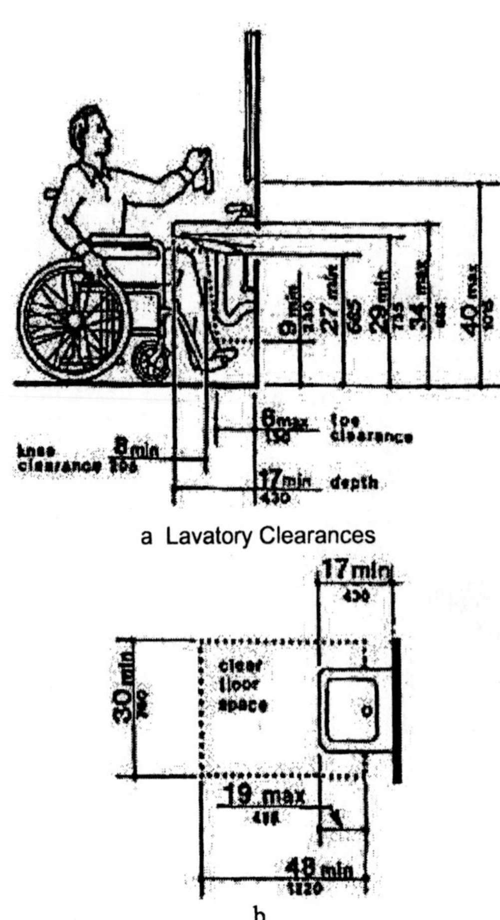

FIGURE 4.27. Lavatory clearances (a); clear floor space at lavatory (b).

Americans with Disabilities Act of 1990, Accessibility Guidelines for Facilities. Federal Register / Vol. 56, No. 144 / Friday, July 26, 1991 / Rules and Regulations, p. 35622. Final Rule Part III CFR 28 Part 36. A copy of the final federal rule should be obtained from American with Disabilities Act's Architectural and Transportation Barriers Compliance Board, U.S. Department of Justice, Civil Rights Division (Washington, DC). A copy of American National Standard Accessible and Usable Building and Facilities, CABO/ANSI A117.1-1992 should be obtained from American National Standards Institute, 11 West 42nd St., New York, NY, 10036

4.20 Bathtubs

Must meet floor space requirements depending on arrangement of bathroom fixtures. They must have the following:

- an in-tub seat or a seat at the head of the tub
- grab bars and controls (5 pounds of pressure maximum pressure to operate) located on near side of tub enclosure
- a shower spray unit with hose at least 60 inches long usable as a hand-held shower or fixed shower spray

4.21 Shower Stalls

Must meet size requirements; have grab bars, controls, and shower hand-held sprayer unit as required for tubs, and provide a seat.

4.22 Toilet Rooms

These must meet requirements as outlined above for doors, toilets, urinals, tubs, and so on. In addition, any medicine cabinet provided must be located so as to have a usable shelf no higher than 44 inches above the floor.

4.23 Bathrooms, Bathing Facilities, and Shower Rooms

Must meet all the above relevant requirements.

4.24 Sinks

Must be accessible and mounted with counter or rim no higher than 34 inches above the finish floor. Knee clearance at least 27 inches high, 30 inches wide, and 19 inches deep under sink. Water depth maximum is 6_ inches. Clear floor space of at least 30 by 48 inches. All exposed pipes covered, faucets easily operated with maximum of 5 pounds of pressure to operate.

4.25 Storage

A clear floor space of 30 by 48 inches, within easy reach ranges, clothes rods a maximum of 54 inches above the finish floor (see Figure 4.28).

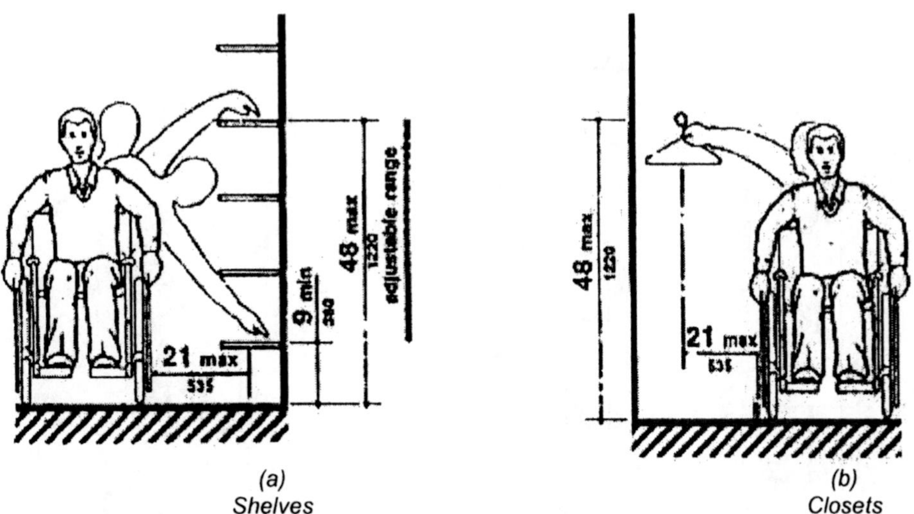

FIGURE 4.28. Shelf placement (a); Closet reach (b).
Americans with Disabilities Act of 1990, Accessibility Guidelines for Facilities. Federal Register / Vol. 56, No. 144 / Friday, July 26, 1991 / Rules and Regulations, p. 35622. Final Rule Part III CFR 28 Part 36. A copy of the final federal rule should be obtained from American with Disabilities Act's Architectural and Transportation Barriers Compliance Board, U.S. Department of Justice, Civil Rights Division (Washington, DC). A copy of American National Standard Accessible and Usable Building and Facilities, CABO/ANSI A117.1-1992 should be obtained from American National Standards Institute, 11 West 42nd St., New York, NY, 10036

4.26 Handrails, Grab Bars, and Tub and Shower Seats

Handrails and grab bars must be 1_ to 1_ inches or provide equivalent gripping surface. If wall mounted, at least 1_ inch space between the grab bar and wall. Bending, sheer stress point: must be 250 pounds of pressure or greater. Must not rotate within fittings and have no sharp edges (minimum radius of edge = 1/8 inch) (see Figure 4.29).

4.27 Controls and Operating Mechanisms

Electrical switches must be located at least 15 inches above the floor.

Clear floor space must allow a forward or parallel approach by a person in a wheelchair.

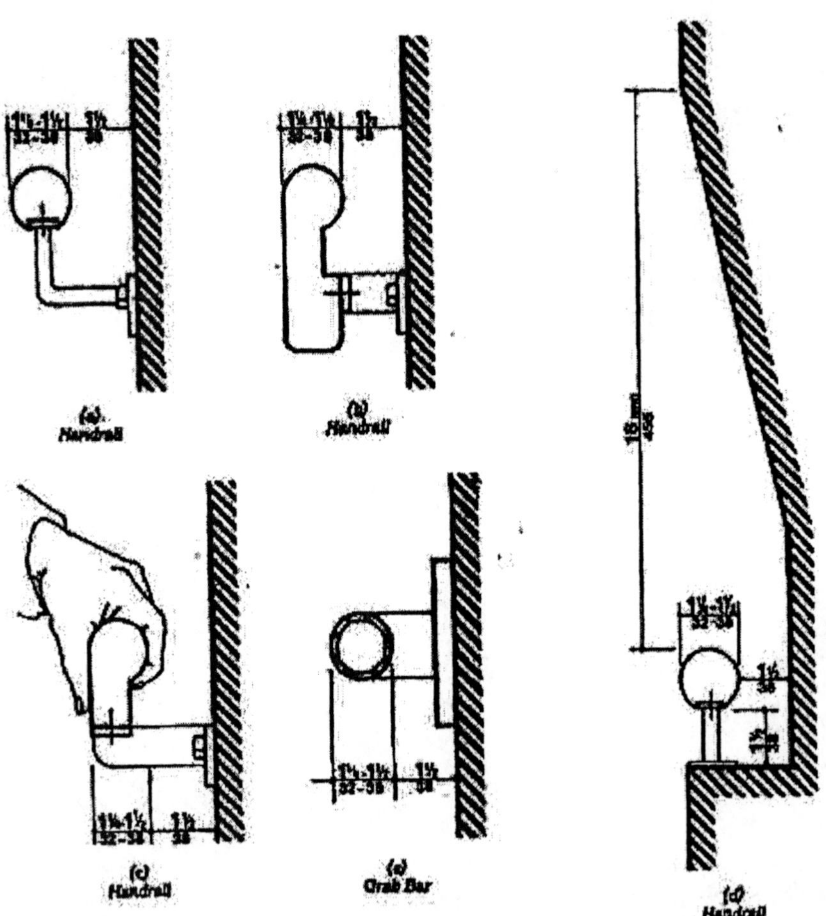

FIGURE 4.29. Size and spacing of handrails and grab bars.

Americans with Disabilities Act of 1990, Accessibility Guidelines for Facilities. Federal Register / Vol. 56, No. 144 / Friday, July 26, 1991 / Rules and Regulations, p. 35622. Final Rule Part III CFR 28 Part 36. A copy of the final federal rule should be obtained from American with Disabilities Act's Architectural and Transportation Barriers Compliance Board, U.S. Department of Justice, Civil Rights Division (Washington, DC). A copy of American National Standard Accessible and Usable Building and Facilities, CABO/ANSI A117.1-1992 should be obtained from American National Standards Institute, 11 West 42nd St., New York, NY, 10036

4.28 Alarms

At least **visual signal appliances** shall be provided in facilities in each of the following areas: restrooms and any other general usage areas (e.g., meeting rooms), hallways, lobbies, and any other area for common use.

Audible Alarms. If provided shall produce a sound that exceeds the prevailing equivalent sound level in the room or space by at least 15 decibels or exceeds any maximum sound level with a duration of 60 seconds by 5 decibels, whichever is louder. Maximum decibel level is 120 decibels.

Visual Alarms. Must be provided; may be integrated into the facility alarm system. Must have following features:

- a xenon strobe-type lamp or equivalent
- color: clear or nominal white
- 0.2 second maximum pulse duration
- minimum 75 candle intensity
- flash rate: minimum of 1 Hz and maximum of 3 Hz
- 80 inches above highest floor level or 6 inches below ceiling, whichever is lower
- no more than 50 feet from all space in a room, 100 feet in large spaces such as auditoriums
- maximum 50 feet apart in hallways and common corridors

Auxiliary alarms. Required in sleeping accommodations and connected to the building emergency alarm system and visible to all areas of the room.

4.29 Detectable Warnings

On walking surfaces shall be 0.9 inch in diameter and 0.2 inch in height with 2.35 inch spacing, contrast visually, and be of material similar to that used on the surface. Shall be provided at hazardous vehicular areas, which are without curbs, and at edges of reflecting pools not having railings, walls, or curbs.

4.30 Signage

Letters must have a width to height ratio between 3:5 and 1:1 and a stroke-width-to-height ratio between 1:5 and 1:10.

Character Height. Sized to viewing distance with a minimum of 3 feet.

Raised and Brailled Characters and Pictorial Symbol Signs. Must meet several size and type specifications.

Symbols of Accessibility. International symbols shall be used and displayed for areas required to be identified as accessible (see Figure 4.30).

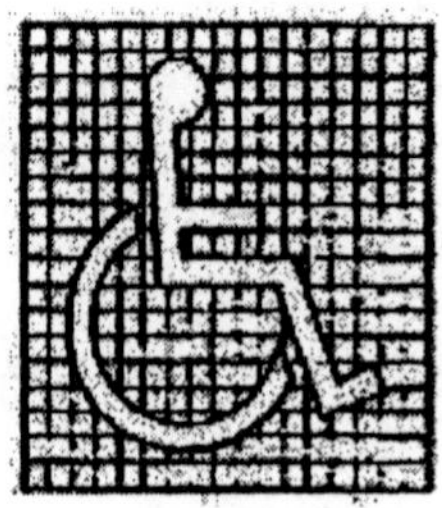

(a)
Proportions
International Symbol of Accessibility

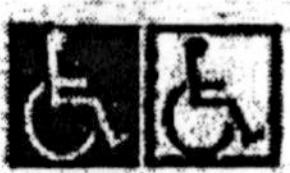

(b)
Display Conditions
International Symbol of Accessibility

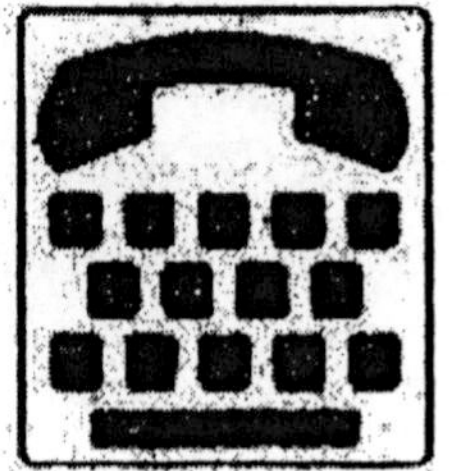

(c)
International TDD Symbol

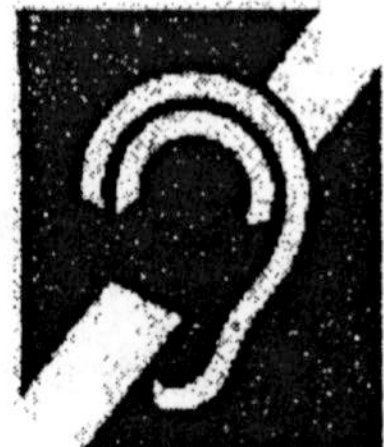

(d)
International Symbol of Access for Hearing Loss

FIGURE 4.30. International symbols.

Americans with Disabilities Act of 1990, Accessibility Guidelines for Facilities. Federal Register / Vol. 56, No. 144 / Friday, July 26, 1991 / Rules and Regulations, p. 35622. Final Rule Part III CFR 28 Part 36. A copy of the final federal rule should be obtained from American with Disabilities Act's Architectural and Transportation Barriers Compliance Board, U.S. Department of Justice, Civil Rights Division (Washington, DC). A copy of American National Standard Accessible and Usable Building and Facilities, CABO/ANSI A117.1-1992 should be obtained from American National Standards Institute, 11 West 42nd St., New York, NY, 10036

4.31 Telephones

Seating/Location. At least 30 inches by 48 inches of clear floor space.

Mounting Heights. Highest part shall be within ranges of 15 to 48 inches of forward reach.

Hearing Aid Compatible and Volume Controllable. Both are required. Volume capable of a minimum of 12 decibels and a maximum of 18 decibels above normal, directories provided within reach and a 29-inch or longer cord. A text telephone may be required.

4.32 Fixed or Built-in Seating and Tables

Knee space of 27 inches high, 30 inches wide, and 19 inches deep must be provided.

Height. Tops of accessible tables and counters shall be from 28 to 34 inches above the floor or ground (see Figure 4.31).

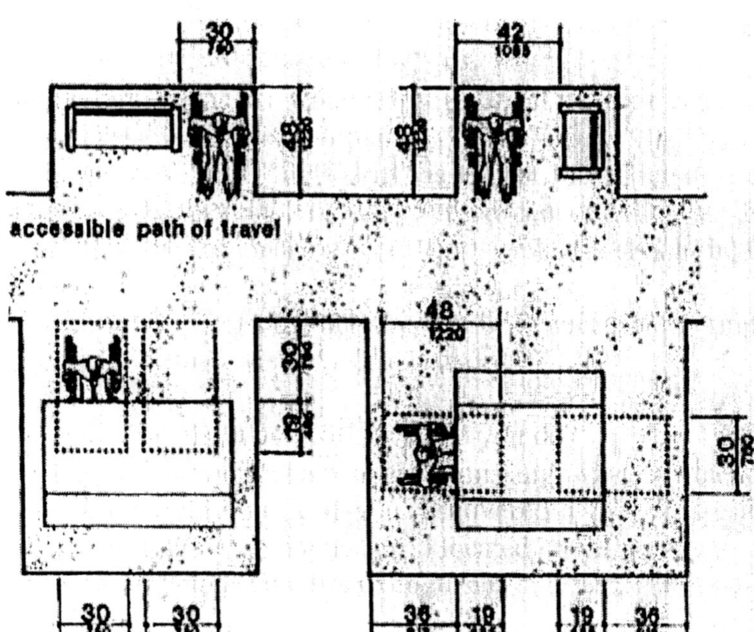

FIGURE 4.31. Minimum clearances for seatings and tables.

Americans with Disabilities Act of 1990, Accessibility Guidelines for Facilities. Federal Register / Vol. 56, No. 144 / Friday, July 26, 1991 / Rules and Regulations, p. 35622. Final Rule Part III CFR 28 Part 36. A copy of the final federal rule should be obtained from American with Disabilities Act's Architectural and Transportation Barriers Compliance Board, U.S. Department of Justice, Civil Rights Division (Washington, DC). A copy of American National Standard Accessible and Usable Building and Facilities, CABO/ANSI A117.1-1992 should be obtained from American National Standards Institute, 11 West 42nd St., New York, NY, 10036

4.33 Assembly Areas

Floor space requirements are provided in Figure 4.32. Wheelchair seating areas must allow a choice of admission prices and lines of sight comparable to those for members of the general public and adjoin an accessible route that serves as a means of egress in case of emergency. At least one companion fixed seat shall be next to each wheelchair space. Readily removable seats may be installed in wheelchair areas when not occupied. Floor surfaces of wheelchair areas must be level. Wheelchair persons must have full access to performing areas. Views of the stage must be complete. Assisted listening systems may be installed.

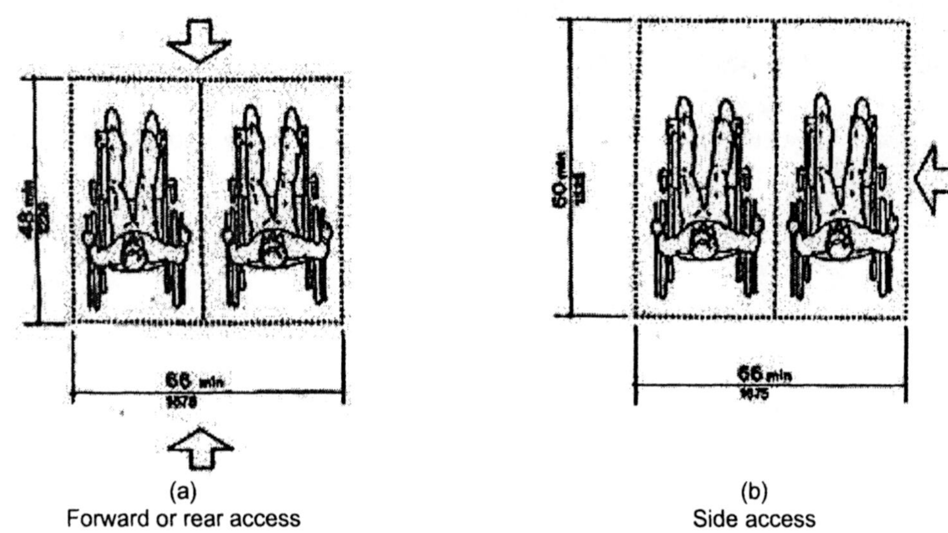

FIGURE 4.32. Space requirements for wheelchair seating spaces in series.

Americans with Disabilities Act of 1990, Accessibility Guidelines for Facilities. Federal Register / Vol. 56, No. 144 / Friday, July 26, 1991 / Rules and Regulations, p. 35622. Final Rule Part III CFR 28 Part 36. A copy of the final federal rule should be obtained from American with Disabilities Act's Architectural and Transportation Barriers Compliance Board, U.S. Department of Justice, Civil Rights Division (Washington, DC). A copy of American National Standard Accessible and Usable Building and Facilities, CABO/ANSI A117.1-1992 should be obtained from American National Standards Institute, 11 West 42nd St., New York, NY, 10036

4.7 Recommended Operating Standards

The following standards are voluntary for assisted living facilities. They are required for nursing facilities. These standards mark the expectations set for providers of long-term care. As residents age in place and receive increasingly sophisticated health-related care in the assisted living facility setting, the assisted living administrator should be aware of the following standards. These recommended standards are found in the *Federal Requirements and Guidelines to Surveyors* (2003) for nursing homes.

Nearly all of these standards are representative of the quality sought by the typical assisted living facility operator. An acquaintance with these industry standards may help the administrator be confident that he or she is providing appropriate quality and can be a tool with which to convince staff of the need for the following quality controls. Acquaintance with these definitions may also be helpful in developing the facility operating standards.

Resident's Environment

The facility should provide a safe, clean, comfortable, and homelike environment, allowing the resident to use his or her personal belongings to the extent possible. A "homelike environment" is one that deemphasizes the institutional character of the setting, to the extent possible, and allows the resident to use those personal belongings that support a homelike environment. A personalized, homelike environment recognizes the individuality and autonomy of the resident, provides an opportunity for self-expression, and encourages links with the past and family members. *Environment* refers to any environment in the facility that is frequented by residents, including the residents' rooms, bathrooms, hallways, activity areas, and any therapy areas.

Necessary Housekeeping and Maintenance Services

This refers to housekeeping and maintenance services necessary to maintain a sanitary, orderly, and comfortable interior.

Sanitary includes, but is not limited to, preventing the spread of disease-causing organisms by keeping resident care equipment clean and properly stored. Resident care equipment includes toothbrushes, dentures, denture cups, glasses and water pitchers, emesis basins, hairbrushes and combs, bed pans, urinals, pads, and positioning devices.

Orderly is defined as an uncluttered physical environment that is neat and well kept.

Balance the resident's need for a homelike environment and the requirements of having a "sanitary" environment in a congregate living situation. For example, a resident may prefer a cluttered room, but does this clutter result in unsanitary or unsafe conditions?

Clean Bed and Bath Linens in Good Condition

Clean bed and bath linens must be kept in good condition.

Adequate and Comfortable Lighting Levels

Adequate lighting is defined as levels of illumination suitable to tasks the resident chooses to perform or the facility staff should perform. For some residents (e.g., those with glaucoma), lower levels of lighting would be more suitable.

Comfortable lighting is defined as lighting that minimizes glare and provides maximum resident control, where feasible, over the intensity, location, and direction of illumination so that visually impaired residents can maintain or enhance independent functioning.

Comfortable and Safe Temperature Levels

Comfortable and safe temperature levels should be maintained. Facilities should maintain a temperature range of 71° to 81° Fahrenheit.

Comfortable and safe temperature levels means that the ambient temperature should be in a relatively narrow range that minimizes residents' susceptibility to loss of body heat and risk of hypothermia or susceptibility to respiratory ailments and colds. (See discussion of hypothermia in Part Five.)

Comfortable Sound Levels

Comfortable sound levels do not interfere with residents' hearing and enhance privacy when privacy is desired. Of particular concern to comfortable sound levels is a resident's control over unwanted noise.

Consider whether residents have difficulty hearing or making themselves heard because of background sounds (e.g., overuse or excessive volume of intercom, shouting, loud TV, cleaning equipment). Consider if it is difficult for residents to concentrate because of distractions or background noise such as traffic, music, equipment, or staff behavior. Consider the comfort of sound levels based on the needs of the residents participating in a particular activity (e.g., the sound levels may have to be turned up for hard-of-hearing individuals watching TV or listening to the radio). Consider the effect of noise on the comfort of residents with dementia.

Disaster and Emergency Preparedness

Preparations include the following:

1. The facility should have detailed written plans and procedures to meet all potential emergencies and disasters, such as fire, severe weather, and missing residents.
2. The facility should train all employees in emergency procedures when they begin to work in the facility, periodically review procedures with existing staff, and carry out unannounced staff drills using those procedures.

The facility should tailor its disaster plan to its geographic location and the types of residents it serves. "Periodic review" is a judgment made by the facility based on its unique circumstances. Changes in physical plant or changes external to the facility can cause a review of a disaster plan.

The purpose of a "staff drill" is to test the efficiency, knowledge, and response of institutional personnel in the event of an emergency. Unannounced staff drills are directed at the responsiveness of staff, and care should be taken not to disturb or excite residents.

To test the extent to which this has been successfully implemented, the assisted living administrator may wish to ask selected staff:

- If the fire alarm goes off, what do you do?
- If you discover that a resident is missing, what do you do?
- What would you do if you discovered a fire in a resident's room? Where are fire alarms and fire extinguisher(s) located on this unit?
- How do you use the fire extinguisher?

Infection Control

The facility should establish and maintain an infection control program designed to provide a safe, sanitary, and comfortable environment and to help prevent the development and transmission of disease and infection.

Infection Control Program. the facility should establish an infection control program under which it

- investigates, controls, and prevents infections in the facility
- Decides what procedures, such as isolation, should be applied to an individual resident
- maintains a record of incidents and corrective actions related to infections

The facility's infection control program should have a system to monitor and investigate causes of infection (nosocomial and community acquired) and manner of spread. A facility, for example, should maintain a separate record on infection that identifies each resident with an infection; states the date of infection, the causative agent, the origin or site of infection, and describes what cautionary measures were taken to prevent the spread of the infection within the facility. The system should enable the facility to analyze clusters, changes in prevalent organisms, or increases in the rate of infection in a timely manner.

Surveillance data should be routinely reviewed and recommendations made for the prevention and control of additional cases.

The written infection control program should be periodically reviewed by the facility and revised as indicated.

Current standards for infection control programs address the following. (The following are not regulatory requirements but provide guidance for evaluating the facility's program.)

- definition of nosocomial/facility-acquired infections and communicable diseases
- risk assessment of occurrence of communicable diseases for both residents and staff

that is reviewed annually, or more frequently if indicated

- methods for identifying, documenting, and investigating nosocomial infections and communicable diseases. The infection control program should be able to identify new infections quickly, paying particular attention to residents at high risk of infection (e.g., residents who are immobilized, have pressure sores, have been recently discharged from a hospital or a long-term care facility, have decreased mental status, or are nutritionally compromised or have altered immune systems)
- early detection of residents who have signs and symptoms of tuberculosis (TB) and a referral protocol to a facility where TB can be evaluated and managed appropriately
- measures for prevention of infections, especially those associated pressure sores, bladder and bowel incontinence, and any other factors that compromise a resident's resistance to infections
- measures for the prevention of communicable disease outbreaks, including tuberculosis, flu, hepatitis, and scabies (see Part Five)
- procedures to inform and involve a local or state epidemiologist, as required by the state for nonsporadic, facility-wide infections that are difficult to control
- use of in-service education regarding standard precautions (e.g., universal precautions/body substance isolation)
- hand washing, respiratory protection, linen handling, housekeeping, needle and hazardous waste disposal, as well as other means for limiting the spread of communicable organisms
- proper use of disinfectants, antiseptics, and germicides in accordance with the manufacturers' instructions and EPA or FDA label specifications to avoid harm to staff, residents, and visitors and to ensure its effectiveness
- orientation of all new facility personnel to the infection control program and periodic updates for all staff
- measures for the screening of the health care workers for communicable diseases, and for the evaluation of workers exposed to residents with communicable diseases, including TB and blood-borne pathogens
- work restriction guidelines for an employee who is infected or ill with a communicable disease
- measures that address prevention of infection common to assisted living residents (e.g., vaccination for influenza and pneumococcal pneumonia as appropriate)
- sanitation of tubs, whirlpools, and multiple use equipment to be performed according to manufacturers' recommendations

The facility should take universal or standard blood and body fluid precautions related to HIV contamination for the following:

- blood
- semen
- vaginal secretions
- cerebrospinal fluid
- synovial fluid
- pleural fluid
- peritoneal fluid

- pericardial fluid
- amniotic fluids
- fluids with visible blood

"Universal precautions" or "standard blood and body fluid precautions" is an approach to infection control where all human blood and certain human body fluids are treated as if known to be infectious for HIV and other blood-borne pathogens.

Employees with Communicable Disease or Infected Skin Lesions

The facility should prohibit employees with a communicable disease or infected skin lesions from direct contact with residents or their food, if direct contact will transmit the disease. The intent of this recommendation is to prevent the spread of communicable diseases from employees to residents when the employee has a communicable disease or an infected skin lesion.

State law defines communicable diseases for purposes of defining facility policies. Skin lesions should be considered infected if they have purulent drainage, or areas hot, indurated without purulent drainage.

Staff Hand Washing After Direct Resident Contact

The facility should require staff to wash their hands after each direct resident contact for which hand washing is indicated by accepted professional practice. The intent of this recommendation is to ensure that staff use appropriate hand-washing techniques to prevent the spread of infection from one resident to another.

Procedures should be followed to prevent cross-contamination, including hand washing or changing gloves after providing personal care, or when performing tasks among individuals that provide the opportunity for cross-contamination to occur. Facilities for hand washing should exist and be readily available to staff. The facility should follow the Centers for Disease Control's *Guideline for Handwashing and Hospital Environmental Control* (1985) for hand washing.

Linens

Personnel should handle, store, process, and transport linens so as to prevent the spread of infection.

Soiled linens should be handled to contain and to minimize aerosolization and exposure of personnel to any waste products. Soiled linen storage areas should be well ventilated and maintained under a relative negative air pressure. The laundry should be designed to eliminate crossing of soiled and clean linen.

Questions the administrator may ask:

- Do staff handle linens on the resident care floors and in the laundry areas to prevent the spread of infection?
- Do staff follow the facility's protocols for handling linens?
- Are linens processed, transported, stored, and handled properly?

Physical Services

The facility should be designed, constructed, equipped, and maintained to protect the health and safety of residents, personnel, and the public.

Fire Safety

Normally, an assisted living facility would seek to meet the *Life Safety Code* current in the year it is built. In any case, the facility should meet the applicable provisions of the 2000 edition of the *Life Safety Code* of the National Fire Protection Association. Incorporation of the 1985 edition of the National Fire Protection Association's *Life Safety Code* (published February 7, 1985; ANSI/NFPA) was approved by the Director of the Federal Register in accordance with 5 U.S.C. 552(a) and 1 CFR Part 51 that govern the use of incorporations by reference. The code is available for inspection at the Office of the Federal Information Center, Room 8301, 1110 L Street N.W., Washington, DC. Copies may be obtained from the National Fire Protection Association, Batterymarch Park, Quincy, MA 02200. If any changes in this code are also to be incorporated by reference, a notice to that effect will be published in the *Federal Register.*

Emergency Power

An emergency electrical power system should supply power adequate at least for lighting all entrances and exits; equipment to maintain the fire detection, alarm, and extinguishing systems; and life support systems in the event the normal electrical supply is interrupted.

Emergency electrical power system includes, at a minimum, battery-operated lighting for all entrances and exits, fire detection and alarm systems, and extinguishing systems. Assisted living facilities, for example, with multiple floors involving an elevator should consider emergency provisions in case of fire causing a power outage.

An *exit* is defined as a means of egress that is lighted and has three components: an exit access (corridor leading to the exit), and exit (a door), and an exit discharge (door to the street or public way). We define an entrance as any door through which people enter the facility. Furthermore, when an entrance also serves as an exit, its components (exit access, exit, and exit discharge) should be lighted. A waiver of lighting requirement for exits and entrances is not permitted.

Additional guidance is available in the National Fire Protection Association's *Life Safety Code* 99 and 101 (NFPA 99 and NFPA 101), 12-5.1.3, which is surveyed in tags K105 and K106 of the *Life Safety Code* survey.

Occasionally, a resident in an assisted living facility may be placed on a life support system. When life support systems are used, the facility should provide emergency electrical power with an emergency generator (as defined in NFPA 99, Health Care Facilities) that is located on the premises.

Life support systems is defined as one or more electromechanical devices necessary to sustain life, without which the resident will have a likelihood of dying (e.g., ventilators, suction machines if necessary to maintain an open airway). The determination of whether a piece of equipment is life support is a medical determination dependent upon the condition of the individual residents of the facility (e.g., a suction machine may be required "life support equipment" in a facility, depending on the needs of its residents).

Sufficient Space and Equipment

The facility should provide sufficient space and equipment in dining, health services, recreation, and program areas to enable staff to provide residents with needed services as required by these standards and as identified in each resident's plan of care.

The intent of this recommendation is to ensure that dining, health services, recreation, activities, and program areas are large enough to comfortably accommodate the needs of the residents who usually occupy this space.

Dining, health services, recreation, and program areas should be large enough to comfortably accommodate the persons who usually occupy that space, including the wheelchairs, walkers, and other ambulation aids used by the many residents who require more than standard movement spaces. *Sufficient space* means the resident can access the area, it is not functionally off-limits, and the resident's functioning is not restricted once access to the space is gained.

Program areas where resident groups engage in activities focused on manipulative skills and hand-eye coordination should have sufficient space for storage of their supplies and "works in progress."

Program areas where residents receive physical therapy should have sufficient space and equipment to meet the needs of the resident's therapy requirement.

Recreation/activities area means any area where residents can participate in those activities identified in their plan of care.

Maintenance of Equipment

Maintain all essential mechanical, electrical, and patient care equipment in safe operating condition.

Questions the administrator may ask:

- Is essential equipment (e.g., boiler room equipment, nursing unit/medication room refrigerators, kitchen refrigerator/freezer and laundry equipment) in safe operating condition?
- Is equipment maintained according to manufacturers' recommendations?

Resident Rooms

Resident rooms should be designed and equipped for adequate ADL care, comfort, and privacy of residents.

Full Visual Privacy for Each Resident

Full visual privacy means that residents have a means of completely withdrawing from public view while occupying their bed (e.g., curtain, moveable screens, private room).

Resident Room Window to the Outside

Each room should have at least one window to the outside.

A facility with resident room windows, as defined by section 13-3.8.1 of the 1985 edition of the *Life Safety Code,* that open to an atrium in accordance with Life Safety Code 6-2.2.3.5 can meet this requirement for a window to the outside.

In addition to conforming with the Life Safety Code, this requirement was included to aid each resident's orientation to day and night, weather, and general awareness of space outside the facility. The facility is required to provide for a "safe, clean, comfortable, and homelike environment" by deemphasizing the institutional character of the setting, to the extent possible. Windows are an important aspect in ensuring the homelike environment of a facility.

Beds

The facility should provide each resident with (1) a separate bed of proper size and height for the convenience of the resident; (2) a clean, comfortable mattress; (3) bedding appropriate to the weather and climate; (4) functional furniture appropriate to the resident's needs, and individual closet space in the resident's bedroom with clothes racks and shelves accessible to the resident.

Shelves accessible to the resident means that the resident, if able, or a staff person at the direction of the resident, can get to the clothes whenever he or she chooses.

Resident Call Systems

A central station should be equipped to receive resident calls through a communication system from (1) resident rooms and (2) toilet and bathing facilities.

The intent is that residents, when in their rooms and toilet and bathing areas, have a means of directly contacting staff at the nurse's station. This communication may be through audible or visual signals and may include wireless systems.

Other Environmental Conditions

The facility should provide a safe, functional, sanitary, and comfortable environment for residents, staff, and the public.

Water Available at All Times

The facility should establish procedures to ensure that water is available to essential areas when there is a loss of normal water supply.

The facility should have a written protocol that defines the source of water provisions for storing the water, both potable and nonpotable, a method for distributing water, and a method for estimating the volume of water required.

Adequate Outside Ventilation

The facility should have adequate outside ventilation by means of windows, or mechanical ventilation, or a combination of the two.

Questions the administrator may ask:

- How well is the space ventilated?
- Is there good air movement?
- Are temperature, humidity, and odor levels all acceptable?

Firmly Secured Handrails in Corridors

The facility should equip corridors with firmly secured handrails on each side. *Secured handrails* means handrails that are firmly affixed to the wall.

Pest Control

The facility should maintain an effective pest control program so that the facility is free of pests and rodents.

An *effective pest control program* is defined as measures to eradicate and contain common household pests (e.g., roaches, ants, mosquitoes, flies, mice, and rats).

REFERENCES

American Hospital Association. (1976). *Taft Hartley Amendments: Implications for the health care field. Report of a symposium.* Chicago: Author.

_____. (1989). *Guide to the health care field.* Chicago: Author.

American National Standards Institute. (1980). *American national standard specifications for making buildings and facilities accessible to and usable by physically handicapped people* (ANSI A117.1–1980). New York: Author.

Argenti, P. A. (1994). *The portable MBA desk reference.* New York: Wiley.

Boling, T. E., Vrooman, D. M., & Sommers, K. M. (1983). *Nursing home management.* Springfield, IL: Charles C Thomas.

Burda, G. (1993). Long term care facts must be addressed. *Modern Healthcare, 23*(44), 36.

Bureau of Labor Statistics. (2002). U.S. Department of Labor, December, 2002

Carley, M. M. (1991, December). New medical devices. Reporting requirements. *Contemporary Long Term Care,* p. 66.

Centers for Medicare and Medicaid Services. (2002). Office of the Actuary, National Health Statistics Group, April 1, 2002.

Cherry, R. L. (1993). Community presence and nursing home quality of care: The ombudsman as a complementary role. *Journal of Health & Social Behavior, 34,* 336–345.

Chruden, J. J., & Sherman, A. W., Jr. (1980). *Personnel management: The utilization of human resource* (6th ed.). Dallas, TX: South-Western.

Clement, P. F. (1985). History of U.S. aged poverty. *Perspectives on Aging, 9*(2), 4–7.

Committee on Nursing Home Regulation, Institute of Medicine. (1986). *Improving the quality of care in nursing homes.* Washington, DC: National Academy Press.

Council on Scientific Affairs. (1990). Home care in the 1990s. *Journal of the American Medical Association, 263,* 1241–1244.

A deregulation report card. (1982, January 11). *Newsweek,* pp. 50–53.

EEOC Notice 915.002. (1994, May 19). *Enforcement guidance* (revised EEOC form 106 [6-91]). Washington, DC: U.S. Government Printing Office.

Enforcing the ADA. (2003). A Status Report from the Department of Justice, January – March, 2003.

Falling short. (1995, July). Austin, TX: SEIO.

Federal requirements and guidelines to surveyors. (19XX). New York: Springer Publishing Co.

Feinleib, S. E., Cunningham, P. J., & Short, P. F. (1994, August). *Use of nursing and personal care homes by the civilian population, 1987* (National medical expenditures survey research findings 23, AHCPR Pub. No. 94-0096). Rockville, MD.

Focus on retirement. (1998, March 9). *The Wall Street Journal,* p. 22.

Freymann, J. G. (1980). *The American health care system: Its genesis and trajectory* Huntington, NY: Robert E. Krieger Publishing.

Greene, V. L., Lovely, M. E., & Ondrich, J. I. (1993). The cost-effectiveness of community services in a frail elderly population. *Gerontologist, 33,* 177–187.

Health Care Financing Administration (HCFA). (1982). Conditions of participation for skilled nursing and intermediate care facilities (a proposed rule), 42 CFR Parts 405, 442, and 483, March 19, 1980. In D. B. Miller (Ed.), *Long term care administrators desk manual* (pp. 7042–7076). Greenvale, NY: Panel Publishers.

Health care labor manual: Vol. 1. (1983). Rockville, MD: Aspen Publishers.

Hogstel, M. O. (1983). *Management of personnel in long-term care.* Bowie, MD: Robert J. Brady Co.

Ivancevich, J. M., & Glueck, W. F. (1983). *Foundations of personnel: Human resource management* (rev. ed.). Plano, TX: Business Publications.

Joint Commission on Accreditation of Hospitals. (1979). *Accreditation manual for hospitals, 1980.* Chicago: Author.

_____. (1982). *Facts about JCAHO.* Chicago: Author.

_____. (1983a). *Accreditation manual for long term care facilities/84.* Chicago: Author.

_____. (1983b). *JCAHO eligibility criteria.* Chicago: Author.

Jonas, S. (1981). *Health care delivery in the United States* (2nd ed.). New York: Springer Publishing Co.

Kaplan, B. (1985). Social Security: 50 years later. *Perspectives on Aging, 9*(2), 4–7.

Kart, C. S. (1981). *The realities of aging.* Boston: Allyn & Bacon.

Lathrop, J. K. (1985). *Life safety code handbook.* Quincy, MA: National Fire Protection Association.

Liu, F., Manton, K., & Allston, W. (1982). Demographic and epidemiological determinants of expenditures. In R. Vogel & H. Palmer (Eds.), *Long term care* (pp. 81–132). Washington, DC: Health Care Financing Administration.

long-term care News (January 1990). p. 22.

Lutz, S. (1994). Hospitals' profit margins jump as costs are adjusted. *Modern Healthcare, 24*(43).

Manton, K. G., Stallard, E., & Woodbury, M. A. (1994). Home health and skilled nursing facility use: 1982–90. *Health Care Financing Review, 16*(1), 155–183.

Miller, D. B. (Ed.). (1982). *Long term care administrator's desk manual.* Greenvale, NY: Panel Publishers.

Miller, D. B., & Barry, J. T. (1979). *Nursing home organization and operation.* Boston: CBI Publishing.

Moore, J. D., Jr. (1995). Hillhaven nurses stage strike. *Modern Healthcare,* p. 12.

Muse, D. N., & Sawyer, D. (1982). *The Medicare and Medicaid handbook* (p. 96). Washington, DC: Health Care Financing Administration.

McCarthy, M. (1994, November 8). Frayed lifeline: Hunger among elderly surges; meal programs just can't keep up, *The Wall Street Journal,* pp. 1, 11.

National Fire Protection Association. (1985). *Life safety code 1985* (NFPA 101 ANSI/NFPA 101). Quincy, MA: Author.

National Fire Protection Association. (1994). *Life safety code 1994* (NFPA 101–1994 ANSI/NFPA 101). Quincy, MA: Author.

National nurse survey. (1995). Washington, DC: Service Employees International Union.
Office of the Actuary. (2000). HCFA, September 27, 2000
Office of the Actuary. (2002). Centers for Medicare and Medicaid, April 1, 2002
Pointer, D., & Metzger, N. (1975). *The National Labor Relations Act: A guidebook for health care facility administrators.* New York: Spectrum Publications.
Raskin, A. H. (1981, December). From sitdowns to solidarity: Passage in the life of American labor. *Across the Board,* pp. 12–32.
Rogers, W. W. (1980). *General administration in the nursing home* (3rd ed.). Boston: CBI Publishing.
Rosenfeld, L. S., Gaylord, S. A., & Allen, J. E. (1983). *Introduction to long-term care for the aging.* Chapel Hill: University of North Carolina Independent Study by Extension.
Rosmann, J. (1975). One year under Taft-Hartley. *Hospitals, 49*(24), 64–68.
Scott, L. (1994). NLRB order against Beverly voided. *Modern Healthcare, 24*(1).
Service Employees International Union (2003). AFL/CIO, CLC www.seiu.org September, 2003
Sharma, S. K., & Fallovolleta, B. S. (1992). *The Older Americans Act: Access to and utilization of the ombudsman program* (GAO-PEMD-92-21). Washington, DC: USGAO Program Evaluation and Methodology Division.
Shriver, K. (1995, October 2). Union can't stop Vencor-Hillhaven deal. *Modern Healthcare,* p. 18.
Simon-Rusinowitz, L., & Hofland, B. F. (1993). Adopting a disability approach to home care services for older adults. *Gerontologist, 33,* 159–166.
Sirocco, A. (1994). *Nursing homes and board and care homes: Data from the 1991 National Health Provider Inventory.* (National Center for Health Statistics: Advance Data, 244, February 23, 1994). Washington, DC: National Center for Health Statistics.
Smith, D. B. (1981). *Long-term care in transition: The regulation of nursing homes.* Washington, DC: Association of University Programs of Health Administration Press.
Staff. (1984, October 1). Perspectives. *Washington Report on Medicine and Health,* pp. 1–4.
Strahan, G. (1994). *An overview of home health and hospice care patients* (National Center for Health Statistics: Advance Data, 256, July 22). Vital and health Statistics, Centers for Disease Control.
The state of health planning. (1984, October 22). *Medical and Health,* Insert.
Thomas, C. (1989, September). *1989 update: CON program changes (State health Notes,* No. 96). Washington, DC: George Washington University, Intergovernmental Health Policy Project.
Twomey, D. W. (1980). *Labor law and legislation.* Cincinnati: South-Western.
U.S. Department of Health, Education and Welfare. (1975). *Interpretive guidelines and survey procedures.* Washington, DC: American Health Care Association. (Originally published in the *Federal Register,* January 17, 1974.)
U.S. Department of Health and Human Services. (1985). *Publication No. 348.* Washington, DC: U.S. Government Printing Office.

U.S. Department of Labor. (1976). *Brief history of the American labor movement* (Bulletin 1000). Washington, DC: U.S. Government Printing Office.

U.S. Department of Labor, Bureau of Labor Statistics. (1977). *U.S. working women: A data book.* Washington, DC: U.S. Government Printing Office.

U.S. Department of Labor, Occupational Safety and Health Administration. (1976). *All about OSHA.* Washington, DC: U.S. Government Printing Office.

U.S. Senate Special Committee on Aging, *Assisted Living Workgroup's final report,* April 29, 2003.

Vladeck, B. C. (1980). *Unloving care: The nursing home tragedy.* New York: Basic Books.

Waxman, H. A. (1986). Consensus calls for nursing home reform. *Provider, 12*(11), 15–16.

Weissert, W. (1985, April). *Estimating the long term care population* (p. 11). Report for the Office of the Assistant Secretary for Planning and Education. Washington, DC: U.S. DHHS.

Weissert, W. G. (1989). Models of adult day care. *Gerontologist, 29,* 648.

Williams, S. J., & Torrens, P. R. (1980). *Introduction to health services.* New York: Wiley.

Wilson, F. A., & Neuhauser, D. (1982). *Health services in the United States* (2d ed.). Cambridge, MA: Ballinger.

PART FIVE

RESIDENT CARE

5.0 The Assisted Living Environment

Caring for the residents is the administrator's greatest challenge, for the administrator must ensure that, to the extent possible, each resident thrives. The "assisted" and "living" in assisted living means helping people make the best use of their remaining abilities and special talents. The goal of assisted living, according to B. Cowdrick (personal communication, 1996), is to create an environment that does as much as possible to promote each individual's best work in old age.

The real task of the assisted living administrator is to create a vibrant, happy, and productive community "where the staff focus on the joyful business of living life to its fullest" (B. Cowdrick, personal communication, 1996). The real purpose of health care treatments, described extensively below, is to liberate each resident to live as fully as possible in spite of health difficulties. The many treatments described below are challenges to be dealt with so that the pleasures and special work of old age become the focus. Health care treatments are only the means to the end: vibrant living in old age.

MINIMIZING INSTITUTIONALIZATION

Congregate living, it must be acknowledged, is institutional living. When in the "residential care" phase of senior housing, residents normally still drive their own cars, get up and eat what they wish when they wish—they are able to perform both the ADLs and IADLs. Life is still relatively free of intrusions by others. Residents are able to sleep, play, and work in different places, without any overall plan imposed on them.

The assisted living setting, in contrast to the residential care setting, is, of necessity, much more institutional. Older persons move into the assisted living facility precisely because they are no longer able to perform most of the IADLs and only some of the ADLs. Life is routine and formally administered.

The assisted living facility administrator can minimize the effects of institutionalization by constantly working to overcome institutionalizing effects, such as dinner being served at a specified time, with each resident assigned a place in the dining room. Residents in this type of prescribed eating arrangement are no longer able to eat what they want, where they want, and when they want. Each aspect of a resident's daily life now takes place in the immediate company of other residents and staff. The typical resident's day is in danger of becoming so routinized that most staff members can predict what a particular resident is likely to be doing day or night. Increasingly, for most assisted living residents, most aspects of life are carried out under one roof under careful supervision of staff. A social chasm may exist between the staff and the residents. A powerful set of forces are in place that can impose the negative aspects of institutional living on the residents. The successful assisted living administrator will understand and mitigate these dangers.

PREVENTING INSTITUTIONALIZATION'S EFFECTS

Institutionalization can be minimized by consciously emphasizing choices, control, and private space for each resident. This can be accomplished in a number of ways.

Think Residential: Develop and Maintain a "Residential" Environment

Assisted living architect Victor Regnier (1995) has observed that it is difficult to convince people that the frail elderly can live in an unrestricted environment. Assisted living has its roots in residential living. To the extent possible, living in an assisted living facility should differ as little as possible from living in one's own private home.

The Dwelling Unit

A successful assisted living facility is a working combination of the physical setting itself, the residents in the facility, and the activities that take place within its boundaries.

The following concepts apply primarily in the design and construction phase. However, these concepts should be kept in mind when renovations or alterations are contemplated in an existing facility. For example, skylights can always be added, and patios outside resident rooms can always be built during a renovation project. If a building which has no balconies for upper-floor residents, similar space could be created on the grounds. There are many ways to achieve equivalent residential feeling tones about the facility and its grounds.

Personal privacy is a fiercely held value for most persons. The assisted living setting typically offers privacy through access to a single occupied, lockable unit. Typically, this unit includes kitchen facilities, which allow the resident to continue previous residential behaviors such as cooking, preparing snacks, and the like. It is a simple matter to disconnect the stove for residents whose behaviors are dangerous. The kitchen can stimulate a range of independent behaviors and be part of rehabilitation programs after an illness.

Adequate and versatile storage can be provided in the assisted living facility. Bathroom items, linens, clothes, hobby materials, computers, and other items require appropriate storage. Storage units can be mobile and sized to individual residents' needs. Fixtures and handles that can be easily grasped and conform to the (ANSI) requirements need not be obvious. It is a simple matter to install large-sized dials for heating and cooling adjustments.

Bathrooms can be made handicapped accessible following ANSI design guidelines. To make a bathroom appear cozy and noninstitutional until such time as a resident requires access room, removable storage units can be installed in the space. Inclusion of a shower or tub in each unit, along with the usual central bathing facilities, continues a sense of residential living whether or not each resident regularly uses the private bathing facility. The issue is choice: to maximize choices available to each resident who seeks an individualized lifestyle.

Unit Size

While costs are associated with increasing size, one- and two-bedroom units in assisted living facilities allow residents an extra "catch-all" room, which can serve a number of functions. Access to the outside is an essential element of an appropriately designed assisted living facility. If at ground level, doors and an individual patio, however small, provide a sense of wholeness and access to the outside world. On upper-level units a balcony, often a screened-in porch, can provide important access to the outside. Lower sill heights allow residents to view the outside from their bed or lounge chair. A gas-fired fireplace in resident rooms can be a valuable symbol of home---whether the gas is turned on or not.

Access to Light

Plants thrive on light. So do people. Construction that allows generous amounts of light contributes to quality of life. Natural sunlight is the most desirable, but indirect light from skylights and other sources can be acceptable substitutes. Carefully discussing light needs with each applicant will assist in placing persons into appropriately oriented units. Some may prefer the morning sun, others the afternoon sun; yet others may prefer the indirect light of a north-facing unit. These are important considerations in long-term satisfaction with units.

Using Residential Materials

Use of finishes found around a typical home can help make the assisted living facility feel less like an institution. Often builders seeking first-time cost savings use materials that scream out "institution" to the resident and the public. Low maintenance, cleanability, and commercial construction often win over more homelike materials. Wood rather than rubber-based trim suggest "home." So do brick and stone. Furniture with washable fabrics are practical, yet each time residents sit in these "practical" chairs they are reminded that they now live in an institution.

Unit Clusters

A number of assisted living builders create natural living units by clustering four or so units built around a common parlor or common dining room. A central kitchen and common laundry are other examples of shared space. Unit clusters let builders create opportunities for fostering group interaction among residents.

Site Design Common Areas

The outdoors and indoors can be continuous in a good building and site design. The use of picture windows, sliding glass doors, appropriate landscaping, and the like can link the inside with the outside, thus extending the living space for each resident, much like the front, side, and backyards of an individual residence. Views of attractively landscaped grounds from inside the building must be carefully planned. The benefits are enormous in terms of reducing the institutional feel of an assisted living facility. If, for example, the administrator and staff wish to encourage the residents to walk and get outdoor exercise, appropriate space that naturally encourages such activities must be provided. Facilities that have sought to encourage gardening activities, for example, have provided raised beds for residents. Such raised planting beds are appreciated not only by residents in wheel chairs but also everyone for whom getting up from the ground is not as easy as it used to be.

The size of common rooms matters. When feasible, size should be limited to that of a large home. Commercial furnishings in large-scale rooms will seldom communicate a homelike feeling. Use of glass in walls to most common areas, in contrast, is a very user-friendly approach, allowing the resident to "preview" what is going on in a room before entering.

Corridors

Corridors that do not communicate an institutional feeling are difficult to design. However, they can be limited to short lengths with frequent offsets or alcoves that allow light and offer additional social functions. When properly designed, hallways can be sources of socialization and planned interactions among residents. Corridors are either single-loaded or double-loaded (i.e. rooms on one or both sides). While more expensive, single-loaded corridors can open onto the outside can create light and warmth. Furniture, skylights, benches, sitting clusters, and such can turn a hallway into a pleasant space.

Architectural Scale

The architectural scale of the assisted living building, that is, its perceived size compared to surrounding buildings, is important. Rather than a high-rise, three or four more intimate buildings on a site can keep the scale more residential.

Facilities that fit into the architectural style of the region also minimize the institutional feel. In the South this might approximate a colonial plantation; in the North a country house; in the West a large ranch house. Each can contribute to blending the assisted living facility into the community.

Creating a Human Habitat

An assisted living facility is a human habitat. To the extent it can be an extension of residents' lives in their own residences over their life history, institutional effects can be minimized. In their homes residents had dogs, cats, plants, children, and other aspects of the diversity that makes up the human habitat. Residents are likely to thrive to the extent these life dimensions can be continued and encouraged by the facility. How this can be achieved is documented by William H. Thomas in his book *Life Worth Living* (1996).

Supporting the Residents' Families

A goal of assisted living administration is to involve residents' families in the day-to-day life of the residents and the facility. This can be fostered by architecture that is user-friendly to families. Guest rooms should be available to family visiting from afar. Kitchens in the units and hospitality areas about the structure in which families can socialize make visiting less institutional and a more homelike experience for children. Common laundry rooms can be designed to encourage family members and residents to socialize while getting the laundry done. Places inside and outside designated for children to play can make the difference in whether the grandkids dread or look forward to a visit with Grandma and Granddad. A well-equipped kids corner in the social rooms and refrigerators well stocked with soda and snacks will tell kids they are welcome.

Occasionally, but not nearly often enough, owners and their architects think of these things. The alert administrator, through improvising and imagination, can often achieve similar results.

Developing a Program of Care

The following ideas are suggestions by Philip Brown (personal communication, 1998), a long-term care administrator with three decades of experience, as important dimensions of providing care in the assisted living setting.

The assisted living facility team will seek to develop a program of care for each resident based upon

- needs of residents being served
- choices of resident and family
- regulations and licensure
- knowledge of the aging process

In the process of developing a program of care, a number of services will be developed and provided that

- meet basic needs such as food, shelter, health care, clothing, and the activities of daily living
- help residents fill in the gaps in their lives such as memory shortfalls and physical disabilities

Parameters of Services

It is important for the facility to spell out the parameters of services provided (e.g., the acuity levels of services, what is provided in-house and what is contracted out, and the choices residents may make).

Residents need the facility to spell out what services are provided, how the facility will handle and meet their health care needs, what the admission and discharge policies are, what the residents' rights are at the facility—in short, how love and human needs will be met. Residents need to be clearly informed on services provided in such areas as

- food
- laundry
- transportation
- housekeeping
- recreation/activities
- maintenance
- heat and air conditioning
- TV
- call system
- fire safety

Emphasizing Quality of Living. Dimensions the assisted living team will want to consider in developing and implementing each resident's program of care include the following.

Privacy—space

- knock before you enter
- respect the need for privacy
- encourage a homelike setting with the residents' own furnishings

Choice—from a range of options, the facility can create resident control over

- when you eat, what you eat
- when you go to bed
- when you get up
- what you do with your time

Use of time—assisting the resident in achieving quality time

- providing activities that relate to resident interests
- offering social programs that create inclusiveness for each resident
- staff understanding and honoring the effects of time and aging

Challenge—to move beyond personal disabilities

- listening devices
- talking books
- tables at wheelchair height
- walking aids

Participation in the community

- family
- friends
- the larger community
- religious and civic group participation

Maintaining connectedness to the outside world via

- telephone
- transportation
- mail
- fax/email
- right to entertain guests

Treatment—which preserves or restores one's sense of personhood

- using proper names and title as desired by the resident
- use of patience and understanding
- honoring resident's choice to refuse treatment
- creating an atmosphere that maintains personal dignity

Staff understanding of typical changes during the aging process physical changes such as

- hearing loss
- muscle strength loss
- diminished eyesight
- chronic conditions

psychological changes such as

- loss of self-image
- lack of purpose in being
- impatience
- changing relationship to the world

sociological changes, as reflected in these questions:

- Where do I belong?
- Who are my friends/family?
- How can I remain a responsible citizen?
- Shall I participate in or withdraw from the world?

These dimensions will require that staff have specialized skills in such areas as

- developing and implementing policies and procedures
- conflict resolution
- understanding and managing grief
- motivating residents
- choosing among support services

5.1 The Aging Process

Providing resident care is a most complex process. How it is achieved will vary from facility to facility and over time within the same facility. The following pages offer background knowledge that may be useful to the assisted living administrator in the process of achieving an atmosphere in which residents thrive.

How many Americans die of old age each year? Depending on the definitions used, the answer could range from more than one million persons to no one. Our answer is, "No one." Old age is not a disease process.

It used to be customary to say that a person died of old age, but this is too imprecise an observation. It seems more functional to approach disease and disabilities and causes of death among older persons as one approaches these concerns in younger persons: to look for causes and seek either cure or relief.

Every older person, just as every younger one, dies of specific causes. Generally, one or more of the body systems becomes overwhelmed for some specific reason, such as a disease or an injury to the person, and death results (Kane, Ouslander, & Abrass, 1989). It is important, to understand that age changes are not in themselves diseases, but rather are natural losses of function (Hayflick, 1965).

RESEARCH ON AGING

The two groups who study aging individuals are identified by different titles. Physicians who specialize in treating the elderly are called geriatricians. Professionals who study the problems of the aging population in society, and usually are not physicians, are called gerontologists.

How much have the geriatricians and gerontologists learned about aging? With the development of medicine over the past century, attention to diseases of aging persons and the aging process itself have become increasingly active areas of scientific investigation. Much has been learned, and some of this knowledge will be discussed below. However, a good deal of uncertainty remains. Much of the so-called knowledge about aging is still being tested and is not yet well established.

GENERAL OBSERVATIONS

One observation that seems safe to make is that aging is highly individualized. In the typical assisted living facility there are individuals whose chronological age is 90, yet their physiologic appearance and strong activity level are more characteristic of a 60-year-old person (Maddox, 2001). Similarly, there are those in their 60s and 70s in the same facility who appear to be more aged than the 90-year-old (Evans, et. al., 2000). The extent to which this is due to genetic inheritance or is influenced by an individual's lifestyle and health behaviors remains a subject of lively debate.

A few additional general observations can be made about aging, none of them entirely safe, because for every such observation the reader may be able to produce valid exceptions.

Take, for example, observations of Alexander Leaf in *Scientific American* (1973, pp. 44–52). Leaf compared 75-year-olds with 30-year-olds and found that among those he studied, a person age 75 has

92% of the former brain weight
84% of the former basal metabolism
70% of the former kidney filtration rate
43% of the former maximum breathing capacity

Those are impressive figures. What do they mean? Does the progressive loss of cortical neurons (brain cells) mean that older persons are that much less smart? Apparently not. There is little substantial evidence that reduction of mental competence accompanies reduction in brain weight.

If Leaf's data are correct—that, on average, when a person reaches 75 the brain weighs about 10% less, the body is burning calories at a reduced rate, the kidneys are filtering about three fourths as fast, and the lungs process oxygen more slowly—what is their significance? Certainly this may be important for the physician and the pharmacist concerned about drug tolerance and dosages, but these data do not make the 75–year-old individual any more or less of a person than the 30–year-old Evans, et. al., 2000).

The main import of Leaf's data to confirm that, in general, aging is a continuous process that begins at birth, that it is a gradual decline of at least some systems of the body that proceed at different rates in different individuals. Kane et al. (1989) suggest the 1% theory: that the majority of body organs lose function at the rate of 1% per year after age 30 (p. 5). They caution, however, that newer findings suggest that functional decreases observed in some groups of persons and not others may point to disease patterns among some groups rather than normal aging in the general population.

5.1.1 Overview of Some Appearance and Functional Changes Believed to Be Associated With Aging

The following observations are discussed at greater length section 5.3. By way of gaining an overall perspective, these phenomena can be observed.

Change in Collagen

Collagen is connective tissue that loses elasticity over time and appears to account for sagging of the skin often observed in the aging person. Sagging can occur around the eyes and jaws and can affect the general body tone of the muscles, especially in the arm.

Reduced Reserve

Leaf's (1973) observation of the lungs' diminished ability to process oxygen tends to be true of several other body systems. Starr (1964) found that after age 20 the heart muscle loses strength every year at the rate of 0.85%. Leaf (1973) discovered that at-rest heart output at age 75 is no more than 70% of at-rest heart output at age 30.

Gradual Changes in the Immune System

Usually, the body rejects foreign cells, but as the body ages, one theory holds that a progressive weakening of the immune response increases susceptibility to respiratory and other illnesses (Kane et al., 1989).

Temperature Response Changes

A reduction of capacity to maintain body temperature within a narrow range appears to lead to a diminished shivering and sweating response, allowing the body temperature of some older individuals to range dangerously. This can lead to the elderly dying in heat waves and cold waves that do not so adversely affect younger people. Ten percent of those over 65, or 2.5 million Americans, are believed to be vulnerable to hypothermia (lowered body heat) due to reduced heat production by the body (Reichel, 1983).

Postural Imbalances

The balancing mechanisms appear to function less well, resulting in some persons age 65 and older being progressively at risk of tripping (Redford, 1989).

Decalcification of the Bones

Many older persons are at increased risk of bone fractures, especially if they fall (Glowacki, 1989).

Decreases in Bowel Function Control

Because the central nervous system tends to function less and less well in some older persons, the ability to control the bowels lessens.

Frequent Anorexia

Anorexia (loss of appetite) among some elderly leads to skipping meals and a reduced level of nutrition (Gibbons & Levy, 1989; Maddox, 2001).

Skin

With the loss of some subcutaneous fat, an older person may feel colder, and the skin may wrinkle. Some pigment (color) cells of the skin enlarge with age, resulting in the pigmented plaques often seen on the skin of aged persons.

Decreased Bone and Muscle Mass

This process among some elderly individuals can result in stooped posture, reduced height, loss of muscle power, misshapen joints, and limitations in mobility.

Renal System

The bladder of some persons appears to reduce to less than half its former capacity, and micturition, the desire to urinate, appears delayed until the bladder is at near capacity instead of triggering at one half of capacity. One researcher (Lindeman, 1989) estimated that the average 80-year-old has about half the glomerular filtration rate of a 30–year-old.

Hearing and Vision

Both hearing and vision appear to become diminished among many aged persons.

5.2 Theories of Aging

Most investigators of the causes of aging agree that there is no one theory that currently explains the aging phenomenon fully (Hayflick, 1965; Meites & Quadri, 1995; Hefti, 1995; Landfield, 1995). Reichel (1983, p. 8), for example, defines aging as a progressive deterioration in functional capacity occurring after reproductive maturity.

Because no one really knows why people age, there are several theories instead of one generally accepted explanation. Hayflick (1965) thinks the question might more usefully be posed as, Why do we live so long? He observes that theorists are increasingly suspecting that the forces that produce age changes are different from those that drive longevity determination.

There has been an explosion of biogerontologic theory about why we age. The main criticism of these theories is that changes such as reduced exercise capacity may be indicative of certain, more fundamental change processes.

A LIMIT TO THE NUMBER OF CELL DIVISIONS?

Some theories of aging relate to the genome, or genetic apparatus, age-related changes in cell metabolism and function. Leonard Hayflick (1965), while doing research at Stanford University, found that normal human fibroblasts (embryonic cells that give rise to connective tissue), when cultured in vitro (in a test tube or other artificial environment), undergo only a limited number of divisions, usually about 50, before they die. His hypothesis is that the life span of a normal human cell is a programmed event under genetic control. Hayflick gained support for his theory by showing that cells from adult human tissue undergo about 20 divisions before they die. Kane et al. (1989) expressed their doubt about his theory, however.

AN ANSWER IN CANCER RESEARCH?

Cancer cells appear to be able to continue reproducing indefinitely (Rimer, 1995). If this is so, what causes noncancerous cells to lose their ability to divide? Some researchers think that the answer to cancer cell divisions may hold information that will reveal the factor that limits the normal human cell's ability to continue dividing.

SOMATIC MUTATION THEORY

Some researchers have speculated that a sufficient level of accumulation of mutations in body cells produces the physiologic decrements we identify as aging (Hayflick, 1995).

THE ERROR THEORY: A LOSS IN GENETIC PROGRAMMING?

At the University of California, Bernard Strehler hypothesized that age-related changes in cell metabolism are a programmed loss of the genetic material found in the DNA molecule (the molecule of heredity in most organisms). Essentially, this is based on the theory that there is increasing inaccuracy in the protein synthesis. The idea is that at the ends of linear chromosomes the telemere length decreases until cell division ceases (Hayflick, 1965).

RANDOM MUTATIONS?

When he was working at the Boston University Medical School, Marott Sinex (1977) proposed that random mutations of cells may produce aging by causing damage to DNA molecules. His theory is that as mutations (changes) accumulate in the body cells, they progressively lose their ability to reproduce and perform their original functions (Maddox, 2001).

PROGRAM THEORY

Proponents of this approach contend that the events we associate with aging are programmed into the genome; that just as progressive maturation is programmed, progressive deterioration is programmed (Hayflick, 1965).

AN AUTOIMMUNE EXPLANATION?

Several investigators (see H. T. Blumenthal, 1968, pp. 3–5) suggest that a progressive failure of the body's immune system, which consists of white blood cells and various antibodies that are our first line of defense against diseases (discussed below), leads to autoimmune responses in older persons. Their idea is that "copying errors" in repeated cell divisions lead to cells that are progressively not recognized by the body, triggering the immune system to attack these cells, thinking foreign cells have invaded.

This is similar to the wear-and-tear theory (see below), which postulates that as mutations progress over time, unrepaired changes of DNA and similar processes result in aging (Medvedev, 1995; Maddox, 2001).

ENTROPY AND AGING

The second law of thermodynamics postulates that ordered systems move toward disorder. In this theory, aging is an inevitable expression of the idea that closed systems, such as our bodies, tend to remain in a state of equilibrium in which nothing more happens.

LONGEVITY ASSURANCE GENES

In this approach, aging is thought to be under the control of hormones and to be genetically based (Meites & Quadri, 1995; Hayflick, 1965).

STRESS THEORY OF AGING: WEAR AND TEAR

Some theorists have suggested that the body simply wears out, or that vital parts wear out, similar to that which occurs in machines (Landfield, 1995; Medvedev, 1995). Hans Selye suggests that the body's response to long-term stress resembles the normal life cycle, leading to the final stage of senescence. In this view, repeated experiences with stress are associated with a speeding up of the aging process. Some researchers have focused on the possible role of adrenal steroids and or stress hormones that appear to accelerate aging of the brain (Landfield, 1995).

NEUROENDOCRINE THEORY OF AGING

Several theorists believe that the brain and the endocrine glands control aging. The concept is that, as derangements in normal functioning occur, tissues and organs are affected in ways we identify with aging. Some of the theory is based on immune-neuroendocrine interactions. Basically, the brain and endocrine glands are believed to affect, for example, the immune system, which leads to impairment of antibody formation (Meites & Quadri, 1995).

Some researchers have focused on caloric restriction being associated with delaying the maturing of the neuroendocrine functions, delaying body growth and puberty, lowering blood temperature, lowering cell division, decreasing body metabolism, and so on, thus delaying what we think of as the aging process.

NEUROTROPHIC FACTORS AND AGING

Neurotrophic factors are observed to control the survival of neurons or nerves over time, and some theorists believe that understanding this phenomenon will lead to a greater understanding of what we identify with the aging process (Hefti, 1995).

FAILURE OF COLLAGEN?

Collagen is a protein fiber that is distributed in the walls of the blood vessels, the heart, and the connective tissue. Some researchers postulate that age is accompanied by a reduction in the elasticity of this protein, possibly leading to heart muscle inefficiency and, because of rigidity, to reduced cell permeability, making cell nutrition more difficult.

Regardless of which, if any, of these explanations of the aging process turns out to be correct, the assisted living facility administrator should deal with the effects of aging in planning the care of residents.

WHAT OF THE FUTURE?

Leonard Hayflick recently observed that even if cures are achieved for Alzheimer's, heart disease, stroke, cancer, diabetes, hepatitis, and Parkinson's disease only about 15 years will be added to current longevity. He and others expect that through the 21st century average longevity will likely not exceed 90 years. To the question, "Can we stop aging?" an insurance executive at the Society of Actuaries meeting observed that right now, we do not know. The title of his talk was "Plastic Omega," suggesting that the maximum life span tables and calculations may have to be revised and even viewed as "plastic," or changeable, in light of current medical research (Hall, 2003, p. 349).

5.3 The Aging Process as it Relates to Diseases Common to the Assisted Living Facility Population

It is useful for the administrator to be familiar with the rudiments of biological processes and human anatomy and to be able to recognize the parts of the body that are most affected by the aging process. In this way, the administrator will be better able to appreciate the special problems with which the facility should cope.

All physical processes in the body may undergo some changes as a result of aging, including a slowing down, a decrease in the overall energy reserve, a breakdown of some of the body functions, and an alteration of some individual cell structures, which ultimately affects the functioning of some body tissues and organs as well.

The systems referred to are groups of structures that perform a specialized function for the body. Below is a list of 10 systems of the body processes and structures as they are most commonly categorized. They are presented to reflect also the prevalence of diseases affecting them in the assisted living facility population.

It is important to remember that these systems or groups of structures are highly interrelated and that most assisted living facility residents typically suffer from multiple chronic diseases that may affect combinations of body systems.

1. **Blood circulation**—the basic processes and structures that enable the body to transport oxygen to the cells and tissues
2. **Breathing**—the system that obtains oxygen from the environment and distributes it throughout the body
3. **Nervous system**—responsible for controlling all of the body functions and ensuring that they are functioning properly; these are the regulatory activities
4. **Digestive System**—system in which the body breaks down food into a form in which the nutrients may be used by the individual cells
5. **Nutrition**—process by which the body takes in nutrients
6. **External and internal defense mechanisms**—the skin and an internal immune system, which play important roles in protecting the body from any harmful invasions

7. **Musculoskeletal system**—the bones, muscles, tendons, and joints used in movement
8. **Excretory system**—the way in which the body relieves itself of fluid and chemical waste products
9. **Reproductive system**—sexuality in the elderly
10. **Emotional and mental well-being**—the psychological status

5.3.1 Blood Circulation

The circulatory system, also called the cardiovascular system, may be thought of as an elaborate pumping mechanism (Rosendorff, 1983). It is powered by the heart, which pumps the blood throughout the body within a network of blood vessels (arteries and veins).

ARTERIES

Arteries are the vessels that carry blood rich in nutrients away from the heart to the remainder of the body cells.

Nutrients obtained from the food are processed in the digestive tract. Combined with oxygen, nutrients permit individual cells to perform the chemical reactions that produce energy.

Oxygen is a colorless, odorless, gaseous chemical element that is found in the air. Oxygen is most plentiful in the arteries, which divide into smaller and smaller branches until they become capillaries. These capillaries are the smallest blood vessels and form a network connecting the smallest arteries to the smallest veins (see Figure 5.1). It is here at the capillaries that the function of oxygenation occurs.

Oxygenation is the transfer of oxygen from the blood cells at the capillary level into the necessary tissues in exchange for carbon dioxide. Carbon dioxide is also a gas. It is produced as a waste product of the chemical reactions in the cells.

VEINS

The blood cells carry carbon dioxide through the vein network and back to the heart. Veins return blood that is carrying carbon dioxide back to the heart through the superior (from upper body) and inferior (lower body) vena cava (see Figure 5.1).

The blood then enters the right side of the heart. When a sufficient amount of blood has collected, the right ventricle of the heart contracts, actually squeezing its contents into the artery that leads to the lungs (pulmonary artery).

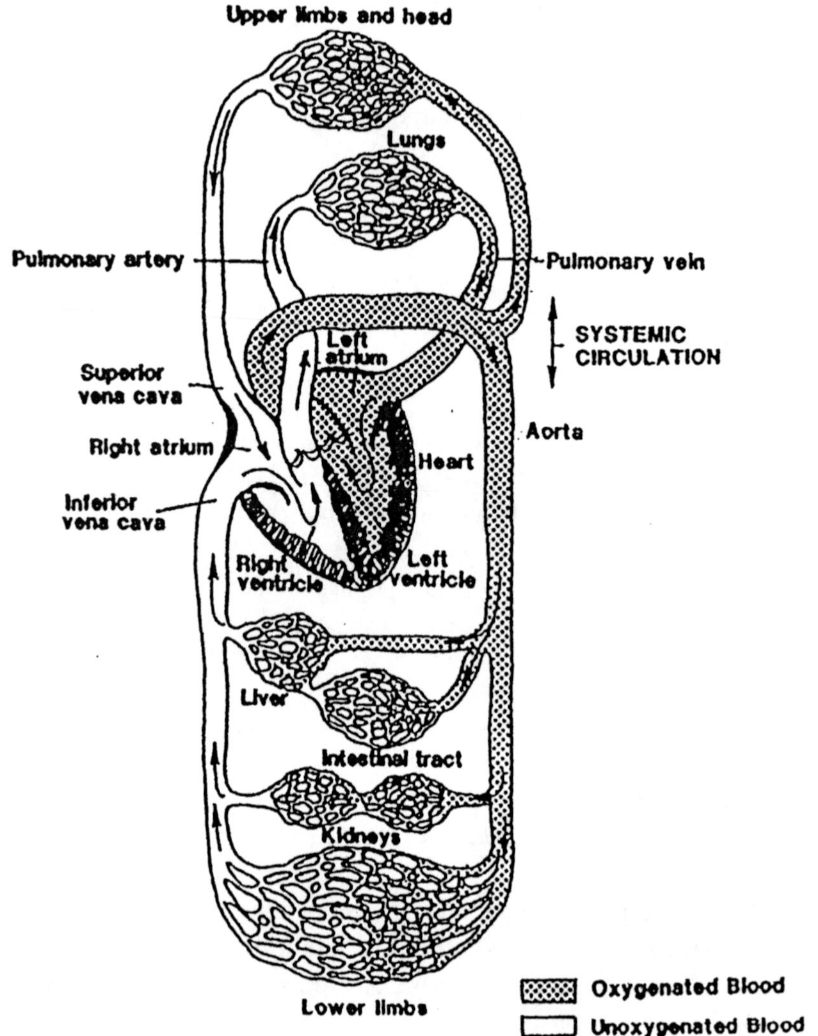

FIGURE 5.1 Representation of the circulatory and oxygenation process.

LUNGS

Within the lungs the carbon dioxide that has been collected by the veins is discarded and exchanged for oxygen. The carbon dioxide is then exhaled into the air as the breath is expelled. It has followed the reverse of the oxygen pathway until it is removed from the body. This is a simplification of the respiratory process (breathing), which will be discussed further in the next section.

The newly oxygenated blood returns to the heart through the pulmonary vein. The blood is then channeled into the left side of the heart. When enough blood has collected, this blood is then pumped forcefully out of the heart into the aorta. The aorta is the largest artery from which all the smaller arteries branch off, carrying blood that is rich in oxygen throughout the rest of the body again. This process occurs with every heartbeat.

THE HEART

The heart itself is a complex organ. It is a muscle composed of various types of cells to facilitate the pumping process. The heart requires oxygen to function and is supplied by a network of coronary arteries that stem from the aorta (see Figure 5.2).

The inner structure of the heart is also very complex, with four distinct chambers and a valve network that regulates blood flow.

CELL CHANGES

Any substantial change in these structures or the circulatory process itself can eventually affect all the body cells. The significance, then, of the oxygenation process is that when the health of cells has deteriorated, it is usually due to a change in the cardiovascular system that interferes with the supply of nutrients to the cells and with the supply of oxygen. This in turn damages the tissues and organs in the body, leading to the decline of other major processes.

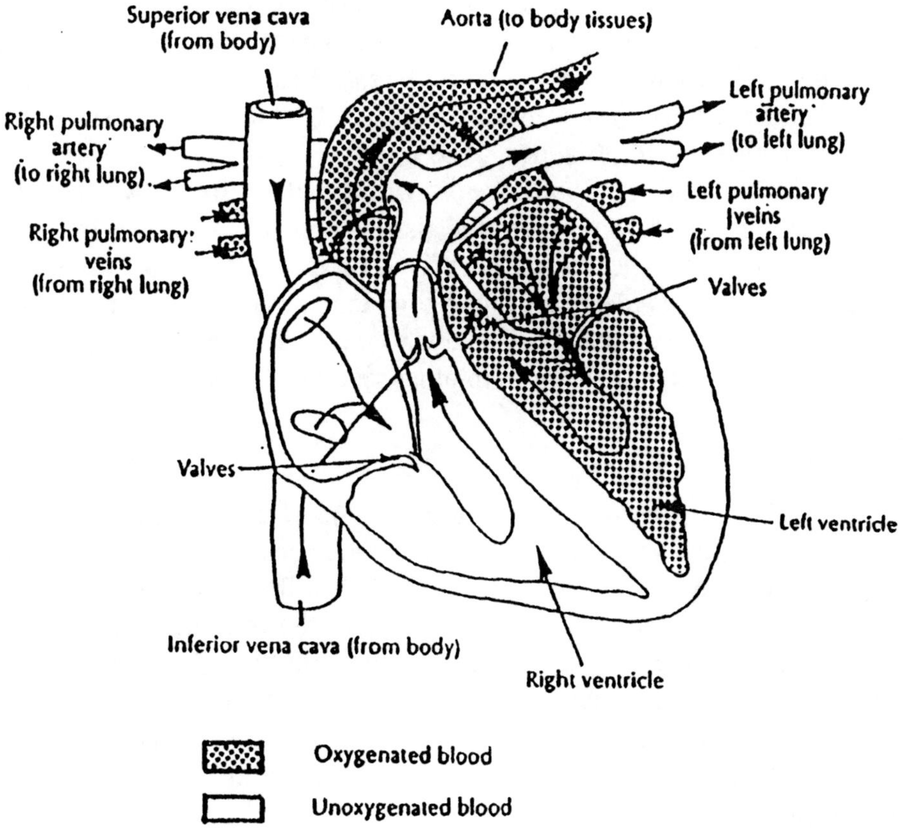

FIGURE 5.2 Schematic representation of blood flow through the heart.

AGING EFFECTS

The extent to which the aging process plays a role in this deterioration is still being argued. It is known that the cardiovascular system (heart and blood vessels) is not designed to last indefinitely. Many of the cells are not capable of dividing and remain part of the system for long periods of time.

Decreased Elasticity

A specific age-related change in the heart may include a lessening of the force of contraction (pumping) due to the decreased elasticity of muscle. Elasticity is the ability of the heart muscle to stretch and return to normal size spontaneously. When this property has been decreased in the heart muscle, the heart becomes stretched. This loss of elasticity reduces the force of contractions by the heart (pumping), which ultimately diminishes the amount of blood pumped by the heart (also termed cardiac output).

Decreased Cardiac Output

The reduced cardiac output is also due to an increased resistance to blood flow within the blood vessels and a loss in the heart's ability to compensate by beating faster. This added resistance to blood flow within the blood vessels may be a direct result of arteriosclerosis (hardening of the arteries) or more specifically atherosclerosis (one type of arteriosclerosis; Golden, 1995; Maddox, 2001).

A change in any one of these components will affect the other two. If the amount of blood circulated is reduced, the organs and tissues will receive fewer nutrients and less oxygen, resulting in some cells dying (if deprived for more than 3 to 5 minutes).

It is estimated that in the elderly the blood flow to the kidneys is reduced by as much as 50%, and to the brain by as much as 20%, due to these same processes (Kenney, 1982, p. 51). These changes can explain changes in other systems associated with age.

Blood Pressure Changes

There is much debate among scientists about the role of the aging process and its effect on blood pressure. In many elderly persons the blood pressure does increase (O'Brien & Bulpitt). This increased pressure may be attributed to the stiffness of the large arteries (arteriosclerosis) and peripheral vascular resistance (the resistance in the blood vessels throughout the body) that are commonly associated with the aging process. Other studies of individuals in isolated areas reveal no changes in blood pressure levels for the elderly. Some investigators feel that there is a strong association of social and environmental factors contributing to the presence of high blood pressure in any individual (Kane et al., 1989; [The] "Best drugs," 1995).

Blood vessel changes due to this progressive stiffening have suggested that they become like rigid tubes (Finch & Haflick, 1977). This promotes the resistance to blood flow throughout the body (peripheral vascular resistance) and may exacerbate an already adversely affected heart function and increased blood pressure.

The vein walls tend to weaken over time with increased deposits of fats, cholesterol, fibrin, platelets, cellular debris, and calcium. The capillary walls become thickened, thus decreasing their ability to exchange oxygen with the cells. This thickening also contributes to the overall decrease in perfusion (flow) of nutrients into the tissues and organs.

COMMON CARDIOVASCULAR/CEREBROVASCULAR DISEASES

Cardiovascular disease is the major cause of death in the elderly population. The distinction between changes related to the aging process and those related to disease is a fine one. This dilemma becomes clear with the discussion of arteriosclerosis. According to the National Center for Health Statistics, heart disease was reported as the third most frequently occurring chronic condition in persons 65 and older, occurring at the rate of 325 per 1,000 individuals ("Retirement checkup," 1998).

Arteriosclerosis

Usually, arteries are smooth inside and can stretch to permit the passage of more blood and oxygen when needed. With arteriosclerosis, the blood vessels are not as responsive as they had been. Everyone has arteriosclerosis to some degree. Almost half of all assisted living facility residents manifest disease changes due to chronic arteriosclerosis. Two forms of this condition (atherosclerosis and aortic stenosis) account for much of the heart disease in the elderly.

Aortic Stenosis. The term describes a narrowing of the aorta, which is the major artery leading from the heart and channeling the oxygenated blood supply to the rest of the body. This stenosis, or narrowing of the vessel, increases the workload specifically for the left ventricle of the heart, since it now has to pump harder to overcome the obstructive resistance to blood flow.

The increased workload eventually is felt by the entire heart, and when combined with the normal changes attributed to the aging process, this disease places considerable stress on the cardiovascular system. It can result in congestive heart failure, which will be discussed at the end of this section.

For many elderly residents, the cause of the disease is either the result of scarring from a childhood outbreak of rheumatic fever or calcified deposits found lining the blood vessels.

Some of the symptoms of aortic stenosis are difficulty in breathing, dizziness, high blood pressure, chest pain, and symptoms associated with congestive heart failure.

Treatment can consist of surgical correction, rest to decrease the workload on the heart, and medication therapy.

Atherosclerosis. In this, the most common form of arteriosclerosis, there is a progressive buildup of fat deposits on the inner lining of blood vessel walls. The disease does not usually manifest itself until the blood vessel becomes completely obstructed or shows a markedly decreased ability to facilitate blood flow. The symptoms can be found affecting the body anywhere that an initial pathology (a disease-related change in a tissue or organ) may be present; this usually includes the main arteries. In 1980 atherosclerosis caused twice the number of deaths as cancer in older groups.

Cerebrovascular Disease

This disease manifests itself through restricted blood flow to the brain, caused by occlusions within the carotid arteries that supply blood to the brain. One of the most important causes of strokes is atherosclerosis. According to the National Center for Health Statistics, in 1995 stroke was the third leading cause of death among persons age 65 and older; 414 deaths per 100,000, or 138,762 actual deaths ("Retirement checkup," 1998).

Assisted living facility residents who may be predisposed to cardiovascular disease are those with high blood pressure and a previous history of heart disease and who are overweight (Birchenall & Streight, 1982). The specific symptoms of the disease depend on the affected location in the brain. Transient ischemic attacks (also termed "mini-strokes") are caused by a temporarily diminished blood supply to the brain. According to the National Center for Health Statistics, in 1995 heart disease was the leading cause of death among persons 65 and older; 1,835 deaths per 100,000, for a total of 615,426 deaths ("Retirement checkup," 1998).

Signs of cerebrovascular disease can be slurred speech, blurred vision, dizziness, numb hands and fingers, and mental confusion. Some of these symptoms could be easily attributed to the aging process rather than this underlying disease pathology.

A much more severe consequence of cerebrovascular disease is a stroke, or cerebrovascular accident. This occurs when the lack of oxygen for a much larger area of the brain causes permanent damage. Again, the resulting damage will depend on the area of the brain affected and may range from temporary loss of taste or smell to paralysis of many of the body parts.

Peripheral Vascular Disease

This actually describes a group of diseases that affect the veins, arteries, and other blood vessels of the extremities (Birchenall & Streight, 1982). The symptoms are a result of decreased blood flow to the affected area. The most frequent symptom is intermittent claudication, which is a complex of symptoms including the following:

- pain on movement of an extremity
- pain that is chronic in a localized area
- cold, numb feet
- changes in skin integrity, such as ulcers or infections that are slow to heal

Coronary Artery Disease

Also known as chronic ischemic heart disease, here the heart muscle itself suffers from a lack of oxygen due to blockages in the coronary arteries that usually supply it.

The current popular coronary artery bypass graft surgery is a common treatment for persons with severe blockages who do not respond to medical therapy. Since this is major surgery, some assisted living facility residents would not be considered good surgical risks for such treatment. This may be increasingly true inasmuch as a growing number of researchers are coming to believe that medical treatment may be as effective as surgery.

Symptoms can include chest pain—commonly called angina—which results from a lack of oxygen to certain areas of the heart muscle. Pain may be located anywhere in the chest, especially in the left arm or neck. This symptom is commonly found in persons over 60 years of age (Kleiger, 1976).

Myocardial infarction (MI) (literally meaning heart muscle death) results when a large enough area of the heart muscle does not receive oxygen for a period of time. With a massive myocardial infarction, the heart can no longer continue to act as a pump and may completely stop beating. There is a greater chance that persons over 60 years old will die from a heart attack than will younger individuals (Kieiger, 1976).

The phases in coronary artery disease range from diffuse, incomplete blockages throughout the arteries, to one or more large blockages that occlude more of the blood flow.

Symptoms can range from none at all to various types of angina or, most serious, to a complete cessation of heart activity that occurs after MI or complete heart block.

Treatments vary. Initially, individuals without severe manifestations of the disease can be treated conservatively with restrictions on sodium and fat in their diet. Medications commonly used in the assisted living facility are nitroglycerin and propranolol.

Nitroglycerin, the most common medication prescribed for persons with angina, is administered sublingually, or under the tongue. This drug lowers the blood pressure by dilating the blood vessels, including the coronary arteries, to decrease resistance to blood flow.

Propranolol hydrochloride (Inderol®) is referred to as a beta blocker because of its action in blocking body chemicals that act to increase the heart rate. This acts to slow down the heart, thereby decreasing blood pressure and lowering the amount of oxygen required by the heart muscle.

There are also a variety of antiarrhythmic medications available, which are prescribed in accordance with the particular type of arrhythmia diagnosed.

A common result of prolonged or diffuse coronary artery disease is the inability of the heart to initiate contractions independently. When this occurs, another type of treatment is often prescribed: permanent pacemaker. The pacemaker is a mechanical device implanted under the skin with its wires attached to the heart muscle to provide a continuous flow of electrical impulses that stimulate the heart to contract with a steady rhythm.

High Blood Pressure

High blood pressure, or hypertension, is usually considered to be present when the blood pressure measurement is consistently greater than 160/95. According to the National Center for Health Statistics, in its most recent survey, hypertension was reported as the second most frequently occurring chronic condition in persons 65 and older, occurring at the rate of 364 per 1,000 individuals ("Retirement checkup," 1998).

The numbers 160/95 are a measurement of the amount of pressure the blood exerts on the walls of the arteries. The first number (160) measures the maximum pressure (systolic) exerted when the heart is fully contracted near the end of the stroke output of the left ventricle. The second number (here, 95) measures the minimum or diastolic pressure occurring when the heart ventricles are in the period of dilation or fully relaxed. This should be monitored for each individual to account for height and weight variations.

There are two types of this disease: essential hypertension and secondary hypertension. The cause of essential hypertension is unknown, and therefore the disease is without a complete cure, but it can be successfully controlled by medication. Secondary hypertension in the elderly results from other underlying diseases, including anemia, fever, endocrine disease or hormonal disruption, arteriosclerosis, and/or kidney disease (Rubin, 1981). These diseases place a greater demand on the heart and may cause the blood pressure to increase during the disease episode or permanently.

The effects of continued high blood pressure, regardless of the cause, may be harmful to various organs within the body, especially the heart, brain, kidney, and eyes. When a person has high blood pressure, the heart should automatically pump harder to circulate the blood throughout the body. As the heart works harder and harder to compensate, eventually it begins to fail after being overworked for such long periods of time. This in turn reduces the blood flow to the vital organs, damaging their functioning as well.

Some signs of hypertension are prolonged, elevated blood pressure greater than 160/95, or the individual's norm, and prolonged presence of risk factors such as overweight, smoking, and high salt intake. Using the 160/95 definition, 40% to 50% of individuals over age 65 are hypertensive and should be actively treated (Kane et al., 1989; Maddox, 2001).

Treatments typically include prescribing weight loss and diet therapy, including restricted salt intake. The goal of medication therapy is to use as few drugs as possible. Some of the most common medications used in an assisted living facility include diuretics, nitroglycerin, and propranolol.

Diuretics are frequently used to get rid of the excess fluids in the body to decrease the workload of the heart by decreasing the blood volume that it should pump. Vasodilators such as nitroglycerin are used to dilate blood vessels and therefore decrease the amount of resistance against which the heart should work. Cardiac drugs such as propranolol may also be used to relieve the workload of the heart by decreasing its rate of contractions.

Congestive Heart Failure

This is not a disease, but is actually a complex set of many symptoms associated with an impaired performance of the heart. A progressively weakening heart results in an increasing inability of the heart to pump enough oxygen to the various tissues of the body. This failure results in a congestion of blood being backed up in the circulatory system. This backup causes fluids to leak out of the bloodstream into the various tissues and organs, most notably the lungs. Taken together, these constitute the disease process called congestive heart failure (CHF) (see Figure 5.3) (Maddox, 2001; Evans, et al., 2000).

The cause of congestive heart failure may be a variety of diseases or conditions, most notably arteriosclerosis, coronary artery disease, uncontrolled high blood pressure and/or a problem with one of the heart valves, heart attack, alcoholism, or chronic exposure to agents harmful to the body tissues.

The symptoms usually are seen in other organs and can be classified according to whether the heart failure primarily affects the left or right side of the heart.

Congested Heart
Congestive heart failure occurs when a healthy heart (*right, top*) loses its ability to contract fully. As a result, too much blood remains in the heart after each pump cycle, and the heart cannot supply the body with an adequate amount of oxygenated blood (*bottom*).

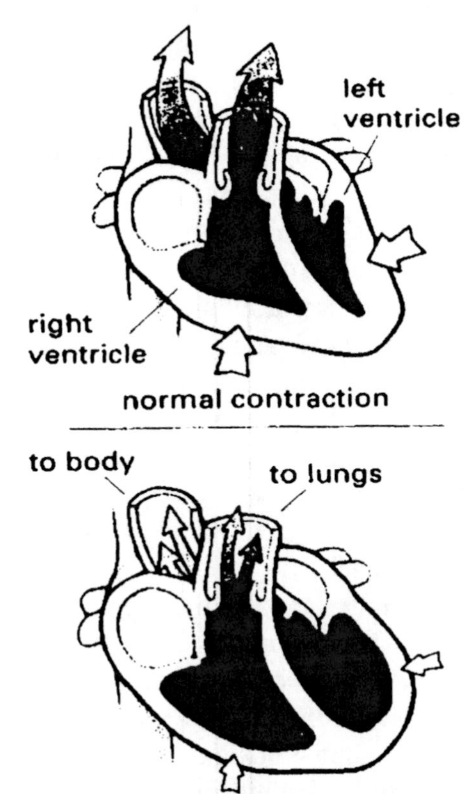

FIGURE 5.3 Congested heart. Reprinted with permission form The Johns Hopkins Medical Letter (1995, December), *Health After 50, 7*(10), 4.

Right-sided failure of the heart:

- edema: a build-up of fluids outside the blood vessels that forces fluid into the tissues; occurs mostly in the ankles
- gradual loss of energy
- anorexia (loss of appetite for food)
- constipation
- weight gain (because kidneys cause the body to keep too much sodium and water)
- grayish or blue color of the skin due to decreased blood flow

Left-sided failure of the heart:

- frequent coughing or wheezing
- shortness of breath (dyspnea), a result of the blood backing up into the lungs, thus decreasing the amount of space in the lungs available to hold air. This is one of the definitive signs of CHF and usually occurs after exercise (Anderson, 1976)
- confusion and loss of memory are severe symptoms that suggest the disease has progressed far enough to damage the brain tissue

Treatment generally consists of rest; monitoring weight to guard against sudden changes; diet therapy, including reducing salt intake and encouraging potassium intake with foods like bananas and oranges; and oxygen therapy to improve the oxygen content of red blood cells, since there is less and less exchange area available in the lungs (Moss, 1989). Liquid oxygen and other innovations are addressing the mobility problem generated by left-sided failure.

Technologic advances are being made in providing oxygen to residents. Machines called oxygen concentrators are available, obviating the constant need for oxygen tanks. The advantage is an ability to use ambient air in the resident's room to produce the required oxygen. The potential disadvantage is that, unlike the bulky and unsightly tanks, the oxygen concentrator should have a continuous supply of electricity.

Medications can include digoxin (Lanoxin®), which acts directly on the heart muscle to increase the force of contraction. This is an extremely powerful medication that may cause severe side effects in the elderly when the level of the medication becomes too high in the blood. Confusion or severe behavioral changes may indicate this is occurring (Gambert, 1983; Kane et al., 1989).

To avoid fluid buildup, diuretics are also often prescribed to aid the body in eliminating toxic wastes and fluids that have accumulated (Crow, 1984). Some of the more powerful diuretics deplete the body's supply of important electrolytes, such as sodium and potassium. Low levels of potassium can be particularly dangerous for the elderly, who are especially vulnerable to such imbalances. Potassium supplements are frequently prescribed, in addition to dietary supplements, to increase the blood level of this naturally occurring mineral.

RESIDENT EXERCISE AND FITNESS

As we will see later, a degradation of function in the cardiovascular system usually interferes with the supply of nutrients and oxygen to the cells (Sullivan, 1995). This, in turn, damages the tissues and organs in the body, leading to the decline of other major organs in the body and of other major processes. It is not surprising, then, that a consensus is emerging: Moderate exercise is important to the cardiovascular system of aged persons (Maddox, 2001). Harris (1989) cites studies by deVries, Frankel, Kraus, Jokl, and others that demonstrate that physical conditioning can improve the cardiovascular system, the respiratory system, the musculature, and the body composition of older persons. The Paffenbarger study of 16,920 Harvard male alumni attributed 1 to 2 years of increased longevity to men 80 years old who had exercised moderately over the years (Paffenbarger, Wing, & Hsieh, 1986).

This all makes sense. The body systems we have mentioned and will describe in more detail below, all depend on oxygen and nutrients from the blood. Exercise increases the blood supplied to the body systems. Improved supplies of oxygen and nutrients lead to improved organ and cell status.

Claims for the benefits of exercise for the elderly are extensive. Beneficial effects on depression, reduction in risk of developing heart disease, improved oxygenation and oxygen transport, greater protection against deterioration of glucose tolerance, improved oxygen transport, and denser bone mass are some of the perceived benefits (Harris, 1989).

Sedentary lifestyle and poor physical fitness are thought to be responsible for some of the typical symptoms, such as headaches, constipation, joint pain, back aches, insomnia, and fatigue. Keeping the cardiovascular system at its peak through regular exercise, then, is seen to have beneficial effects upon many of the body's systems. Inclusion of a level of aerobic exercise (i.e., exercise sustaining the heart rate at an elevated level, delivering increased oxygen for specified minimum period of time each week) matched to each resident's capabilities in the plan of health care seems appropriate as a facility policy (Maddox, 2001).

5.3.2 Respiratory System

The chief function of the respiratory process is providing the body with oxygen while removing excess carbon dioxide. These processes occur during breathing, when air enters and exits the body through the nose and mouth. The air that enters the body is rich in oxygen, the gas necessary for many of the cells' basic chemical functions. The respiratory and circulatory systems are very closely related, because both are involved with the oxygenation process.

THE OXYGENATION PROCESS

The circulatory system can be envisioned as a train carrying the oxygen in each car, or blood cell. The lungs, then, are the depot terminals where the blood cells pick up oxygen and deposit carbon dioxide. The structures in the body that help the respiratory system do its work include the mouth, nose, pharynx, trachea, bronchi, bronchioles, lungs, alveoli, diaphragm, and various respiratory muscles. The respiratory process involves all of these structures to promote the inhalation and exhalation of air that transports gases to the blood cells and diffuses oxygen into the body (Rosendorff, 1983).

After the air is inhaled through either the nose or the mouth, it travels through the trachea, which leads to the bronchi of the lungs. There, the two bronchi, the main airways leading into the lungs, divide and subdivide numerous times before ultimately forming the bronchioles (see Figure 5.4). The bronchioles are the smallest airways in the lungs and eventually terminate in the numerous alveoli that are the basic respiratory units (see Figure 5.5).

Alveoli are the many air-filled sacs that are the site of the actual oxygen–carbon dioxide exchange. In this transaction oxygen is absorbed by the blood, and carbon dioxide is released into the air as the breath is exhaled. Much of the volume within the lungs is taken up by blood undergoing this stage of the oxygenation process.

Because the respiratory and cardiovascular systems are closely related, any damage to one of these systems is likely to directly affect the other (Kart, Metress, & Metress, 1978). A number of other structures are essential for breathing, including the diaphragm and associated respiratory muscles of the chest. These structures aid the lungs in expanding and contracting with each inhalation and exhalation.

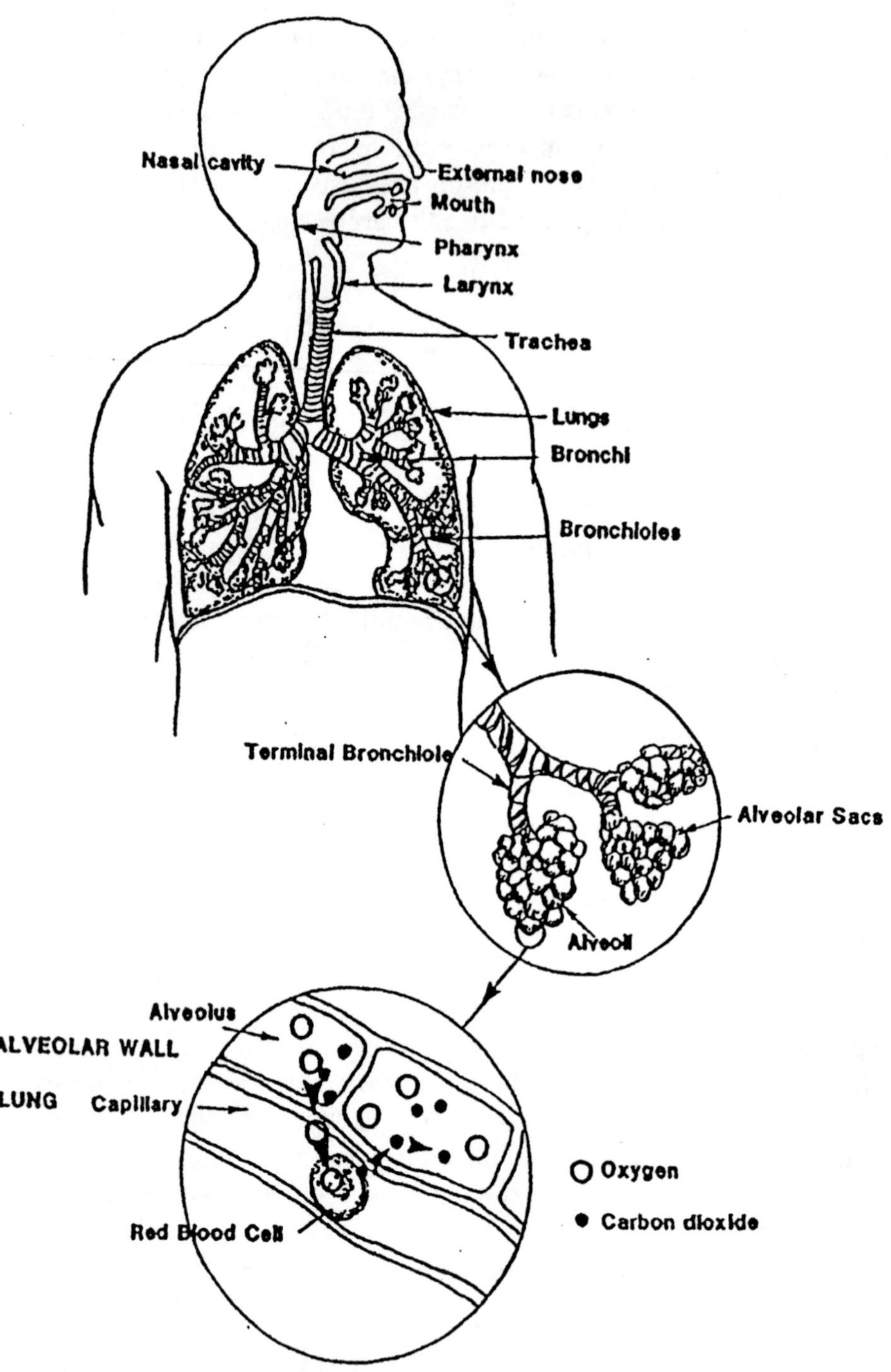

FIGURE 5.4 The respiratory tract. Oxygen-carbon dioxide exchange at alveolar wall where permeation of oxygen and carbon dioxide cells occurs.

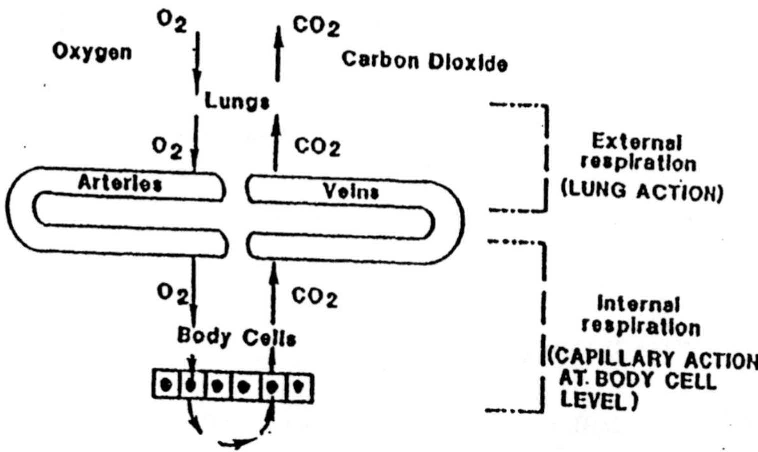

FIGURE 5.5 Diagram of events occurring simultaneously during respiration.

AGE-ASSOCIATED CHANGES

Changes associated with the aging process do occur. However, in the elderly person without any significant disease, the overall result of these changes should not be incapacitating or prevent him or her from carrying on the activities of daily living (Kart et al., 1978).

One of the reasons for this is that the lung, unlike the heart, has a remarkable ability to repair itself after infection or damage. These repairs usually leave only minor traces that could later be mistaken for degenerative changes (Woodruff & Birren, 1975). Changes due to aging that do affect the respiratory system include the following (Kenney, 1982):

- decreasing size (and therefore capacity) of the alveoli
- loss of elasticity of lung tissue
- stiffening of the ribs (requiring muscles to work harder to pump air in and out of the lungs)
- changes in the shape of the chest
- decreased resistance to infection

The decreased capacity of the alveoli is not in itself enough to cause any dramatic changes in the breathing process. However, this does reduce the efficiency of the breathing mechanism and may lead to disability and respiratory problems over time (Weg, 1983).

The elderly are more prone to infections than the rest of the population. When these additional factors are coupled with the fact that the lungs receive foreign materials continuously from the air, it is not surprising that many elderly persons suffer from some form of lung disease.

INFLUENCE OF THE ENVIRONMENT ON THE LUNGS

Because the lungs are in almost direct contact with the air outside, the environment may play a more important role in the development of lung disease than in any other body system. Environmental exposure to a lung irritant over a prolonged period of time often produces the type of changes that result in respiratory disease. Some examples are miners' exposure to coal dust, welders' to asbestos, and chronic cigarette smokers' to tar and nicotine. Lung infection is one of the more common causes of death among older persons (Garagusi, 1989).

CHRONIC RESPIRATORY DISEASE

The most common classification of lung disease is chronic obstructive lung disease (COLD) or chronic obstructive pulmonary disease (COPD). The COPD diagnosis includes chronic bronchitis, asthma, and emphysema (Shashaty, 1989). There is no cure for these diseases, but there are a variety of treatments available ("Best drugs," 1994, p. 6). New diagnostic instruments are becoming available such as a pulse oximeter that uses infrared light through the finger to read the oxygen level within 30 seconds. Spirometers are used to detect the amount of lung volume the individual can exhale; then results are compared with predicted curves.

The main complication brought on by COPD is that the body is unable to rid itself of the air containing carbon dioxide. This may be because of a disruption of the alveoli or because the bronchial tubes are not expanding and permitting the gases to escape during respiration.

Chronic bronchitis and emphysema are two diseases of this type that are most commonly seen in the assisted living facility resident. The signs, symptoms, and treatment of the respiratory diseases mentioned are very similar. The symptoms listed following the discussion of the next two diseases will apply to all the diseases in the remainder of this section.

Chronic Bronchitis

As the name suggests, chronic bronchitis is caused by a continuing irritation of the bronchi (the two airways into the lungs). The inside of these airways swell and become clogged with mucus secretions, making it more difficult to breathe. This may be due to something irritating from the environment or a recurrent infection. Chronic smokers are most likely to develop bronchitis. This disease is the most common respiratory condition found in the elderly and is defined as a chronic productive cough in more than 3 months of 2 successive years, unexplained by another diagnosis (Shashaty, 1989, p. 101).

Asthma is characterized by bronchial reactions to internal or external stimulants. It is generalized reversible airway obstruction. Usually a bronchodialator is administered orally, by inhalation or both (Shashaty, 1989).

Emphysema

Emphysema results in a loss of elasticity in all of the lung tissue. As a consequence, the lung is less able to hold as much air, but the alveoli tend to have air trapped inside, causing carbon dioxide to build up. The increasing amount of carbon dioxide only worsens the respiratory condition, because the body is triggered to obtain more and more oxygen to compensate for this imbalance. Continuous oxygen therapy may be supplied from large oxygen tanks, liquid oxygen reservoirs, or an oxygen concentrator. Oxygen therapy reduces lung hypertension and promotes oxygenation of the other body systems (Shashaty, 1989). According to the National Center for Health Statistics, in 1995 emphysema was the fourth leading cause of death among persons age 65 and older: 264 deaths per 100,000, or 88,478 actual deaths ("Retirement checkup," 1998).

The causes of emphysema are similar to those of bronchitis, the most common one being a recurrent infection or chronic irritant to the lung. Emphysema is much more serious than bronchitis, and usually persons with this disease die from heart failure as a result of prolonged stress on the cardiovascular system.

Symptoms common for most lung diseases are chronic cough, increased production of thick white mucus, and some shortness of breath. These symptoms are a result of the body attempting to rid itself of whatever is irritating the respiratory tract. Irritation of the inner lining of the respiratory tract results in the increased production of mucus, which is intended to coat the cause of the irritation and assist its excretion from the body.

A cough is another way the body has of rejecting whatever is causing the irritation. When this irritation is chronic, these mechanisms are continually being triggered.

These lung disease symptoms can be found in more severe forms:

- stress on the entire cardiovascular system with related symptoms
- enlarged heart
- heart failure (with emphysema)
- thick mucus plugs blocking the smaller airways within the lung
- alveoli that have become overinflated and eventually burst, decreasing the amount of space available for oxygen exchange
- barrel-shaped chest
- poor appetite
- weight loss
- dizziness

Treatments include medications to minimize airway irritation and obstruction, such as bronchodilators (to relax the breathing tubes, widening them, and thus improving air flow) and expectorants (to thin the mucus so that coughing is more successful).

Pneumonia

Pneumonia is an infection in the lungs caused by either a virus or bacteria. Residents with chronic obstructive lung disease are much more susceptible to this infection because bacteria grow in stagnant areas like those where the mucus is collecting. This infection further complicates the elderly person's ability to breathe and causes disruptions in other systems. According to the National Center for Health Statistics, in 1995 pneumonia was the fifth leading cause of death among persons age 65 and older: 222 deaths per 100,000, or 74,297 actual deaths ("Retirement checkup," 1998).

The signs and **symptoms** are very similar to those already described and may include a fever or very weak condition resulting from the infection. **Treatment** generally includes some type of antibiotic therapy when bacteria are the cause of this infection.

Chronic Tuberculosis

Tuberculosis is an infectious disease more commonly found among assisted living facility residents because of their higher risk of infection, resulting from multiple chronic diseases (Cohan, 1989).

Tuberculosis may infect a person while he or she is young, but oftentimes a healthy immune system wards off the disease, which goes into a dormant state. As a person ages, this immunity may break down and the dormant disease may become active ("Tuberculosis," 1995).

Signs and **symptoms** are similar to those listed for COLD, except that the secretions contain the tuberculosis bacteria. The disease is termed infectious because it may easily be transmitted through the secretions or when a resident coughs.

One of the most important **treatments,** then, is to isolate the person as long as he or she is coughing and producing sputum. To prevent the spread of infection, staff and visitors generally are required to wear masks and gloves when in contact with the resident or in his or her room.

Lung Cancer

Lung cancer is a chronic lung disease and is among the leading causes of death for American men. It is also the most prevalent from of cancer found among assisted living facility residents. Because the disease affects the lung, symptoms are similar to those of COLD.

Generally, the assisted living facility resident is receiving palliative treatment (just enough therapy to make him or her comfortable). Other types of treatment include radiation, chemotherapy, or surgery, depending on the size and location of the tumor. With improved understanding of this disease process, new drug regimens and improved radiation treatments, lung cancer is becoming treatable (Tuberculosis Letter, August, 1995, p. 1; Evans et.al, 2000).

5.3.3 Nervous System

One of the body's most important mechanisms is the nervous system, which acts as its control center by coordinating functions and maintaining order. The brain can be thought of as a computer system, with the nerves and spinal cord transferring input and output messages to and from each part of the body (Brody, 1995).

Some specific nervous systems functions for control of the body include responding to events outside the body through the five senses, performing voluntary activities such as walking, and storing memories, ideas, and emotions so they may be used at a later time for various thought processes. The nervous system also performs automatic responses such as breathing, maintaining heart rate, and controlling temperature.

COMPONENTS OF THE CENTRAL NERVOUS SYSTEM

The central nervous is composed of the brain, spinal cord, and nerves. The brain is considered to be the most important organ in the body because it is accorded a high level of priority among body functions. When the body is undergoing a great deal of stress, other organs will reduce nutrient intake so that more nutrients can be directed to the brain.

The brain is protected by the skull and surrounded inside by a protective layer of cerebrospinal fluid. This organ is very specialized, with different areas responsible for different body functions.

The cranial nerves connect the brain with the areas of the body responsible for sensory perception (identifying what is outside the body through the senses, including taste, smell, and hearing). The base of the brain is called the medulla. It is primarily responsible for controlling motor activity or movement. It is this area that connects the brain to the spinal cord.

The spinal cord looks like a tree trunk, with the nerves representing the branches of the tree and eventually leading to the blood vessels, muscles, and/or organs throughout the body.

The brain itself is made up of many specialized cells that are unique to the individual areas of the brain in which they are found. Because the brain cells perform complex processes, they need large amounts of oxygen to function continually. A lack of oxygen to the brain causes the cells and their tissues to die within minutes.

The nerves are composed of many individual fibers that are encased in a fatty substance called myelin for the same reason that electrical wires are covered with a plastic coating: to prevent them from "shorting out." These individual fibers are composed of neurons, which are the nerve cells. Unlike the heart cells, nerve cells can be replaced or regenerate themselves, although at a very slow rate.

The nerve fibers form an intricate network that is responsible for carrying a variety of messages to the brain. These messages are carried in the form of electrical impulses that stimulate the appropriate area of the brain, triggering either an involuntary response reaction (reflex) or a thought (cognitive) process.

The nerve fibers form a complex series of pathways that impulses travel along to reach the brain. It is important to remember that the left side of the brain controls the functions on the right side of the body, and the right side of the brain controls functions on the left side of the body.

POSSIBLE EFFECTS OF AGING

The effects of aging on the nervous system are most commonly believed to be the result of a change in the system that reduces the oxygen supply to the brain cells. This can lead to permanent alterations to those cells which are so sensitive to the level of the oxygen supply (Chui, 1995b; Hefti, 1995; Woodruff & Birren, 1975).

Apparently the weight of the brain, as mentioned above, decreases with age, possibly because of some loss of brain cells and nerve fibers (Kenney, 1982).

Researchers, using refined instruments, have been able to detect changes in the neurological system of the elderly when observing the speed with which impulses are transmitted to the brain. But this change is not directly associated with a slowing down of functioning in the thought process. It is probably a myth that older people's thought or cognitive process is much slower than other age groups.

PERCEPTUAL CHANGES

One of the perceptual changes commonly attributed to the aging process is a decreased sensitivity to touch (Kenney, 1982).

Some of the visual changes associated with age include loss of range of vision for near objects, decreased flexibility of the lens of the eye, and reduced clarity of vision, or the "dusty windshield" effect of the lens of the eye, accompanied by a loss in ability to distinguish pastels.

There may be a change in the central processing of sound in the inner ear. This has not been proven as yet, so residents who are hard of hearing are not necessarily that way just because of age. There does appear to be a loss of ability to hear high-pitched sounds; speaking to residents in deep tones can help compensate for this loss.

In many elderly individuals the taste buds appear to have degenerated, and the amount of saliva produced also appears to be diminished, producing a change in the capacity to taste different flavors. Abuse of salt may result from efforts to "improve" or increase taste sensations. Ability to taste sweets is apparently unaffected, which may explain the preference of many elderly residents for eating dessert first.

There may also be an age-related decrease in neurons responsible for smell, resulting in the loss of smell for different odors.

Some of the elderly also appear to dream less and have increased periods of wakefulness throughout the night (Libow, 1981).

Diseases associated with the nervous system include those that affect sensory components, impair mobility and communication processes, and affect the ability to distinguish reality from fantasy (Steffl, 1984).

THE EYE

The eye is a complicated structure, with muscles holding it in place. The retina is the innermost layer of the eye and contains receptor cells that actually generate electrical nerve impulses when hit by light. These impulses are carried to the brain on the nerve fibers that leave the retina and form the optic nerve. This nerve leads to the area of the brain responsible for vision. The retina is protected by the lens covering the eye.

The lens can be thought of as a layer of skin, except that all of the old cells on the lens cannot be discarded like old layers of skin, and they are continually compacted within the eye (Corso, 1981). The aqueous humor is a substance that bathes the eye and protects it.

Presence of Eye Problems

The aging process may result in an overproduction of aqueous humor, resulting in a large amount within the eye. When this happens, glaucoma may result.

Glaucoma. Glaucoma is a chronic condition that is actually a complex of many different symptoms. This condition is not a direct result of the aging process, but the incidence of the disease is definitely greater among older individuals (Corso, 1981; Kane et al., 1989).

There are four different types of glaucoma: chronic, acute, secondary, and congenital. In each of these, the primary problem is that fluids within the eye undergo increasing pressure changes. These fluids are continually being formed, but not draining from the eye chamber, because of some disruption in the drainage system (Kasper, 1989). As a result, the eyeball itself becomes very hard. This also causes an extremely painful pressure in the eye, which can lead to a range of other conditions.

Symptoms of glaucoma can induce acute pain in the eye, elevated blood pressure, blurred vision, and halos seen around lights. Untreated glaucoma can lead to blindness.

Treatment usually varies with the form or state of disease, but initially medical therapy is used to promote the drainage of excess fluids from the eye. As a rule, medications are the critical variable in preventing blindness from glaucoma (Steffl, 1984).

Mydriatics usually come in the form of eyedrops and act to dilate the pupil of the eye, helping to drain off some of the excess fluid.

Cataracts. A cataract is a cloudiness that affects the transparency of the lens to the extent that light cannot get through to the retina of the eye. The retina is the area of the eye that transforms light into the objects seen. Usually cataracts form in both eyes.

The major symptom of cataracts is increasingly blurred vision, with perceptions of "shadows." Treatment usually consists of eyeglasses or contact lenses. The lens can be surgically removed and replaced with a new manufactured one (lens implant).

According to the National Center for Health Statistics, a cataract was reported as the fourth most frequently occurring chronic condition in persons age 65 and older, occurring at the rate of 166 cases per 1,000 individuals ("Retirement checkup," 1998).

Importance of Vision Among Residents

When older persons with visual impairments are assisted to see better through intervention, they adapt better to the area around them. Interventions do not need to be complex. They can include providing large-type books, magazines, and newspapers; painting color-coded boundaries and walkways throughout the facility for easy identification (e.g., a painted baseboard in the hallway helps distinguish spatial location); and using large letters and numbers in all visual displays such as doors, elevators, and clocks. According to the American Foundation for the Blind, the percentage of the older population with severe visual impairment is

Age 65–74	5.9%
Age 75–84	11.9%
Age 85+	21.5% ("Retirement checkup," 1998, p. 22).

According to the National Center for Health Statistics, visual impairment was the 10th most frequently occurring chronic condition, occurring at the rate of 82 cases per 1,000 persons age 65 and older ("Retirement checkup," 1998).

HEARING

The structures of the outer ear include those portions of the ear external to the eardrum (tympanic membrane). The middle ear contains three small bones that conduct the sound waves; they are called the incus (anvil), the malleus (hammer), and the stapes (stirrup).

The inner ear contains the cochlea, which transmits sound waves to nerve impulses that travel down the auditory nerve (the eighth cranial nerve) to the auditory center of the brain.

Hearing Impairments

Presbycusis is the term used to describe any hearing impairment in old age. According to the National Center for Health Statistics, hearing impairment was reported as the fourth most frequently occurring chronic condition in persons age 65 and older, occurring at the rate of 286 cases per 1,000 individuals ("Retirement checkup," 1998).

Hearing impairments can also be due to a buildup of wax in the ear or to what is known as a conductive or sensorineural hearing loss. Conductive disorders and ear wax are the only ones that may be treated effectively. Usually surgery or hearing aids are prescribed for those with a conductive loss. The sensorineural disturbances result from a disruption in the structure of the inner ear or the nerve pathway to the brain stem.

Symptoms of hearing impairment can include tinnitus (an intermittent, sometimes constant, ringing in the ears), progressive hearing loss, and increased inability to hear high-frequency sounds, including shouting, warning bells, or buzzers (Yoder, 1989).

Treatment can include a hearing aid when appropriate; sign language; lip reading; speech reading; slow, well-enunciated communication; always facing the resident when speaking to him or her; and providing appropriate warning signals to communicate the presence of fires or other dangerous occurrences within the facility.

MOBILITY AND COMMUNICATION

A cerebrovascular accident (CVA), also known as a stroke, can be one of the most debilitating conditions that an elderly person faces. The cause of stroke is lack of oxygen to the brain, usually resulting from the blockage of a major blood vessel or the leakage of blood from a vessel that has ruptured. Sixty percent of cerebral vascular accidents are due to arterial thrombosis (Grob, 1989, p. 299).

Warning signs can include weakness of some muscle, depression, and a tingling in the arm or leg.

Degrees of Disability

The degree of disability resulting from a stroke may range from only a slight impairment to complete immobility and loss of voluntary muscle control (Van Vilet, 1995a). Signs following a stroke are usually specifically related to the area of the brain affected. These symptoms may include the following:

- muscle weakness on one side of the body (hemiplegia)
- difficulty standing or walking
- poor balance
- pain in arms and legs
- fatigue
- poor vision
- confusion
- difficulty in spatial judgment, distortion
- complete loss of muscle control (quadriplegia)
- paralysis of the body below the upper extremities (paraplegia)
- difficulty speaking (aphasia)
- dysphasia

Aphasia

Aphasia is the term used to describe an inability to interpret and formulate language. Specifically, such problems may be seen as a slowdown in ability to retrieve vocabulary and inappropriate use of grammar or words, as well as problems in understanding what is being said.

Usually this occurs because the area of the brain responsible for speech is damaged during the stroke. There are many different types of aphasia, with the most severe resulting in an individual being unable to understand what others are saying to him or her (receptive aphasia).

Other types of aphasia result in an inability to express in words what the individual really wants to communicate (expressive aphasia). Other times, inappropriate words or vulgar language is uttered as if the individual had no control of what he or she says.

Dysarthria

Dysarthria (literally, imperfect articulation of speech) is a speech rather than a language abnormality that may accompany paralysis, weakness, or lack of coordination. This deficit can be a frustrating experience for the resident who has all other mental capacities intact. This frustration often leads to emotional upset. The most important need that residents have at this time is the ability to communicate.

Individually designed rehabilitative therapy is the most usual form of treatment. The ability of a person to recover from a stroke is best correlated with the cause. Lower brain stem damage from a stroke has a more favorable prognosis than an assault on the upper part of the brain.

Rehabilitation therapy usually focuses on standing, ambulating, taking initial steps, and walking with a cane or other appliance. Physical and occupational therapists are integral members of the rehabilitation team for these residents.

Parkinson's Disease

Parkinson's disease is actually a group of symptoms that can progressively lead to complete disability in those severely affected. Scientists believe that selected groups of neurons (nerve cells) in the brain are lost as a result of this disease, but the cause of this loss remains a mystery.

Symptoms of Parkinson's disease can include tremor, or trembling, of any of the limbs while at rest, rigidity or muscle stiffness, and bradykinesia (a slowness in body movements). Additional symptoms may include the following:

- stooped posture while standing
- walking with short, shuffling steps
- garbled speech
- illegible handwriting
- sad, lifeless facial expression
- facial droop
- mood swings
- dementia (an impairment in intellectual ability)

There is no cure for Parkinson's disease, so the treatment is determined by the specific symptoms and degree of physical impairment in functioning (Cohan, 1989).

Often residents with Parkinson's disease suffer from mental disturbances similar to those seen in residents with Alzheimer's disease, and physicians are finding it difficult to distinguish one from the other. Alzheimer's residents have the additional diagnosis of dementia (Ripich, Wykle, & Niles, 1995).

Dementia

Dementia is a broad, nonspecific term denoting cognitive loss (Reichel & Rabins, 1989). The diagnosis and understanding of mental deterioration among some elderly is still in its early stages.

Reichel and Rabins (1989) identified three major causes of senile dementia. About 60% is due to Alzheimer's type, 25% to infarction of brain tissue due to cerebrovascular disease, and 15% to several other diseases such as paresis, Huntington's chorea, Pick's disease, Parkinsonism, acquired immune deficiency syndrome, and Wilson's disease.

Dementia is usually thought of as senility in an elderly person and may include behavior such as forgetfulness, a deterioration in personality, and a decrease in intellectual functioning (Reisberg, 1995).

A common misperception is that these behaviors are all a normal result of the aging process. But none of these senile behaviors are considered to be normal aging effects and are instead due to some type of disease or disruption (Kane et al., 1989).

Hardening of the arteries due to arteriosclerosis is a disease that may lead to dementia in the elderly person. In this situation, the arteries do not allow enough oxygen to pass through to the brain, with the result that areas of the brain die. The only way physicians currently have of distinguishing between multi-infarct dementia and Alzheimer's disease is to perform a computer automated tomograph (CAT scan). The treatment, however, is no different for either diagnosis.

Alzheimer's Disease

Alzheimer's disease is the most common form of dementia seen in persons over 60 years old; its incidence increases dramatically after that age. The Alzheimer's resident displays an intellectual impairment that is irreversible. The disease progression varies from 1 resident to another and can extend from one year to over a decade (Schneck et al., 1982). Alzheimer's type of dementia is also known as primary degenerative dementia, a disorder that involves alteration in the structure, number, and functions of neurons in some areas of the brain's cerebral cortex.

Three distinct phases of Alzheimer's disease have been identified: Stage I—forgetfulness or early stage; Stage II—confusion or mild stage; and Stage III—dementia or terminal stage (Schneck et al., 1982).

The signs and symptoms of the disease vary with each stage, but some, including memory loss and behavioral changes, progress in severity until they become profound in the final stage. The following list of signs and symptoms reveals the progressive nature of the disease:

Stage I

- memory loss
- time disorientation
- anxiety
- irritability
- lack of spontaneity
- behavior and personality change
- agitation
- inability to concentrate for long periods of time

Stage II

- excessive hunger
- aphasia
- temper tantrums
- restlessness
- muscle twitching
- aimless wandering, sometimes getting lost
- inability to read, write, or do arithmetic calculations
- obsession behavior (e.g., constant washing and rewashing of hands)
- repetitive movements (e.g., tapping, chewing, lip smacking)

Stage III

- bedridden
- unable to perform purposeful movement (i.e., walk)
- poor appetite
- poor articulation
- incontinence
- emaciation
- frequent seizures

The goal of treatment is to achieve the highest quality of life while maintaining physical function. Several assisted living facility chains as well as individual facilities have installed special Alzheimer's units, usually characterized by enclosed outdoor areas and indoor gates of various types to control wandering (e.g., coded key pads on doors). Typically, it is the Stage II resident who is the primary type of resident in these units due to the special management needs created by this stage of the disease process.

Medications are palliative, often being tranquilizers to relax the resident and relieve any agitation or violence. Antidepressants are also used to improve the overall mood. Over 250 pharmaceutical companies as well as other researchers are racing to find breakthrough drugs or cures for Alzheimer's (Dewey, 1995)

Breaking New Ground. Research into treatments appears promising, but no breakthroughs have been achieved. It seems likely that as more is learned, new disease patterns will be identified within the current broad categories of (1) Alzheimer's type, (2) infarction of the brain tissue due to cerebrovascular disease, or (3) other. Researchers at the Harvard Medical School studied 3,623 elderly Bostonians and found Alzheimer's present in 3% of those age 65 to 74, 19% of the 75 to 84-year-olds and 47% of those 85 and older. According to the National Center for Health Statistics, in 1995 Alzheimer's disease was the eighth leading cause of death among persons age 65 and older: 60 deaths per 100,000, or 20,230 actual deaths ("Retirement checkup," 1998).

Cognitive losses are being identified more successfully and, it is hoped, will become more treatable. Persons 85 and older make up the fastest growing segment of the U.S. population. The assisted living facility is often the institution of choice to care for persons of that age diagnosed as having dementia.

Articles and research reports concerning Alzheimer's disease abound. See, for example, Bennett and Knopman (1994); Sterritt and Pokorny (1994); Zinn and Mor (1994); McCaddon and Kelly (1994); Swanson, Maas, and Buckwalter (1993); "Best drugs," (1995); Karcher (1993); and Office of Technology Assessment (1994).

5.3.4 Digestive System

Digestion is the process by which the body breaks down food into needed nutrients. These nutrients are further broken down into particles small enough to pass through tissues and enter the bloodstream for delivery to the appropriate tissues and organs. After absorbing necessary nutrients, the leftover materials or waste products are discarded from the body.

The digestive system is commonly referred to as the gastrointestinal or alimentary tract in reference to the various organs that participate in the digestive process (see Figure 5.6).

MOUTH

Digestion begins when food enters the mouth. Chewing the food is an important step in preparing it for digestion. Saliva, produced by salivary glands in the mouth, contains enzymes that begin breaking down food substances while they are still in the mouth.

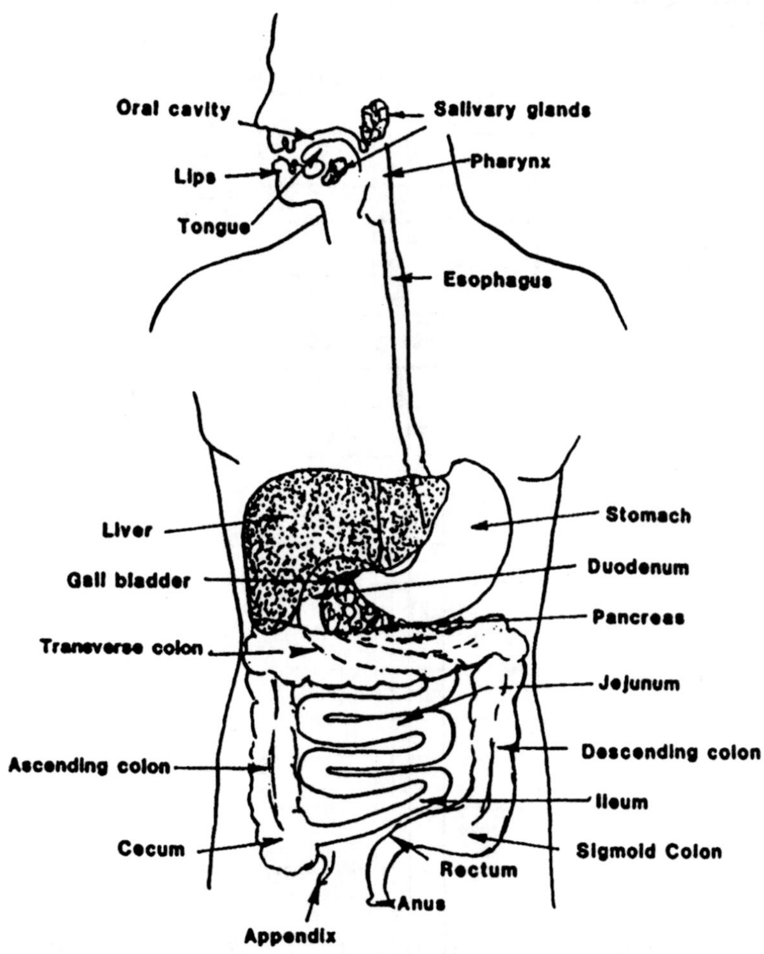

FIGURE 5.6 Organs involved in the digestive processes.

ESOPHAGUS

After food is swallowed, it enters the esophagus. The esophagus is the tube (made of smooth muscle) connecting the mouth to the stomach. When food is swallowed, the gastric (stomach) sphincter relaxes to allow food into the stomach. Swallowing initiates a wavelike movement of the esophagus (called peristalsis) that propels food toward the stomach (see Figure 5.7).

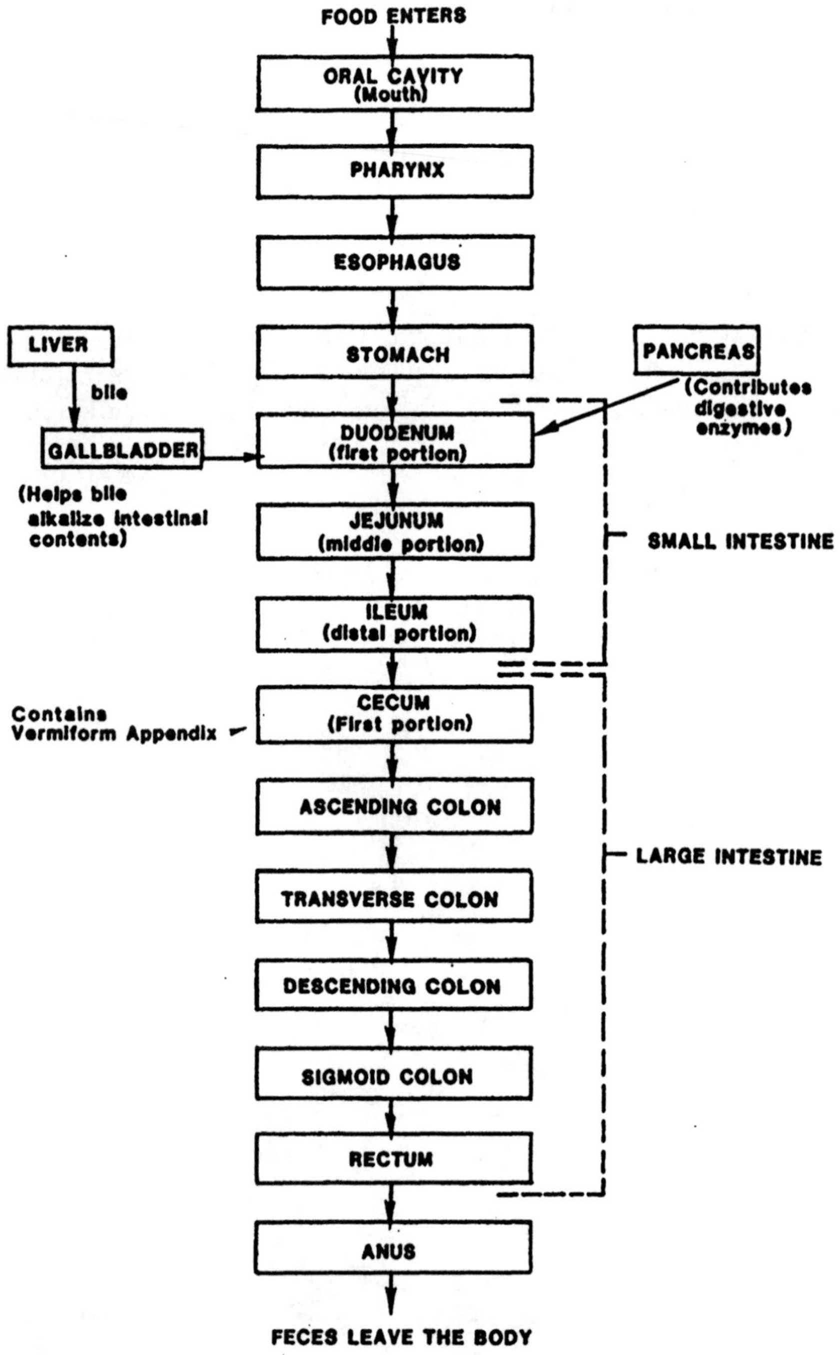

FIGURE 5.7 Diagrammatic representation of the path of food through the digestive system.

STOMACH

The next phase of digestion begins in the stomach. The stomach has sphincters (muscles) at both ends that close when the stomach is full, enabling the stomach acids to have sufficient time to break down the food.

The digestive process in the stomach is controlled by the brain through the nerves, which constantly carry impulses directing the digestion process.

INTESTINES

The intestines, small and large, may be thought of as a long tube. The intestines are also referred to as the bowels or lower gastrointestinal tract (lower GI). Despite its name, the small intestine is actually much longer than the large intestine.

When the digestive contents enter the small intestine (duodenum), further chemical digestive actions occur. The food is in liquid form at this stage and contains powerful enzymes that break down certain substances. The intestines are also filled with a supply of bacteria that help to digest some of the food substances. These same bacteria are very harmful to any other part of the body if allowed to escape.

Like the stomach, the intestines also have nerves carrying impulses to and from the brain. These nerves are especially important in stimulating the bowel to move the waste materials along the intestinal tract. As in the esophagus, the intestine contracts in snakelike movements, propelling the food along the digestive tract.

If, for some reason the brain does not send the appropriate impulses to the intestines, the waste moves much more slowly though these organs. Unlike the esophagus, the intestines do not have the added force of gravity to assist in this process.

LARGE INTESTINE

The large intestine is a continuation of the small intestine and plays its own role in the digestive process. One function of the large intestine is to store the waste so that the body can absorb excess fluids and nutrients before elimination.

By the time waste materials are excreted from the body, they are in a solid form, often referred to as feces or stool. It is important to note that usually persons have voluntary control over when they choose to eliminate these waste materials because the sphincters at the very end of the digestive tract are within the realm of voluntary control.

POSSIBLE EFFECTS OF AGING

Mouth

The amount of saliva secreted by the salivary glands may decrease. The saliva also may become thicker, until it is almost like mucus (MacHudis, 1983). The loss of teeth may also cause digestive complications (Libow, 1981).

Esophagus

In some elderly persons food may not travel as quickly through the esophagus. Causes for this appear to be (1) a reduction in the effectiveness of the swallowing mechanism helping foods move toward the stomach and (2) the gastric sphincter failing to close as quickly as before (Kenney, 1982).

Stomach

The lining of the stomach can decrease in thickness with age. This decreased thickness of the lining may allow the size of the stomach to increase. The amount of acid produced by the stomach may decrease (Kenney, 1982; Sklar, 1983).

DIGESTIVE DISEASES

The digestive tract is an area of the body about which elderly assisted living facility residents often complain. Physicians use the general diagnosis "gastrointestinal distress" to describe a range of diseases affecting this system.

Esophagus

The esophagus may be a common site of discomfort for the elderly resident. Esophagitis (inflammation or irritation of the esophagus) is another name for heartburn, a frequent problem for elderly individuals. Often this sharp, burning pain may be confused with chest pain and may become worse when the person lies flat, allowing stomach contents to reenter the esophagus.

Dysphagia is difficulty in swallowing or transferring food from the mouth to the esophagus (Gibbons & Levy, 1989; Logeman, 1995). Persons with neurological damage may be subject to this problem. Persons who have recently suffered a stroke can be at increased risk because without this function they may aspirate (inhale particles of) food into their lungs.

Stomach

Peptic ulcers may occur anywhere in the gastrointestinal tract. Two of the most common types are gastric ulcers that affect the mid-stomach and duodenal ulcers that involve the lower stomach.

An ulcer is a wearing away of the inner lining of the stomach wall and is due to a chronic buildup of excessive levels of acid. Excessive stress, inactivity, prolonged bed rest, severe trauma, and irritating drugs may all serve to cause or irritate this condition. On examination at death 35% of persons under 50 years of age had gastric ulcers, whereas 80% of those over 80 years of age (i.e., typical assisted living facility residents) had gastric ulcers (Gibbons & Levy, 1989, p. 191).

Ulcer symptoms can include sharp burning abdominal pain 1 to 4 hours after eating, nausea, weight loss, blood in vomitus, and blood in stools.

The goal of treatment is to prevent any complications arising from the initial ulceration, thus allowing it to heal. Medications, including antacids, are prescribed to relieve the condition. Long-term treatment for peptic ulcers remains controversial. The preferred approach appears to be to treat for 12 months; others prefer intermittent courses of treatment (Gibbons & Levy, 1989, p. 191). Recently, it has been demonstrated that many stomach ulcers are actually due to a disease organism that is treatable with drugs.

Intestines

Constipation is an irregularity in or lack of elimination of waste materials from the body. "Normal" bowel habits studied in 1,500 older residents indicated 99% reported anywhere from 3 bowel movements daily to 3 per week (Gibbons & Levy, 1989, p. 196).

Constipation may initially be a decrease in the number of stools passed, progressing to a complete lack of stool or bowel movements. When the person has not been able to pass stool for a long period of time, an impaction (blockage) has probably occurred. The waste in the large intestine has accumulated in one area and become hard because much of the fluid content has been reabsorbed by the body.

Treatment of constipation can include laxative medications, which are commonly prescribed for assisted living facility residents. Bulk laxatives, osmotic laxatives, suppositories, and enemas are the different forms of medications that may be prescribed. Increased activity is one of the best treatments.

Hemorrhoids are another painful disturbance that can affect the elimination of waste materials from the body. A hemorrhoid is a vein either in the rectum (internal) or around the anus (external) that becomes enlarged.

The external type is usually more painful for the resident. Hemorrhoids may either be the causes or result of chronic constipation.

Incontinence is the inability to control the timing of elimination. Some of the causes of this dysfunction may be a neurological disturbance due to disease or trauma to the brain and spinal cord, anal surgery, chronic diarrhea, or mental disturbance. Urinary incontinence is often caused by impaction. Bacteriuria is also prevalent in this group and the two conditions are commonly found together (Ouslander et al., 1995). A number of researchers feel that urinary incontinence is generally manageable (Palmer, Bennett, Marks, McCormick, & Engel, 1994). Incontinence care, however, is a major disruptor of the ability of assisted living facility residents to "get a good night's sleep" (Engel, 1995; Schnelle, Ouslander, Simmons, Alessi, & Gravel, 1993).

5.3.5 Nutrition

Food provides the body with the nutrients necessary to cell functioning. Adequate nutrition can be of value in the maintenance of fitness and independence as well as prevention of disease (Franz, 1981).

In the preceding section on digestion, the digestive process was described as the time when foods are initially broken down into nutrients so they can be absorbed by the body. The next phase of nutrition is the metabolic process, whereby the remainder of the nutrients are absorbed, helping to produce energy and/or control the various body functions.

Metabolism is the transformation process in which nutrients undergo various chemical reactions throughout the body, producing energy while also helping cells perform necessary functions. Calories are the units of measurement for determining the amount of energy that is contained in foods or used by the body. Below is a list of some the nutrients considered essential to the body. All of them occur naturally in foods and can be obtained from a well-balanced diet.

Protein is a nutrient that can be broken down into components called amino acids. Protein is necessary for growth, repair of damaged tissues, transporting nutrients and chemicals throughout the body, and producing various hormones and enzymes.

Carbohydrates can be broken down quickly into readily available fuel for the body. Two common sources are starches and sugars. The brain is especially sensitive to any decreased levels of carbohydrates in the body and may be permanently damaged whenever the level is reduced for a period of time.

Fats are considered to be the body's source of energy reserve. Fat forms a protective padding around the major organs, prevents heat loss from the body, and carries vitamins A, D, E, and K, helping with their absorption.

Minerals needed by the body include:

Calcium—used to build bones and teeth, giving them their hard structure; also helps to clot blood

Iron—important in building healthy red blood cells that are able to carry oxygen

Sodium—acts as a buffering mechanism, helps dissolve substances in the bloodstream, and monitors the amount of fluid in the body

Potassium—contained in fluids and tissues; important in muscle contraction; maintains the body fluid balance and acts as a buffering mechanism in the bloodstream

Vitamins act to control certain body functions and regulate the body's utilization of other foods.

FLUIDS

Internally, the body is bathed in fluids that help to eliminate wastes and assist the cells with chemical reactions. Fluids help maintain the integrity of the body by protecting the skin and distributing nutrients to promote healing.

Some major body fluids include:

- **Plasma**—carries red blood cells and essential nutrients throughout the body
- **Cerebrospinal fluid**—protects the brain and spinal cord
- **Lymphatic fluid**—carries white blood cells and fluids from the tissues

In all phases of life, adequate nutrition sustains the building-up processes of the body and impedes the wearing-out processes (Albanese, 1980). However, elderly persons suffering from multiple chronic diseases may need even more nutrients than other healthy adults.

POSSIBLE EFFECTS OF AGING

The elderly are believed by some researcher to require fewer calories because of a reduction in body weight, a decrease in the metabolic rate, and often a decline in physical activity (Albanese, 1980; Franz, 1981). However, at the same time that it may be desirable to reduce the amount of carbohydrates and fats, the elderly person has an increased demand for nutrients to enable him or her to resist the effects of disease. Thus the appropriate diet for an older person is complex.

Osteoporosis, a softening of the bones, is a concern among numerous elderly persons. It has been observed frequently in women over 40 (V. Barzel, 1983). A lack of sufficient calcium may contribute to a softening of the bones, making some assisted living facility residents especially susceptible to bone breakage in falls or other accidents.

Dehydration may occur more easily among older persons if they reduce their fluid intake. Smaller proportions of fat under the skin may permit body fluids to evaporate more readily than previously. Dehydration can occur quickly when an elderly person has a fever (Beattie & Louie, 1989).

Aging may affect other structures that aid in digestion. Loss of teeth can result in changes in the types of foods eaten. Loss of weight generally causes problems with the fitting of dentures; refitting is often necessary.

A loss in the overall number of cells and muscle mass may decrease body weight. In this situation the body may no longer need as many calories to provide sufficient energy.

As with any person, consumption of more calories than needed while remaining relatively inactive can lead to obesity—more and more fat being stored in the tissues as reserve energy. Obesity has been referred to as a frequent form of malnutrition in the elderly (Foley, 1981; Kane et al., 1989).

PRESCRIBED DIETS

Although the majority of assisted living facility residents will eat normal diets, some residents will have special nutritional needs. Chronic disease and the effects of institutionalization on appetite pose a challenge.

Physicians often prescribe special therapeutic diets for this group. The following are among the most common:

- **Soft diet**—for residents who need a diet that is low in fiber, soft in texture, and mild in flavors
- **Mechanical soft diet**—same as above, except texture is either chopped, pureed, or ground to make foods easier to ingest

- **Strict full-liquid diet**—consists of foods and liquids that are liquid at body temperature, but can include cold ice cream and hot soups
- **High-fiber diet**—to provide bulk; similar to regular diet, but with foods that are difficult to digest (e.g., fruits, vegetables, whole-grain breads and cereals, nuts, and brans)
- **High-calorie-high-protein diet**—may include milk shakes, meats, and similar foods, to provide additional sources of proteins

Aspiration Issues

Reduced capacity to swallow can lead to aspiration of thinner liquids. Aspiration is the inspiratory sucking into the airways of fluid or foreign bodies such as food. Often the resident aspirates saliva when the swallowing function is compromised. Aspiration can lead to pneumonia and sometimes death; hence it is a matter requiring attention.

Occasionally a physician will prescribe thickened liquids for residents at risk of aspiration. Also, a swallowing evaluation may be in order, for example, if a resident returns from the hospital on thickened liquids. The purchase of prethickened liquids from food suppliers is preferred to having kitchen employees attempt to thicken liquids.

Frequently, residents whose physicians prescribe thickened liquids as a cautionary measure will (perhaps rightly) insist on drinking water and other liquids instead to maintain both their hydration and their sense of well-being. This is clearly within their right to do so. In such situations the facility will want to obtain from each resident a written release from liability.

When residents cannot eat normally, nasogastric, esophagostomy, or gastrostomy tube feeding may be prescribed by the physician.

Nasogastric tubes are inserted through the nose and enter the stomach. Esophagostic tubes pass through the neck into the esophagus. Gastrostomy tubes are surgically inserted directly into the stomach.

Gastrostomy tubes may be preferred for residents needing long-term tube feeding, (e.g., cancer residents), because they can be more comfortable and there is no chance for fluids to flow into the lungs. This often leads to aspiration pneumonia. These tubes also will not irritate the lining of the upper gastrointestinal tract, as may nasogastric tubes.

Enteral feeding uses such products as Osmolite and Ensure. In this case, the feeding tube is inserted nasogastrically but continues into the duodenum (past the stomach into the opening of the small intestine). A pump feeding tube similar to an IV arrangement delivers the nutrients to enter the duodenum. The obvious advantage is to reduce the possibility of aspiration occurring, since the nutrients are introduced into the small intestine itself. The disadvantage is that a permanently inserted tube between the stomach and the duodenum should be reinserted with the use of an X-ray machine, usually in a hospital setting.

ANEMIA AND DIABETES: TWO METABOLIC DISEASE PROCESSES

Two of the most common diseases that disrupt the metabolism of important nutrients are anemia and diabetes. According to the National Center for Health Statistics, in 1995 diabetes was the fifth leading cause of death among persons age 65 and older: 133 deaths per 100,000, or 44,452 actual deaths ("Retirement checkup," 1998). It was also the eighth most frequently occurring chronic condition, occurring at the rate of 101 cases per 1,000 individuals.

Anemia is a condition in which hemoglobin is deficient, resulting in the body not getting enough oxygen. The red blood cells contain a substance called hemoglobin, which carries the oxygen. Diabetes occurs when the body is unable to metabolize glucose (sugar) because of a problem with a hormone, insulin, that is produced by a ductless gland, the pancreas.

Anemia

Various types of anemia are found in the elderly population. It is thought to be due to disease, not old age (Freedman, 1982; Kane et al., 1989), and therapy for each type of anemia is varied.

Anemia is the result of a significant decrease in the number of red blood cells produced. Having multiple chronic diseases can lead to anemia. Symptoms of anemia are similar to those for heart disease because they also result in a problem with oxygenation (Kravitz, 1989). When anemia is combined with other diseases, such as peripheral vascular disease or coronary artery disease, it may be very serious as well as painful.

Diabetes

Diabetes results from an inability to convert carbohydrates to forms the body can utilize.

Usually, the pancreas produces the hormone insulin, which helps the cells convert sugar (or glucose) into a form of energy for use or storage. Diabetics either produce insufficient amounts of this hormone or have some difficulty in utilizing insulin. The result is large amounts of sugar continually circulating in the bloodstream, causing the condition known as hyperglycemia (high blood sugar).

Chronic hyperglycemia can damage many of the body tissues. Hyperglycemia can cause complications and disabilities in other systems in the body. In its more extreme form diabetes is a factor in the cause of blindness and amputation.

There are two different classifications of persons with diabetes: insulin dependent and noninsulin dependent. Insulin-dependent diabetes mellitus (IDDM) individuals generally have had the disease since childhood and require daily doses (or the equivalent) for the control of the disease. Almost all of the long-term assisted living facility diabetic population fall into this category (Bazzare, 1983, p. 257). Noninsulin-dependent diabetes mellitus (NIDDM) is usually diagnosed in adults, who are generally able to control the disease by dietary restrictions and the use of oral hypoglycemics (Bazzare, 1983; Beattie & Louie, 1989).

Much of the treatment provided to assisted living facility residents involves monitoring the blood sugar level. It is often unclear who is truly a diabetic. Glucose tolerance progressively deteriorates with each decade of life. One researcher, Andres (1989), formulated a percentile system demonstrating decreasing glucose tolerance with age. Thus the physician practicing in an assisted living facility should guard against treating a laboratory value that represents an altered physiologic state as a true case of diabetes (Reichel, 1983).

5.3.6 External and Internal Defense Mechanisms

The body is equipped with special defense mechanisms to protect it from harmful disruptions in the environment, through the use of two different types of defense mechanisms.

THE BARRIER SYSTEM OF DEFENSE

The first type acts as a barrier preventing harmful substances from entering the body, the largest such organ being the skin. While protecting the body from harmful organisms, the skin also seals in essential body fluids and regulates the body temperature. The respiratory, intestinal, and urinary tracts also have barrier-like components to protect the body from foreign materials that may enter through their systems.

In the respiratory tract, thousands of cilia (small hairlike elements) line the passageways and help propel outward any foreign materials that may be inhaled from the air. Coughing expels these particles from the body and back into the environment.

Two additional barrier-like protections are the acid composition of gastric juices and urine, which also act to protect the digestive system and the urinary tract from the entrance of harmful organisms.

THE CHEMICAL DEFENSE SYSTEM

The immune system is often referred to as the second line of defense; it protects the internal structures of the body. Whenever foreign material or an antigen enters the body, the components of the immune system recognize this and mobilize for an attack response. Most often, the foreign material is a small bacterial or viral microorganism. Different types of antibodies have various means of fighting an infection and use a much more complex interaction than that seen in the cell-mediated response.

INFECTIONS

When bacteria or viruses are successful in penetrating the defense mechanisms in large numbers or are allowed to enter the areas of the body where they are not usually found, the resulting disruption is known as an infection.. Assisted living facility residents may be more prone to infections than other population groups because of

- age-related changes in their bodies
- the presence of multiple chronic diseases
- associated use of multiple medications with side effects that may compromise the body

- increased incidence of immobility and incontinence
- use of invasive devices such as indwelling urinary catheters

These factors all increase assisted living facility residents' susceptibility to infections and also serve to weaken their natural defense mechanisms. Kane et al. (1989) remain unconvinced, however, that alterations in defense mechanisms predispose the elderly to certain infections. They speculate that environmental factors, specific diseases, and physiological changes other than the immune system may account for increased frequency of certain infections in the elderly (see also Goldrick & Larson, 1992).

New infectious processes are being identified in assisted living facilities. More recently documented infections include bacteremia (bacteria in the bloodstream occurring with intravascular catheters), conjunctivitis, AIDS, streptococcal infection, Legionnaires' disease, and methicillin-resistant staphylococcus aureus (MRSA). More and more nursing facilities are being asked to care for and accept MRSA residents, which requires special guidelines for enforcing the universal precautions when providing care. Of particular concern is whether the MRSA is colonized or noncolonized upon admission. A colonized MRSA means the infectious agents are encapsulated and much less likely to spread infection. Noncolonized MRSA can spread infection via airborne particles and by touching objects in the resident's physical vicinity.

Nosocomial Infections

Infections that are associated with institutionalization or acquired while in a health care facility are called nosocomial infections. Assisted living facility residents are considered to be at a particular risk of developing these infections because of the levels of group interaction and activities among residents (Garibaldi, Brodine, & Matsumiya, 1981).

Farber, Brennen, Punteri, and Brody (1982) found that half of all infections in the chronic care facility they studied may be due to nosocomially acquired pneumonia or urinary tract infections and that these two infections are commonly responsible for morbidity (illness) in the elderly population. Some of the other types of nosocomial infections often seen in the assisted living facility include infections of the skin, soft tissues, and gastrointestinal tract (Farber et al., 1982; Nicolle, McIntyre, Zacharias, & MacDonald, 1961). Because of more frequent and longer hospitalizations assisted living facility residents are at increased risk for staphylococcus and gram negative infections (Kane et al., 1989). Infection control generally has improved in recent years, according to research by Raymond Otero (1993) who focused on MRSA.

The Inflammation Response

Inflammation occurs in the physical responses by the other body systems when fighting off infection of some external threat. The blood vessels dilate (expand), bringing more cells to combat the unwanted component. This is often the cause of redness surrounding areas of skin that may have become infected. The debris from the antigen often becomes pus, which may drain from the infection.

Special Difficulties in Identifying Infections

Infections in the elderly may be more difficult to diagnose because it is possible to confuse the symptoms with those of other chronic diseases. Also, even when symptoms are present, the elderly resident may be reluctant to complain about these disruptions, so they are less likely to be reported (Beck & Smith, 1983).

Most infections are not considered to be chronic diseases because they respond to treatment, and their damage to the body can often be reversed. Some of the possible effects of aging on the immune system are discussed below.

Possible Effects of Aging

The skin contains fibers that change as a person ages. These changes may make the skin and other connective tissue drier and less resilient (Balin & Lin, 1995; Kenney, 1982; Tonna, 1995).

Skin, nail, and hair cells, which are among the fastest to grow during younger years, often do not replace themselves as quickly when persons age (Carter & Balin, 1983). Together, these changes help explain why many elderly people have some degree of tough, dry, wrinkled skin (Kenney, 1982). Kligman (1979) also suggests that these types of changes work to diminish the barrier function of the skin as a person ages.

A study by Tindall and Smith (1963) of 163 persons 64 years of age and older showed that 94% of them had "lax" skin, secondary to changes in connective tissue, which contributed to wrinkling and other related manifestations.

The greatest alteration in the internal immune system is the involution (decrease in size) of the thymus gland (Felser & Raff, 1983; Smith, 1982; Weksler, 1981). This change is suspected to influence the function of the immune system, but it is still too early to determine the full range of implications this may have on the health of elderly individuals. However, Weksler (1981) notes, in contrast to Kane et al. (1989), that some impairment of the immune response makes elderly individuals more susceptible to infection.

DISEASE PROCESSES

Some of the more prevalent diseases or disruptions that affect either of the body's defense mechanisms are discussed below.

Facility Responses to the Presence of Infections: The Infection Control Program

Depending on the nature of the infection, various isolation precautions need to be taken to protect other residents, staff, and visitors from acquiring the infection. The administrator should also make sure that residents with certain communicable diseases are reported to the state health department. Each state, in cooperation with the U.S. Public Health Service, specifies diseases that should be reported to the state health department.

Infections complicate the elderly residents' disease status and may even increase their chance of death. Besides this risk, infections may increase the likelihood that a resident will need to be transferred to a hospital for more intensive care (Irvine, VanBuren, & Crossley, 1984).

The risk of an epidemic is always present in the assisted living facility. An epidemic is a cluster of infections involving multiple individuals. Assisted living facility epidemics include influenza, staphylococcal skin infections, antibiotic-resistant bacteria, infectious diarrhea, scabies, and tuberculosis. A careful following of the Department of Labor's Universal Precautions (Bloodborne Pathogens) rules will do much to reduce epidemics.

Skin Disease

Herpes zoster (shingles) that primarily affects elderly individuals. This infection is caused by the herpes varicella virus (not to be confused with herpes simplex) which travels along nerve pathways to infect skin cells (Becker, 1979). Skin covering the chest region and surrounding the eye are among the areas more commonly infected by this disease. Residents who suffer from a debilitating disease, such as cancer, are also at greater risk of developing this infection.

Signs and symptoms include itching, usually preceding a rash, reddened areas of the skin (usually along a nerve pathway), vesicles (fluid-filled pimples) often erupting over reddened areas, and burning accompanied by stabbing pain.

At present, there is no cure for this form of herpes infection, so treatment consists of attempts to alleviate the associated symptoms rather than effect a cure. Steroids are often used to reduce inflammation, which may shorten the length of the infection and provide comfort. Antibiotics are sometimes prescribed to prevent secondary infections and analgesics to relieve pain (Beacham, 1989).

Pressure Ulcers

Pressure sores is the federal government's preferred term for these infections, known also as bedsores, decubitus ulcers, and stasis ulcers (ulcers resulting from tissue death due to reduced blood flow, all terms for the same process—tissue breakdown; Bergstrin, 1995). Stasis ulcers are the sores that result from extremely poor peripheral circulation or peripheral vascular disease (Garagusi, 1989).

Tissue breakdown often occurs over a bony prominence (buttocks, elbow, heel, hip, shoulder). These ulcers do not develop from an infection, but rather from some form of constant unrelieved pressure on one area of the body.

With all of these ulcers the end result is the same: Tissues do not receive an adequate amount of oxygen, so they break down and begin to die. This process is similar to what happens to the heart muscle in coronary artery disease.

Residents at most risk for developing these ulcers are those chronically immobile (paralyzed) because of a stroke or some other incapacitating illness and those experiencing poor nutritional status, constant pain, incontinence, or dementia (Husain, 1953). These ulcers often enlarge to form cavities of dead tissue prone to the development of infection and once enlarged, are more difficult to heal (Collier, 1997; Kart et al., 1978).

Decubitus Ulcer Formation. The formation of an ulcer usually occurs when the weight of the body exerts pressure on internal soft tissues by compressing them between skeletal bone and another hard surface. Residents who are immobilized or unable to move by themselves are particularly at risk for developing bedsores. Because these residents cannot, on their own, change position frequently, there is the danger of continuous pressure on one area of the body.

Many of these residents spend much of their time lying on their back, also known as the decubitus position (*decubitus* means "lying down"). When this occurs, the areas most likely to develop sores are the buttocks, hips, heels, shoulders, ears, and elbows. Similarly, residents who spend long periods sitting up in a chair without moving are also at risk of developing these sores (Gallagher, 1997).

Signs and symptoms of decubitus ulcers include:

- tingling, pale skin color, or other signs that there is a loss of circulation to an area
- reddened area of skin over a bony prominence
- a sore that will not heal
- edema (swelling) of the lower legs and shiny skin

However, these signs are often difficult to recognize before tissue has already died and the ulcer itself has already developed (Rowe & Besdine, 1982; Fletcher, 1997).

Pressure sores are typically classed as Stage I, I, III, and IV.

Stage I: acute inflammatory response, often over a bony prominence; skin red but unbroken
Stage II: extension of the acute inflammatory response through the dermis to subcutaneous fat
Stage III: extension through fat to deep fascia; base of ulcer infected
Stage IV: deep ulceration reaching the bone

Following are some of the main treatments the facility may use:

- providing special equipment, such as a water mattress
- keeping the resident clean and dry
- eliminating the source of pressure
- working to improve the resident's circulation
- ensuring frequent position change (at least every 2 hours) for those who are unable or unlikely to do so themselves
- padding feet, elbows, and other areas at high risk of tissue breakdown (e.g., using "bunny boots" on the feet)
- frequently assessing the integrity of a resident's skin
- changing diet to include foods higher in protein, vitamin C, and calorie content to promote healing
- preventing infection by applying dressings and dispensing antibiotic medications as prescribed
- using elastic stockings or Ace wrap bandages, which are often prescribed for the person with peripheral vascular insufficiency (poor blood circulation in the arms and legs)
- experimental treatments (e.g., use of a hypobaric chamber, which facilitates the flow of oxygen to injured areas).

Both pressure sores and stasis ulcers are significant disruptions of the skin's protective barrier defense. A study by Garibaldi et al. (1981) concluded that 32% of infections originated from this source. One of the most severe types of infections that may result is called sepsis, a condition in which the circulating bloodstream carries infectious organisms throughout the body.

Attention of the Administrator. The in-house acquired preventable decubitus ulcer rate is one of the three or four yardsticks by which the quality of the care given in the facility is judged. Good health care is the best form of overall treatment. Lehman (1983) identifies the administrator's roles as ensuring that evaluation and screening for residents at high risk for developing these ulcers is done routinely. Approximately two thirds of ulcers develop within the first weeks that a resident is institutionalized (p. 22). In light of this, it is important that the assisted living staff pay attention to this possibility during the early weeks of each new resident's admission.

The Department of Health and Human Services' Agency for Health Care Policy and Research has developed health practice guidelines for the management of pressure sores (AHCPR, 1995).

Hypothermia

Hypothermia (low body temperature) is an issue of special concern to assisted living facility staff. Usually, the body temperature is maintained between 97° and 99° Fahrenheit. Residents in an assisted living facility may be endangered by subtle changes in temperature (Collins et al., 1977). The elderly resident often may have less insulation from body fat, increasing the risk of hypothermia.

Hypothermia is the sudden appearance of a low body temperature (less than 95° F). Often it is difficult to diagnose hypothermia because symptoms may be similar to those of a minor stroke.

When the body temperature drops below 95° F, residents are no longer able to feel cold and may be suffering from confusion, so they are often unable to complain of other symptoms, such as skin that is pale, dry, and cool, with low pulse or blood pressure.

Many complications may result from hypothermia, including dehydration, renal failure, pneumonia, and cardiac arrhythmias. Treatment is aimed at slowly bringing the resident back to a normal body temperature, usually with blankets. Residents with multiple chronic diseases may not survive an episode of hypothermia.

Because of the threat of hypothermia, loss of heat in the assisted living facility can be a life-threatening situation for the residents.

Cancer

Cancer is actually a group of chronic diseases that affect different areas of the body. Cancer is discussed here as a disorder of the immune system because cancer cells act as antigens and are known to attack many organs or cells throughout the body.

The growth of cancer cells is markedly different from that of normal cells. They grow much more rapidly and are often released or break out from their initial area of growth (tumor) and travel into the bloodstream or lymphatic channels, then throughout the body.

Damage may result either from this rapid cell growth, depleting normal cell food supply, or from actual expansion and crushing of the organ affected.

Another mode for cancer growth occurs when cancerous cells travel from the initial growth to new sites, forming metastases or other cancer sites throughout the body. Metastasis is the transfer of disease from one organ or part of the body to another not directly connected with it, due either to the transfer of pathogenic microorganisms or the transfer of cells.

The cause of cancer is still unknown, but among the different factors believed to play possible roles in this disease are environmental exposure to harmful substances, chronic chemical or biologic irritation (drugs, alcohol, smoking, viral infections, radiation), inherited genetic predisposition to the disease, diet, and even behavior.

It has been suggested that some combination of these factors probably best explains the cause of cancer (Fraumeni, 1979). Often these factors may expose the body to a substance known as a carcinogen, which alters the body's immune response capabilities and allows these substances to enter the body and promote the growth of cancerous cells.

According to Birchenall and Streight (1982), the leading types of cancer seen in assisted living facility residents, listed in order of prevalence by sex, are as follows:

Males: lung, colon, rectum, and prostate
Females: breast, colon, rectum, and lung

According to the National Center for Health Statistics, in 1995 cancer was the second leading cause of death among persons 65 and older: 1,137 deaths per 100,000, or 381,142 actual deaths ("Retirement checkup," 1998).

Variations in Cancer Treatments. Physicians may choose to manage cancer residents with different forms of treatments, depending on the specifics of the disease. Surgery, radiation, and use of chemical therapy are the three most common forms of cancer treatment. There are more than 250 different kinds of cancer. Forms of treatment will vary for individual residents according to the severity of their illness.

Problems Associated With Cancer Treatments. There are many problems associated with cancer treatment. The resident with colon cancer, for example, may have undergone surgery to remove the diseased portion of the bowel. If a large enough area has been removed, then the resident will usually also have a colostomy, which is an opening in the abdomen where the end of the bowel is brought to the surface and digestive waste materials are collected in a bag attached to an appliance surrounding the site. Depending on the level of independence, residents with colostomies may require additional assistance with this special type of elimination process.

The two other types of cancer treatment (radiation and chemotherapy) may be quite painful for residents because of their associated side effects. One of these is anorexia (continual lack of appetite). When this persists, physicians may prescribe special high-calorie food supplements to maintain the resident's strength and energy, as well as treatments for pain and nausea.

5.3.7 Musculoskeletal System

The muscles and skeleton working together provide two important functions: a supporting framework for all of the other body structures and mobility, which is closely related to the assisted living facility resident's degree of independence and autonomy.

THE SKELETON AND MUSCLES

One of the basic elements of the supporting framework of the body is the skeleton, which is composed of the many bones that meet to form joints. The muscles are attached to the skeleton. The skeleton also protects soft tissues and organs inside the body. This framework dictates an individual's posture, directly affecting personal appearance. According to the U.S. Census Bureau and the National Council on Aging, 31% of Americans age 60 and over reported taking medications to relieve chronic pain from bones and joints ("Retirement checkup," 1998).

JOINTS

In the body there are 68 joints, which are the points at which the ends of two bones meet. These joint bones are covered by cartilage and surrounded by a capsule containing fluid that lubricates the area to enhance movement. The joint is held in place by ligaments.

MOVEMENT

In order for movement to occur, the muscles should first receive a nerve impulse from the brain directing them to contract, then relax. Because the muscles are attached to the bones, when they move, the bone moves also. The joints respond like mechanical levers to assist in completing this movement. Thus mobility requires coordination between both the nervous and the musculoskeletal systems.

POSSIBLE EFFECTS OF AGING

The individual bones contain an inner component, bone marrow, that produces the red blood cells. The remainder of bone consists of a network of fibrous tissue containing salts, which are primarily minerals, such as calcium, that serve to harden and strengthen the bone.

There is some consensus that during the aging process the total amount of bone in the body decreases. However, to determine the loss, one needs to have measured the amount of bone the individual had at age 35 (Heaney, 1982).

Higher Risk for Women

Women are at a high risk of experiencing some degree of bone loss following menopause. It has been established that this loss results from a withdrawal of estrogen, which apparently helps promote the body's use of dietary calcium for the purpose of bone growth.

When bone loss occurs, some of the observable changes are shortened stature and a slumped posture due to a compression of the vertebrae (bones in the spine) and the cartilage discs between them. Often, because of these changes, elderly individuals become stooped and appear to have a hump back. They are also more likely to fracture one of their bones (Glowacki, 1989; Grob, 1983, 1989).

While a certain amount of bone loss is associated with aging, much of it in the elderly is a result of osteoporosis. There is considerable controversy over the extent to which these changes in the bone can be attributed to normal aging rather than to osteoporosis, which will be described below.

Both muscles and bones are made up of connective tissue and collagen. Similar to the collagen-related changes associated with age, muscles also become less elastic as a result of this same process. The most significant age-related muscle change for the elderly is a decrease in the amount throughout the body. In addition, degenerative changes in the nervous system may disturb impulses, decreasing muscle skills. However, it is unclear to what extent, if any, these changes in bone and muscle size and strength are related to age, rather than to the possible effects of decreased activity (Weg, 1983).

DISEASE PROCESSES

The discussion of age-related changes in the musculoskeletal system reflects the considerable uncertainty as to whether the changes in bones are a manifestation of the aging process or a distinct disease process (Barzel, 1983).

The term *rheumatism* has often been used to describe any painful disorder of the muscles, joints, and their surrounding areas (Agate, 1979). Following is a discussion of some of the common disruptions of musculoskeletal functioning as experienced in the assisted living facility population.

Osteoporosis

Osteoporosis has already been described as a condition of decreased skeletal mass without alteration of any chemical components of bone (Rossman, 1979, p. 285). Thus, while there may be less total amount of bone, the components of bone are still present in necessary proportions.

The cause of osteoporosis remains unclear, but the mechanism of bone loss apparently is through increased resorption of bone tissue by the body. Osteoporosis may result from prolonged use of medication, immobility, or some other underlying disease (Spencer, 1977).

Symptoms of osteoporosis include bone pain, often in the lower back, recurrent bone fractures, and frequent falls and related injuries.

Treatment can include managing the symptoms of pain, treating complications such as fractures, rehabilitation to correct physical inactivity, and increasing protein and vitamin intake. Medications often used are calcium supplements and hormones, usually estrogen, to improve the body's ability to absorb calcium.

Simply taking extra calcium without estrogen replacement appears to be dramatically less effective, according to Glowacki (1989), who also maintains that reports that estrogen replacement therapy causes endometrial (inner lining of the uterine wall) cancer are exaggerated. There is no evidence, he asserts further, that estrogen replacement therapy causes breast cancer.

Arthritis

Arthritis is an inflammation of a joint. There are many different types of arthritis. According to the U.S. Census Bureau and the National Council on Aging, 43% of Americans age 60 and over reported taking medications to relieve chronic pain from arthritis (WSJ, 1998). Two that commonly afflict assisted living facility residents are listed below. Arthritis was reported as the most frequently occurring chronic condition in persons age 65 and older, occurring at the rate of 502 per 1,000 individuals (WSJ, 1998).

Osteoarthritis. Also called degenerative joint disease, this is the most prevalent form of arthritis. As the disease progresses, the cartilage and other components of the joint begin to wear away or degenerate. The joints that bear most of the weight on a continual basis are most commonly affected, including the knees, hips, and ankles.

Symptoms include aching pain in the affected joint, most often a backache, and decreased mobility because the pain becomes worse following exercise.

Treatment consists of relieving symptoms. Use of an anti-inflammatory agent such as enteric-coated aspirin is usually recommended (Kane et al., 1989, p. 224). Continual degeneration of the hip or knee joint may require surgical replacement if the resident still has good walking skills.

Rheumatoid Arthritis

This is a much more serious form of arthritis. It can affect any age group and is considered an autoimmune disease, because it is thought the body begins to attack its own cells in the joint, causing an inflammatory reaction.

Signs and symptoms include

- symmetric inflammation of joints on both sides of the body
- frequent flare-ups and remissions of pain
- stiffness and joint swelling, usually in the hands
- pain, often occurring in the morning hours and decreasing with exercise

Treatments include

- a balance of rest and exercise
- physical therapy
- heat and cold applications
- whirlpool baths

Medications include

- aspirin, to decrease the inflammation
- analgesics, to relieve the pain

FALLS

More than 70% of deaths that result from all falls occur among persons over 65 years of age. Falling is a major cause of disability and death in the elderly and may be due to factors such as chronic illness or orthostatic hypotension (decreased blood pressure upon standing) ("Best drugs," 1994; Kennie & Warshaw, 1989; Kippenbrock & Soja, 1993; Tideiksaar, 1995).

Residents in the facility dining room who have just finished a large meal are especially vulnerable to falls. It appears that, following a meal, the blood supply is routed to the digestive system, causing even lower blood pressure when the resident stands up (Cohan, 1989).

Osteoporosis, gait disorders, and decreased blood supply to the brain also leave residents more prone to falls than the noninstitutionalized elderly population (Rodstein, 1983).

It is estimated that only 25% of falls in institutions are witnessed and that 25% to 50% of residents fall each year (Kallman & Kallman, p. 553). The number of resident falls in assisted living facilities is unknown, but, as the current assisted living residents age, falls should be of concern to the staff. Eighty percent of all individuals falling are age 75 or older.

The facility environment can often be unsafe (Kane et al., 1989). An emphasized and smoothly running risk management program focusing on incident reports can identify changes needed in the facility environment to reduce falls.

FRACTURES

Frequently, when facility residents fall, they fracture one of the bones in their body. Often this is in either the spine or the hip. When an assisted living facility resident fractures the hip, two treatment approaches are used.

One is to place the resident on bed rest. Lyon and Nevins (1984) suggest that this conservative form of treatment is safer and less likely to lead to further mental decline or other complications. The other approach is for the resident to have surgery to repair the hip. Often the resident is provided with an artificial prosthesis. Gordon (1989) argues for definitive treatment within the first 24 to 72 hours, as well as early ambulation with physical therapy.

The danger of hip fracture increases dramatically with age: in women age 75 to 79 the incidence of hip fracture is 6 of 1,000 falls; for those 85 to 89 the incidence of hip fracture rises to 48.6 per 1,000 falls (Kallman & Kallman, p. 551; Pousada, 1995).

AMPUTATION

Amputees are another group of assisted living facility residents who need special assistance when walking.

Three fourths of all amputations are performed on residents 65 years of age and older (Vallarino & Sherman, 1981, p. 148). The most common type of amputation is the removal of the leg either above or below the knee. An amputation is the treatment of last resort for residents with a severe infection, peripheral vascular disease, or injury that is often related to diabetes. Many devices are available to restore lost function. In the absence of suitable prosthetic devices, the environment can be changed to accommodate the resident's skills (Redford, 1989, pp. 186–187).

CONTRACTURES

Often residents with chronic rheumatoid arthritis develop contractures in their hands. Contractures are a deformity that result when the muscle has shortened and pulls the adjacent joint into a flexed position. After a period of time the joint becomes fixed in this position and results in a permanent deformity in which the joint cannot be straightened. Contractures are another disruption likely to occur in the immobilized resident.

Other joints that are likely to develop contractures, besides those in the hand and wrist, include the feet, hips, and legs.

The best form of treatment for contractures is to help prevent them by exercising the joints of those who are unable to do so for themselves. These are called passive range of motion exercises and can be taught to the resident's family. Proper positioning in bed helps prevent the development of these contractures. Special devices and splints are available for that purpose.

5.3.8 Genitourinary (Renal) System

The renal system consists of the two kidneys, which filter wastes from the blood, and two ureters, which transmit the filtered materials (urine) from the kidneys to the bladder, where the urine is stored until discharged through the urethra.

In addition to removing waste materials from the bloodstream, the kidneys help regulate the amount of fluid in the body. At the same time, the kidneys also monitor the level of important electrolytes including sodium, potassium, and calcium.

Channels within the kidney filter the blood and collect a concentration of waste products and excess fluids. The newly filtered blood supply is returned to the general circulation by the renal vein, and the concentration of waste materials or urine travels from within the kidney to the bladder by connecting tubes (ureters).

The bladder is a balloonlike muscular structure that serves as a holding tank for the continuous stream of urine produced by the kidneys. When a sufficient amount of urine has collected in the bladder, signals are sent to the brain identifying the need to urinate.

Individuals have voluntary control over the bladder in responding to this need to urinate. A nerve impulse sent back to the bladder signals it to contract and expel urine through the urethra, at which point it leaves the body. See Figure 5.8 for an illustration of the location of the renal system for both men and women.

EFFECTS OF AGING ON THE RENAL SYSTEM

The average 80-year-old adult, according to some studies, has approximately one half of the renal function of a normal 30-year-old (Lindeman, 1989, p. 286). According to the National Center for Health Statistics, in 1995 kidney disease was the ninth leading cause of death among persons age 65 and older: 60 deaths per 100,000, or 20,182 actual deaths ("Retirement checkup," 1998).

Because the kidneys are so closely linked with the circulatory system, age-associated atherosclerotic (hardening) changes in blood vessels can also affect the kidneys. Because of the location of the renal organs, age-related changes in the reproductive organs also influence their ability to function.

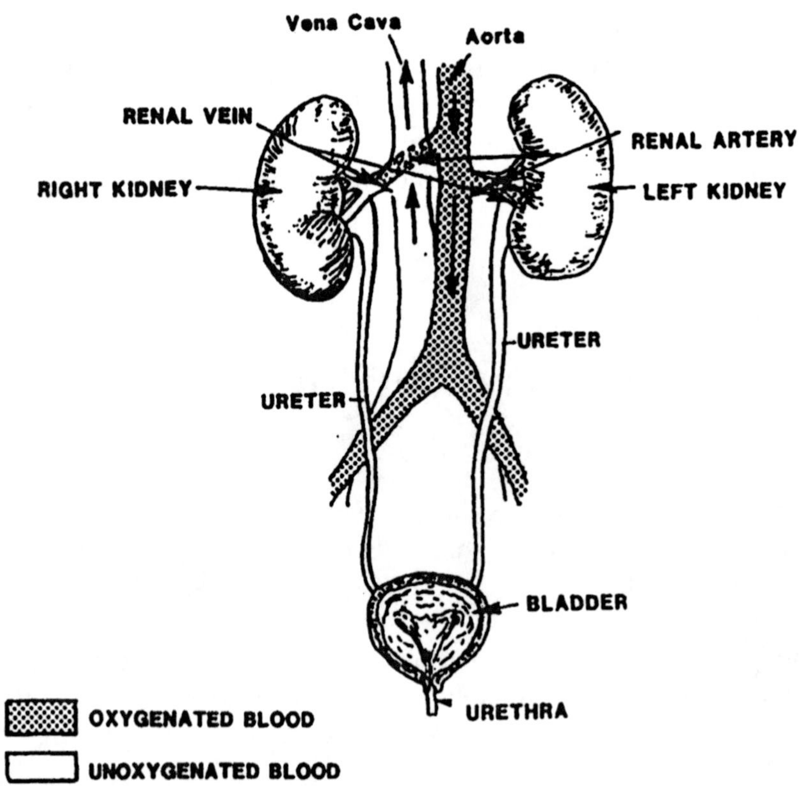

FIGURE 5.8 Diagram of the urinary system.

Studies have shown that the ability of the kidneys to concentrate urine probably decreases with age (McLachlan, 1978). A progressive loss of renal mass (size) is also believed to occur (Rowe, 1982). However, these changes have not been associated with an overall decline in kidney function. Because the bladder is a muscle, its capacity to hold large amounts of urine also seems to decrease with age.

Alterations in Renal Function

Disruptions in renal function may be caused by problems in an associated system or systems, such as arteriosclerotic changes in blood vessels and changes in body nutrients, as in diabetes, leading to renal failure.

A disruption may also be due to a malfunction of a kidney or to some type of internal blockage within the kidneys and ureters, as with kidney stones or tumors.

Chronic Renal Failure

Renal failure is the inability of the kidneys to filter out body waste products. This can be either an acute (short-term) or, more likely, a chronic (long-term) process.

Chronic renal failure may be caused by cardiovascular changes leading to a decreasing amount of blood being filtered through the kidneys. This decrease in blood flow can result in permanent damage to some of the kidneys' internal filtering mechanisms (nephrons) that require continual use for optimal functioning. The most obvious physical sign of renal failure is uremia, or a decrease in urine output, which may progressively lead to oliguria, or no urine output.

The symptoms of chronic renal failure, much like the disease itself, develop gradually. Some of the initial symptoms include dehydration, electrolyte imbalance, osteoporosis, nocturia (producing much urine at night), and anemia.

When little or no urine is produced by the body, toxic waste materials may build up, which could damage other organs and cause painful symptoms, including itching and dry skin, mental confusion, weakness, muscle cramps, nausea, vomiting, and diarrhea. The elderly are particularly prone to developing end-stage renal disease and are the largest group entering kidney dialysis programs (Faubert, Shapiro, Porush, & Kahn, 1989).

End-Stage Renal Disease. Chronic renal failure that has progressed to the stage at which little or no urine is being produced is called end-stage renal disease (ESRD). The two most common forms of treatment are kidney transplantation and dialysis.

Kidney dialysis (hemodialysis, i.e., filtering the blood) requires special equipment that performs much like the kidneys in filtering unwanted waste materials and fluids from the blood. The process is usually performed in special clinics and takes several hours. The resident's blood is circulated externally through a small machine that filters the blood in much the same fashion as the kidneys themselves. Feinstein and Friedman (1979) report that from its inception hemodialysis has been successful when used for older residents.

Peritoneal dialysis may be performed for the bedridden resident; it involves filtering out excess fluids from the peritoneum, which lines the abdominal organs (i.e., the membrane lining the walls of the abdominal and pelvic cavities, containing the viscera). This procedure is similar to kidney dialysis. The waste products are filtered out by dialyzing the peritoneal cavity instead of the kidneys themselves.

Renal Calculi

Kidney stones, or renal calculi, are formed in the kidney as a result of an imbalance in body chemistry. These stones are crystalline, stonelike substances that become a problem when they block urine flow out of the kidneys or block any other area of the renal system.

The group of residents most at risk for developing kidney stones are those unable to move or who are on chronic bed rest. In the preceding section we discussed how these residents are likely to suffer from increased osteoporosis. The extra calcium that the body absorbs may also form kidney stones when enough of this mineral is filtered.

Symptoms are blood in urine, decrease in urine outflow, and pain in the back or side. Treatment consists of relief of pain symptoms and medications to relax ureters, allowing the stones to pass. If retrieved, the stones are analyzed to determine their composition and the necessity for any further treatment. In recent years, the need for surgical removal of kidney stones has been greatly reduced by the use of a machine called a lithotripter, which bombards and breaks the kidney stones into small fragments by directing electrical shock waves that pass harmlessly through body tissue to break up the kidney stones.

Urinary Incontinence

Urinary incontinence is the inability to control the timing of urination. There are many reasons why a resident may become incontinent, including neurologic damage, chronic constipation, and impactions. A defect in the nervous system (stroke residents who lose nervous control of the bladder), urinary tract infections, and constant pressure on the bladder from other disorders such as constipation may cause incontinence (Kane et al., 1989).

Problems in mobility that prevent the resident from reaching the toilet in time may also lead to incontinence (Keegan & McNichols, 1982; Williams & Fitzhugh, 1982). The health care staff should be prompt in assisting the resident to the bathroom on a regular schedule. The resident is more able to empty the bladder if placed on the commode.

Bladder retraining is used to assist the resident in using the bathroom at appropriate times. There are several types of bladder retraining programs (Kane et al., 1989, pp. 172–173). Once assurance has been obtained that there is no impaction, the nurses monitor the amount of fluid consumed by the resident and help the resident to use the toilet about 2 hours afterwards (or per each resident's need pattern).

Residents who are unable to use a bathroom may be catheterized. Urine is released intermittently about every 2 hours following fluid intake. Special devices are also used to assist the resident in voiding (urinating). These include bed pans, urinals for men, and bedside commodes for the resident who can get up out of bed. In the assisted living setting frequent use is made of adult briefs for residents who experience incontinence.

If none of the above treatments is successful, some type of drainage system can be ordered for the resident. Men may use either a condomlike or an indwelling type of catheter. Women may use only the indwelling catheter, which is inserted into the urethra and threaded up into the bladder. Urine flows out of the bladder and through the catheter. It is then collected in a clear plastic drainage bag. This is a closed system to attempt to control the introduction of bacteria or other harmful microorganisms into the urinary tract, but it is a last choice because urinary tract infections are associated with this approach (Kane et al., 1989, p. 179).

Urinary Tract Infections

According to Kurtz (1982), of all age groups, the elderly most frequently have urinary tract infections (UTI) and associated illnesses. Together, urinary tract infections and pneumonia were found to be responsible for more than half of all infections in one chronic care facility studied (Farber et al., 1982, p. 518). Sterile catheter insertions tend to become infected within 3 weeks regardless of preventive efforts.

Infection from urinary catheters, therefore, is usually impossible to prevent. The bladder is usually sterile. Urinary tract infections are the most common form of catheter-related infections and account for 30% of all nosocomial infections. The female rate of urinary tract infections is higher than the male rate because pathogenic organisms traveling up the outside of the catheter have a shorter distance to travel in women (2 inches) compared to men (6 to 8 inches). When urinary catheters are used for extended periods of time the risk for acute UTI complicated by pyelonephritis (inflammation of the kidney) occurs. Sepsis from pyelonephritis is a major cause of death in residents with long-term indwelling catheters.

The most commonly associated causes of UTI, as identified by Bjork and Tight (1983), include lack of handwashing between resident contacts (an example of poor infection control practices by staff), close proximity of residents with catheters, and the prevalence of residents who have indwelling urinary catheters. Other causes, such as poor insertion techniques and poor positioning of drainage bags, have been identified.

Since all indwelling catheters are assumed to eventually cause UTI, residents with catheters are especially at risk of infection. Residents with urinary catheters often show no symptoms associated with the initial stages of this infection. Residents who do not have indwelling catheters may complain of symptoms, including burning and painful urination, cloudy and foul-smelling urine, fever, and chills (Garagusi, 1989, p. 202). The indwelling catheter should be cleaned daily with soap and water where it enters the urethra and the catheter itself changed aseptically every month.

An initial form of treatment is to obtain a sample of urine, which may be studied to determine the organisms present. Antibiotic therapy is usually held off for as long as possible. There is only a limited number of antibiotics available to treat UTI, and residents with chronic indwelling catheters are likely to become resistant to these antibiotics quickly, at which point there is little alternative treatment available. As many as half of all urinary tract infections are recurrent.

A frequently encountered assisted living facility problem is that many elderly women have asymptomatic bacteriuria. Treatment protocols may indicate a constant need for treatment in these cases. However, chronic suppressive antibiotic administration to these residents can be counterproductive because it can lead to development of antibiotic-resistant organisms, leading in turn to a superinfection (Garagusi, 1989, p. 202).

In an effort to avoid overuse of antibiotics, a new trend among geriatric physicians is to treat UTI only if it is symptomatic (i.e., exhibiting burning discomfort or pain), not when the culture is positive but the resident is asympotomatic.

UTI is an ongoing treatment challenge in the assisted living facility. New approaches are constantly being sought. Practical experience suggests that no matter how careful or sterile the procedures, infection often spreads. Despite every staff effort an incontinent female resident may be at risk of infection within minutes after incontinence occurs.

5.3.9 Reproductive System

The reproductive system in the younger adult has the capacity to promote the creation of new life and facilitate the expression of intimacy through human contact. Some of the most notable changes in the elderly involve the woman's loss of reproductive capabilities following menopause (change of life), whereas a man retains reproductive capabilities. However, both sexes have continued needs to express their sexuality throughout the life span (Wallace, 1992).

The first part of this section is a description of the reproductive organs and age-associated changes for each sex; the second is a discussion of sexuality and the assisted living facility resident.

WOMEN

The reproductive organs in women include the ovaries, which produce eggs that travel down the fallopian tubes to the uterus about once every month. Hormones act to control these reproductive cycles. Estrogen is the female sex hormone that directs most of these processes.

The organs of the lower reproductive tract are the cervix, the uterus, and the vagina. The cervix is the opening of the uterus leading into the vagina. The vagina is a barrel-shaped organ that leads to the external genitals in the female reproductive tract, such as the labia and the clitoris. During midlife women go through menopause (cessation of egg production and therefore of menstruation) and are no longer fertile.

Diseases of the uterus tend to decrease with age (Rossman, 1979, p. 334). Changes in the reproductive system are closely related to decreases in secretions of the hormone estrogen.

Some of the physical changes that may be experienced by elderly women include a loss of tone and elasticity in the breast, uterus, cervix, and vagina; a thinning and drying of the vaginal walls, which may cause uncomfortable irritations, infections, and bleeding; decrease in size of the uterus, fallopian tubes, and vagina (U.S. Barzel, 1989); loss of pubic hair; and decrease in the number of ducts or milk glands of the breasts (Butler & Lewis, 1977; Goldfarb, 1979; Kart et al., 1978; Kay & Neeley, 1982; Stilwell & O'Conner, 1989).

Elderly women do not tend to suffer from diseases of the uterus or reproductive tract per se (Rossman, 1979, p. 334). However, the incidence of breast cancer does continue to rise with age, and it remains the most common type of cancer affecting elderly women. The signs and symptoms of breast cancer are a hardened lump or thickening in the breast and a change in the size of the breast and the nipples. Treatment depends on the extent of the disease and may include surgery, radiation, and chemotherapy, as well as the relief of associated symptoms.

Another age-related change is genital prolapse. This occurs when the tone of the genital organs becomes so weakened that they begin to drop and may seem to fall out of the vagina. Women with weak muscles are at risk. Some of the signs and symptoms associated with genital prolapse include constant pressure on the bladder, incontinence of

urine, and a sense of weight in the pelvis. Usually this disorder can be repaired surgically.
Decrease in the production of the female sex hormone estrogen may also lead to osteoporosis (discussed in section 5.3.7).

MEN

The primary organs of the male reproductive tract are the testes, scrotum, prostate, and penis.

The testes are encased within the scrotum and produce the male hormone testosterone and sperm cells. These cells mature as they travel through the surrounding epididymis until released into the vas deferens. The sperm travel through the vas deferens until they are released from the ejaculatory ducts into the urethra. Nearby ducts secrete seminal fluid from the prostate gland, which provides food for the sperm as well as enhancing their motility. When the male ejaculates, the sperm travel down the urethra through the penis and are emitted from the body.

Some of the age-related changes in the male reproductive tract are an enlargement of the prostate gland, decreased production of testosterone, which may result in a slight decrease in sexual desire and a reduction in muscle bulk and strength. Sperm production continues into advanced old age, so males continue with the ability to impregnate into old age (Barzel, 1989; Kay & Neeley, 1982).

Problems with the prostate gland are a major concern for many elderly men (Kart et al., 1978, p. 152). Enlargement of the prostate is a common age-related change in men (Kart et al., 1978, p. 152; Reichel, 1983, pp. 304, 596; Rossman, 1979, p. 328). For some men, this enlargement may interfere with the ability to urinate or may cause incontinence. Prostatitis is an inflammation of this gland that often develops following the initial enlargement of the prostate gland and can be very painful. Other symptoms include painful urination and blood in the urine.

This enlargement may develop into cancer of the prostate, which is the second most common type of cancer in elderly men. Cancer of the prostate is considered a "geriatric disease," with 95% of all cases seen in elderly men (Rowe, 1982). The initial symptoms for this disease are the same as those experienced with prostatitis, including a decrease in urination and discomfort. Surgery is usually performed to remove the cancerous or extremely large prostate. Chemotherapy or hormone treatments may also be used.

COPING WITH SEXUALITY

Sexual needs persist into old age, with continued activity considered healthy and health-preserving (Griggs, 1978; Snowden, 1983). The elderly assisted living facility resident, continues to have needs for a positive self-image and self-esteem, which are closely associated with the needs for intimacy and sexuality (Butler, 1975; Griggs, 1978). Too often, society and individuals discourage sexual activity in the assisted living facility because of existing stereotypes and misunderstandings about sex and old age (Huntley, 1989; Wasow & Loeb, 1979).

Sexuality is not achieved exclusively by sexual intercourse, but may also incorporate a variety of activities related to touch and displays of affection. Older people may be more likely to express their sexuality in these more diffuse and varied terms (Boyer & Boyer, 1982; Huntley, 1989).

The sexual partners of those who have confirmed HIV antibody tests are themselves at risk for developing AIDS. Education to prevent disease transmission in the facility may become important (O'Connor & Stilwell, 1989).

Impotence, or the inability to perform sexually, is more often attributed to the male. The extent of this disorder in old age is not known, but an early American Medical Association report revealed that, rather than organic problems, anxiety and internalization of societal pressures account for most of the problems related to impotence (Kay & Neeley, 1982, p. 40). Assisted living facilities are often perceived as disapproving and as actively discouraging displays of love or affection among residents. A frequent suggestion in the literature is that assisted living facility staff be educated concerning sexuality in old age and that more efforts be made to deal with problems of morality that may arise.

Stillwell and O'Connor (1989) attempt to dispel some of the myths concerning sexuality with the observation that

- older people do remain interested in sex
- older people find each other physically attractive
- sexuality contributes to overall well-being

Contrary to public perceptions, the incidence of a heart attack or stroke during sexual intercourse is actually very low, and sexual activity is sometimes recommended for residents with diseases such as arthritis because of the therapeutic effects of exercise and intimacy (Huntley, 1989).

One research study suggests allowing for privacy of some residents to develop closer relationships (Kay & Neeley, 1982, p. 45). Another encourages the development of programs to deal with quality of life issues such as loneliness and isolation that are important to residents. Sexual expression would be only one component of this effort (Huntley, 1989; Kahana, 1995).

5.3.10 Emotional and Mental Well-Being

A number of the physical system disruptions discussed above can have profound effects on the mental well-being of the assisted living facility resident.

EFFECTS OF AGING

Differences of opinion exist as to whether intelligence declines with age. One difficulty is the use of tests that may not be appropriate measures for the elderly (Botwinick, 1978).

Aging is associated with special problems that may not be as disruptive for younger individuals. Burnside (1981) identifies two of these as behavioral problems and mental illness. The range of behaviors residents employ to cope with these problems will vary, but studies often show that many of the recurrent problems in an assisted living facility are related to behavioral problems (Stotsky, 1973).

When residents are admitted to the facility, they may display initial symptoms of anxiety and apprehension regarding their new surroundings (Trella, 1994). Chronic illness and the process of dying are anxiety-provoking and necessarily are an aspect of life with which assisted living facility residents must constantly cope.

Anxiety may be experienced by most individuals, and each deals with it in a particular way. Some manifestations of anxiety include fantasizing, hostile or dependent behavior, avoidance of eye contact, fidgeting, insomnia, and isolation from others.

INSOMNIA

Insomnia, or sleep disorder, is common among the elderly. Studies of human sleep patterns have shown that the elderly spend more time in bed, have more difficulty getting to sleep, and tend to awaken during sleep periods (Busse & Pfeiffer, 1973; Dement, Miles, & Bliwise, 1982).

Sleep problems may result from the use of multiple medications as well as from anxiety. To help the residents cope, sleeping medications may be prescribed, along with increases in daily activities and attempts to alleviate the source of anxiety.

LONELINESS

Behaviors associated with loneliness are similar to those of a mild depressive mood and include isolation, constipation, weight loss, insomnia, fatigue, and loss of appetite. Depression is often associated with losses, some of which are depicted in Figure 5.9, which focuses on admission to a long-term care facility. It is precisely these kinds of losses that the assisted facility attempts to minimize or eliminate.

Treatment for these residents is to discern the cause of depression and try to help them cope effectively with those feelings (Aller & Coeling, 1995; Moore & Gilbert, 1995). If these behaviors persist and worsen, the resident may be progressing toward mental illness. Antidepressive medications may also be prescribed in these cases (see Ade-Ridder & Kaplan, 1993; Engle & Graney, 1993).

LOSSES →	ADJUSTMENTS →	GAINS
FAMILIAR SURROUNDINGS—"home" whatever it was.	ADAPT TO NEW ROOM, ROOMMATE(S)	AN ENVIRONMENT ADAPTED TO THEIR NEEDS
LOSS OF FAMILY CONTACTS or caregiver contact pattern	ACCEPT NEW CAREGIVERS AS NEW "FAMILY"	PERSONNEL AVAILABLE 24 HOURS, WHO TRY TO CARE
LOSS OF CONTACT PATTERN WITH FRIENDS	REDUCED CONTACT, ESPECIALLY IF FRAIL	NEW FRIENDS ONE'S OWN AGE AND CONDITION
LOSS OF CONTROL OVER ONE'S LIFE, INCLUDING		EXPERT CAREGIVERS WHO TAKE OVER THIS FUNCTION
meal timing choice of snacks	ACCEPT THE FACILITY FOOD CHOICES	PREDICTABLE MEALS, SNACKS, 24 HRS.
RANGE OF DECISION MAKING LOSSES Independence, e.g., eat or not, take medicines or not	ACCEPT PHYSICIAN'S NEARLY TOTAL CONTROL OVER DIET, ACTIVITIES	AN ARRAY OF CONCERNED STAFF, ASSISTING DECISION MAKING
PERSONALIZATION LOSSES in clothing, life style, timing, activities or daily living	CONFORMITY TO TIME SCHEDULE, FOOD CHOICES, DAILY SCHEDULE	NOT MUCH—AN INTENSE STRUGGLE TO REPERSONALIZE ONESELF IN A POTENTIALLY DEPERSONALIZING INSTITUTIONAL ENVIRONMENT

FIGURE 5.9 Losses, adjustments, and gains of resident admitted for long term care.

MENTAL ILLNESS

Some studies have revealed that about 10% of elderly citizens have severe mental illness (Palmore, 1973), and the incidence of mental illness tends to increase as people age (Butler, 1975).

Often the term senile is used to describe a variety of behaviors in mental illness, ranging from slight to forgetfulness to a generalized decline in mental functioning of the elderly. Butler and Lewis (1977) describe two different groups of older personal suffering from mental illness as those with a history of mental illness and those who develop mental illness for the first time later in life.

Those with a history of mental illness, often by default, have ended up moving to an assisted living facility from a psychiatric facility, a phenomenon brought about by the development of psychotropic drugs in the 1950s and 1960s. This population may also be suffering from mental retardation (Kahana, 1995a).

Psychotrophic drugs are those that exert an effect on the mind. They are usually used to calm and control resident behavior. Equipped with these new medications and a belief that mentally ill persons are better cared for in the community setting, most states dramatically reduced the number of persons held in the state mental hospitals. It is believed that a significant portion of persons who were deinstitutionalized during this movement have entered the assisted living facility as a substitute for the mental hospital.

As time passes and the states continue to keep lower the number of hospital beds available for the mentally ill, this phenomenon is likely to continue (Mosher-Ashley & Henrikson, 1993).

The second group of mentally ill residents often become emotionally disturbed because they are no longer able to cope with the physical and social changes associated with the aging process (Miller, 1994).

Who is mentally ill? What is mental illness? These are difficult questions in the setting of the assisted living facility (Scott, Bramble, & Goodyear, 1991; Haight, 1995). The changes brought about by chronic physical illnesses and by the "normal" social changes faced by older persons are sometimes powerful enough to overwhelm even a well-adjusted person. The line between disabling mental illnesses and the day-to-day effects of attempting to cope with aging, especially in the institutionalized setting of the assisted living facility, is often blurred.

ORGANIC BRAIN SYNDROME

Organic brain syndrome, brain failure, and *senility* are all different terms describing the same disorder (Burnside, 1981; Gwyther, 1983; Golden & Cohen, 1995). Dementia and Alzheimer's disease have already been discussed as problems of the nervous system.

The two most common causes of organic brain syndrome are Alzheimer's disease and cerebrovascular insufficiency, or reduced blood flow to the brain. The brain tissue responds to any impairments resulting from these disorders with a variety of symptoms that initially can involve memory loss, leading to levels of disorientation and confusion and to difficulty following even simple directions. These symptoms of confusion progress until the resident is no longer aware of reality (Blustein, 1993; Emanuel & Emanuel, 1992).

Affected residents may engage in such problematic behaviors as suicidal threats or attempts, destructiveness, hostility, nosiness, and wandering off (Busse & Pfeiffer, 1973; Rantz & McShane, 1995). These behaviors can become especially troublesome in the group setting of an assisted living facility. Psychiatric consultation is usually desirable in these instances.

Treatment can include

- reality orientation (continually reminding residents of the date, time, and place to keep the residents oriented to their environment)
- choosing compatible roommates and company for these residents
- avoiding sudden changes or surprises
- increasing the amount of assistance available to these residents to perform the activities of daily living
- providing a supportive environment

DEPRESSION

Depression is probably the most common mental illness in the elderly (Blazer, 1995; M. Blumenthal, 1980; Buffum & Buffum, 1997; Kurlowicz, 1997; Tueth, 1995). Residents should be assessed to determine whether they are merely in a depressed mood or the disease has progressed to a mental illness (Kane et al., 1989; Lazar & Karasu, 1980). Often depression may be associated with another underlying chronic disease (e.g., arthritis or Parkinson's disease) or may be a result of a reaction to medications (M. Blumenthal, 1980; Lazar & Karasu, 1980). Busse and Pfeiffer (1973) also implicated depression as a symptom or precursor of other chronic diseases.

Additional signs of depression include loss of appetite resulting in weight loss, feelings of sadness, loss of interest in people, and a sense of great effort needed to perform daily activities (M. Blumenthal, 1980). The elderly may also complain of symptoms that are actually attributable to depression. Often the real problem is loss of control over their daily lives, along with a lack of decision-making opportunities.

Treatment of depression can include the use of antidepressant medications, usually tricyclic antidepressant drugs or newer ones such as Prozac and Paxil ("Listening to depression," January, 1995). These drugs themselves, however also have strong side effects (Kane et al., 1989, p. 134).

Electrocortical shock treatment (ECT) is a powerful form of treatment used to stimulate a specified area of the brain. M. Blumenthal (1980) suggested that ECT may be safer than drug therapy. However, use of electric shock treatments for depression and other mental disorders has been a subject of intense controversy for decades (Kane et al., 1989).

Counseling, group activities, and social functions appear to be productive therapeutic techniques available to the assisted living facility staff (Busse & Pfeiffer, 1973; Shore, 1978).

In essence, efforts by the staff to restore a sense of worth and importance to the resident may be among the most powerful tools available. Some of these include daily exercise, such as aerobics geared to the resident's level of physical capacity, dance therapy, recreation therapy, work therapy, and bibliotherapy (reading books) (see Kane et al., 1989; Kennie & Warshaw, 1989; Osgood, 1995; Waldo, Ide & Thomas, 1995).

5.4 The Scope-of-Care Issue

HEALTH CARE SERVICES IN THE ASSISTED LIVING SETTING

Health care is the most hotly debated aspect of the emerging assisted living facility industry. To what extent should the assisted living facility be engaged in providing health care? Increasingly, the reality is that all assisted living facilities are engaged in providing health care: The only variable is intensity. Intensity varies from no more than assisting residents take their medications and make and keep health care appointments in the community to providing a well-qualified health care staff that works closely with each resident's medical caregivers (whether personal physician or health maintenance organization).

What Is Health Care?

The World Health Organization defines health as a state of complete mental, social, and physical well-being, and not just the absence of disease. It is this more global concept of "health care" that the residents expect the assisted living facility to provide.

Given that the typical assisted living facility resident is in his or her 80s, physical health is a matter of intense concern for most residents. Understandably, physical well-being becomes more and more important to residents as they age in place. Residents enter assisted living facilities seeking social, mental, and physical well-being. Providing assistance to residents as they cope with failing health may be of equal importance with providing assistance with social well-being.

Scope of Care

The range of care assisted living facilities are permitted to provide varies widely from state to state. Most states limit assisted living facilities to providing assistance with the activities of daily living and with self-administration of medications. This model, however, is changing. As the health care system seeks less expensive sites of care for aging individuals who do not need the increasingly more intense level of nursing care provided by nursing homes, states will likely turn to assisted living facilities for help in providing health care.

A New Model Is Emerging. Several states are clearly moving in the direction of both permitting and seeking the services of assisted living facilities to provide a level of health care less intense than that provided in the nursing facility, but more intense than currently permitted in most states. Florida, Montana, Nevada, New Hampshire, New Jersey, New Mexico, Ohio, Oregon, and Vermont are moving in the direction of permitting assisted living facilities to go beyond personal services. Florida has had more years of experience with large retiree populations than most states and has had several years more experience in developing care models than most states. The Florida Extended Congregate Care Facility (ECCF) could well be the model for the future. In essence, Florida permits the ECCF to provide health care similar to that provided by nursing facilities. In the Florida model the ECCF should provide:

- a plan of health care which includes ongoing social and medical evaluation
- nursing diagnoses, monitoring for change in condition
- care of residents needing assistance with up to three of the activities of daily living
- medication administration
- dietary care including special diets and, if needed, input and output monitoring
- pressure sore prevention
- infection control

To distinguish the ECCF from the nursing facility, Florida does not permit ECCFs to offer advanced nursing care such as tube feeding, suctioning, blood gas checks, and intensive rehabilitation services for strokes. Nor does Florida permit the ECCF to provide 24-hour per day nursing care. Over time, as the health care system needs change and as assisted living facilities gain experience and proficiency in providing health care, the scope of health care services permitted the ECCF will likely increase just as the scope of nursing services permitted home health care agencies has increased in response to technological capabilities and the health care system needs. The following discussion of health care options the assisted living facility may wish to consider is based on the assumption that something resembling the Florida model will likely become the national model over the next few years.

The Health Care Staff

The assisted living industry, as mentioned earlier, is evolving the concept of "aging in place." In this model the typical resident expects to consider the assisted living facility his or her new home for life. The expectation is that if he or she has a catastrophic health care event such as a stroke or breaking a hip, he or she will be taken to the hospital for treatment and perhaps follow this by going to a local nursing facility for intensive stroke or mobility rehabilitation, then return to the assisted living facility once he or she has reached the highest functional level possible through rehabilitation programs.

Temporary Transfers Out. In this model some assisted living facility residents will be transferred permanently to a higher level of care if this becomes necessary (e.g. a lifelong need for complex medical care available only at a nursing facility). In general, however, the assisted living resident expects to return to his or her assisted living facility after necessary acute or rehabilitative care. In this model, the resident would expect to be able to die, using the services of the local hospice, in the assisted living facility, and not in a hospital or nursing facility.

This model seems to be what residents want and what the society wants. The resident wants to avoid having to go to a nursing home to live or to die in a hospital bed at the end of an extended hospital stay. Society wants to have residents cared for in the most cost-effective setting. Acute care in the hospital and restorative care in the nursing facility is intensive health care provided at high cost to both the individual and society. An increasing capacity for providing health care in the assisted living setting makes emotional and economic sense.

Health Care Work Area Tasks

The health care service has the following responsibilities:

- ensuring that health care to residents as ordered by the physician is accomplished
- completing and implementing a plan of health care
- assisting with or administering medications to the residents
- keeping resident records
- monitoring residents for changes in condition and notifying the responsible physician—in short, serving as the physician's eyes and ears on a 24-hour basis
- achieving optimal quality of care and quality of life for residents
- making certain that every resident is functioning at the highest possible level
- playing a coordinating role with other staff (e.g., coordinating planned physical therapy, activities, and physician office visits)

In short, health care workers are involved in a myriad of activities such as

assessments
wound care
range of motion
toileting
feeding
counseling
friendship
comfort
ambulating
transferring from bed to toilet
assistance with the activities of daily living
changing the diapers and sheets
turning residents
use of assistive devices
bathing
toileting
dressing
ambulating
cleaning up spills
washing hands
room tidiness
ice water
hospice
recruiting
training
disciplining
evaluating staff
interfacing with the other work areas
observing the infection control precautions
interfacing with physicians, pharmacists, numerous health care professionals
counseling
reassuring families and significant others
washing hands
coping with volunteers
cooperating with the police, fire department, and disaster control
doing infection control
working short
conducting in-services
charting
bowel and bladder programs
fire safety
disaster preparedness
answering call bells

checking on the residents hundreds of times each day
participating in lengthy health care planning sessions
afternoon and evening snacks
getting food substitutes from the kitchen
mediating disputes among residents
washing hands
coping with dementia
avoiding learned helplessness
death and dying
emergencies
morticians
admissions
lost clothing
lost teeth
lost jewelry
running out of bed pads
hazardous waste rules
electrical outages
failing equipment
room transfers
roommate dissatisfaction
refusal to eat
missing oxygen tank wrenches
snippy staff
arrogant physicians
dissatisfied residents
troublesome visitors
unresponsive decubitus ulcers
unresponsive attending physicians
overflowing linen bins
broken wheelchairs
epidemics among staff and residents
wandering residents
misplaced charts
constant phone calls
late lab reports
physicians who don't sign orders or visit

Quality of Resident Life

There are unwritten dimensions to care performed by the health care service. It is not possible, and perhaps not desirable, to set them all down, for many of the health care acts that increase the quality of life cannot be fully spelled out in policy statements. The quality of life enjoyed is directly proportional to the quality of the effort given by the health care staff.

Organizational Interdependencies

Organizational interdependencies between health care and virtually every other area exist within the facility. Health care is dependent on dietary, housekeeping, laundry, maintenance, the business office, the social worker, and the allied health professionals: They must be a single team when it comes to achieving resident care. No health care provider can function effectively unless the administrator is able to create and lead teams. In sum, for health care to do its tasks properly, nearly every other work area and functional area within the organization should also be doing its tasks in a cooperative manner.

Staffing

Three health care–related shifts, 24 hours a day, 365 days a year, offer a staffing challenge. The proportional ratios between nurses and aides will vary with the staffing philosophy of the facility administrator and the resident profile. As acuity level increases in many facilities, the proportion of professionally trained health caregivers increases.

A HEALTH CARE STAFF HEADED BY A REGISTERED NURSE?

A registered nurse is needed in the health care services because a person licensed to do assessments and health care planning is required in order to provide day-to-day care for residents and to establish and implement a plan of health care. Licensed nurse practitioners, in most states, are not allowed to do assessments or develop a plan of health care. A physician or a nurse practitioner, however, may do assessments and develop plans of care for residents. The registered nurse is the least expensive health care professional allowed to assess residents' health care changes and initiate plans of care. A registered nurse is an independent health care practitioner. A licensed practical nurse is a dependent health care practitioner and may only assist in such processes such as developing a health care plan or assessing a resident for change in health care status.

NATIONAL STANDARDS OF PRACTICE FOR NURSING STAFF

Most states specify in their guidelines that assisted living facilities must have sufficient staff to serve residents' needs identified in the plan of health care. The federal guideline for nursing care is: "The facility should have sufficient nursing staff to provide nursing and related services to attain or maintain the highest practicable physical, mental, and psychosocial well-being of each resident, as determined by resident assessments and individual plans of care." The intention is to ensure that sufficient qualified nursing staff are available on a daily basis to meet residents' needs for nursing care in a manner and in an environment that promotes each resident's physical, mental, and psychosocial well-being, thus enhancing quality of life.

At a minimum, *staff* is defined as licensed nurses (RNs and/or LPNs/LVNs) and nurse's aides. Nurse's aides should meet the training and competency guidelines.

In assessing whether sufficient staff are in place, the administrator of the assisted living facility may ask:

- Is there adequate staff to meet direct care needs, assessments, planning, evaluation, and supervision?
- Do workloads for direct care staff appear reasonable?
- Do residents, family, and ombudspersons report insufficient staff to meet residents' needs?
- Are staff responsive to residents' needs for assistance, and are call bells answered promptly?
- Do residents call out repeatedly for assistance?
- Are residents, who are unable to call for help, checked frequently (e.g., every half hour) for safety, comfort, positioning, and to offer fluids and provision of care?
- Are identified care problems associated with a specific unit or tour of duty?
- What does the registered nurse do to correct problems in nurse staff performance?
- How does the facility ensure that each resident receives nursing care in accordance with his or her plan of health care on weekends, nights, and holidays?
- How does the sufficiency (numbers and categories) of nursing staff contribute to identified quality of care, residents' rights, quality of life, and facility practices problems?

5.5 Resident Care Policies: Establishing and Maintaining Quality Care

Each assisted living facility must develop policies stating whether and how it will provide health care for its residents. Policies and practices of facilities providing health care to residents have been the subject of national debate for several decades. Over the past four decades a national consensus has emerged that defines the professional standards expected of facilities that offer health-related care to elderly Americans. The following are the nationally accepted guidelines for facilities to take into account as they formulate their own resident care policies.

QUALITY OF CARE GUIDELINES

Each resident should receive and the facility should provide the necessary care and services to attain or maintain the highest practicable physical, mental, and psychosocial well-being, in accordance with the plan of health care.

Highest practicable is defined as the highest level of functioning and well-being possible, limited only to the individual's presenting functional status and potential for improvement or reduced rate of functional decline.

The facility should ensure that the resident obtains optimal improvement or does not deteriorate within the limits of a resident's right to refuse treatment, and within the limits of recognized pathology and the normal aging process.

When the facility health care team notes a lack of improvement or a decline, the team should determine if the occurrence was unavoidable or avoidable. A determination of unavoidable decline or failure to reach highest practicable well-being can be made if the following are present:

- a health care plan that is implemented consistently and based on information from the resident
- evaluation of the results of the interventions and revising the interventions as necessary

Activities of Daily Living

The following is a detailed discussion of national guidelines on how assisted living facilities and similar providers can achieve satisfactory results in their effort to ensure that the residents are being properly helped in their activities of daily living.

Based on the health care plan of a resident, the facility should ensure that a resident's ability in activities of daily living do not diminish unless circumstances of the individual's health condition demonstrate that diminution was unavoidable. The goal is that the facility should ensure that a resident's abilities in ADLs do not deteriorate unless the deterioration was unavoidable.

The health care staff and the administrator may use the following concepts in judging their level of success in assisting residents with their activities of daily living.

The mere presence of a health diagnosis, in itself, justifies a decline in a resident's ability to perform ADLs. Conditions that may demonstrate unavoidable diminution in ADLs include the natural progression of the resident's disease:

- deterioration of the resident's physical condition associated with the onset of a physical or mental disability while receiving care to restore or maintain functional abilities
- the resident's refusal of care and treatment to restore or maintain functional abilities after aggressive efforts by the facility to counsel and/or offer alternatives to the resident, surrogate, or representative. (Refusal of such care and treatment should be documented in the resident's record.)

Appropriate treatment and services includes all care provided to residents by employees, contractors, or volunteers of the facility to maximize the individual's functional abilities. This includes pain relief and control, especially when it is causing a decline or a decrease in the quality of life of the resident.

How Well Are Residents Maintaining ADL Skills?

The following are useful guidelines in judging the extent to which, over a specified time period (typically a year), residents have been enabled to maintain their activities of daily living to the appropriate degree.

For evaluating a resident's ADLs and determining whether a resident's abilities have declined, improved, or stayed the same within the last 12 months, the facility can use the following definitions:

1. **Independent:** no help or staff oversight; or staff help/oversight provided only 1 or 2 times during prior 7 days.
2. **Supervision:** oversight encouragement or cueing provided 3 or more times during the last 7 days, or supervision plus physical assistance provided only 1 or 2 times during the last 7 days.
3. **Limited assistance:** resident highly involved in activity, received physical help in guided maneuvering of limbs, and/or other non-weight-bearing assistance 3 or more times; or more help provided only 1 or 2 times over 7-day period.
4. **Extensive assistance:** while resident performed part of activity, over prior 7-day period, help of the following types was provided 3 or more times;
   a. Weight-bearing support
   b. Full staff performance during part (but not all) of week
5. **Total dependence:** full staff performance of activity over entire 7-day period.

The Individual Activities of Daily Living

The following is a discussion of the guidelines recommended as standards of practice for evaluating the individual activities of daily living.

Bathing, Dressing, Grooming. *Bathing* means how the resident takes full-body bath, sponge bath, and transfers into and out of the tub or shower. Excludes washing of back and hair.

Dressing means how resident puts on, fastens, and takes off all items of clothing, including donning and removing prosthesis.

Grooming means how resident maintains personal hygiene, including preparatory activities, combing hair, brushing teeth, shaving, applying makeup, and washing and drying face, hands, and perineum. Excludes baths and showers.

For each resident on at least an annual basis determine

1. whether the resident's ability to bathe, dress, and/or groom has changed since admission or over the past 12 months
2. whether the resident's ability to bathe, dress, and groom has improved, declined, or stayed the same
3. whether any deterioration or lack of improvement was avoidable or unavoidable

The staff should ask whether individual objectives of the plan of health care are periodically evaluated, and if the objectives were not met, if alternative approaches were developed to encourage maintenance of bathing, dressing, and/or grooming abilities.

Continuous Quality Improvement Questions:

- What care did the resident receive to address unique needs to maintain his or her bathing, dressing, and/or grooming abilities (e.g., resident needs a button hook to button his shirt; staff teaches the resident how to use it; staff provides resident with dementia with cues that allow him or her to dress himself or herself)?

- If the resident's abilities in bathing, dressing, and grooming have only been maintained, what evidence is there that the resident could have improved if appropriate treatment and services were provided?
- Are there physical and psychosocial deficits that could affect improvement in functional abilities?
- Was the health care plan consistently implemented? What changes were made in treatment if the resident failed to progress or when initial rehabilitation goals were achieved, but additional progress might have been possible?

Transfer and Ambulation. *Transfer* means how resident moves between surfaces—to/from bed, chair, wheelchair, standing position.

Ambulation means how resident moves between locations in his or her room and adjacent corridor on same floor. If in wheelchair, involves self-sufficiency once in chair.

Determine for each resident whether the resident's ability to transfer and ambulate has declined, improved or stayed the same and whether any deterioration or decline in function was avoidable or unavoidable.

Continuous Quality Improvement Questions:

- If the resident's transferring and ambulating abilities have declined, what evidence is there that the decline was unavoidable?
- What risk factors for decline of transferring or ambulating abilities did the facility identify (e.g., red area of foot becoming larger, postural hypotension)?
- What care did the resident receive to address risk factors and unique needs to maintain transferring or ambulating abilities?
- What evidence is there that sufficient staff time and assistance are provided to maintain transferring and ambulating abilities?
- Has resident been involved in activities that enhance mobility skills?
- Were individual objectives of the plan of health care periodically evaluated, and if goals were not met, were alternative approaches developed to encourage maintenance of transferring and ambulation abilities (e.g., resident remains unsteady when using a cane, returns to walker, with staff encouraging the walker's consistent use)?
- If the resident's abilities in transferring and ambulating have only been maintained, is there evidence that the resident could have improved if appropriate treatment and services were provided?
- Are there physical and psychosocial deficits that could affect improvement in functional abilities?
- Was the health care plan driven by the resident's strengths?
- Was the health care plan consistently implemented? What changes were made in treatment if the resident failed to progress or when initial rehabilitation goals were achieved but additional progress seemed possible?

Toileting. *Toilet use* means how the resident uses the toilet room (or commode, bedpan, or urinal), transfers on and off the toilet, cleanses self, changes pad, manages ostomy or catheter, and adjusts clothes.

Determine for each resident whether the resident's ability to use the toilet has improved, declined, or stayed the same and whether any deterioration or decline in improvement was avoidable or unavoidable.

Continuous Quality Improvement Questions:

- If the resident's toilet use abilities have declined, what evidence is there that the decline was unavoidable?
- What risk factors for the decline of toilet use abilities did the staff identify (e.g., severe arthritis in hands makes use of toilet paper difficult)?
- What care did resident receive to address risk factors and unique needs to maintain toilet use abilities (e.g., assistive devices to maintain ability to use the toilet such as using a removable elevated toilet seat or wall grab bar to facilitate rising from seated position to standing position)?
- Is there sufficient staff time and assistance provided to maintain toilet use abilities (e.g., allowing resident enough time to use the toilet independently or with limited assistance)?
- Were individual objectives of the plan of health care periodically evaluated, and if objectives were not met, were alternative approaches developed to encourage maintaining toilet use abilities (e.g., if resident has not increased sitting stability, seek occupational therapy consult to determine the need for therapy to increase sitting balance, ability to transfer safely, and manipulate clothing during the toileting process)?
- If the resident's toilet use abilities have only been maintained, what evidence is there that the resident could have improved if appropriate treatment and services were provided?
- Are there physical and psychosocial deficits that could affect improvement in functional abilities?
- Was the health care plan driven by the resident's strengths?
- Was the health care plan consistently implemented? What changes were made to treatment if the resident failed to progress or when initial rehabilitation goals were achieved but additional progress seemed possible?

Eating. *Eating* means how resident ingests and drinks (regardless of self-feeding skill).

Determine whether the resident's ability to eat or eating skills have improved, declined, or stayed the same and whether any deterioration or lack of improvement was avoidable or unavoidable.

Continuous Quality Improvement Questions

- If the resident's eating ability has declined, is there any evidence that the decline was unavoidable?
- What risk factors for decline of eating skills did the health care staff identify?
  1. a decrease in the ability to chew and swallow food
  2. deficit in neurological and muscular status necessary for moving food onto a utensil and into the mouth

3. oral health status affecting eating ability
4. depression or confused mental state

- What care did the resident receive to address risk factors and unique needs to maintain eating abilities?
  1. assistive devices to improve resident's grasp or coordination
  2. seating arrangements to improve sociability
  3. seating in a calm, quiet setting for residents with dementia
- Is there sufficient staff time and assistance provided to maintain eating abilities (e.g., allowing residents enough time to eat independently or with limited assistance)?
- Were individual objectives of the plan of health care periodically evaluated, and if the objectives were not met, were alternative approaches developed to encourage maintaining eating abilities?
- If the resident's eating abilities have only been maintained, what evidence is there that the resident could have improved if appropriate treatment and services were provided?
- Are there physical and psychosocial deficits that could affect improvement in functional abilities?
- Was the health care plan driven by the resident's strengths identified?
- Was the health care plan consistently implemented? What changes were made to treatment if the resident failed to progress or when initial rehabilitation goals were achieved but additional progress seemed possible?

Communicating: Using speech, language, or other functional communication systems. *Speech, language or other functional communication systems* is defined as the ability to effectively communicate requests, needs, opinions, and urgent problems; to express emotion; to listen to others; and to participate in social conversation whether in speech, writing, gesture, or a combination of these (e.g., a communication board or electronic augmentative communication device).

Determine for each resident if the resident's ability to communicate has declined, improved, or stayed the same and whether any deterioration or lack of improvement was avoidable or unavoidable.

Continuous Quality Improvement Questions:

- If the resident's communication abilities have diminished, is there any evidence that the decline was unavoidable?
- What risk factors for decline of communication abilities did the health care staff members identify and how did they address them (e.g., dysarthria, poor fitting dentures, few visitors, poor relationships with staff, Alzheimer's disease)?
- Has the resident received audiologic and vision evaluation that may have seemed needed? If not, did the resident refuse such services?
- What unique needs and risk factors did the staff identify (e.g., does the resident have specific difficulties in transmitting messages, comprehending messages, and/or using a variety of communication skills such as questions and commands; does the resident receive evaluation and training in the use of assistive devices to increase and/or maintain writing skills)?

- What care does the resident receive to improve communication abilities (e.g., nurse's aides communicate in writing with deaf residents or residents with severe hearing problems; practice exercises with residents receiving speech-language pathology services; increase number of residents' communication opportunities; offer nonverbal means of communication; initiate review of the effect of medications on communication ability)?
- Is there sufficient staff time and assistance provided to maintain communication abilities?
- Were individual objectives of the plan of health care periodically evaluated, and if the objectives were not met, were alternative approaches developed to encourage maintenance of communication abilities (e.g., if drill-oriented therapy is frustrating a resident, should a less didactic approach be attempted)?
- If the resident's speech, language, and other communication abilities have only been maintained, what evidence is there that the resident could have improved if appropriate treatment and services were provided?
- Are there physical and psychosocial deficits that could affect improvement in functional abilities?
- Was the health care plan driven by the resident's strengths as identified in the health care plan?
- Was the health care plan consistently implemented? What changes were made to treatment if the resident failed to progress or when initial rehabilitation goals were achieved but additional progress seemed possible?

For Residents Unable to Carry Out Some of the ADLs

Unable to carry out ADLs means those residents who need extensive or total assistance with maintenance of nutrition, grooming, and personal and oral hygiene.

Methods for maintenance of good nutrition may include hand feeding of foods served on dishes.

Oral hygiene means maintaining the mouth in a clean and intact condition and treating oral pathology such as ulcers of the mucosa. Services to maintain oral hygiene may include brushing the teeth, cleaning dentures, cleaning the mouth and tongue either by assisting the resident with a mouth wash or by manual cleaning with a gauze sponge, and application of medication as prescribed.

Vision and hearing. To ensure that residents receive proper treatment and assistive devices to maintain vision and hearing abilities, the facility should, if necessary, assist the resident (1) in making appointments and (2) arrange for transportation to and from the office of a practitioner specializing in the treatment of vision or hearing impairment or the office of a professional specializing in the provision of vision or hearing assistive devices.

The goal is to assist residents in gaining access to vision and hearing services by making appointments and arranging for transportation and assistance with the use of any devices needed to maintain vision and hearing.

Assistive devices to maintain vision include glasses, contact lenses, and magnifying glasses. Assistive devices to maintain hearing include hearing aids.

This guideline does not mean that the assisted living facility should providerefractions, glasses, contact lenses, or provide hearing aids. The facility's responsibility is to assist residents in locating and utilizing any available resources for the provision of needed services. This includes making appointments and arranging transportation to obtain needed services.

Continuous Quality Improvement Questions:

- If the resident needs and/or requests and does not have vision and/or hearing assistive devices, what has the facility done to assist the resident in making appointments and obtaining transportation to obtain those services?
- If the resident has assistive devices but is not using them, why not (e.g., are repairs or batteries needed)?

MAJOR POLICY ISSUES BEYOND THE ACTIVITIES OF DAILY LIVING

Restraints

Restraints is a highly controversial area for facilities that provide health care assistance to elderly persons over long periods of time. Hospitals and nursing facilities, during the 1960s to 1990s, became progressively involved in placing physical and chemical restraints. The use of restraints in nursing homes is being discarded as a practice that does not meet professional standards of care. Hospitals continue to unnecessarily restrain elderly residents.

Just say no? Cogent arguments against restraints can be marshaled (Aller & Coeling, 1995; Brooke, 1991; Burger, 1994; Jenelli, Kanski, & Neary, 1994; Johnson, 1995; Magee et al., 1993; Menscher, 1993; Moss & Puma, 1991; Scherer, Janelli, Kanski, Neary, & Morth, 1994; Stolley, et al., 1993; Watzke & Wister, 1993; Werner, Cohen-Mansfield, Koroknay, & Braun, 1994; Maddox, 2001). Reducing chemical restraints has also been of concern (Burger, 1992) and is a source of contention.

It has been the author's observation that restraints kill the human spirit, and sometimes the human. Restraints have no place in the assisted living facility environment. The best restraints policy is a no restraints policy.

A "no physical restraints policy" is observable as one moves down the hallway. No chemical restraints is another matter. The use of drugs to restrain residents may sometimes be for the betterment of the entire assisted living facility's quality of life. However, this is a complex area with which ach assisted living facility must grapple. The following observations are made regarding restraints in the nationally recommended guidelines.

Pressure From Families. It is important for the assisted living facility administrator and health staff to be familiar with the restraint issue because it is unavoidable: Some family member (possibly a well-meaning spouse) will ask the assisted living facility staff to okay a restraint or some attending physician will order the assisted living facility staff to apply a restraint. Residents will too often come back from an acute care episode in the local hospital in restraints. How should the facility staff respond? In reading through the national guidelines, it will become clear that the practice of using restraints is under considerable negative pressures.

At the very minimum, the resident has the right to be free from any physical or chemical restraints imposed for purposes of discipline or convenience, and not required to treat the resident's medical symptoms.

Physical restraints are defined as any manual method or physical or mechanical device, material, or equipment attached or adjacent to the resident's body that the individual cannot remove easily and that restricts freedom of movement or normal access to one's body.

Chemical restraint is defined as a psychopharmacological drug that is used for discipline or convenience and not required to treat medical symptoms.

Discipline is defined as any action taken by the facility for the purpose of punishing or penalizing residents.

Convenience is defined as any action taken by the facility to control resident behavior or maintain residents with a lesser amount of effort by the facility and not in the residents' best interest.

Restraints = Accident Hazard. Restraint use may constitute an accident hazard, and professional standards of practice have eliminated the need for physical restraints except under limited medical circumstances. Therefore, medical symptoms that would warrant the use of restraints should be reflected in the health care planning. It is further expected that for those residents whose health care plans indicate the need for restraints that the facility engage in a systematic and gradual process toward reducing restraints (e.g., gradually increasing the time for ambulating and muscle-strengthening activities).

For the resident to make an informed choice about the use of restraints, the facility should explain to the resident the negative outcomes of restraint use. Potential negative outcomes include incontinence, decreased range of motion, decreased ability to ambulate, symptoms of withdrawal or depression, and reduced social contact.

Physical restraints include, but are not limited to, leg restraints, arm restraints, hand mitts, soft ties or vests, lap cushions, and lap trays the resident cannot remove. Also included as restraints are facility practices that meet the definition of a restraint, such as

- using bed rails to keep a resident from voluntarily getting out of bed as opposed to enhancing mobility while in bed
- tucking in a sheet so tightly that a bed-bound resident cannot move
- using wheelchair safety bars to prevent a resident from rising out of a chair
- placing a resident in a chair that prevents rising
- placing a resident who uses a wheelchair so close to a wall that the wall prevents the resident from rising

Orthotic body devices may be used solely for therapeutic purposes to improve overall functional capacity of the resident.

Bed rails are not be used to restrain residents or to assist in mobility and transfer of residents. The use of bed rails as restraints is prohibited unless they are necessary to treat a resident's medical symptoms. Bed rails used as restraints add risk to the resident. They potentially increase the risk of more significant injury from a fall from a bed with raised bed rails than from a fall from a bed without bed rails. They also potentially increase the likelihood that the resident will spend more time in bed and fall when attempting to transfer from bed. Other interventions that the facility might incorporate in health care planning include

- providing restorative care to enhance abilities to stand safely and to walk
- adding a trapeze to increase bed mobility
- placing the bed lower to the floor and surrounding the bed with a soft mat
- equipping the resident with a device that monitors attempts to arise
- providing frequent staff monitoring at night with periodic assisted toileting for residents attempting to arise to use the bathroom
- furnishing visual and verbal reminders to use the call bell for residents who are able to comprehend this information

When used for mobility or transfer, assessment should include a review of the resident's

- bed mobility (e.g., would the use of the bed rail help the resident turn from side to side? Or is the resident totally immobile and cannot shift without assistance?)
- ability to transfer between positions and to and from a bed or chair, as well as to stand and toilet (e.g., does the raised bed rail add risk to the resident's ability to transfer?)

Continuous Quality Improvement Questions:

Since continued restraint usage is associated with a potential for a decline in functioning if the risk is not addressed, determine if the health care team addressed the risk of decline at the time restraint use was initiated and that the health care plan reflected measures to minimize a decline. Also determine if the plan of health care was consistently implemented. Determine whether the decline can be attributable to unavoidable disease progression, versus inappropriate use of restraints.

In thinking through ways to eliminate any need for restraints, the assisted living facility staff can ask:

- What are the symptoms that led to the consideration of the use of restraints (e.g., a resident returned from the hospital restrained)?
- Are these symptoms caused by failure to
  1. meet individual needs
  2. use aggressive rehabilitative/restorative care
  3. provide meaningful activities
  4. improve the resident's environment, including seating
- Can the cause(s) be removed?
- If the cause(s) cannot be removed, has the facility staff attempted to use alternatives in order to avoid a decline in physical functioning associated with restraint use?

- If the alternatives have been tried and found wanting, does the facility use the least restrictive restraint for the least amount of time? Does the facility monitor and adjust care to reduce negative outcomes while continually trying to find and use less restrictive alternatives?
- Did the resident make an informed choice about the use of restraints? Were risks, benefits, and alternatives explained?
- Has the facility reevaluated the need for the restraint, made efforts to eliminate its use, and maintained the resident's strength and mobility?

Pressure Sores

This discussion of pressure sores enlarges our earlier discussion and presents the standards of practice definitions used nationally. As mentioned earlier, pressure sores are a serious risk when using restraints. The assisted living facility health care staff must understand pressure sores, how to prevent them, how to treat them, and when to send the resident out for more intensive treatment.

The goal is that a resident who enters the assisted living facility without sores does not develop pressure sores unless the individual's health condition demonstrates that they were unavoidable.

For additional information on prevention, staging, and treatment, refer to the staging system found in the booklet *Pressure Ulcers in Adults: Prevention and Treatment,* from the Public Health Service Agency for Health Care Policy and Research.

Pressure sore means ischemic ulceration and/or necrosis of tissues overlying a bony prominence that has been subjected to pressure, friction, or shear. The staging system presented below is one method of describing the extent of tissue damage in the pressure sore. Pressure sores cannot be adequately staged when covered with eschar or necrotic tissue. Staging should be done after the eschar has sloughed off or the wound has been debrided. Vascular ulcers due to peripheral vascular disease have to be considered separately. They usually occur on the lower legs and feet and are very persistent even with aggressive treatment.

Stage I: A persistent area of skin redness (without a break in the skin) that is nonblanchable. Redness can be expected to be present for one half to three fourths as long as the pressure applied that has occluded blood flow to the areas. For example, if a resident is lying on his right side for 30 minutes and turned onto his back, redness may be noticed over the right hip bone. Redness in that area can be expected to remain for up to 20 minutes. The health care staff can then check to see if the area is nonblanchable. Just having the redness does not indicate Stage I. To identify the presence of Stage I pressure ulcers in residents with darkly pigmented skin, look for changes in skin color (grayish hue), temperature, swelling, and tenderness or texture.

Stage II: A partial thickness loss of skin layers, either dermis or epidermis, that presents clinically as an abrasion, blister, or shallow crater.

Stage III: A full thickness of skin is lost, exposing the subcutaneous tissues—presents as a deep crater with or without undermining adjacent tissue.

Stage IV: A full thickness of skin and subcutaneous tissue is lost, exposing muscle and/or bone.

If the resident is receiving hospice care and life-sustaining measures have been withdrawn or discouraged as documented in the record, pressure sores may be clinically difficult to prevent.

A determination that development of a pressure sore was unavoidable may be made only if routine preventive and daily care was provided. Routine preventive care means turning and proper positioning, application of pressure reduction or relief devices, providing good skin care (i.e., keeping the skin clean, instituting measures to reduce excessive moisture), providing clean and dry bed linens, and maintaining adequate nutrition and hydration as possible.

At some point many assisted living facility residents may become at risk for developing pressure sores. Health conditions that are the primary risk factors for developing pressure sores include, but are not limited to, resident immobility and the following:

1. The resident has two or more of the following diagnoses:
   - continuous urinary incontinence or chronic voiding dysfunction
   - severe peripheral vascular disease
   - diabetes
   - severe chronic pulmonary obstructive disease
   - severe peripheral disease
   - chronic bowel incontinence
   - continuous urinary incontinence or chronic voiding dysfunction
   - paraplegia
   - quadriplegia
   - sepsis
   - terminal cancer
   - chronic or end stage renal, liver, and/or heart disease
   - disease or drug-related immunosupression; or
   - full body cast
2. The resident receives (usually on an out-resident basis at a local hospital or ambulatory care center) two or more of the following treatments:
   - steroid therapy
   - radiation therapy
   - chemotherapy
   - renal dialysis; or
   - head of bed elevated the majority of the day due to medical necessity
3. Malnutrition/dehydration, whether secondary to poor appetite or another disease process, places residents at risk for poor healing, and may be indicated by the following lab values:
   - serum albumin below 3.4 g/dl
   - weight loss of more than 10% during last month
   - serum transferrin level below 180 mg per dl
   - Hgb less than 12 mg per dl
4. If laboratory data are not available, health signs and symptoms of malnutrition/dehydration may be
   - pale skin
   - red, swollen lips

- swollen and/or dry tongue with scarlet or magenta hue
- poor skin turgor
- cachexia
- bilateral edema
- muscle wasting
- calf tenderness
- reduced urinary output

Urinary Incontinence

Assisted living facilities are increasingly involved in dealing with urinary incontinence. The following is a discussion of current guidelines and expands on our discussion earlier. Some assisted living facilities will include catheter care within its plans of care; others may exclude catheter care as an offered health care service.

The intent is to ensure that an indwelling catheter is used only when there is a valid medical justification. The resident should be assessed for and provided the care and treatment needed to reach his or her highest level of continence possible.

Examples of resident conditions demonstrating that catheterization may be unavoidable include

- urinary retention that (1) is causing persistent overflow incontinence, symptomatic infections, and/or renal dysfunction; (2) cannot be corrected surgically; or (3) cannot be managed practically with intermittent catheter use
- skin wounds, pressure sores, or irritations that are being contaminated by urine
- terminal illness or severe impairment, which makes bed and clothing changes uncomfortable or disruptive (as in the case of intractable pain)

Because most older males in assisted living facilities will have benign prostatic hyperplasia, which normally leads to urine retention, the above concerns will affect nearly all assisted living facilities.

Continuous Quality Improvement Questions:

- If continent at admission, was the resident identified as having risk factors of incontinence (e.g., frequency of urination, with limited mobility)?
- What care did the resident receive to promote maintenance of continence?
- Did the facility attempt to manage the incontinence and increase bladder function without the use of an indwelling catheter (e.g., a bladder training program, repeated voiding schedule, external catheter)?

If the resident has an indwelling catheter:

- Is the staff following the facility's protocol and/or written procedures for catheterization?
- Do all personnel wash their hands before and after caring for the catheter/tubing/collecting bag?

- Does the health care team assess for continued need for use of the catheter, as appropriate, utilizing the evaluative data as described and implemented in the health care plan?

UTI Treatment, Restoration of Function

Guidelines on urinary tract infection (UTI) include the following. For purposes of these guidelines, *urinary tract infection (UTI)* is defined as colonization (growth of bacteria) of the urinary tract with signs or symptoms of UTI. Asymptomatic colonization is not a UTI. Care should be provided based on the type, severity, and cause (if known) of urinary incontinence. Antibiotic therapy should be reserved for residents with active symptoms of UTI. Routine and overzealous use could lead to resistance of organisms.

Continuous Quality Improvement Questions:
For each incontinent resident ask:

- Has the health care team identified (or attempted to identify) the cause of the incontinence?
- Is the resident adequately hydrated?
- How many residents currently have a UTI? One should differentiate between bacterial colonization vs. acute infection.
- Are risk factors for UTI monitored and managed (e.g., poor fluid intake, previous UTIs)? Are residents with a history of UTI adequately assessed and provided care and treatment to prevent UTI?
- Are infection control procedures in place (e.g., adequate fluid intake)?
  What care did the resident receive to restore or improve bladder functioning (e.g., pelvic floor exercises, habit training, or maintaining adequate hydration)?
- Have the individualized goals of this treatment program been evaluated periodically, and if goals were not reached, have alternative goals and approaches been developed?
- If staff determine that continence cannot be improved or maintained, has a plan been implemented to prevent incontinent-related complications and to maintain resident dignity (e.g., skin care will be provided after each episode of incontinence, adult sanitary padding will be worn at all times when the resident is out of bed)?

Range of Motion

As the acuity level of residents intensifies, the need for constant staff attention to range of motion increases.

The goal is that a resident who enters the assisted living facility without a limited range of motion should not experience reduction in range of motion (ROM) unless the resident's health condition demonstrates that a reduction in range of motion is unavoidable.

Range of Motion (ROM) is defined as the extent of movement of a joint. The health condition that may demonstrate that a reduction in ROM is unavoidable is limbs or digits immobilized because of injury or surgical procedures (e.g., surgical adhesions).

Adequate preventive care may include active ROM performed by the resident or passive ROM performed by staff; active-assistive ROM exercise performed by the resident and staff; and application of splints and braces, if necessary.

Examples of conditions in the typical assisted living facility that are the primary risk factors for a decreased range of motion are

- immobilization (e.g., bedfast for a period of time)
- deformities arising out of neurological deficits (e.g., strokes, multiple sclerosis, cerebral palsy, and polio)
- pain, spasms, and immobility associated with arthritis or late-stage Alzheimer's disease

When residents are identified as experiencing a range of motion problem, the health care staff is expected to take initiatives to provide or obtain care for the condition.

Continuous Quality Improvement Questions:

- Are passive ROM exercises provided and active ROM exercises supervised per the plan of health care?
- Have health care plan objectives identified resident's needs and has progress been evaluated?
- Is there evidence that health care planning is changed as the resident's condition changes?

Mental and Psychosocial Functioning

It is believed that at least half of residents in assisted living facilities have decreased psychosocial functioning due to various health conditions. Increasingly, the assisted living facility staff will deal with ensuring that residents are able to maintain the highest psychosocial functioning feasible.

It is a guideline of practice that a resident who displays mental or psychosocial adjustment difficulty receive appropriate treatment and services to correct the addressed problem. The intent of this guideline is that the resident receives care and services to help him or her to reach and maintain the highest level of mental and psychosocial functioning.

Mental and psychosocial adjustment difficulties refer to problems residents have in adapting to changes in life's circumstances. The former focuses on internal thought processes; the latter, on the external manifestations of these thought patterns. Mental and psychosocial adjustment difficulties are characterized primarily by an overwhelming sense of loss of one's capabilities, of family and friends, of the ability to continue to pursue activities and hobbies, and of one's possessions. This sense of loss is perceived as global and uncontrollable and is supported by thinking patterns that focus on helplessness and hopelessness; that all learning and essentially all meaningful living ceases once one enters the facility. A resident with a mental adjustment disorder will have a sad or anxious mood or a behavioral symptom such as aggression.

The *Diagnostic and Statistical Manual of Mental Disorders,* 4th edition (*DSM/IV;* American Psychiatric Association, 1994), suggests that adjustment disorders develop within 3 months of a stressor (e.g., moving from one's home in the community into an assisted living or similar type of facility) and are evidenced by significant functional impairment. Bereavement over the death of a loved one is not associated with adjustment disorders developed within 3 months of a stressor.

Other manifestations of mental and psychosocial adjustment difficulties may, over a period of time, include

- impaired verbal communication
- social isolation (e.g., loss or failure to have relationships)
- sleep pattern disturbance (e.g., disruptive change in sleep/rest pattern as related to one's biological and emotional needs)
- spiritual distress (disturbances in one's belief system)
- inability to control behavior and potential for violence (aggressive behavior directed at self or others)
- stereotyped response to any stressor (i.e., the same characteristic response, regardless of the stimulus)

Appropriate treatment and services for psychosocial adjustment difficulties include precisely the types of activities and programming emphasized by assisted living facilities (e.g., providing residents with opportunities for self-governance; systematic orientation programs; arrangements to keep residents in touch with their communities, cultural heritage, former lifestyles, and religious practices; and maintaining contact with friends and family).

Appropriate treatment for mental adjustment difficulties may include crisis intervention services; individual, group, or family psychotherapy; drug therapy and training in monitoring of drug therapy; and other rehabilitative services.

Health conditions that may produce apathy, malaise, and decreased energy levels that can be mistaken for depression associated with mental or psychosocial adjustment difficulty are (this list is not all-inclusive):

- metabolic diseases (e.g., abnormalities of serum glucose, potassium, calcium, and blood urea nitrogen; hepatic dysfunction)
- endocrine diseases (e.g., hypothyroidism, hyperthyroidism, diabetes, hypoparathyroidism, hyperparathyroidism, Cushing's disease, Addison's disease)
- central nervous system diseases (e.g., tumors and other mass lesions, Parkinson's disease, multiple sclerosis, Alzheimer's disease, vascular disease)
- miscellaneous diseases (e.g., pernicious anemia, pancreatic disease, malignancy, infections, congestive heart failure)
- overmedication with antihypertensive drugs
- presence of restraints

Continuous Quality Improvement Questions:

- Is there a complete and accurate understanding by the health care staff of the resident's usual and customary routines?
- Is the facility making sufficient accommodations for the resident's usual and customary routines?
- What programs/activities is the resident receiving to improve and maintain maximum mental and psychosocial functioning?
- Has the resident's mental and psychosocial functioning been maintained or improved (e.g., fewer symptoms of distress)? Have any treatment plans and objectives been reevaluated?
- Has the resident received a psychological or psychiatric evaluation to evaluate, diagnose, or treat his or her condition, if necessary?
- How are mental and psychosocial adjustment difficulties addressed in the health care plan?

Avoidance of Pattern of Decreased Social Interaction

The health care plan goal needs to ensure that a resident whose health care plan did not reveal a mental or psychosocial adjustment difficulty does not display a pattern of decreased social interaction and/or increased withdrawn, angry, or depressive behaviors, unless the resident's health condition demonstrates that such a pattern is unavoidable.

Continuous Quality Improvement Questions:

- Is the facility attempting to evaluate whether this behavior was attributable to organic causes or other risk factors not associated with adjusting to living in the assisted living facility?
- Were individual objectives of the plan of health care periodically evaluated, and if progress was not made in maintaining, or increasing behaviors that help the resident have his or her needs met, were alternative treatment approaches developed to maintain mental or psychosocial functioning?

Nutritional Status for Each Resident

Resident nutrition is a key to optimizing residents' health. The assisted living facility staff should ensure that appropriate nutritional levels are maintained for each resident.

The goal is that each resident maintains acceptable parameters of nutritional status, such as body weight and protein levels, unless the resident's health condition demonstrates that this is not possible, and receives an appropriate diet when there is a nutritional problem.

Parameters of nutritional status that the facility staff should seek to avoid include unplanned weight loss as well as other indices such as peripheral edema, cachexia, and laboratory tests indicating malnourishment (e.g., serum albumin levels).

Because ideal body weight charts have not yet been validated for the institutionalized elderly, weight loss (or gain) is a guide in determining nutritional status. An analysis of weight loss or gain should be examined in light of the individual's former lifestyle as well as the current diagnosis.

When a Resident's Weight Demonstrates Significant Change. Assisted living facility staff can monitor residents' weight losses. The facility may or may not wish to attempt a weight-monitoring program for every resident. However, residents who appear to be at risk of a health-affecting weight loss can be formally or informally monitored by the staff using the following suggestions.

Interval	Significant loss	Severe loss
1 month	5%	Greater than 5%
3 months	7.5%	Greater than 7.5%
6 months	10%	Greater than 10%

The following formula determines percentage of loss:

$$\% \text{ of body weight loss} = \frac{\text{usual weight - actual weight}}{\text{usual weight}} \times 100$$

In evaluating weight loss, consider the resident's usual weight through adult life; the assessment of potential for weight loss, and the health care plan for weight management. Also, was the resident on a calorie-restricted diet, or if newly admitted and obese and on a normal diet, are fewer calories provided than prior to admission? Was the resident edematous when initially weighed, and with treatment, no longer has edema? Has the resident refused food?

When residents have laboratory work done, the health care staff may wish to examine results for indicators of good nutrition status. These include:

Albumin >60 yr.: 3.4–4.8 g/dl (good for examining marginal protein depletion). Plasma transferrin >60 yr.: 180–380 g/dl (rises with iron deficiency anemia, more persistent indicator of protein status)
Hemoglobin, males: 14–17 g/dl; females: 12–15 g/dl
Hematocrit, males: 41–53 females: 36–46
Potassium: 3.5–5.0 mEq/L
Magnesium 1.3–2.0 mEq/L

Some laboratories may have different "normals." Determine the range for the specific laboratory.

Because some healthy elderly people have abnormal laboratory values, and because abnormal values can be expected in some disease processes, do not expect laboratory values to be within normal ranges for all residents. Consider abnormal values in conjunction with each resident's health condition and baseline normal values.

Health Observation. Potential indicators of malnutrition are pale skin, dull eyes, swollen lips, swollen gums, swollen and/or dry tongue with scarlet or magenta hue, poor skin turgor, cachexia, bilateral edema, and muscle wasting.

Malnutrition. Malnutrition is a condition that can quickly develop among the older population served by assisted living facilities. Despite the presence of a nutritionally balanced diet served by the kitchen staff, some residents' eating behaviors may result in malnutrition.

Risk Factors

1. The pharmacy consultant can help the assisted living facility staff look for drug therapy that may contribute to nutritional deficiencies such as
   - cardiac glycosides
   - diuretics
   - anti-inflammatory drugs
   - antacids (antacid overuse)
   - laxatives (laxative overuse)
   - psychotropic drug overuse
   - anticonvulsants
   - antineoplastic drugs
   - phenothiazines
   - oral hypoglycemics
2. Poor oral health status or hygiene, eyesight, motor coordination, or taste alterations
3. Depression or dementia
4. Therapeutic or mechanically altered diet
5. Lack of access to culturally acceptable foods
6. Slow eating pace resulting in food becoming unpalatable, or in staff removing the tray before resident has finished eating; and
7. Cancer

Sometimes it will not be possible to maintain adequate nutritional status. In this situation, the assisted living facility staff should be aware of this circumstance and note the situation in the resident's records.

Health conditions demonstrating that the maintenance of acceptable nutritional status may not be possible include, but are not limited to

- refusal to eat and refusal of other methods of nourishment
- advanced disease (i.e. cancer, malabsorption syndrome)
- increased nutritional/caloric needs associated with pressure sores and wound healing (e.g., fractures, burns)
- radiation or chemotherapy
- kidney disease, alcohol/drug abuse, chronic blood loss, and hyperthyroidism
- gastrointestinal surgery
- prolonged nausea, vomiting, and diarrhea not relieved by treatment given according to accepted standards of practice

Some assisted living facilities may choose to offer therapeutic diets to residents. *Therapeutic diet* means a diet ordered by a physician as part of a treatment for a disease or health condition, to eliminate or decrease certain substances in the diet (e.g., sodium), to increase certain substances in the diet (e.g., potassium), or to provide food the resident is able to eat (e.g., a mechanically altered diet).

Resident hydration

Make sure the facility staff keep water and liquids constantly available to residents. While the typical assisted living facility staff may not distribute water to each resident each day, the staff can help the residents make sure they drink enough liquids. Dehydration often appears among the elderly who are unaware of not drinking enough liquids. Making sure that liquid refreshments are available and consumed at resident functions is a step the staff can take toward ensuring resident hydration. Suggestion: Stock a refrigerator fully accessible to all residents on each wing 24-hours a day with tasty drinks. Expensive? No. This intervention will build good will and pay for itself in improved resident self-hydration status.

Sufficient fluid means the amount of fluid needed to prevent dehydration (output of fluids far exceeds fluid intake) and maintain health. The amount needed is specific for each resident and fluctuates as the resident's condition fluctuates (e.g., increase fluids if resident has fever or diarrhea).

Risk factors for the resident becoming dehydrated are

- coma/decreased sensorium
- fluid loss and increased fluid needs (e.g., diarrhea, fever, uncontrolled diabetes)
- fluid restriction secondary to renal dialysis
- functional impairments that make it difficult to drink, reach fluids, or communicate fluid needs (e.g., aphasia)
- dementia in which the resident forgets to drink or forgets how to drink
- refusal of fluids

A general guideline for determining baseline daily fluid needs is to multiply the resident's body weight in kg times 30 cc (2.2 lbs = 1 kg), except for residents with renal or cardiac distress. An excess of fluids can be detrimental for these residents.

PHYSICIAN SERVICES

The following is a list of some of the types of medical specializations residents of the assisted living facility might be seeing.

Specialization is typically a 3-year training program taken beyond the medical school curriculum, which itself is usually 4 years. By professional custom, physicians usually place only "M.D." after their names, omitting any reference to any certification they may hold as a specialist. The following is not a list of all the prominent specialists; rather, it is a list of those more commonly seen in or consulted by residents in the assisted living facility.

Cardiologist—a physician who specializes in the diagnosis and treatment of heart diseases.

Chiropodist—see Podiatrist.

Dermatologist—a physician who diagnoses and treats diseases of the skin.

Endocrinologist—a physician who specializes in disorders affecting the endocrine (ductless gland) system. This system includes the pituitary, thyroid, pancreas, and adrenal glands, which secrete hormones into the blood stream.

Family medicine specialist or practitioner—in 1879 80% of physicians were general practitioners (GPs), 20% were specialists. With the proliferation of medical knowledge the reverse is true today: 80% of physicians are specialists, 20% are general practitioners. The general practitioner of yesteryear, since the late 1980s, has gone full circle and is itself a specialty requiring 3 years of internship beyond medical school. In this sense, nearly all physicians are now specialists. They specialize in diagnosing diseases and making referrals to specialists when appropriate.

Gastroenterologist—a physician who treats and diagnoses diseases of the digestive tract.

General surgeon—a physician who specializes in operative procedures to treat illnesses or various injuries.

Geriatrician—a physician who concentrates on the treatment of elderly persons. Gerontology became a specialization only in 1987. Note: There are currently a number of physicians who, during the late 1980s, by taking the written exam only, became certified gerontologists without doing the required 3-year specialization. Still at issue, and an important question for the assisted living facility industry, is whether gerontology will be a subspecialty or cover all treatment of elderly patients. Current expert opinion is that gerontology will move toward being a subspecialty because the typical needs of older persons, especially assisted living facility residents, will best be met by other specialists, regardless of the residents' age. Persons with hip fracture, prostate problems, cardiac problems, etc., will require the care of a specialist.

Internist—a physician who specializes in diagnostic procedures and treatment of nonsurgical cases.

Neurologist—a physician who diagnoses and treats diseases of the brain, nervous system, and spinal cord.

Ophthalmologist—a physician who diagnoses and treats eye diseases and disorders, performs eye surgery, refracts the eyes, and prescribes corrective eyeglasses and lenses.

Optician—a technician, not a physician, trained to grind lenses and to fit eyeglasses.

Orthopedist—a physician who specializes in diseases and injuries to bones, muscles, joints, and tendons. An orthopedic surgeon is a physician who specializes in surgical procedures relating to the bones, muscles, joints, and tendons.

Osteopath—a doctor of osteopathy, not an allopathic trained medical doctor, who uses methods of diagnosis and treatment that are similar to those of a medical doctor, but who places special emphasis on the interrelationship of the musculoskeletal to the other body systems.

Physiatrist—a physician who specializes in physical medicine, body movements, and conditioning much like the focus of a physical therapist; often associated with sports medicine.

Podiatrist—a trained professional, who is not a medical doctor, concerned with care of the feet, including clipping of toenails for diabetics, and who treats ailments such as corns and bunions.

Proctologist—a physician specializing in the diagnosis and treatment of the large intestine, particularly the rectum and anus.

Psychiatrist—a physician who specializes in the diagnosis and treatment of mental disorders.

Psychoanalyst—a psychiatrist who specializes in the use of the psychoanalytic therapy technique.

Psychologist—one, not a physician, who studies the function of the mind and behavioral patterns and administers psychological tests.

Pulmonologist—a physician specializing in treatment of the lungs.

Radiologist—a physician specializing in the use of X-ray and similar medical diagnostic machines such as magnetic resonance imaging (MRI), computer automated tomography (CAT) scans, and other medical techniques or modalities.

Rheumatologist—a physician who specializes in the treatment of rheumatic and arthritic diseases.

Urologist—a physician specializing in the diagnosis and treatment of diseases of the kidney, bladder, and reproductive organs.

A MEDICAL DIRECTOR?

Should each assisted living facility appoint a medical director? Ideally, yes. As the residents age in place and the assisted living facility staff are called on for more and more health care-related functions, the need for a medical director emerges.

Finding a medical director may not be easy. Even nursing facilities have difficulty finding and retaining physicians who are willing to serve as medical directors. As the population ages and as the number of physicians graduating from medical school approaches an oversupply, more physicians are taking an interest in the field of aging. This may mean that more physicians will be interested in becoming medical directors to assisted living facilities.

Ideal Description of a Medical Director's Role:

The following is the national standard sought for medical direction in assisted living facilities.

The facility should designate a physician to serve as medical director. The medical director is responsible for implementation of resident care policies.

Resident care policies include admissions, infection control, use of restraints, physician privileges and practices, and responsibilities of nonphysician health care workers (e.g., nursing, rehabilitation therapies, and dietary services in resident care, emergency care, and resident assessment and health care planning).

The medical director is also responsible for policies related to accidents and incidents; ancillary services such as laboratory, radiology, and pharmacy; use of medications; use and release of clinical information; and overall quality of care. The medical director is responsible for ensuring that these care policies are implemented.

The Coordination of Medical Care in the Facility

The medical director's "coordination role" means that the medical director is responsible for ensuring that the facility is providing appropriate care. This involves monitoring and ensuring implementation of resident care policies and providing oversight and supervision of physician services and the medical care of residents. It also includes having a significant role in overseeing the overall health care of residents to ensure that care is adequate. When the medical director identifies or receives a report of possible inadequate medical care, including drug irregularities, he or she is responsible for evaluating the situation and taking appropriate steps to try to correct the problem. This may include any necessary consultation with the resident and his or her physician concerning care and treatment. The medical director's coordinating role also includes ensuring the support of essential medical consultants as needed.

As a matter of practical reality, even a nursing facility cannot afford such heavy physician services, much less an assisted living facility. Nevertheless, it is desirable to contract with a physician to provide some type of medical oversight for the facility health care staff.

DENTAL CARE

Dental care is a major, often neglected, aspect of services delivered in the assisted living facility. Local dentists normally do not own the portable equipment needed to provide dental care inside an assisted living facility. Beyond this lack is perhaps the dental practitioner's insecurity about functioning outside his or her office and dealing with the sometimes complex health care histories of residents.

No one in the typical facility is trained in oral care. The mouth is not included in any significant way in the health care curriculum; physicians do not focus on the mouth.

While the majority of current residents in assisted living facilities may have dentures, the introduction of fluoride and other dental care efforts after World War II is resulting in increasingly larger proportions of residents having teeth rather than dentures. So long as any residents have dentures, the use of an inexpensive denture label kit will simplify life for the residents and staff of the facility. The need for periodic dental care does not change because one enters an assisted living facility.

PHYSICAL THERAPY (PT)/OCCUPATIONAL THERAPY (OT)/SPEECH THERAPY (ST)

A facility of 100 residents will not likely have in-house physical, occupational, and speech therapy services. Typically, these are provided by a home health care agency or contracted services group.

These therapists' work is not fully accomplished unless the health care and other staff are involved in the process of helping the residents achieve the desired level of function in their activities of daily living and not merely during the therapy period. This implies cooperation between the therapists who provide care (whether in-house or at another site) and the regular staff who, in effect, are doing "habilitative" therapy for some residents.

FOOT AND EYE CARE

There is need for a podiatrist -- a trained professional, who is not a health care doctor and who is concerned with care of the feet, including clipping of toenails for diabetics and others, and treats ailments such as corns and bunions.

As the assisted living facility population becomes less and less able to make health care visits outside the facility, a periodic visit by a podiatrist, who normally brings an assistant, may become a routine need of resident care. The podiatrist and assistant may arrange their work area in a room or a separate area on a monthly basis and provide care to a large portion of the residents over the course of a morning or afternoon.

Eye care needs are similar to those for teeth and feet. As the population's mobility becomes more and more restricted, arrangements for a local optician to make periodic visits is becoming a routine health care need to be arranged for by the facility staff.

LABORATORY AND OTHER DIAGNOSTIC SERVICES

On an attending physician's order, laboratory and X-ray or other diagnostic services normally should be obtained. These may be on the premises or contracted for in a local hospital or private office. Portable X-ray and, increasingly, additional diagnostic services are generally available on an on-call basis to provide services when a fall or other event occurs that might have injured a resident.

Delayed or inaccurate laboratory work is often a concern among health care staff. Telephone calls placed by frustrated caregivers inquiring about results that should have been received may indicate a need for examining the current procedures or contracts to emphasize timely communication.

5.6 Health Care Records

Assisted living facilities need to keep some kind of records of its health care services to residents. In most states there are no formal requirements for clinical records like those expected in hospitals, nursing homes and home health agencies. However, as a practical matter, and in the interests of both good caregiving and risk management, each assisted living facility must face the issue of how to adequately record their efforts.

A complete health record contains an accurate and functional representation of the actual experience of the individual in the facility. It contains enough information to show that the facility knows the status of the individual, has an adequate plan of health care, and provides sufficient evidence of the effects of the care provided. Documentation should provide a picture of the resident's progress, including response to treatment, change in condition, and changes in treatment. New HIPAA regulations are making patient privacy increasing complex and important.

RETENTION OF HEALTH RECORDS

Although there typically are no requirements for assisted living facilities to retain any health records for specific periods of time, the following national guideline may be useful information.

Health records should be retained for the period of time required by state law or 5 years from the date the resident permanently leaves the facility when there is no guideline in state law.

COMPUTERIZATION OF RECORDS

Increasingly, facility records will be kept, for the most part, on computers. In cases in which facilities have created the option for an individual's record to be maintained by computer, rather than hard copy, electronic signatures are acceptable. In cases when such attestation is done on computer records, safeguards to prevent unauthorized access and reconstruction of information should be in place. The following guideline is an example of how such a system may be set up:

- There is a written policy, describing the attestation policy(ies) in force at the facility.
- The computer has built-in safeguards to minimize the possibility of fraud.
- Each person responsible for an attestation has an individualized identifier.
- The date and time are recorded from the computer's internal clock at the time of entry.
- An entry is not to be changed after it has been recorded.
- The computer program controls in what sections/areas any individual can access or enter data, based on the individual's personal identifier (and, therefore his or her level of professional qualifications).

Questions the assisted living facility administrator may ask in reviewing sampled resident health records:

- Is there enough record documentation for staff to conduct the care program and to revise the program, as necessary, to respond to the changing status of the resident as a result of the interventions?
- How is the health record used in managing the resident's progress in maintaining or improving functional abilities and mental and psychosocial status?

The facility should safeguard health record information against loss, destruction, or unauthorized use. The facility should keep confidential all information contained in the resident's records, regardless of the form or storage method of the records, except when release is required by transfer to another health care institution, law, or third-party payment contract.

Points the assisted living facility administrator may keep in mind:

- *Keep confidential* is defined as safeguarding the content of information including video, audio, or other computer-stored information from unauthorized disclosure without the consent of the individual and/or the individual's surrogate or representative.
- If there is information considered too confidential to place in the record used by all staff, such as the family's financial assets or sensitive medical data, it may be retained in a secure place in the facility, such as a locked cabinet in the administrator's office. The record should show the location of this confidential information.
- The health record should contain (1) sufficient information to identify the resident, (2) a record of the resident's plan of health care, (3) services provided, (4) the results of any preadmission screening, and (5) progress notes.

ABBREVIATIONS

Health records normally contain many abbreviations used by health care personnel. The following set of abbreviations are often found in such records. Each facility should assure that the health care staff all agree on the meanings of the abbreviations they commonly use.

aa	of each
Abd	abdomen
Ad lib	as much as desired, at pleasure
ac	before meals
A/G	albumin/globulin ratio
AIDS	acquired immune deficiency syndrome
aq	water
aq dist	distilled water
ASHD	arteriosclerotic heart disease
amp	ampule
amt	amount
B E	barium enema
bid	twice a day
BMR	basal metabolic rate
BP or B/P	blood pressure
BRP	bathroom privileges
Ca	carcinoma
CAD	cornary artery disease
caps	capsules
cath	catheter
c	with
cc	cubic centimeter
CBC	complete blood count
cf	compare

comp	compound
COLD	chronic obstructive lung disease
COPD	chronic obstructive pulmonary disease
CNS	central nervous system
CVA	cerebral vascular accident
d/c	discontinued
decub	lying down
Diab	diabetic
Diag or Dx	diagnosis
Diff	differential blood count
Dil	dilute
Disc	discontinue
Disch or D/C	discharge
dx	diagnosis
EEG	electroencephalogram
EKG or ECG	electrocardiogram
exam	examination
fl or fld	fluid
FUO	fever of unknown origin
Fx	fracture
GI	gastrointestinal
gm	gram
gr	grain
gtt gtts	drop(s)
H or hr	hour
hs	at bedtime
hypo	hypodermically
IDDM	insulin-dependent diabetes mellitus
IM	intramuscular
inf	infusion
IV	intravenous
KUB	kidney-ureter-bladder
l	liter
lab	laboratory
Lat	lateral
lb	pound
liq	liquid
mg	milligram
min	minute
ml	milliliter
mm	millimeter
MN	midnight
MRSA	methicillin-resistant staphylococcus aureus

N	noon
NIDDM	non-insulin-dependent diabetes mellitus
no	number
noct.	at night
NPO	nothing by mouth
NV	nausea and vomiting
pt	pint
od	right eye
os	left eye
ou	each eye
OT	occupational therapy
oz	ounce
p	pulse
pc	after meal
PEARL	pupils equal and reactive to light
po	by mouth
prn	as needed
prog	prognosis
PROM	passive range of motion
PT	physical therapy
PX	physical examination
qd	every day
qh	every hour
qhs	each bedtime
qid	four times a day
qn	every night
qod	every other day
qs	sufficient quantity
ROM	range of motion
Rx	prescription
s	without
sol	solution
SOB	shortness of breath
sos	one dose, if necessary
spec	specimen
SS	soap solution
ss	half
stat	immediately
surg	surgery
T	temperature
tab	tablet
TB	tuberculosis
tid	three times a day
tinct or tr	tincture

TO	telephone order
TPR	temperature, pulse, and respiration
u	unit
ung	ointment
URI	upper respiratory infection
UTI	urinary tract infection
vol	volume
VO	verbal order
vs	vital signs
WBC	white blood cells
W/C	wheelchair
wt	weight

5.7 Pharmaceutical Services

As persons age, they typically take more and more drugs. The number of drugs being taking by the resident population of the typical assisted living facility will be of increasing concern to assisted living facility administrators and health care staff. In Part Two, we recommend that the assisted living facility contract with a pharmacist for at least 8 hours a month to do drug regimen reviews for residents.

The consulting or the facility pharmacist is responsible for ensuring that

- all medications are available as ordered by the residents' physicians
- all medications handled by staff are within expiration date and properly labeled and handled
- all reorders and stop orders for drugs handled by staff are implemented
- each resident's medications are reviewed periodically for possible adverse reactions and/or interactions
- appropriate pharmacy policy and procedures are followed

ROUTES USED IN DRUG ADMINISTRATION

Drugs typically function in the body after being absorbed, usually through the digestive tract, into the bloodstream, following a pathway similar to that traveled by nutrients from food.

Drugs may be administered several ways in addition to orally (by mouth): intramuscularly (IM) by an injection; directly on skin (topically); on membranes or other tissue, such as being held under the tongue (sublingually); or as suppositories. Usually medications eventually become inactive in the liver and are removed from the body by the kidneys.

FIVE BASIC DRUG ACTIONS

The following are the five basic types of actions drugs will produce (Poe & Holloway, 1980, pp. 14–15):

- blocking nerve impulses
- stimulating nerve impulses
- working directly on living cells
- working to replace body deficiencies
- any combination of the above

Every person is affected by drugs differently because of individual body chemistries, so every resident should be monitored to determine the appropriateness of different dosages (Jones, 1989).

As a result of age-related changes in the liver, kidneys, and other organs throughout the body that alter the normal utilization of drugs, the elderly are at much greater risk of suffering from drug reactions, which are often the result of a buildup or excess amount of drugs in the body. In addition, there may be an increase in the occurrence of side effects that are commonly associated with most medications (Jones, 1989).

POLICY IMPLICATIONS

Because assisted living facility residents are more likely to suffer from multiple diseases and, as suggested above, use multiple medications, these drug combinations can produce dangerous drug interactions (Roberts & Snyder, 1995). The same residents are also at a much greater risk of suffering from an adverse drug reaction, many of which are the result of chemical incompatibilities among the different medications.

For these reasons, the assisted living facility administrator should ensure that drug regimens in the facility are appropriately monitored by a consulting pharmacist with properly in-depth periodic reports to the facility management. Special precautions can be mounted to prevent the consequences of illness or disability from drug reactions.

The five rights of medication administration include identifying

- the right medication
- the right dose
- the right time for administration
- the right route (oral, shot, etc.)
- the right resident

Some practitioners add a sixth "right": good documentation.

GENERIC AND BRAND NAMES

Familiarity with some of the more commonly prescribed medications by both the generic (chemical) and brand (manufacturing) names can be useful. In the following discussion the generic names are mentioned first, with the brand names following in parentheses. Brand names are often used among health professionals unless a particular medication (e.g., aspirin) is produced by a number of companies. Some of the more frequently prescribed medications are discussed below.

ANTIANXIETY AND ANTIPSYCHOTIC (PSYCHOACTIVE) MEDICATIONS

Antianxiety and antipsychotic medications act on the central nervous system to enable residents to deal with changes in their own behavior or stressful and anxiety-provoking changes in their environment. The two major classes of this type of drug are tranquilizers and sedatives/hypnotics.

These medications act directly on the major control center—the brain—and should be administered very cautiously. Many of the drug-related fatalities among the elderly are associated with these medications (Basen, 1977).

Some of the most commonly prescribed tranquilizers and sedatives/hypnotics used in the assisted living facility are thioridazine and chlordiazepoxide. Thioridazine (Mellaril®) is a major tranquilizer and/or antipsychotic drug prescribed for mild to moderate anxiety relief. This medication has been used for long-term alcoholics to control their illness. Chlordiazepoxide hydrochloride (Librium®) is a minor tranquilizer prescribed for relief of anxiety. Two new drugs for the management of psychotic disorders are available. Risperdal® is an antipsychotic agent belonging to the benzisoxazole derivatives (*Physician's Desk Reference,* 1998). Zyprexa® is an antipsychotic agent belonging to the thienobenzodiazepine class. Both appear to be better tolerated by the elderly than the above drugs (*Physician's Desk Reference,* 1998). For residents with a generalized anxiety disorder (GSA), the new drug Buspar® appears effective. Buspar® is not chemically or pharmacologically related to the benzodiazepines, barbiturates, or other sedative/anxiolytic drugs.

The side effects associated with these medications include drowsiness, dizziness, disorientation, and allergic reactions. An extensive and apparently successful effort has been made over the past few years to reduce the number of antipsychotic drugs used in the typical nursing facility (Ray et al., 1993; Selma, Palla, Poddig, & Brauner, 1994). The assisted living facility staff would do well to emulate this success.

VITAMINS AND MINERALS

Vitamins and minerals are the most common classes of medications prescribed for the elderly assisted living facility resident, according to one national long-term care survey (Hing, 1977). Ferrous sulfate, which is an iron supplement, and multivitamins are among the most popular in this category.

A common side effect of iron supplements is irritation of the gastrointestinal tract, which may cause some stomach upset. Too much iron is suspected of contributing to heart attacks. Other frequently prescribed minerals include calcium and potassium supplement.

ANALGESICS

Analgesics are often administered for pain relief. Acetylsalicylic acid, or aspirin, may be relatively safe, except for assisted living facility residents with kidney problems and ulcers. Aspirin may also act as an anti-inflammatory agent for arthritic residents. Such medications serve to reduce the amount of damage to the joints and to lessen the painful side effects associated with the inflammatory process.

Some of the side effects associated with aspirin include stomach upset, ringing in the ears, deafness, dizziness, confusion, and irritability (Gotz & Gotz, 1978).

Acetaminophen (Tylenol®) is an analgesic similar to aspirin, but without anti-inflammatory properties; hence it may serve only as a pain reliever. Some side effects associated with it are redness and itching of the skin and possible liver damage.

Another group of much stronger analgesics are the narcotics. Federal guidelines require that they be kept under lock and key in a safe place because of their potential for abuse. A dangerous side effect with these drugs is the potential to depress breathing and respiratory functions that are controlled by the central nervous system. Alterations in consciousness or blood pressure may also occur. Some of the more commonly prescribed narcotic analgesics include codeine (Methylmorphine®), meperidine (Demerol®), morphine sulfate, and oxycodone terephthalate (Percodan®).

LAXATIVES AND GASTROINTESTINAL AGENTS

Gastrointestinal agents are among some of the more commonly prescribed medications for assisted living facility residents. Laxatives are also referred to as cathartics. This category includes suppositories, such as bisacodyl (Dulcolax®), bulk laxatives like plantago seed (Metamucil®), and stool softeners such as milk of magnesia (Cooper, 1978).

Often these agents are prescribed with other medications to neutralize their irritating effects on the gastrointestinal tract. Antacids, one of the most commonly indicated for this purpose, unfortunately may also cause side effects such as diarrhea. Milk of magnesia is frequently prescribed for gastrointestinal problems.

CARDIOVASCULAR AGENTS

Various groups of cardiovascular agents work to reduce blood pressure by different actions.

Methyldopa (Aldomet®) is an antihypertensive that works directly on the central nervous system to lower blood pressure. Orthostatic hypotension, or decreased blood pressure on standing, may be associated with this medication and increases the likelihood of residents' falling (Gotz & Gotz, 1978).

Diuretics work by forcing the body to excrete excess fluids. Furosemide (Lasix®) and hydrochlorothiazide (Esidrix®) are commonly prescribed. But, as noted earlier, they cause the body to excrete potassium, and this may result in muscle weakness, lethargy, and muscle cramping.

Other medications, also mentioned earlier, act directly on the heart muscle. Digoxin (Lanoxin®) acts to slow down the heart rate by decreasing the speed of impulses traveling along muscle fibers. Propranolol hydrochloride (Inderal®) is another medication that works to block chemicals from increasing the heart rate. Some side effects from these medications include a loss of appetite, nausea, vomiting, confusion, blurred vision, and arrhythmias (irregular heartbeats).

Antianginal medications work to alleviate the pain associated with a decreased oxygen supply to the heart muscle. Nitroglycerin works as a vasodilator to increase the size of blood vessels so they will carry more oxygen. This medication is administered sublingually (under the tongue).

ANTIDEPRESSANTS

Amitriptyline hydrochloride (Elavil®) is one of the most commonly prescribed drugs for elderly residents in an assisted living facility. This medication also acts as a tranquilizer. The extent of its use is not surprising, considering that depression is one of the most common forms of illness (Jones, 1989). Depression is also common among residents suffering from other chronic ailments, especially Alzheimer's and Parkinson's diseases (Kaszniak, 1995; Maddox, 2001).

Some of the side effects associated with antidepressant medications such as Elavil® include confusion, drowsiness, decreased blood pressure, constipation, dry mouth, heart flutter, rashes, and retention of urine.

ANTIINFECTIVES

Antiinfectives kill or decrease the growth of infectious organisms, complementing the natural body defense mechanisms.

Antibiotics are one of the more notable groups of medications within this class. Among the different types are the penicillins, cephalosporins, and tetracyclines. One of the most important side effects associated with these medications is allergic reactions, which are often identified by skin rashes.

Some antibiotics may be used to combat fungal and viral infections. Intravenous (IV) therapy is introduced when dealing with the more resistant organisms.

MISCELLANEOUS MEDICATIONS

Respiratory Agents

Expectorants, including ammonium chloride (Robitussin®), terpin hydrate, and acetylcysteine (Mucomyst®) are used to break up and expel mucus from the respiratory tract. The first two medications are taken orally; the third is usually administered by inhaling it in the form of a vapor. Tetracycline and ampicillin can be effective antibiotics for residents with respiratory tract infections due to chronic bronchitis (Rodman & Smith, 1977; Evans, et. al., 2000).

Optical Medications

Mydriatics are often used for residents with glaucoma. Pilocarpine and physostigmine are two often prescribed medications. They act to decrease the fluid buildup in the eye resulting from glaucoma. These medications are administered as eyedrops. Some of their more common side effects are headaches, diarrhea, and sweating.

CONTROLLED DRUGS SCHEDULES

Federal guidelines require all drugs and biologicals to be stored in locked compartments. Separately locked, permanently affixed compartments are required for Schedule II drugs listed in the Comprehensive Drug Abuse Prevention and Control Act of 1970. The typical assisted living facility will not have controlled Schedule II drugs in-house.

Formerly, drugs were regulated under the 1914 Harrison Narcotic Act, which placed them into classes A, B, X and M narcotics. Subsequently, each state passed drug acts.

Today assisted living facilities should meet the individual state drug laws and the federal drug law. Most states have passed a "State Uniform Controlled Substances Act," some with six instead of five drug group classifications.

The federal government has classified drugs into the following five schedules.

Schedule I Drugs: drugs with a high abuse potential and no accepted medical use in the United States (e.g., heroin, marijuana, LSD, peyote, mescaline, and certain other opiates and hallucinogenic substances).

Schedule II Drugs: drugs with accepted medical use in the United States but having high abuse and dependency potential (e.g., opium, morphine, codeine, methadone, cocaine, amphetamine, secobarbital, methaqualone (Quaalude), and phencyclidine ("angel dust")). These were formerly Class A narcotics.

Schedule III Drugs: drugs with less abuse potential than schedules I and II drugs. Several compounds are included (e.g., Empirin compound with codeine, Tylenol® with codeine, and Phenaphen® with codeine). These were formerly Class B drugs.

Schedule IV Drugs: drugs with less abuse potential than Schedule III drugs (e.g., barbital, Librium,® diazepam (Valium®), and Dalmane®).

Schedule V Drugs: drugs with less abuse potential than Schedule IV drugs. These typically are compounds containing limited quantities of narcotic drugs for antitussive (anticough) and antidiarrheal purposes. Examples are Lomotil®, Phenergan,® expectorant with codeine, and Robitussin® A-C syrup. These were formerly Class X (exempt narcotics) under the Harrison Act.

THERAPEUTIC ACTIONS OF DRUGS

Analgesic-reduces pain (e.g., aspirin).
Antacid-neutralizes the acid in the stomach (e.g., Maalox®).
Antianemic-used in treatment of anemia (e.g., liver extract).
Antibiotic-destroys microorganisms in the body (e.g., penicillin).
Anticoagulant-depresses (slows) the clotting of blood.
Antidote-used to counteract poisons.
Antiseptic-slows down growth of bacteria, but does not kill all of the bacteria (e.g., hydrogen peroxide).
Antispasmodic-relieves smooth muscle spasm (e.g., Valium® (diazepam).
Antitoxin-neutralizes bacterial toxins in infections (e.g., tetanus antitoxin).
Astringent-used to constrict skin and mucous membranes by withdrawing water (e.g., alum).
Carminative-an agent that reduces flatulence (gas) in the stomach or intestinal tract.
Cathartic-laxative, purgative, inducing bowel movements (e.g., cascara sagrada).
Caustic-destroys tissue by local application (e.g., silver nitrate).
Chemotherapeutics-chemicals used to treat illness (e.g., sulfanilamide for streptococcal infection).
Coagulant-stimulates clotting of the blood.
Diaphoretic-used to induce perspiration.
Disinfectant-destroys pathogenic organisms (e.g., Zephiran® chloride).
Diuretic-stimulates elimination of urine, often used with medications prescribed to reduce hypertension (e.g., diazide).
Emetic-induces vomiting (e.g., warm salt water).
Emollient-used to soften and soothe tissue (e.g., cold cream, petroleum jelly).
Expectorant-used to induce coughing; an agent that increases bronchial secretion and facilitates its expulsion (coughing) (e.g., Robitussin®).
Hypertensive-helps raise blood pressure.
Hypnotic-aids in sleeping (e.g., Nembutal®).
Miotic-constricts the pupil of the eye.
Mydriatic-dilates the pupil of the eye.
Sedative-relieves anxiety and emotional tensions (e.g., Seconal®).
Tonic or stimulant-used to stimulate body activity (e.g., Eldertonic® or Ritalin®).
Vasoconstrictor-causes blood vessels to narrow or constrict.
Vasodilator-expands or dilates blood vessels.
Vitamins-used in replacement therapy (e.g., vitamin C).

Drugs and biologicals used in the facility should be labeled in accordance with currently accepted professional principles and include the appropriate accessory and cautionary instructions, and the expiration date when applicable.

The critical elements of the drug label are the name of the drug and its strength. The names of the resident and the physician do not have to be on the label of the package, but they should be identified with the package in such a manner as to ensure that the drug is administered to the right resident.

All drugs approved by the Food and Drug Administration should have expiration dates on the manufacturer's container. "When applicable" means that expiration dates should be on the labels of drugs unless state law stipulates otherwise.

During the years 1988 to 1998 drug costs to all payers increased at a 10% growth rate: $50 billion in 1988, to $122 billion in 1998 (Office of the Actuary. HCFA, September 27, 2000).

MEDICATION MANAGEMENT

The Assisted Living Workgroup Report to the U.S. Senate Special Committee on Aging (April, 2003) recommends that policies and procedures of the residence address the following issues:

1. Medication orders, including telephone orders
2. Pharmacy services
3. Medication packaging
4. Medication ordering and receipt
5. Medication storage
6. Disposal of medications
7. Medication self-administration
8. Medication reminders
9. Medication administration by the resident
10. Medication administration specific procedures
11. Documentation of medication administration
12. Medication error detection and reporting
13. Quality improvement systems
14. Monitoring and reporting adverse drug reactions
15. Review of medications
16. Storage and accountability of controlled drugs
17. Training, qualifications, and supervision of staff involved

MEDICATION ERRORS

To help ensure that residents being assisted by the health care staff are free of significant medication errors, a rate of no more than 5% medication pass errors has been practiced. It is useful for the assisted living facility administrator and staff to understand differences between significant and insignificant medication errors and such matters.

Medication error means a discrepancy between what the physician ordered and what the resident receives.

Significant medication error means one that causes the resident discomfort or jeopardizes his or her health and safety. Criteria for judging significant medication errors as well as examples are provided under significant and nonsignificant medication errors.

Medication error rate is determined by calculating the percentage of errors. The numerator in the ratio is the total number of errors observed, both significant and nonsignificant. The denominator is called "opportunities for errors" and includes all the doses the observer saw being administered plus the doses ordered but not administered. The equation for calculating a medication error rate is as follows:

$$\text{medication error rate} = \frac{\text{number of errors observed}}{\text{opportunities for errors}} \times 100$$

A medication error rate of 5% or greater includes both significant and nonsignificant medication errors. It indicates that the facility has systematic problems with its drug distribution system and a deficiency should be written.

Significant and Nonsignificant Medication Errors

The relative significance of medication errors is a matter of professional judgment. Three general guidelines may be employed in determining whether a medication error is significant or not:

1. **Resident Condition.** The resident's condition is an important factor to take into consideration. For example, a potent diuretic erroneously administered to a dehydrated resident may have serious consequences, but if administered to a resident with a normal fluid balance may not. If the resident's condition requires rigid control, a single missed or wrong dose can be highly significant.
2. **Drug Category.** If the drug is from a category that usually requires the resident to be titrated to a specific blood level, a single medication error could alter that level and precipitate a recurrence of symptoms or toxicity. This is especially important if the half-life of the drug is short. Examples of drug categories that require titration of resident blood levels include anticonvulsants, anticoagulants, and antiarrhythmic, antianginal, and antiglaucoma agents.
3. **Frequency of Error.** If an error is occurring with any frequency, there is more reason to classify the error as significant. For example, if a resident's drug was omitted several times, as verified by reconciling the number of tablets delivered with the number administered, classifying that error as significant would be more in order. This conclusion should be considered in concert with the resident's condition and the drug category.

Examples of Significant and Non-Significant Medication Errors

Examples of medication errors that have actually occurred in long term care facilities are presented below. Some of these errors are identified as significant. This designation is based on expert opinion without regard to the status of the resident. Most experts concluded that the significance of these errors, in and of themselves, have a high potential for creating problems for the typical resident. Those errors identified as nonsignificant have also been designated primarily on the basis of the nature of the drug. Resident status and frequency of error could classify these errors as significant.

Omissions (Drug ordered but not administered at least once):

Drug Order	*Significance*
Haldol (1 mg BID)	NS*
Motrin (400 mg TID)	NS
Quinidine (200 mg TID)	S**
Tearisol drops (2 both eyes TID)	NS
Indocin (25 mg TID pc)	NS
Lioresal (10 mg TID)	NS
Thorazine (25 mg BID)	NS
Ampicillin (500 mg TID)	NS
Metamucil (one packet BID)	NS
Inderal (20 mg once every 6 hours)	S
Multivitamin (one daily)	NS
Mylanta Susp. (1 oz TID AC)	NS
Nitrol Oint. (1 inch)	S
Librium (10 mg one TID)	NS
Cortisporin otic drop (4 to 5 left ear QID)	NS
Aldactone (25 mg QID)	NS

* Not significant
**Significant

Unauthorized Drug (Drugs administered without a physician's order):

Drug Order	*Significance*
Feosol	NS
Coumadin (4 mg)	S
Lasix (40 mg)	S
Zyloprim (100 mg)	NS
Tylenol (5 gr)	NS
Triavil (4-25)	NS
Multivitamins	NS
Motrin (400 mg)	NS

Wrong Dose:

Drug Order	*Administered*	*Significance*
isoptocarpine 1% (one drop in the left eye, TID)	Three drops in each eye	NS
Epinal (1% one drop in eyes, BID)	Three drops in each eye	NS
Digoxin (0.125 mg QD)	0.25 mg	S
Lasix (20 mg QD)	40 mg	NS
Amphojel (30 cc QID)	15 cc	NS
Slow K (two TID)	one	NS
Dilantin 125 Susp (12 cc)	2 cc	S
Lasix (40 mg QD)	20 mg	NS

Wrong Route of Administration:

Drug Order	*Administered*	*Significance*
Hydergine (0.5 SL.L BID)	Resident swallowed	NS
Cortisporin Otic drops (4 to 5 left ear QID)	Left eye	S

Wrong Dosage Form:

Drug Order	*Administered*	*Significance*
Colace Liquid (100 mg BID)	Capsule	NS
Mellaril (10 mg)	Concentrate	NS*
Kapseals po HS	capsules po	S**

* If correct dose was given.
** Parke Davis Kapseals have an extended rate of absorption.

Wrong Drug:

Drug Order	*Administered*	*Significance*
Tylenol 325 mg (routinely)	Ascriptin	S

Wrong Time:

Drug Order	*Administered*	*Significance*
Indocin (25 mg PC)	AC	NS
Periactin (4 mg PC)	AC	NS
Digoxin (0.25 daily at 8 a.m.)	at 9:15 a.m.	NS
Tetracycline (250 mg QID AC and HS)	PC	S

Determining Medication Errors

Timing Errors. If a drug is ordered before meals (AC) and administered after meals (PC), always count this as a medication error. Likewise, if a drug is ordered PC and is given AC, count as a medication error. Count a wrong time error if the drug is administered 60 minutes earlier or later than its scheduled time of administration, but only if that wrong time error can cause the resident discomfort or jeopardize the resident's health and safety. Counting a drug with a long half-life (e.g., Digoxin) as a wrong time error when it is 15 minutes late is improper because this drug has a long half-life (beyond 24 hours) and 15 minutes has no significant impact on the resident. The same is true for many other wrong time errors (except AC and PC errors) in long-term care facilities.

Final Observations

The hospital administrator was right when she responded to the prospective medical director's elaborate and expensive proposals: "Doctor, no margin, no mission." Assuming a margin, what is the essence of the assisted living administrator's mission?

A highly respected long-term care administrator, Philip Brown (1998), when asked this question while lecturing to a long-term care class, answered that the essence of the assisted living administrator's mission is to

- guarantee privacy of the resident
- guarantee resident freedom of choice
- provide a setting aesthetically pleasing to the eyes
- deliver the highest quality of health care

Personal privacy is cherished. Yet the forces of society and the institutional setting of the assisted living facility are natural enemies of personal privacy. Personal privacy will be guaranteed only to the extent it is nourished and enforced by the administrator.

Loss of control as one ages, loss of a living environment in which one has freedom to make and enforce one's personal choices, is perhaps the greatest fear experienced by aging persons. Ironically, the greatest single threat to freedom of choice in the assisted living facility is the professionally trained and highly motivated staff who have spent years learning what is "best" for residents. Without incessant intervention by the administrator on residents' behalf, the staff will make decisions for the residents.

Adults of all ages and conditions thrive best in settings in which they feel comfortable. The assisted living facility is home. In our homes we strive to achieve a comfortable and aesthetically pleasing environment. The assisted living administrator is the new head of household—make it a household that is easy on the eyes and comforting to the spirit.

Quality care is job one. A pleasant, professionally competent caregiving team enables residents to live confidently. The assisted living administrator is the team leader.

FIX IT (THE FACILITY) ALL THE TIME

Nobel laureate Albert Szent-Gyorgyi observed that there is a tendency for all living things to keep growing, changing, evolving (Kriegel, 1991). Everything around us is constantly changing: the health system, the economic system, the aging population itself and its relationship to everything else. The relationships among hospitals, assisted living facilities, home health care agencies, third-party payers, health maintenance organizations, managed care processes, and government guidelines are always in flux. If the assisted living facility does not change and grow, improve and evolve, it will face extinction. The assisted living facility is a living organism. Treat it as alive, and you and it will survive.

FIX IT (YOUR OWN CAREER) ALL THE TIME

In the unlikely event that at some point in your career in assisted living facility administration you feel yourself on a plateau, having achieved all you had hoped in your facility, consider the following.

An aboriginal tribe made it a practice to move on whenever the food was plentiful from lush harvests. When life was this easy, they knew they were in danger of becoming fat, lazy, and unprepared for the inevitable seasons of scarcity, when their survival skills would be needed.

FINISHED NEVER IS

The Japanese concept of *kaizen* means continuous improvement, a commitment to the idea that "finished never is."

David Harrington, a violinist with the avant-guard Kronos Quartet, finds being an artist a source of perpetual renewal because it is a task that has no ending point (Kriegel, 1991).

Pablo Casals, the cellist, was asked why, at the age of 94, he continued to practice as hard each day as he had decades earlier, since he remained clearly the preeminent cellist in the world. He replied that he practiced because he hoped to improve.

REFERENCES

Adams, G. (1981). *Essentials of geriatric medicine* (2nd ed.). Oxford: Oxford University Press.

Ade-Ridder, L., & Kaplan, L. (1993). Marriage, spousal care giving, and a husband's move to a nursing home. *Journal of Gerontological Nursing,* 19(10), 13–23.

Agate, J. (1979). *Geriatrics for nurses and social workers* (2nd ed.). London: Heinemann Medical Books.

Agency for Health Care Policy and Research. (1995, March-April). Guidelines on pressure sores released. *Research Activities* (Agency for Health Care Policy and Research, No. 183, AHCPR Pub. No. 95-0051), p. 15.

Albanese, A. A. (1980). *Nutrition for the elderly.* New York: A. R. Liss.

Albert, M. (1995). Alzheimer's disease: Clinical. In G. L. Maddox (Ed.), *The encyclopedia of aging* (2nd ed., pp. 56–57). New York: Springer Publishing Co.

Allen, J. E. (1994). *Key federal requirements for nursing facilities* (2nd ed., Appendix A). New York: Springer Publishing Co.

Aller, L. J., & Van Ess Coeling, H. (1995). Quality of life: Its meaning to the long term care resident. *Journal of Gerontological Nursing, 21*(2), 20–25.

American Medical Association. (1967). *The extended care facility: a handbook for the medical society.* Chicago: American Medical Association.

American Psychiatric Association. (1994). *Diagnostic and statistical manual of mental disorders* (4th ed.). Washington, DC: American Psychiatric Press.

Anderson, W. F. (1976). *Practical management of the elderly* (3rd ed.). Oxford: Blackwell Scientific Publications.

Andres, R. (1989). Relation of physiologic changing in aging to medical changes of disease in the aged. In W. Reichel (Ed.), *Clinical aspects of aging* (3rd ed.). Baltimore: Williams & Wilkins.

Austin (1981). In Haley & Keenan (Ed.), *Health care of the aging.* Charlottesville: University Press of Virginia.

Balin, A. K., & Lin, A. N. (1995). Connective tissues. In G. L. Maddox (Ed.), *The encyclopedia of aging* (2nd ed., pp. 220–222). New York: Springer Publishing Co.

Barzel, U.S. (1989). Endocrinology and aging. In W. Reichel (Ed.), *Clinical aspects of aging* (3rd ed.). Baltimore: Williams & Wilkins.

Barzel, V. (1983). Common metabolic disorders of the skeleton. In W. Reichel (Ed.), *Clinical aspects of aging* (2nd ed.). Baltimore: Williams & Wilkins.

Basen, M. (1977). The elderly and drugs - problem overview and program strategy. *Public Health Reports, 92*(1), 43–48.

Bazzare, T. (1983). Nutritional requirements of the elderly. In McCue (Ed.), *Medical care of the elderly: A practical approach.* Lexington, MA: Callamore Press.

Beacham, B. E. (1989). Geriatric dermatology. In W. Reichel (Ed.), *Clinical aspects of aging* (3rd ed.). Baltimore: Williams & Wilkins.

Beattie, B. L., & Louie, V. Y. (1989). Nutrition and health in the elderly. In W. Reichel (Ed.), *Clinical aspects of aging* (3rd ed.). Baltimore: Williams & Wilkins.

Beck, S., & Smith, J. (1983). Infectious diseases in the elderly. *Medical Clinics of North America, 67*(2), 273–289.

Becker, L. (1979). Herpes zoster: A geriatric disease. *Geriatrics, 34*(9), 41–47.

Berlowitz, D. R., Brandeis, G. H., Anderson, J., & Brand, H. K. (1997). Predictors of pressure ulcer healing among long-term care residents. *Journal of the American Geriatrics Society, 45*(1), 30–34.

Bennett, D. A., & Knopman, D. S. (1994). Alzheimer's disease: A comprehensive approach to patient management. *Geriatrics, 43*(8), 20–26.

Bergstrom, N. (1995). Pressure ulcers. In G. L. Maddox (Ed.), *The encyclopedia of aging* (2nd ed., pp. 751–752). New York: Springer Publishing Co.

[The] best drugs for hypertension. (1995). *Johns Hopkins Medical Letter, 7*(4), 1.

Birchenall, J. M., & Streight, M. E. (1982). *Care of the older adults* (2nd ed.). Philadelphia: Lippincott.

Birkmayer, W., & Riederer, P. (1983). *Parkinson's disease: Biochemical, clinical, pathology and treatment.* New York: Springer Verlag-Wein.

Birren, J. (1964). *The psychology of aging.* Englewood Cliffs, NJ: Prentice-Hall.

Bjork, D., & Tight, R. (1983). Nursing home hazard of chronic indwelling urinary catheters. *Archives of Internal Medicine, 143*(9), 1675–1676.

Blazer, D. G. (1995). Depression. In G. L. Maddox (Ed.), *The encyclopedia of aging* (2nd ed., pp. 265–266). New York: Springer Publishing Co.

Bleckner, M. The place of the nursing home among community resources. *Journal of Geriatric Psychiatry, 1*(67), 135–144.

Blumenthal, H. T. (1968). Some biomedical aspects of aging. *Gerontologist,* 8.

Blumenthal, M. (1980). Depressive illness in old age: Getting behind the mark. *Geriatrics, 35*(4), 34–43.

Blustein, J. (1993). The family in medical decision making. *Hastings Center Report, 23*(3), 6–13.

Botwinick, C. (1978). *Aging and behavior: A comprehensive integration of research findings.* New York: Springer Publishing Co.

Boyer, G., & Boyer, J. (1982). Sexuality and the elderly. *Nursing Clinics of North America, 17*(3), 421–427.

Bozzetti, L. (1977, March). Contemporary concepts in aging. *Psychiatric Annals, 7,* pp. 16–43.

Breschi, L. (1983). Common lower urinary tract problems in the elderly. In W. Reichel (Ed.), *Clinical aspects of aging* (2nd ed.). Baltimore: Williams & Wilkins.

______. (1989). Common lower urinary tract problems in the elderly. In W. Reichel (Ed.), *Clinical aspects of aging* (3rd ed.). Baltimore: Williams & Wilkins.

Brocklehurst, J. (1971). Dysuria in old age. *Journal of the American Geriatrics Society, 19,* 582.

Brocklehurst, J. (1979). The urinary tract. In Rossman (Ed.), *Clinical geriatrics* (2nd ed.). Philadelphia: Lippincott.

Brocklehurst, J., & Hanley, T. (1981). *Geriatric medicine for students.* London: Churchill Livingstone.

Brody, H. (1995). Central nervous system (brain and spinal cord). In G. L. Maddox (Ed.), *The encyclopedia of aging* (2nd ed., pp. 166–171). New York: Springer Publishing Co.

Brooke, V. (1991–1992, Winter). Meeting the challenge: Involuntary restraints in the nursing home. *Journal of Long Term Care Administration,* pp. 9–14.

Bruns, H. J. (1995). Gastrointestinal system. In G. L. Maddox (Ed.), *The encyclopedia of aging* (2nd ed., pp. 390–392). New York: Springer Publishing Co.

Bryant, J., & Tuttle, K. (1989). Setting up top facility policies and procedures. *Provider, 15*(12), 13–14.

Buffum, M. D., & Buffum, J. C. (1997, July/August). The psychopharmacologic treatment of depression in elders. *Geriatric Nursing 18,* 144–149.

Burch, G. E. (1983). Interesting aspects of the aging process. *Journal of American Geriatrics Society, 31*(12), 766–779.

Burger, S. G. (1994). Avoiding physical restraint use: New standards in care. *Long Term Care Advances* (Duke University Center for the Study of Aging and Human Development), *5*(2), 1–9.

Burnside, I. (Ed.). (1981). *Nursing and the aged.* New York: McGraw-Hill.

Busse, E., & Pfeiffer, E. (1973). *Mental illness in later life.* Washington, DC: American Psychological Association.

Butler, R., & Lewis, M. (1977). *Aging and mental health* (2nd ed.). St. Louis: Mosby.

Butler, W. (1975, September). Psychology and the elderly: An overview. *American Journal of Psychiatry, 132,* pp. 893–900.

Caird, F. I. (1979). *Assessment of the elderly patient* (2nd ed.). Philadelphia: Lippincott.

Callahan, D. (1987). *Setting limits: Medical goals in an aging society.* New York: Simon & Schuster.

Cape, R. D. (Ed.). (1983). *Fundamentals of geriatric medicine.* New York: Raven Press.

Carter, D., & Balin, A. (1983). Dermatological aspects of aging. *Medical Clinics of North America, 67*(2), 531–534.

Chui, H. (1995a). Cerebrovascular disease. In G. L. Maddox (Ed.), *The encyclopedia of aging* (2nd ed., pp. 171–172). New York: Springer Publishing Co.

Chui, H. (1995b). Vascular dementia. In G. L. Maddox (Ed.), *The encyclopedia of aging* (2nd ed., pp. 173–174). New York: Springer Publishing Co.

Cohan, S. L. (1989). Neurologic diseases in the elderly. In W. Reichel (Ed.), *Clinical aspects of aging* (3rd ed., pp. 163–174). Baltimore: Williams & Wilkins.

Collins, K., Dore, C., et al. (1977). Accidental hypothermia and impaired temperature homeostasis in the elderly. *British Medical Journal.*

Collier, M. (1997). Know how: Vacuum-assisted closure. *Nursing Times, 93*(5), 32–33.

Cooper, J. (1978). Drug therapy in the elderly: Is it all it could be? *American Pharmacist, 18*(7), 25–33.

Corso, J. (1981). *Aging: Sensory systems and perception.* New York: Praeger.

Crow, (1984). *Pharmacology for the elderly.* New York: Teachers College Press.

Dement, W. Miles, L., & Bliwise, D. (1982, April). Physiological markers of aging: human sleep patterns. In Reff and Schneider (Ed.), *Biological markers of aging* (pp. 177–187). Washington, DC: U.S. Department of Health and Human Services, National Institutes of Health, Public Health Service.

DeVita, V. (1982, June). *Cancer treatment* (Publication No. 82-1807). Washington, DC: Medicine for the Layman Services, U.S. Department of Health and Human Services, Public Health Service.

deVries, H. A. (1989a). Physiological effects of an exercise training regimen upon men aged 52 to 88. In W. Reichel (Ed.), *Clinical aspects of aging* (3rd ed.). Baltimore: Williams & Wilkins.

_____. (1989b). Physiology of physical conditioning for the elderly. In W. Reichel (Ed.), *Clinical aspects of aging* (3rd ed.). Baltimore: Williams & Wilkins.

_____. (1989). *Vigor regained.* In W. Reichel (Ed.), *Clinical aspects of aging* (3rd ed.). Baltimore: Williams & Wilkins.

Dewey, J. (1995, January). New drug options spur a focus on outcomes. *Provider,* pp. 45–56.

Dimond, M., & Jones, S. L. (1983). *Chronic illness across the life span.* Norwalk, CT: Appleton-Century-Crofts.

Duvoisin, R. (1984). *Parkinson's disease: A guide for patient and family.* New York: Raven Press.

Emanuel, E. J., & Emanuel, L. L. (1992). Proxy decision making for incompetent patients. *Journal of the American Medical Association, 267,* 2067–2071.

Engel, B. T. (1995). Incontinence. In G. L. Maddox (Ed.), *The encyclopedia of aging* (2nd ed., pp. 501–502). New York. Springer Publishing Co.

Engel, V. F., & Graney, M. J. (1993). Stability and improvement of health after nursing home admission. *Journal of Gerontology,* 48(1), S17–S23.

Ernst, N. S., & Glazer-Waldman, H. R. (1983). *The aged patient: A sourcebook for allied health professionals.* Chicago: Year Book Medical Publishers.

Evans, J.G., Williams, T.F., Beattie, B.L., Michael, J.P., & Wilcock, G.K. (2000). *Oxford textbook of geriatric medicine* (2nd ed.). New York: Oxford University Press.

Everad, K., Rowles, G. D., & High, D. (1994). Nursing home room changes: Toward a decision-making model. *Gerontologist, 34,* 520–527.

Farber, B., Brennen, C., Punteri, A., & Brody, J. (1982). Nosocomial infections in a chronic care facility. *Journal of the American Geriatric Society, 32*(7), 513–519.

Faubert, P. F., Shapiro, W. B., Porush, J. G., & Kahn, A. I. (1989). Medical renal disease in aged. In W. Reichel (Ed.), *Clinical aspects of aging* (3rd ed.). Baltimore: Williams & Wilkins.

Feinstein, E., & Friedman, E. (1979). Renal disease in the elderly. In Rossman (Ed.), *Clinical geriatrics* (2nd ed.). Philadelphia: Lippincott.

Felser, J., & Raff, M. (1983). Infectious diseases and aging. *Journal of the American Geriatrics Society, 13*(12), 802–806.

Finch, C., & Hayflick, L. (1977). *Handbook of the biology of aging.* New York: Van Nostrand Reinhold.

Fletcher, J. (1997, March 27–April 9). Pressure relieving equipment: Criteria and selection. *British Journal of Nursing,* pp. 323, 326–328.

Focus on retirement. (1998, March 9). *The Wall Street Journal,* p. 22.

Foley, C. (1981). Nutrition and the elderly. In Libow (Ed.), *The core of geriatric medicine: A guide for students and practitioners.* St. Louis: Mosby.

Fowler, M. (1984). Appointing an agent to make medical treatment choices. *Columbia Law Review, 84,* 985.

Franker, L. J., & Richard, B. B. (1989). Be alive as long as you live. In W. Reichel (Ed.), *Clinical aspects of aging* (3rd ed.). Baltimore: Williams & Wilkins.

Franz, M. (1981, Summer). Nutritional requirements of the elderly. *Journal of Nutrition for the Elderly.*

Fraumeni, J. (1979). Epidemiological studies of cancer. In Griffen and Shaw (Eds.), *Carcinogens: Identification and mechanism of action.* New York: Raven Press.

Freedman, M. (1982). Anemias in the elderly: Physiological or pathological? *Hospital Practice, 17*(5), 121–136.

Freeman, J. (1979). *Aging: Its history and literature.* New York: Human Sciences Press.

Fylling, C. P. (1989, Spring). Comprehensive wound management with topical growth factors. *Ostomy/Wound Management.*

Gallagher, S. M. (1997). Outcomes in clinical practice: Pressure ulcer prevalence and incidence studies. *Ostomy Wound Management, 43*(1), 28–32, 34–35, 38.

Gallis, H. (1984). Infectious diseases in the elderly. In Covington and Walker (Eds.), *Current geriatric therapy.* Philadelphia: Saunders.

Gambert, S. R. (1983). A clinician's guide to the physiology of aging. *Wisconsin Medical Journal, 82*(8), 13–15.

Garagusi, V. F. (1989). Infectious disease problems in the elderly. In W. Reichel (Ed.), *Clinical aspects of aging* (3rd ed.). Baltimore: Williams & Wilkins.

Garibaldi, R., Brodine, S., & Matsumiya, S. (1981). Infections among patients in nursing homes. *New England Journal of Medicine, 305*(13), 731–735.

Gibbons, J. C., & Levy, S. M. (1989). Gastrointestinal diseases in the aged. In W. Reichel (Ed.), *Clinical aspects of aging* (3rd ed.). Baltimore: Williams & Wilkins.

Glowacki, G. A. (1989). Geriatric gynecology. In W. Reichel (Ed.), *Clinical aspects of aging* (3rd ed.). Baltimore: Williams & Wilkins.

Goffman, E. (1961). *Asylums: Essays on the social situation of mental patients and other inmates.* Garden City, NY: Anchor Books.

Golden, C. J., & Cohen, D. I. (1995). Organic brain syndrome. In G. L. Maddox (Ed.), *The encyclopedia of aging* (2nd ed., pp. 686–687). New York: Springer Publishing Co.

Goldfarb, A. (1979). Geriatric gynecology. In Rossman (Ed.), *Clinical geriatrics* (2nd ed.). Philadelphia: Lippincott.

Goldrick, B. A., & Larson, E. (1992). Assessing the need for infection control programs: A diagnostic approach. *Journal of Long Term Care Administration, 20*(1), 20–23.

Gordon, J. C. (1989). Musculoskeletal injuries in the elderly. In W. Reichel (Ed.), *Clinical aspects of aging* (3rd ed.). Baltimore: Williams & Wilkins.

Gotz, B., & Gotz, V. (1978). Drugs and the elderly. *American Journal of Nursing, 78*(8), 1347–1350.

Griggs, W. (1978). Sex and the elderly. *American Journal of Nursing, 78*(8), 1352–1354.

Grob, D. (1983). Prevalent joint diseases in older persons. In W. Reichel (Ed.), *Clinical aspects of aging* (2nd ed.). Baltimore: Williams & Wilkins.

______. (1989). Common disorders of muscles in the aged. In W. Reichel (Ed.), *Clinical aspects of aging* (3rd ed., pp. 314–330). Baltimore: Williams & Wilkins.

Grocer, M., & Shekleton, M. (1979). *Basic pathophysiology—a conceptual approach.* St. Louis: Mosby.

Groenwald, S. (1980). Physiology of the immune system. *Journal of the Heart and Lung, 9*(4), 645–650.

Gwyther, L. (1983). Alzheimer's disease. *North Carolina Medical Journal, 44*(7), 435–436.

Gwyther, L., & Matteson, M. A. (1983). Care for the caregivers. *Journal of*

Gerontological Nursing, 9(2).

Haight, B. K. (1995). Suicide risk in frail elderly people relocated to nursing homes. *Geriatric Nursing, 16,* 104–107.

Hall, Stephen S. (2003). *Merchants of Immortality: chasing the dream of human life extension.* Boston: Houghton Mifflin.

Harris, R. (1989). Exercise and physical fitness for the elderly. In W. Reichel (Ed.), *Clinical aspects of aging* (3rd ed.). Baltimore: Williams & Wilkins.

Hayflick, L. (1965). The limited in vitro lifetime of human diploid cell strains. *Experimental Cell Research, 37*(3), 614–636.

Hayflick, L. (1995). Biological aging theories. In G. L. Maddox (Ed.), *The encyclopedia of aging* (2nd ed., pp. 113–118). New York: Springer Publishing Co.

Heaney, R. (1982, April). Age related bone loss. In Reff and Schneider (Ed.), *Biological markers of aging.* Washington, DC: USDHHS, NIH, Public Health Service.

Hefti, F. (1995). Neurotrophic factors and aging. In G. L. Maddox (Ed.). *The encyclopedia of aging* (2nd ed., pp. 686–687). New York: Springer Publishing Co.

Hickey, T. (1982). *Health and aging.* Monterey, CA: Brooks-Cole.

Hiller, M. D. (1987). Ethical decision making and the health administrator. In G. R. Anderson & V. A. Glesnes-Anderson (Eds.), *Health care ethics: A guide for decision makers.* Rockville, MD: Aspen.

Hing, E. (1977). Characteristics of nursing home residents' health status and care received (Series 13, No. 51). Washington, DC: USDHHS, PHS, Office of Health Research Survey, and Testing, National Center for Health Statistics.

Hogstel, M. (1981). *Nursing care of the older adult.* New York: Wiley.

Horstman, B. (1981). Importance of physical therapy in fostering independence. *American Health Care Association Journal, 9*(3), 51–57.

Huntley, R. R. (1989). Common complaints of the elderly. In W. Reichel (Ed.), *Clinical aspects of aging* (3rd ed.). Baltimore: Williams & Wilkins.

Husain, T. (1953). An experimental study of some pressure effects on tissues with reference to the bed sore problem. *Journal of Pathology and Bacteriology, 66,* 347.

Hutchison, T. A., et al. (1989). Post-menopausal estrogens protect against fractures of hip and distal radius: A case control study. In W. Reichel (Ed.), *Clinical aspects of aging* (3rd ed.). Baltimore: Williams & Wilkins.

Irvine, P., VanBuren, N., & Crossley, K. (1984). Causes for hospitalization of nursing home residents: The role of infection. *Journal of the American Geriatrics Society, 32*(2), 103–107.

Janelli, L. M., Kanski, G. W., & Neary, M. A. (1996, June). Physical restraints; Has OBRA made a difference? *Journal of Gerontological Nursing,* pp. 17–21.

Jarvik, L., & Greenblatt, D. (1981). *Clinical pharmacology and the aged patient.* New York: Raven Press.

Johnson, S. H. (1995, Fall). Law and quality in long term care. *Journal of Long Term Care Administration,* pp. 75–77.

Jokl, E. (1989). Abstract, XII International Congress of Gerontology, Hamburg, July 12–17. In W. Reichel (Ed.), *Clinical aspects of aging* (3rd ed.). Baltimore: Williams & Wilkins.

Jones, J. K. (1989). Drugs and the elderly. In W. Reichel (Ed.), *Clinical aspects of aging* (3rd ed.). Baltimore: Williams & Wilkins.

Kahana, B. (1995a). Isolation. In G. L. Maddox (Ed.), *The encyclopedia of aging* (2nd ed., pp. 526–527). New York: Springer Publishing Co.

Kahana, E. (1995b). Deinstitutionalization. In G. L. Maddox (Ed.), *The encyclopedia of aging* (2nd ed., p. 254–256). New York: Springer Publishing Co.

Kamen, & Shermany. (1981). In Libow (Ed.), *The core of geriatric medicine: A guide for students and practitioners.* St. Louis: Mosby.

Kane, R. L., Ouslander, J. G., & Abrass, I. B. (1989). *Essentials of clinical geriatrics.* (2nd ed.). New York: McGraw-Hill.

Kapp, M. B. (1987). *Preventing malpractice in long-term care: Strategies for risk management.* New York: Springer Publishing Co.

Katz, P. R., & Calkins, E. (1989). *Principles and practice of nursing home care.* New York: Springer Publishing Co.

Karasu, T., & Lazar, I. (1980). Evaluation and management of depression in the elderly. *Geriatrics, 35*(12), 47–56.

Karcher, K. A. (1993, March). Is your risk management program designed to deal with Alzheimer's disease? *Nursing Homes,* pp. 34–36.

Kart, C., Metress, E., & Metress, J. (1978) *Aging and health: Biological and social perspectives.* Menlo Park, CA: Addison-Wesley.

Kasper, R. L. (1989). Eye problems of the aged. In W. Reichel (Ed.), *Clinical aspects of aging* (3rd ed., p. 448). Baltimore: Williams & Wilkins.

Kaszniak, A. W. (1995). Parkinson's disease. In G. L. Maddox (Ed.), *The encyclopedia of aging* (2nd ed., pp. 727–729). New York: Springer Publishing Co.

Kay, B., & Neeley, J. (1982). Sexuality and aging: A review of current literature. *Sexuality and Disability, 5*(1), 38–46.

Keegan, G., & McNichols, D. (1982). The evaluation and treatment of urinary incontinence in the elderly. *Surgical Clinics of North America, 62*(2), 261–269.

Kenney, M. (1982). *Physiology of aging: A synopsis.* Chicago: Year Book Medical Publishers.

Kennie, D. S., & Warshaw, G. (1989). Health maintenance and health screening in the elderly. In W. Reichel (Ed.), *Clinical aspects of aging* (3rd ed.). Baltimore: Williams & Wilkins.

Kippenbrock, T., & Soja, M. E. (1993). Preventing falls in the elderly: Interviewing patients who have fallen. *Geriatric Nursing, 14,* 205–209.

Kleiger, R. (1976). Cardiovascular disorders. In Steinberg (Ed.), *Cowdry's: The care of the geriatric patient* (5th ed.). St. Louis: Mosby.

Kligman, A. (1979). Perspectives and problems in cutaneous gerontology. *Journal of Investigative Dermatology, 73*(1), 39–46.

Knighton, D. R., et al. (1989, April). The use of topically applied platelet growth factors in chronic nonhealing sounds: A review. *Wounds: A compendium of Clinical Research and Practice.*

Kraus, H. (1977). Preservation of physical fitness. In R. Harris & L. J. Frankel (Eds.), *Guide to fitness after 50* (p. 35). New York: Plenum Press.

Kravitz, S. C. (1989). Anemia in the elderly. In W. Reichel (Ed.), *Clinical aspects of aging* (3rd ed.). Baltimore: Williams & Wilkins.

Kriegel, R. J. (1991). *If it ain't broke.* New York: Warner.

Kurlowicz, L. H. (1997, September/October). Nursing standard of practice protocol:

Depression in elderly patients. *Geriatric Nursing,* 192–200.

Kurtz, S. (1982). Urinary tract infection in older persons. *Comprehensive Therapy, 8*(2), 54–58.

Lanzar, I., & Karasu, T. (1980). Evaluation and management of depression in the elderly. *Geriatrics, 35*(12).

Landfield, P. W. (1995). Stress theory of aging. In G. L. Maddox (Ed.), *The encyclopedia of aging* (2nd ed., pp. 903–905). New York: Springer Publishing Co.

Leaf, A. (1973). Getting old. *Scientific American, 229*(3), 44–52.

Lehman, K. (1983). Administrator's role in prevention and care of decubitus ulcers. *Journal of Long term Care Administration, 11*(2), 2.

Leone & Siegenthaler. (1994). Alzheimer disease and associated disorders *AHCPR, 8*(Suppl. 1 [AHCPR Pub. No. 94–0106]), S58–S71.

Levine, A. (1984). The elderly amputee. *American Family Physician, 29*(5), 177–182.

Libow, L. (1981). *The core of geriatric medicine: A guide for students and practitioners.* St. Lewis: Mosby.

Lindeman, R. D. (1989). Application of fluid and electrolyte balance principles to the older patient. In W. Reichel (Ed.), *Clinical aspects of aging* (3rd ed.). Baltimore: Williams & Wilkins.

Linley, M. (1971, October). *Good eating: Meeting the nutritional needs for aged persons in residential care homes.* State of California, Human Relations Agency, Department of Social Services.

Lipson, S., & Pattee, J. J. (1989). Medical care in the nursing home. In W. Reichel (Ed.), *Clinical aspects of aging* (3rd ed.). Baltimore: Williams & Wilkins.

Listening to depression: The new medicine. (1995). *Johns Hopkins Medical Letter, 6*(11), 4.

Lo, B., & Dornbrand, L. (1986). The case of Claire Conroy: Will administrative review safeguard incompetent patients? *Annals of Internal Medicine, 104,* 869–873.

Logemann, J. A. (1995). Dysphagia. In G. L. Maddox (Ed.), *The encyclopedia of aging* (2nd ed., pp. 297–298). New York: Springer Publishing Co.

Lotzkar, S. (1977). Dental care of the aged. *Journal of Public Health Dentistry, 37*(3), 201–207.

Louis, M. (1977). Falls and their causes. *Journal of Geriatric Nursing, 4*(6), 143–144.

Lyon, L., & Nevins, M. (1984). Management of hip fracture in nursing home patients: To treat or not to treat? *Journal of the American Geriatrics Society, 32*(5), 391–395.

MacHudis, M. (1983). In W. Reichel (Ed.), *Clinical aspects of aging: A comprehensive text* (2nd ed.). Baltimore: Williams & Wilkins.

Maddox, G.L. (2001). *The encyclopedia of aging* (3rd ed.). New York: Springer.

Magee, R. et al. (1993, April). Institutional policy use of restraints in extended care and nursing homes. *Journal of Gerontological Nursing,* pp. 31–39.

McCaddon, A., & Kelly, C. L. (1994). Familial Alzheimer's disease and vitamin B12 deficiency. *Age and Aging, 23,* 334–337.

McCullough, L. B., & Lipson, L. B. (1989a). Informed consent. In W. Reichel (Ed.), *Clinical aspects of aging* (3rd ed.). Baltimore: Williams & Wilkins.

McCullough, L. B., & Lipson, S. (1989b). Termination of treatment. In W. Reichel (Ed.), *Clinical aspects of aging* (3rd ed.). Baltimore: Williams & Wilkins.

McCullough, L. B., & Lipson, S. (1989c). Termination of food and water. In W. Reichel

(Ed.), *Clinical aspects of aging* (3rd ed.). Baltimore: Williams & Wilkins.

McLachlan, M. (1978). The aging kidney. *Lancet, 2,* 43.

Medvedev, Z. A. (1995). Wear-and-tear theories. In G. L. Maddox (Ed.), *The encyclopedia of aging* (2nd ed., pp. 964–965). New York: Springer Publishing Co.

Meites, J., & Quadri, S. K. (1995). Neuroendocrine theory of aging. In G. L. Maddox (Ed.), *The encyclopedia of aging* (2nd ed., pp. 677–681). New York: Springer Publishing Co.

Menscer, D. (1993). Let the people go: Caring for the demented elderly without using restraints. *North Carolina Medical Journal, 54,* 145–150.

Meza, J., Peggs, J., & O'Brien, J. (1984). Constipation in the elderly patient. *Journal of Family Practice, 18*(5), 695–703.

Miller, R. I. (1994). Managing disruptive responses to bathing by elderly residents. *Journal of Gerontological Nursing, 20*(11), 35–39.

Moore, J. R., & Gilbert, D. A. (1995). Elderly residents: Perceptions of nurses' comforting touch. *Journal of Gerontological Nursing, 21*(1), 6–13.

Mosher-Ashley, P. E., & Henrikson, N. M. (1993, July-August). Long-term care alternatives for the mentally ill. *Nursing Homes,* pp. 34–36.

Moss, A. J. (1989). Diagnosis and management of heart disease in the elderly. In W. Reichel (Ed.), *Clinical aspects of aging* (3rd ed., p. 65). Baltimore: Williams & Wilkins.

Moss, R. J., & La Puma, J. (1991, January-February). The ethics of mechanical restraints. *Hastings Center Report,* pp. 22–24.

National Center for Health Services Research and Health Care Technology Assessment. (March, 1989). *Research activities.* Rockville, MD: National Center for Health Services, no. 115.

National Center for Health Services Research and Health Care Technology Assessment. (1989, September). *Research activities* (no. 121). Rockville, MD: National Center for Health Services.

Nicolle, L., McIntyre, M., Zacharias, H., & MacDonald, J. (1961). Twelve months of surveillance of infections in institutionalized elderly men. *Journal of the American Geriatrics Society, 9*(4), 654–680.

O'Connor, C. E., & Stilwell, E. M. (1989). Sexuality, intimacy and touch in older adults. In W. Reichel (Ed.), *Clinical aspects of aging* (3rd ed.). Baltimore: Williams & Wilkins.

Osgood, N. J. (1995). Leisure programs. In G. L. Maddox (Ed.), *The encyclopedia of aging* (2nd ed., pp. 546–548). New York: Springer Publishing Co.

Ostfeld, A., & Gibson, D. (Eds.). (1972). *Epidemiology of aging* (Publication No. 75-7111). Washington, DC: USDHEW, PHS, NIH.

Otero, R. B. (1993, May). Current approaches to infection, control. *Nursing Homes,* pp. 48–49.

Ouslander, J. G., Schapira, Schnelle, Uman, Fingold, Tuico, & Nigam. (1995). Does eradicating bacteriuria affect the severity of chronic urinary incontinence in nursing home residents? *Annals of Internal Medicine, 122,* 749–754.

Paffenbarger, R. S., Wing, A. L., & Hsieh, C. (1986). Physical activity, all-cause mortality and longevity of college alumni. New England Journal of Medicine, 314(605).

Palmore, J. (1973). In Busse and Lewis (Eds.), *Mental illness in later life.* Washington, DC: American Psychological Association.

Palmer, M. H., Bennett, Marks, McCormick, & Engel. (1994). Urinary incontinence: A program that works. *Journal of Long Term Care Administration,* 19–25.

Phair, J. P. (1979). Aging and infection: A review. *Journal of Chronic Disease, 32,* 535–540.

Physician's desk reference. (1998). Montvale, NJ: Medical Economics.

Poe, W., & Holloway, D. (1980). *Drugs and the aged.* New York: McGraw-Hill.

Pousada, L. (1995). Hip fracture. In G. L. Maddox (Ed.), *The encyclopedia of aging* (2nd ed., pp. 456–457). New York: Springer Publishing Co.

Rantz, M. (1994). Managing behaviors of chronically confused residents. *Journal of Long Term Care Administration,* 16–19.

Ray, W. A., et al. (1993). Reducing antipsychotic drug use in nursing homes. *Archives of Internal Medicine, 153,* 713–720.

Redford, J. B. (1989). Rehabilitation and the aged. In W. Reichel (Ed.), *Clinical aspects of aging* (3rd ed.). Baltimore: Williams & Wilkins.

Regnier, V. (1995). *Assisted living for the aged and frail.* New York: Columbia University Press.

Reichel, W. (Ed.). (1983). *Clinical aspects of aging: A comprehensive text* (2nd ed.). New York: Williams & Wilkins.

Reichel, W., & Rabins, E. V. (1989). Evaluation and management of the confused, disoriented or demented elderly patient. In W. Reichel (Ed.), *Clinical aspects of aging* (3rd ed., pp. 137–153). Baltimore: Williams & Wilkins.

Reisberg, B. (1995). Senile dementia. In G. L. Maddox (Ed.), *The encyclopedia of aging* (2nd ed., pp. 837–847). New York: Springer Publishing Co.

Research activities, National Center for Health Services research and health care technology assessment. (1989, March). Publication No. 115. Rockville, MD: National Center for Health Services.

Research activities, National Center for Health Services research and health care technology assessment. (1989, September). Publication No. 121. Rockville, MD: National Center for Health Services.

Retirement checkup (1998, March 9). *Wall Street Journal,* p. 22.

Rimer, B. K. (1995). Cancer control and aging. In G. L. Maddox (Ed.), *The encyclopedia of aging* (2nd ed., pp. 130–131). New York: Springer Publishing Co.

Ripich, D. N., Wykle, M., & Niles, S. (1995). Alzheimer's disease caregivers: The focused program. *Geriatric Nursing, 76*(1), 15–19.

Roberts, J., & Snyder, D. L. (1995). Drug interactions. In G. L. Maddox (Ed.), *The encyclopedia of aging* (2nd ed., pp. 289–291). New York: Springer Publishing Co.

Rodman, M., & Smith, D. (1977). *Clinical pharmacology in nursing.* Philadelphia: J. B. Lippincott.

Rodstein, E. (1983). Falls by the aged. In Rossman (Ed.), *Fundamentals of geriatric medicine.* New York: Raven Press.

Rosendorff, C. (1983). *Clinical cardiovascular and pulmonary physiology.* New York: Raven Press.

Rossman, I. (Ed.). (1979). *Clinical geriatrics* (2nd ed.). Philadelphia: Lippincott.

Rowe, J. (1982). Renal function and aging. In Reff and Schneider (Eds.), *Biological*

markers of aging. Washington, DC: USDHHS, NIH, Public Health Service.
Rowe, J., & Besdine, R. (1982). *Health and disease in old age.* Boston: Little, Brown.
Rubin, P. (1981). Management of hypertension in the elderly. In F. Ebaugh (Ed.), *Management of common problems in geriatric medicine.* Menlo Park, CA: Addison-Wesley.
Rux, J. (1981, Fall-Winter). Thoughts on culture, nutrition, and the aged. *Journal of Nutrition for the Elderly, 1.*
Sartor, & Nuzum. (1983). In McCue (Ed.), *Medical care of the elderly: A practical approach.* Lexington, MA: Collamore Press.
Satterifield, N. (1989). New regulations bring changes to facilities. *Provider, 15*(12), 10–11.
Schneck, M., et al. (1982). An overview of current concepts of Alzheimer's disease. *Psychiatry, 139*(2).
Schnelle, J. F., Ouslander, J. G., Simmons, Alessi, & Gravel. (1993). The nighttime environment, incontinence care and sleep disruption in nursing homes. *Journal of the American Geriatrics Society, 41,* 910–914.
Schwartz, R. L. (1987). Refusal of treatment: Rights, reasons, responses. In G. R. Anderson & V. A. Glesnes-Anderson (Eds.), *Health care ethics: A guide for decision makers.* Rockville, MD: Aspen.
Scott, R. R., Bramble, K. J., & Goodyear, N. (1991). How knowledge and labeling of dementia affect nurses' expectations. *Journal of Gerontological Nursing, 17*(1), 21–24.
Segal, J., Thompson, J., & Floyd, R. (1979). Drug utilization and prescribing patterns in a skilled nursing facility: The need for a rational approach to therapeutics. *Journal of the American Geriatrics Society, 27*(3), 117–122.
Selma, T. P., Palla, K., Padding, B., & Brauner, D. J. (1994). Effect of OBRA 1987 on antipsychotic prescribing in nursing home residents. *Journal of the American Geriatrics Society, 42,* 648–652.
Shashaty, G. G. (1989). Thromboembolism in the elderly. In W. Reichel (Ed.), *Clinical aspects of aging* (3rd ed.). Baltimore: Williams & Wilkins.
Shinnar, S. (1983). Use of adaptive feeding equipment in feeding the elderly. *Journal of the American Dietetic Association, 83*(3), 321–322.
Shore, H. (1978). Group programs in long term care facilities. In Burnside (Ed.), *Working with the elderly: Group process and techniques.* North Scituate, MA: Duxbury Press.
Sinex, F. M. (1977). The molecular genetics of aging. In C. Finch & L. Hayflick (Eds.), *Handbook of the biology of aging.* New York: Van Nostrand Reinhold.
Sklar (1983). Gastrointestinal diseases in the aged. In W. Reichel (Ed.), *Clinical aspects of aging: A comprehensive text* (2nd ed.). Baltimore: Williams & Wilkins.
Smith, P. W. (1989). Making infection control an art. *Provider, 15*(12), 7–9.
Smith, W. (1982). Infections in the elderly. *Hospital Practice, 17,* 69–85.
Snowden, J. (1983). Sex in nursing homes. *Australian Nurse's Journal, 12*(8), 55–56.
Spencer, H. (1977). The skeletal system. In Rossman (Ed.), *Clinical geriatrics* (2nd ed.). Philadelphia: Lippincott.
Starr, I. (1964). An essay on the strength of the heart. *American Journal of Cardiology, 14*(6), 771–783.
Steffen, G., & Franklin, C. (1985). Who speaks for the patient with locked-in syndrome?

Hastings Center Report 15(13).
Steffl, B. (Ed.). (1984). *Handbook of gerontological nursing*. New York: Van Nostrand Reinhold.
Sterritt, P. F., & Pokorny, M. E. (1994). Art activities for patients with Alzheimer's and related disorders. *Geriatric Nursing, 15,* 155–159.
Stillwell, E., & O'Conner, C. (1989). Sexuality, intimacy, and touch. In W. Reichel (Ed.), *Clinical aspects of aging* (2nd ed.). Baltimore: Williams & Wilkins.
Stolley, J. M., et al. (1993). Developing a restraint use policy for acute care. *Journal of Nursing, 23*(12), 49–54.
[The] stopgap benefits of taurine for Alzheimer's. (1995). *Johns Hopkins Medical Letter, 7*(3), 3.
Stotsky, B. (1973). In Busse & Pfeiffer (Eds.), *Mental illness in later life*. Washington, DC: American Psychological Association.
Strehler, B. (1962). *Time, cells, and aging*. New York: Academic Press.
Strumpf, N., & Gamroth, L. (1989). Ethics and research in teaching nursing homes. In M. D. Mezey, J. E. Lynaugh, & M. M. Cartier (Eds.), *Nursing homes and nursing care: Lessons from the teaching nursing homes*. New York: Springer Publishing Co.
Sullivan, R. J. (1995). Cardiovascular system. In G. L. Maddox (Ed.), *The encyclopedia of aging* (2nd ed., pp. 133–138). New York: Springer Publishing Co.
Swanson, E. A., Maas, M. S., & Buckwalter, K. C. (1993). Catastrophic reactions and other behaviors of Alzheimer's residents: Special unit compared with traditional units. *Archives of Psychiatric Nursing, 7,* 292–299.
Talbott, J. (1985). Clinical and policy issues. *Bulletin of the New York Academy of Medicine, 61,* 445.
Teuth, M. J. (1995). How to manage depression and psychosis in Alzheimer's disease. *Geriatrics, 50*(1), 43–49.
Thomas, W. H. (1996). *Life worth living*. Acton, MA: VanderWyk & Burnham.
Tideiksaar, R. (1995). Falls. In G. L. Maddox (Ed.), *The encyclopedia of aging* (2nd ed., pp. 359–361). New York: Springer Publishing Co.
Tindall, J., & Smith, J. (1963). Skin lesions of the aged. *Journal of the American Medical Association, 186,* 1037–1040.
Tonna, E. (1995). Collagen. In G. L. Maddox (Ed.), *The encyclopedia of aging* (2nd ed., pp. 146–147). New York: Springer Publishing Co.
Trella, R. (1994). From hospital to nursing home: Bridging the gaps in care. *Geriatric Nursing, 15,* 313–316.
Tuberculosis. (1995). *Johns Hopkins Medical Letter, 7*(9), 8.
Uhlman, R. F., et al. (1987). Medical management decisions in nursing home patients: principles and policy recommendations. *Annals of Internal medicine, 106,* 879–885.
U.S. Department of Health Education and Welfare, Public Health Service, Office of Long Term Care. (1976, June). *Physician prescribing patterns in skilled nursing facilities* (Long Term Care Facility Improvement Campaign Monograph No. 2). Washington, DC.
U.S. Senate Special Committee on Aging. (2003). *Assisted Living Workgroup's Final Report,* April 29, 2003.
Vallarino, & Sherman. (1981). Stroke, hip fractures, amputations, pressure sores, and incontinence. In Libow (Ed.), *The core of geriatric medicine: A guide for students*

and practitioners. St. Louis: Mosby.

Van Vliet, L. (1995a). Aphasia. In G. L. Maddox (Ed.), *The encyclopedia of aging* (2nd ed., pp. 75–76). New York: Springer Publishing Co.

Van Vliet, L. (1995b). Communication disorders. In G. L. Maddox (Ed.), *The encyclopedia of aging* (2nd ed., pp. 198–200). New York: Springer Publishing Co.

Wainwright, H. (1978). Feeding problems in the elderly disabled patient. *Nursing Times,* 74.

Waldo, M. J., Ide, B. A., & Thomas, D. P. (1995, February). Postcardiac-event elderly: Effect of exercise on cardiopulmonary function. *Journal of Gerontological Nursing,* pp. 12–19.

Wallace, M. (1992). Management of sexual relationships among elderly residents of long term care facilities. *Geriatric Nursing,* 308–322.

Walsh, D. B., & Nauta, R. J. (Ed.). (1980). *Clinical aspects of aging* (3rd ed.). Baltimore: Williams & Wilkins.

Wasow, M., & Loeb, M. (1979). Sexuality in nursing homes. *Journal of the American Geriatrics Society, 27,* 73–79.

Watzke, J. R., & Wister, A. V. (1993, November). Staff attitudes: Monitoring technology in long term care. *Journal of Gerontological Nursing,* pp. 23–29.

Weg, P. (1983). Changing physiology of aging. In Woodruff & Biren (Eds.), *Aging: Scientific perspectives and social issues* (2nd ed.). Monterey, CA: Brooks/Cole.

Weksler, E. (1981). The senescence of the immune system. *Hospital Practice, 16,* 53–58.

Wenston, S. R. (1987). Applying philosophy to ethical dilemmas. In G. R. Anderson & V. A. Glesnes-Anderson (Eds.), *Health care ethics: A guide for decision makers.* Rockville, MD Aspen.

Werner, P., et al. (1994). Reducing restraints: Impact on staff. *Journal of Gerontological Nursing,* 19–24.

Williams, M., & Fitzhugh, C. (1982). Urinary incontinence in the elderly. *Annals of Internal Medicine, 97,* 895–907.

Woodruff, D., & Birren, J. (1975). *Aging—scientific perspectives and social issues.* New York: Van Nostrand.

Wylie, C. M. (1989). Hospitalization for fractures and bone loss in adults. In W. Reichel (Ed.), *Clinical aspects of aging* (3rd ed.). Baltimore: Williams & Wilkins.

Yoder, M. G. (1989). Geriatric ear nose and throat problems. In W. Reichel (Ed.), *Clinical aspects of aging* (3rd ed.). Baltimore: Williams & Wilkins.

Zinn, J. S., & Mor, V. (1994). Nursing home special care units: Distribution by type, state, and facility characteristics. *Geriatrics, 34,* 371–376.

CPSIA information can be obtained
at www.ICGtesting.com
Printed in the USA
FFOW03n1317040615
13832FF

9 780826 11516